PHARMACEUTICAL DOSAGE FORMS

PHARMACEUTICAL DOSAGE FORMS

Tablets

SECOND EDITION, REVISED AND EXPANDED

In Three Volumes
VOLUME 1

EDITED BY

Herbert A. Lieberman

H.H. Lieberman Associates, Inc.
Consultant Services
Livingston, New Jersey

Leon Lachman

Lachman Consultant Services
Westbury, New York

Joseph B. Schwartz

Philadelphia College of Pharmacy and Science
Philadelphia, Pennsylvania

MARCEL DEKKER, INC.   New York and Basel

Library of Congress Cataloging-in-Publication Data

Pharmaceutical dosage forms--tablets / edited by Herbert A. Lieberman,
   Leon Lachman, Joseph B. Schwartz. -- 2nd ed., rev. and expanded.
      p.   cm.
   Includes index.
   ISBN 0-8247-8044-2 (v. 1 : alk. paper)
   1. Tablets (Medicine) 2. Drugs--Dosage forms. I. Lieberman,
Herbert A. II. Lachman, Leon. III. Schwartz, Joseph B.
   [DNLM: 1. Dosage Forms. 2. Drugs--administration & dosage. QV
785 P535]
RS 201.T2P46   1989
615'.191--dc19
DNLM/DLC   89-1629
for Library of Congress   CIP

6100973666

MARCEL DEKKER, INC.
270 Madison Avenue, New York, New York 10016

Current printing (last digit):
10 9 8 7 6 5 4 3 2 1

PRINTED IN THE UNITED STATES OF AMERICA

Preface

Several years have passed since the first edition of *Pharmaceutical Dosage Forms: Tablets* was published. During this time, considerable advances have been made in the science and technology of tablet formulation, manufacture, and testing. These changes are reflected in this updated, revised and expanded second edition.

The tablet dosage form continues to be the most widely used drug delivery system for both over-the-counter and prescription drugs. The term *tablet* encompasses: the usual compressed tablet; the compressed tablet that is sugar- or film-coated to provide dissolution in either the stomach or the intestine, or partially in the stomach and partially in the intestine; layered tablets for gastric and intestinal release; effervescent tablets; sustained-release tablets; compressed coated tablets; sublingual and buccal tablets; chewable tablets; and medicated lozenges. These various dosage forms are described in depth in the three volumes of this series.

In the first volume, the various types of tablet products are discussed; the second volume is concerned with the processes involved in producing tablets, their bioavailability and pharmacokinetics; and in the third volume, additional processes in tablet production are discussed, as well as sustained drug release, stability, kinetics, automation, pilot plant, and quality assurance.

The first chapter in Volume 1 describes "Preformulation Testing." This second edition of the chapter contains an extensive amount of new material on substance purity, dissolution, the concept of permeability, and some of the pharmaceutical properties of solids. In the second chapter, "Tablet Formulation and Design," the plan for developing prototype formulas has been revised and an approach, using statistical design, is presented. There is consideration given to those elements in tablet formulation that are of importance to the operation of tablet presses with microprocessor controls.

There have been so many advances in the technology of wet granulation and direct compression methods since the first edition that what had previously been one chapter has now been expanded into two chapters.

"Compressed Tablets by Wet Granulation" has been updated, and a new section on unit operations has been added. Information on the formulations of sustained-release tablets by wet granulation is included in the chapter. "Compressed Tablets by Direct Compression," a separate chapter new to this edition, contains: a table comparing all aspects of direct compression versus wet granulation; an extensive glossary of trade names and manufacturers of tableting excipients; a section on morphology of pharmaceutical excipients, including scanning electron photomicrographs; a discussion of direct compression of example active ingredients; and a considerably expanded section on prototype or guide formulations.

The chapter entitled "Compression-Coated and Layered Tablets" describes the current technology for making these types of tablets. The chapter "Effervescent Tablets" has been expanded to include fluid-bed granulation techniques, updating on stability testing methods, new packaging materials, and methodologies for checking airtightness of sealed packets. The chapter on "Special Tablets" now contains information on long-acting and controlled-release buccal tablets as well as new sections on vaginal and rectal tablets. The chapter "Chewable Tablets" has increased its coverage to include microencapsulation and spray coating techniques. This chapter includes an update of the information concerned with excipients, colorants, direct-compression chewable tablets, and current manufacturing and product evaluation procedures related to these tablets. "Medicated Lozenges," the final chapter in Volume 1, has increased its scope to include liquid-center medicated lozenges and chewy-based medicated tablets.

Each of the tablet forms discussed requires special formulation procedures. Knowing how to make a particular type does not guarantee knowledge of how to make another. Since considerable expertise is required for the myriad tablet dosage forms, a multiauthored text seemed to be the only way to accomplish the editors' goals of providing knowledgeable and complete coverage of the subject. The editors chose authors to describe particular types of tablets on the basis of their experience, training, and high degree of knowledge of their subjects.

The authors were charged with the task of covering their technology in a way that would not be merely a review of the literature. Each chapter begins by assuming the reader is not very familiar with the subject. Gradually, as each chapter develops, the discussion becomes more advanced and specific. Following this format, we have intended the text to be a teaching source for undergraduate and graduate students as well as experienced and inexperienced industrial pharmaceutical scientists. The book can also act as a ready reference to all those interested in tablet technology. This includes students, product development pharmacists, hospital pharmacists, drug patent attorneys, governmental and regulatory scientists, quality control personnel, pharmaceutical production personnel, and those concerned with production equipment for making tablets.

The authors are to be commended for the manner in which they cover their subjects as well as for their patience with the editors' comments concerning their manuscripts. The editors wish to express their special thanks to the contributors for the excellence of their works, as well as for their continued forbearance with our attempts to achieve our desired level of quality for this text. Although there has been a great deal written about various types of tablets, it is only in this multivolume treatment that this subject is completely described. The acceptability and usefulness of these volumes is attributable to the efforts and skills of all of the contributing authors.

The topics, format, and choice of authors are the responsibilities of the editors. Any multiauthor book has problems of coordination and minimizing repetition. Some repetition was purposely retained because, in the editors' opinions, it helped the authors to develop their themes and because each individual treatment is sufficiently different so as to be valuable as a teaching aid. The editors hope that the labors of the contributors and our mutual judgments of subject matter have resulted in an up-to-date expanded reference that will facilitate the work of the many people who use it.

Herbert A. Lieberman
Leon Lachman
Joseph B. Schwartz

Contents

Chapter 7. Special Tablets   329

James W. Conine and Michael J. Pikal

Chapter 8. Chewable Tablets   367

*Robert W. Mendes, Aloysius O. Anaebonam, and
Jahan B. Daruwala*

Chapter 9. Medicated Lozenges   419

David Peters

Contributors

Aloysius O. Anaebonam Section Head, Pharmaceutical Development, Fisons Corporation, Rochester, New York

George J. Baley Vice President, Manufacturing and Distribution, The Upjohn Company, Inc., Kalamazoo, Michigan

Fred J. Bandelin Consultant, Schering-Plough Corporation, and Assistant Professor, Department of Pharmaceutics, University of Tennessee, Memphis, Tennessee

Gilbert S. Banker Dean, College of Pharmacy, University of Minnesota Health Sciences Center, Minneapolis, Minnesota

James W. Conine Research Scientist, Lilly Research Laboratories, Eli Lilly and Company, Indianapolis, Indiana, Retired

Jahan B. Daruwala Manager, Macturing Planning and Sourcing, Medical Products Department, E. I. du Pont de Nemours & Company, Wilmington, Delaware

Robert G. Dusel Associate, Lachman Consultant Services, Inc. Westbury, New York

William C. Gunsel Ciba-Geigy Corporation, Summit, New Jersey, Retired

Harold Jacobson Director, Regulatory Affairs, E. R. Squibb & Sons, New Brunswick, New Jersey

Vincent E. McCurdy Scientist, Drug Delivery R&D–Drug Products The Upjohn Company, Kalamazoo, Michigan

Robert W. Mendes   Professor and Chairman, Pharmaceutics and Industrial Pharmacy, Massachusetts College of Pharmacy and Allied Health Sciences, Boston, Massachusetts

Raymond Mohrle   Section Director, OTC Pharmaceutical Development, Consumer Products R&D Division, Warner-Lambert Company, Morris Plains, New Jersey

Garnet E. Peck   Professor of Industrial Pharmacy and Director of the Industrial Pharmacy Laboratory, Purdue University, West Lafayette, Indiana

David Peters*   Senior Research Associate, Consumer Products Development, Warner-Lambert Company, Morris Plains, New Jersey

Michael J. Pikal   Senior Research Scientist, Lilly Research Laboratories, Eli Lilly and Company, Indianapolis, Indiana

Abu T. M. Serajuddin   Section Head and Senior Laboratory Supervisor, Department of Pharmaceutical Research and Development, E. R. Squibb & Sons, New Brunswick, New Jersey

Ralph F. Shangraw   Professor and Chairman, Department of Pharmaceutics, The University of Maryland School of Pharmacy, Baltimore, Maryland

Deodatt A. Wadke   Director, Product Development, Department of Pharmaceutical Research and Development, E. R. Squibb & Sons, New Brunswick, New Jersey

---

Current affiliation: Pharmacist, Treworgy Pharmacy, Calais, Maine

Contents of Pharmaceutical Dosage Forms: Tablets, Second Edition, Revised and Expanded, Volumes 2 and 3

edited by Herbert A. Lieberman, Leon Lachman, and Joseph B. Schwartz

Contents of Pharmaceutical Dosage Forms: Parenteral Medications, Volumes 1 and 2

edited by Kenneth E. Avis, Leon Lachman,
and Herbert A. Lieberman

VOLUME 1

Contents of Pharmaceutical Dosage Forms: Disperse Systems, Volumes 1 and 2

edited by Herbert A. Lieberman, Martin M. Rieger, and Gilbert S. Banker

VOLUME 2

PHARMACEUTICAL DOSAGE FORMS

1

Preformulation Testing

Deodatt A. Wadke, Abu T. M. Serajuddin, and Harold Jacobson

E. R. Squibb & Sons, New Brunswick, New Jersey

I. INTRODUCTION

Preformulation testing is the first step in the rational development of dosage forms of a drug substance. It can be defined as an investigation of physical and chemical properties of a drug substance alone and when combined with excipients. The overall objective of preformulation testing is to generate information useful to the formulator in developing stable and bioavailable dosage forms that can be mass produced. Obviously, the type of information needed will depend on the dosage form to be developed. This chapter will describe a preformulation program needed to support the development of tablets and granulations as dosage forms.

During the early development of a new drug substance, the synthetic chemist, alone or in cooperation with specialists in other disciplines (including preformulation), may record some data that can be appropriately considered as preformulation data. This early data collection may include such information as gross particle size, melting point, infrared analysis, chromatographic purity, and other such characterizations of different laboratory scale batches. These data are useful in guiding, and becoming part of, the main body of preformulation work. Interactions between the responsible preformulation scientist, medicinal chemist, and pharmacologist at the very early stages of drug development are to be encouraged and must also focus on the biological data. Review of such data for a series of compounds when available, and review of the physical chemical properties of the compounds with some additional probing studies if necessary, would help in the early selection of the correct physical and chemical form of the drug entity for further development.

The formal preformulation study should start at the point after biological screening, when a decision is made for further development of the compound in clinical trials. Before embarking on a formal program, the preformulation scientist must consider the following:

Available physicochemical data (including chemical structure, different
   salts available)
Anticipated dose
Supply situation and development schedule (i.e., time available)
Availability of stability-indicating assay
Nature of the information the formulator should have or would like
   to have

The above considerations will offer the preformulation scientist some
quidance in deciding the types and the urgency of studies that need attention.   Selectivity is very critical to the success of the preformulation
program.   Not all the preformulation parameters are determined for every
new compound.   Data, as they are generated, must be reviewed to decide
what additional studies must be undertaken.   For example, a detailed investigation of dissolution is not warranted for a very soluble compound.   On
the other hand, particle size, surface area, dissolution, and the means of
enhancing rate of dissolution are important considerations in the preformulation evaluation of a sparingly soluble drug.

II. ORGANOLEPTIC PROPERTIES

A typical preformulation program should begin with the description of the
drug substance.   The color, odor, and taste of the new drug must be recorded using descriptive terminology.   It is important to establish a standard terminology to describe these properties in order to avoid confusion
among scientists using different terms to describe the same property.   A
list of some descriptive terms to describe the most commonly encountered
colors, tastes, and odors of pharmaceutical powders is provided in Table 1.
   The color of all the early batches of the new drug must be recorded
using the descriptive terminology.   A record of color of the early batches
is very useful in establishing appropriate specifications for later production.
When the color attributes are undesirable or variable, incorporation of a
dye in the body or coating of the final product could be recommended.

Table 1   Suggested Terminology to Describe
Organoleptic Properties of Pharmaceutical
Powders

Color	Odor	Taste
Off-white	Pungent	Acidic
Cream yellow	Sulfurous	Bitter
Tan	Fruity	Bland
Shiny	Aromatic	Intense
	Odorless	Sweet
		Tasteless

Drug substances, in general, have characteristic odors and tastes. In tasting the new drug, due caution must be exerted. If taste is considered as unpalatable, consideration ought to be given to the use of a less soluble chemical form of the drug, if one is available—provided, of course, the bioavailability is not unacceptably compromised. The odor and taste may be suppressed by using appropriate flavors and excipients or by coating the final product. The flavors, dyes, and other excipients selected to alleviate the problems of unsightly or variable color, and unpleasant odor and taste must be screened for their influence on the stability and bio-availability of the active drug.

Many drug substances are irritating to skin or sternutatory. Such information may already be available or developed during the course of pre-formulation studies. Where available, this information must be highlighted such that appropriate procedures for material handling and personnel protection can be developed.

III. PURITY

The preformulation scientists must have some perception of the purity of a drug substance. It is not this individual's primary responsibility to rigor-ously establish and investigate the purity (Notwithstanding that this is an important subject). Such studies are most often performed in an analytical research and development group. But some early knowledge is necessary so that subsequent preformulation and/or early safety and clinical studies are not compromised as to their validity. This is not to mean necessarily that relatively inhomogeneous material or material showing some impurity be rejected for preformulation studies. It does mean that such properties be recognized and be acceptable. It is another control parameter that allows for comparison with subsequent batches.

There are also more direct concerns. Occasionally an impurity can affect stability. Metal contamination at the level of a few parts per million is a relatively common example in which certain classes of compounds are deleteriously affected. Appearance is another area where a slight impurity can have a large effect. Off-color materials upon recystallization can become white in many instances. Further, some impurities require circumspection because they are potentially toxic. The presence of aromatic amines, suspected of being carcinogenic, is an example. In these instances, discussions must be initiated with the chemist preparing the material so that re-medial action can be taken. Very often a problem batch can be made satis-factory by a simple recrystallization.

Fortunately, the techniques used for characterizing the purity of a drug are the same as those used for other purposes in a preformulation study. Most of the techniques mentioned below are described in greater detail elsewhere in the chapter and are used to characterize the solid state, or as an analytical tool in stability or solubility studies.

Thin-layer chromatography (TLC) and high-pressure liquid chromato-graphy (HPLC) are of very wide-ranging applicability and are excellent tools for characterizing the chemical homogeneity of very many types of materials. Paper chromatography and gas chromatography are also useful in the deter-mination of chemical homogeneity.

All of these techniques can be designed to give a quantitative estimate of purity. Measures such as impurity index (II) and homogeneity index

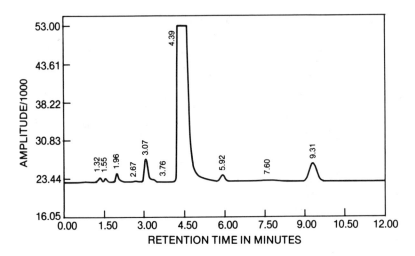

Figure 1   HPLC chromatograph of a typical batch of an experimental drug.

(HI) are useful and easy to calculate, especially from the HPLC chromato-
graphs. The II of a batch is defined as the ratio of all responses due to
components other than the main one to the total response. Typically, the
responses are obtained as area measurements in the chromatographic procedure. The obverse of the II is HI, which is the ratio of the response due
to the main component to the total response. Figure 1, which shows an
HPLC chromatograph for an experimental drug, illustrates determination
of II and HI. The chromatograph was generated using a UV detector. In
Figure 1, peak due to the main component occurs at a retention time of
4.39 with an area response of 4620. The seven other minor peaks are due
to the UV-absorbing impurities with total area response of 251. Thus, II
in this case is 251/(4620 + 251) = 0.0515, and the HI is 1 − 0.0515 =
0.9485.

The United States Pharmacopeia (USP) has proposed a related procedure
called ordinary impurities test that estimates impurities using TLC. In
this test impurity index is defined as a ratio of responses due to impurities
to that response due to a defined concentration of a standard of the main
component. The USP is proposing a general limit of 2% impurities [1,2].

The II, HI, and the impurity index as proposed by the USP are not
absolute measures of impurity since the specific response (i.e., molecular
absorbances or extinction coefficients) due to each impurity is assumed to
be the same as that of the main component. A more accurate analysis requires the identification of each individual impurity followed by preparation
of standards for each one of them. Such information is almost always unavailable at the early stages of development.

Other tools useful in the assessment of purity are differential and
gravimetric thermal analyses. These techniques often provide a qualitative
picture of homogeneity and also give direct evidence of the presence of solvates. Since these methods are simple and are used in characterizing the
material, their use for purity information is incidental. The appearance
of several peaks or the acuteness of an endotherm can often be indicative
of the purity. Similar information may sometimes also be generated by

observing the melting point, especially with a hot-stage microscope. More quantitative information can be obtained by using quantitative differential scanning calorimetry or by phase-rule solubility analysis.

As important to a compound's chemical characteristic are its physical ones. Crystalline form (including existence of solvates) is of fundamental importance, and for complete documentation of the compound X-ray powder diffraction patterns for each batch is desirable. This is simple to execute and provides useful information for later comparison and correlation to other properties.

IV. PARTICLE SIZE, SHAPE, AND SURFACE AREA

Various chemical and physical properties of drug substances are affected by their particle size distribution and shapes. The effect is not only on the physical properties of solid drugs but also, in some instances, on their biopharmaceutical behavior. For example, the bioavailability of griseofulvin and phenacetin is directly related to the particle size distributions of these drugs [3,4]. It is now generally recognized that poorly soluble drugs showing a dissolution rate-limiting step in the absorption process will be more readily bioavailable when administered in a finely subdivided state than as a coarse material. Very fine materials are difficult to handle [5]; but many difficulties can be overcome by creating solid solution of a material of interest in a carrier, such as a water-soluble polymer. This represents the ultimate in size reduction, since in a (solid) solution, the dispersed material of interest exists as discrete molecules or agglomerated molecular bundles of very small dimensions indeed.

Size also plays a role in the homogeneity of the final tablet. When large differences in size exist between the active components and excipients, mutual sieving (demixing) effects can occur making thorough mixing difficult or, if attained, difficult to maintain during the subsequent processing steps. This effect is greatest when the diluents and active raw materials are of significantly different sizes. Other things being equal, reasonably fine materials interdisperse more readily and randomly. However, if materials become too fine, then undersirable properties such as electrostatic effects and other surface active properties causing undue stickiness and lack of flowability manifest. Not only size but shape too influences the flow and mixing efficiency of powders and granules.

Size can also be a factor in stability; fine materials are relatively more open to attack from atmospheric oxygen, heat, light, humidity, and interacting exipients than coarse materials. Weng and Parrott [6] investigated influence of particle size of sulfacetamide on its reaction with phthalic anhydride in 1:2 molar compacts after 3 hr at 95°C. Their data, presented in Table 2, clarly demonstrate greater reactivity of sulfacetamide with decreasing particle size.

Because of these significant roles, it is important to decide on a desired size range, and thence to maintain and control it. It is probably safest to grind most new drugs having particles that are above approximately 100 μm in diameter. If the material consists of particles primarily 30 μm or less in diameter, then grinding is unnecessary, except if the material exists as needles—where grinding may improve flow and handling properties, or if the material is poorly water-soluble where grinding increases dissolution rate. Grinding should reduce coarse material to, preferably, the 10- to

Table 2   Influence of Particle Size
on Conversion of Sulfacetamide

Particle size of sulfacetamide (μm)	% Conversion ± SD
128	21.54 ± 2.74
164	19.43 ± 3.25
214	17.25 ± 2.88
302	15.69 ± 7.90
387	9.34 ± 4.41

Source: Modified from Weng, H.,
and Parrott, E. L., *J. Pharm. Sci.*,
73:1059 (1984). Reproduced with
the permission of copyright owner.

40-μm range. Once this is accomplished, controlled testing can be performed both for subsequent in vivo studies and for in-depth preformulation
studies. As the studies proceed, it may become apparent that grinding is
not required and that coarser materials are acceptable. At that time, it
is conceptually simpler to omit that step without jeopardizing the information
already developed. The governing concept is to stage the material so that
challenges are maximized.
    There are several drawbacks to grinding that may make it inadvisable.
Some are of lesser importance. For example, there are material losses when
grinding is done. Sometimes a static electricity buildup occurs, making the
material difficult to handle. Often, however, this problem, if it exists, may
be circumvented by mixing with excipients such as lactose prior to grinding.
Reduction of the particle size to too small a dimension often leads to aggregation and an apparent increase in hydrophobicity, possibly lowering the
dissolution rate and making handling more troublesome. When materials are
ground, they should be monitored not only for changes in the particle size
and surface area, but also for any inadvertent polymorphic or chemical
transformations. Undue grinding can destory solvates and thereby change
some of the important characteristics of a substance. Some materials can
also undergo a chemical reaction.

A.   General Techniques for Determining Particle Size

Several tools are commonly employed to monitor the particle size. The most
rapid technique allowing for a quick appraisal is microscopy. Microscopy,
since it requires counting of a large number of particles when quantitative
information is desired, is not suited for rapid, quantitative size determinations. However, it is very useful in estimating the range of sizes and the
shapes. The preliminary data can then be used to determine if grinding is
needed. A photomicrograph should be taken both before and after grinding.
The range of sizes observable by microscopy is from about 1 μm upward.

For optical microscopy, the material is best observed by suspending it in a nondissolving fluid (often water or mineral oil) and using polarizing lenses to observe birefringence as an aid to detecting a change to an amorphous state after grinding.

For a quantitative particle size distribution analysis of materials that range upward from about 50 μm, sieving or screening is appropriate, although shape has a strong influence on the results. Most pharmaceutical powders, however, range in size from 1 to 120 μm. To encompass these ranges, a variety of instrumentation has been developed. There are instruments based on lasers (Malvern), light scattering (Royco), light blockage (HIAC), and blockage of an electrical conductivity path (Coulter Counter). The instrument based on light blockade has been adopted by the USP to monitor the level of foreign particulates in parenteral products. The instrument will measure particle size distribution of any powder properly dispersed in a suspending medium. The concentration of sample suspension should be such that only a single particle is presented to the sensor in unit time, thus avoiding coincidence counting.

Other techniques based on centrifugation and air suspension are also available. Most of these instruments measure the numbers of particles, but the distributions are readily converted to weight and size distributions. The latter way of expressing the data is more meaningful. A number of classical techniques based on sedimentation methods, utilizing devices such as the Andreasen pipet or recording balances that continuously collect a settling suspension, are also known. However, these methods are now in general disfavor because of their tedious nature. Table 3 lists some of the common techniques useful for measurement of different size ranges [7].

There are many mathematical expressions that can be used to characterize an average size. These refer to average volumes or weights, geometric mean diameters, and relationships reflecting shapes, such as the ratio of an area to a volume or weight factor [8].

Table 3   Common Techniques for
Measuring Fine Particles of
Various Sizes

Technique	Particle size (μm)
Microscopic	1−100
Sieve	>50
Sedimentation	>1
Elutriation	1−50
Centrifugal	<50
Permeability	>1
light scattering	0.5−50

Source: Parrott, E. L., *Pharm. Mfg.*,
4:31 (1985). Reproduced with the
permission of copyright owner.

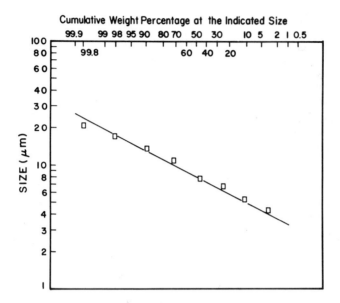

Figure 2   Log probability plot of the size distribution of a sample of triamcinolone acetonide.

A convenient way to characterize a particle size distribution is to construct a log probability plot. Log probability graph paper is commercially available, and particle size distributions resulting from a grinding operation with no cut being discarded will give a linear plot. An example is illustrated in Figure 2 for a powder sample of triamcinolone acetonide. The data used in the construction of Figure 2 are presented in Table 4.

The numbers of particles in Table 4 are converted into weight fractions by assuming them to be spheres and multiplying by the volume of a single sphere (particle) calculated from the geometric relationship:

$$V = \frac{\pi}{6} d^3$$

where V is the volume and d the particle diameter (using the average value of the range given in the first column of Table 4). The result is the total volume occupied by particles in each of the size ranges and is given in the third column of the table. The volume is directly related to a mass term by the reciprocal of the density. However, since the density is constant for all particles of a single species and is rarely known accurately, it is sufficient to use the volume terms to calculate the weight percentages in each size range by dividing the total volume of all the particles into the volumes in each range (column 4 of Table 4). If densities were used, it is obvious that they would cancel out in this calculation. The cumulative weight percentage in each size range is shown in the last column.

Statistical descriptions of distributions most often give a measure of central tendency. However, with powders the distributions are skewed in the direction of increasing size. This type of distribution can be described by the Hatch-Choate equation:

$$f = \frac{\Sigma n}{\sqrt{2\pi} \ln \sigma_g} \exp \left[- \frac{(\ln d - \ln M)^2}{2 \ln^2 \sigma_g} \right] \qquad (1)$$

where f is the frequency with which a particle of diameter d occurs, and n is the total number of particles in a powder in which the geometric mean particle size is M and the geometric standard deviation is σ_g. Equation (1) is succinctly discussed by Orr and Dalla Valle [9].

The two measures M and σ_g uniquely characterize a distribution, and are readily obtained graphically from a log probability plot in which cumulative weight percentage is plotted against the particle size (Fig. 2). The geometric mean diameter corresponds to the 50% value of the abscissa, and the geometric standard deviation is given by the following ratios, the values for which are taken from the graph.

$$\sigma_g = \frac{84.13\% \text{ size}}{50\% \text{ size}} = \frac{50\% \text{ size}}{15.87\% \text{ size}}$$

For the example, the values are 8.2 and 1.5 μm for the geometric mean particle size and its standard deviation, respectively. The latter is also a slope term. For particle size distributions resulting from a crystallization, a linear plot can often be obtained using linear probability paper.

B.   Determination of Surface Area

The determination of the surface areas of powders has been getting increasing attention in recent years. The techniques employed are relatively simple and convenient to use, and the data obtained reflect the particle

Table 4   Particle Size Distribution of a Ground Sample of Triamcinolone Acetonide

Size range (μm)	No. of particles	Volume of particles $\times 10^{-3}$ (μm^3)	Weight percent in range	Cumulative weight percent
22.5−26.5	5	38	0.2	100.0
18.6−22.0	54	237	1.7	99.8
14.9−18.6	488	1212	8.8	98.1
11.8−14.9	2072	2552	18.5	·89.3
9.4−11.8	5376	3352	24.3	70.8
7.4−9.4	9632	2989	21.7	46.5
5.9−7.4	12,544	1888	13.7	24.8
4.7−5.9	12,928	1008	7.3	11.1
3.7−4.7	13,568	526	3.8	3.8

size. The relationship between the two parameters is an inverse one, in that a grinding operation that reduces the particle size leads to an increase in the surface area.

The most common approach for determining the surface area is based on the Brunauer—Emmett—Teller (BET) theory of adsorption. An excellent discussion of the principles and techniques involved has been given by Gregg and Sing [10]. Briefly, the theory states that most substances will adsorb a monomolecular layer of a gas under certain conditions of partial pressure (of the gas) and temperature. Knowing the monolayer capacity of an adsorbent (i.e., the quantity of adsorbate that can be accommodated as a monolayer on the surface of a solid, the adsorbent) and the area of the adsorbate molecule, the surface area can, in principle, be calculated.

Most commonly, nitrogen is used as the adsorbate at a specific partial pressure established by mixing it with an inert gas, typically helium. The adsorption process is carried out at liquid nitrogen temperatures ($-195°C$). It has been demonstrated that, at a partial pressure of nitrogen attainable when it is in a 30% mixture with an inert gas and at $-195°C$, a monolayer is adsorbed onto most solids. Apparently, under these conditions the polarity of nitrogen is sufficient for van der Waals forces of attraction between the adsorbate and the adsorbents to be manifest. The kinetic energy present under these conditions overwhelms the intermolecular attraction between nitrogen atoms. However, it is not sufficient to break the bonding between the nitrogen and dissimilar atoms. The latter are most often more polar and prone to van der Waals forces of attraction. The nitrogen molecule does not readily enter into chemical combinations, and thus its binding is of a nonspecific nature (i.e., it enters into a physical adsorption); consequently, the nitrogen molecule is well suited for this role.

The BET equation is

$$\frac{1}{\lambda(P_0/P - 1)} = \frac{C - 1}{\lambda_m C} \frac{P}{P_0} + \frac{1}{\lambda_m C} \tag{2}$$

where λ is the grams of adsorbate per gram of adsorbent, λ_m the value of that ratio for a monolayer, P the partial pressure of the absorbate gas, P_0 the vapor pressure of the pure adsorbate gas, and C a constant. The constant C is temperature-dependent, as are P and P_0; consequently, measurements are made under isothermal conditions. The equation is that of a straight line, and the inverse of the sum of both the slope [$(C - 1)/\lambda_m C$] and the y intercept ($1/\lambda_m C$) gives λ_m. In an experiment it is necessary to measure at various values of P; P_0 can be obtained from the literature. The other values are then readily calculated. Often the constant C is large and Equation (2) then simplifies to:

$$\lambda_m = \lambda\left(1 - \frac{P}{P_0}\right)$$

A single-point determination (e.e., using only one value of P) is then possible. Knowing the specific weight of adsorbate (λ_m) in a monolayer, it is possible to calculate the specific surface area (SSA) of the sample using the following equation:

$$SAA = \frac{\lambda_m N A_{N_2}}{M_{N_2}}$$

where N is the Avogadro number, A_{N_2} the area of the adsorbate molecule (generally taken to be, for nitrogen, 16.2×10^{-20} m^2 per molecule), and M_{N_2} the molecular weight of the adsorbate.

Several experimental approaches are available that enable rapidity and convenience as well as accuracy and precision. Volumetric techniques represent the classic approach, and the modern instrumentation available has made the procedure convenient. Gravimetric and dynamic methods are also available. The latter methods measure the adsorption process by monitoring the gas streams, using devices such as thermal conductivity detectors and transducers.

An example using a dynamic method is illustrated in the data given in Table 5 for a sample of sodium epicillin. In addition to the instrument, the requirements are a supply of liquid nitrogen, several gas compositions, a barometer, and several gas-tight syringes. Briefly, the procedure entails passing the gas over an accurately weighed sample contained in an appropriate container immersed in liquid nitrogen, removing the liquid nitrogen when the adsorption is complete (as signaled by the instrument), warming the sample to about room temperature, and measuring (via the instrument) the adsorbate gas released (column 3 of Table 5). Calibration is simply performed by injecting known amounts of adsorbate gas into the proper instrument port (columns 4 and 5 of Table 5). The other terms in the table are calculable; P is the product of the fraction of nitrogen in the gas mixture (column 1) and the ambient pressure. The weight of nitrogen adsorbed is calculated from the ideal gas law. Slight adjustments of these values are made in actual practice as outlined by the various instrument manufacturers. Plotting the second column against the last column gives

Table 5 Specific Surface Area of a Sample of Sodium Epicillin[a]

%N$_2$ in He	P/P$_0$	Signal (area)	Vol N$_2$ used (ml)	Signal (area)	Wt N$_2$ absorbed $\times 10^{-4}$ (g)	$[\lambda(P_0/P - 1)]^{-1}$
			Standardization			
4.9	0.0483	178	0.050	137	0.576	677.5
9.7	0.0956	152	0.080	150	0.922	1130.9
20.0	0.1972	248	0.100	238	1.153	2043.6
29.9	0.2948	312	0.130	331	1.499	2957.5

[a]Sample weight: 0.1244 g. Atmospheric pressure: 762.7 mmHg. Temperature: 297 K. Results: Slope, 9210; y Intercept, 238.2; correlation coefficient, 0.99995; specific surface area, 3.0 m^2 g^{-1}.

Table 6   Relationship Between
Diameter of a Particle and
Specific Surface Area

Diameter (μm)	Specific surface area ($m^2\ g^{-1}$)
0.25	24
0.50	12
1.0	6
2.0	3
4.0	1.5
10.0	0.63
15.0	0.4
20.0	0.3
40.0	0.15

the necessary slope and intercept values for calculating the specific surface area.   For the sample of sodium epicillin a single-point determination (using the gas containing 29.9% nitrogen) gives a value of 2.8 $m^2\ g^{-1}$ for the surface area, which agrees well with the value of 3.0 obtained using the multipoint procedure.

It is of interest to note the relationship between a diameter and the surface area of a gram of material of hypothetical monosized particles shown in Table 6.   At relatively large diameters, the specific surface area is insensitive to an increase in diameter, whereas at very small diameters the surface area is comparatively very sensitive.   If there is little difference in the properties of pharmaceutical interest between particles of about 1 μm to those of about 0.5 μm, measurement of surface area is of little value.   In the contrary instance, where a pharmaceutical property changes significantly for small particle-size changes, such measurements would be meaningful.

Some further prudence is necessary when interpreting surface area data.   Thus, although a relatively high surface area most often reflects a relatively small particle size, it is not always true.   A porous or a strongly agglomerated mass would be exceptional.   Also, as implied previously, small particles (thus of high surface area) agglomerate more readily, and often in such a manner as to render the inner pores and surfaces inaccessible to water (as in a dissolution experiment).   Thus, they act as if they are of much larger diameter than they actually are.

V.   SOLUBILITY

Solid drugs administered orally for systemic activity must dissolve in the gastrointestinal fluids prior to their absorption.   Thus, the rate of dissolution of drugs in gastrointestinal fluids could influence the rate and extent of their absorption. Inasmuch as the rate of dissolution of a solid is a function of its solubility in the dissolution medium, the latter could influence absorption of the relatively insoluble drugs. As a rule of thumb, compounds with an aqueous solubility of greater than 1% w/v are not expected to present dissolution-related absorption problems. In the application of this rule, however, one must consider the anticipated dose of the drug and its stability in the gastrointestinal fluids. A highly insoluble drug administered in small doses may exhibit good absorption. For a drug that is unstable in the highly acidic environment of the stomach, high solubility and consequent rapid dissolution could result in a decreased bioavailability. For these reasons, aqueous solubility is a useful biopharmaceutical parameter. The solubility of every new drug must be determined as a function of pH over the physiological pH range of 1 to 8. If the solubility is considered too low or too high, efforts to alter it may be undertaken.

A. Determination of Solubility

A semiquantitative determination of the solubility can be made by adding the solute in small incremental amounts to a fixed volume of the solvent. After each addition, the system is vigorously shaken and examined visually for any undissolved solute particles. When some solute remains undissolved, the total amount added up to that point serves as a good and rapid estimate of solubility. When more quantitative data are needed, a suspension of the solute in the solvent is shaken at constant temperature. Samples are withdrawn periodically, filtered, and the concentration of the solute in the filtrates is determined by a suitable method. Sampling is continued until consecutive samples show the same concentration. In the clarification of the suspension samples, it should be borne in mind that many filter media have a tendency to adsorb solute molecules. It is therefore advisable to discard the first few milliliters of the filtrates.

Solubility of an acidic or basic drug is pH-dependent and, as mentioned earlier, must be determined over the pH range 1 to 8. Since such compounds favor their own pH environment dictated by their pK_a values, it becomes necessary to adjust the pH values of their saturated solution. There is no general method for this pH adjustment. In some reported studies, authors used buffers of appropriate pH values [11–13], whereas others used hydrochloric acid or sodium hydroxide solutions [14–17]. Since the pH of an equilibrated suspension of an ionizable compound in a buffered system may not be the same as that of the starting buffer, it is essential to determine pH of the system after equilibration.

Solubility determinations of poorly soluble compounds present their own unique problems. Higuchi and coworkers [18] demonstrated that the solubilities of such compounds could be overestimated due to the presence of soluble impurities. The saturation solubility of a poorly soluble compound is not reached in a reasonable length of time unless the amount of solid used is greatly in excess of that needed to saturate a given volume of solvent. This is because the final rate of approach to saturation is almost exclusively dictated by the surface area of the dissolving solid. For example, equilibrium solubilities of benzoic acid and norethindrone are 3.4 mg/ml and 6 μg/ml, respectively. In solubility experiments initiated using twice the amount of each compound needed to saturate the medium, the amount of benzoic acid remaining undissolved at near saturation would be approximately 500 times that for norethindrone. As a result, equilibrium solubility of benzoic acid would be reached faster. If one uses a disproportionately greater amount of norethindrone to compensate for its lower solubility, the contribution of soluble impurities present to the total mass dissolved would become significant. Suspending a 500-fold excess of a solid with 1% soluble impurities would show a fivefold increase in the apparent solubility. To overcome this problem one must use a specific assay for the estimation of dissolved chemical of interest. Alternately, one could use the facilitated dissolution method as developed by Higuchi and coworkers [18]. Here, the drug is dissolved in a water-immiscible solvent and then partitioned into the aqueous phase which in turn is assayed. The method is rapid and provides a fairly good estimate of true solubility.

Many compounds in solution degrade, thus making an accurate determination of the solubility difficult. For such compounds, Ohnishi and Tanabe [19] proposed a kinetic method. It consists of the determination of rate constants and orders of reactions for degradation of the solute in a solution and a suspension. If V_s is the velocity of the overall degradation of the solute from the suspension, then

$$V_s = \sum_i k_i [S]^i$$

where i is the order of the reaction in solution, k_i is the rate constant for the ith-order reaction, and [S] is the saturation concentration. The quantities V_s, k_i, and i are measurable kinetic parameters that lead to the determination of [S]. Ohnishi and Tanable used this approach to determine the solubility of benzyl chloride. In an aqueous solution, benzyl chloride hydrolyzes. At 20°C, the authors found that V_s, the velocity of hydrolysis of benzyl chloride in suspension, was 1.67×10^{-6} mole min^{-1}. Analysis of degradation from solutions showed that benzyl chloride in solution degraded by first- and second-order reactions. At 20°C, k_1 and k_2, the first- and second-order rate constants, were determined to be 2.9×10^{-4}/min^{-1} and 3.6×10^{-1} M^{-1} min^{-1}, respectively. The equation describing degradation of benzyl chloride from suspension at 20°C would be

$$1.67 \times 10^{-6} = 2.9 \times 10^{-4}[S] + 3.6 \times 10^{-2}[S]^2$$

which can be solved to yield a value of 3.9×10^{-3} M for [S], the solubility of benzyl chloride at 20°C. The method presupposes that the rate of dissolution of the drug in suspension is much greater than its rate of degradation from solution. It is also essential to determine all the kinetic parameters under identical conditions of temperature, pH, etc.

Difficulty is also encountered in the determination of solubility of metastable forms that transform to more stable forms when exposed to solvents. Here a method based on the determination of intrinsic dissolution rates is applicable [20]. For many compounds exhibiting polymorphism, the metastable forms, when exposed to solvents, are sufficiently stable to permit measurement of initial dissolution rates. These initial dissolution rates, according to the Noyes—Nernst equation, are proportional to the respective solubilities of the polymorphic forms. The proportionality constant for the stable and metastable forms of a given compound is the same. Thus, determination of the intrinsic dissolution rates of the stable and metastable forms and the solubility of the stable form permits calculation of the solubility of the metastable form.

B. pH-Solubility Profile

The degree of ionization and therefore the solubility of acidic and basic compounds depends on the pH of the medium. The saturation solubility for such compounds at a particular pH is the sum total of solubility of ionized and unionized forms. Kramer and Flynn [11] investigated relative contributions of the protonated and free basic forms of several drugs to their total solubilities under different pH conditions. For ionizable compounds a solution may be saturated with respect to one species or the other depending on pH. The pH at which the solution is saturated with respect to both the ionized and unionized forms is defined as pH_{max} — the pH of maximum solubility. For a base, the equation relating total solubility (S_T) to solubilities of protonated (BH^+) and free (BP forms is

$$S_T, pH < pH_{max} = [BH^+]_s \left(1 + \frac{K_a}{[H_3O^+]} \right)$$

where the subscript $pH < pH_{max}$ indicates that the equation is valid only at pH values below the pH_{max}, subscript s denotes saturation species, K_a is the apparent dissociation constant, and $[H_3O^+]$ is the hydronium ion concentration. The equation applicable at pH values higher than the pH_{max} is

$$S_T, pH > pH_{max} = [B_s] \left(1 + \frac{[H_3O^+]}{K_a} \right)$$

The corresponding equations for an acidic compound are

$$S_T, pH < pH_{max} = [AH]_s \left(1 + \frac{K_a}{[H_3O^+]} \right)$$

and

$$S_T, pH > pH_{max} = [A^-]_s \left(1 + \frac{[H_3O^+]}{K_a} \right)$$

where $[A^-]$ and $[AH]$ denote concentrations of ionized and unionized forms.
   Since ionizable compounds may be available in free or salt forms, one could use either in solubility experiments. For example, Serajuddin and Jarowski [17] studied the solubility behavior of phenazopyridine free base and its hydrochloride salt over the pH range 1 to 10. Their findings are presented in Figure 3. Phenazopyridine, a base with a pK_a of 5.2, exhibits maximum solubility at pH 3.45 (pH_{max}). It should be noted here that, depending on the starting material, in the region of pH_{max} experimentally determined solubilities are higher than the equilibrium solubilities. This

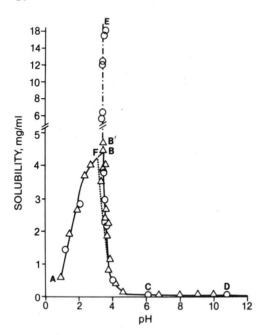

Figure 3   pH-Solubility profiles of phenazopyridine hydrochloride (△) and phenazopyridine base (○) at 37°C. Solubilities are expressed as hydrochloride salt equivalents. Lower pH values than that of a saturated solution of the salt in water (point B) were adjusted by stepwise addition of HCl solution (curve BA); higher pH values were obtained by addition of NaOH solution (curve B'D). Similarly, pH values lower and higher than that of a saturated solution of base in water (point C) were also adjusted by the addition of HCl and NaOH solutions, respectively. Curve BE represents supersaturation of phenazopyridine base solution. Curve DF was fitted theoretically by using 0.037 mg ml^{-1} as base solubility and 5.20 as the pK_a. Points B and F are, respectively, apparent and theoretical pH_{max}. [From Serajuddin, A. T. M., and Jarowski, C. I., *J. Pharm. Sci.*, 74:142 (1985). Reproduced with the permission of copyright owner.]

phenomenon is described as supersaturation. Supersaturated solutions are metastable and will precipitate excess solute in due course on standing.

C. Solubility Product

In a saturated solution of a salt with some undissolved solid, there exists an equilibrium between the excess solid and the ions resulting from the dissociation of the salt in solution. For a hydrochloride salt represented as BH^+Cl^-, the equilibrium is

$$BH^+CL^- (s) \longrightarrow BH^+ + Cl^-$$

where BH^+ and Cl^- represent the hydrated ions in solution. The corresponding equilibrium constant K is given by

$$K = \frac{a_{BH^+} a_{Cl^-}}{a_{BH^+Cl^-}} \qquad (3)$$

where each subscripted "a" denotes the appropriate activity. As a solid the activity of BH^+Cl^- is constant. Equation (3), therefore, reduces to

$$K_{sp} = a_{BH^+} a_{Cl^-} \qquad (4)$$

The constant K_{sp} is known as the solubility product and determines the solubility of a salt.

In practice Equation (4) can be modified substituting concentration for activity. For an ionizable drug as mentioned earlier total solubility S_T is the sum total of $[BH^+]_s$ and $[B]$. Since $[BH^+]_s \gg [B]$, equation (4) for a hydrochloride salt reduces to

$$K_{sp} = S_T[Cl^-] \qquad (5)$$

Equation (5) dictates that total solubility of a hydrochloride salt would decrease with an increase in the chloride ion concentration. This phenomenon is known as *common ion effect*. In Figure 3, the observed decrease in the total solubility of phenazopyridine at pH values below pH_{max} was due to common ion effect.

Since the gastric contents are high in chloride ion concentration, the common ion effect phenomenon suggests that one should use salts other than the hydrochloride to benefit fully from the enhanced solubility due to a salt form. Despite this, many drugs are used as hydrochloride salts. This is because solubilities of most hydrochloride salts in the presence of chloride ion concentration normally encountered in vivo are sufficiently high. The suppression of solubility due to common ion effect under these conditions is not of sufficient magnitude to affect dissolution or bioavailability of these compounds.

D. Solubilization

When the drug substance under consideration is not an acidic or basic compound, or when the acidic or basic character of the compound is not amenable to the formation of a stable salt, other means of enhancing the solubility may be explored. The use of a more soluble metastable polymorph to enhance bioavailability of orally administered solids is one way to approach the problem. Other approaches to improve solubility or rate of dissolution include use of complexation and high-energy coprecipitates that are mixtures of solid solutions and dispersions. Riboflavin in solution complexes with xanthines, resulting in an increase in the apparent solubility of the vitamin [21,22]. The approach, however, has practical limitations. The primary requirement is that the complexing or solubilizing agent be physiologically inert. Thus, unless the solubilizer is an approved excipient, this approach is not recommended. In this regard, the use of water-soluble polymers to form high-energy coprecipitates is more acceptable. Griseofulvin is a water-insoluble, neutral polyethylene glycol antifungal antibiotic. Dispersions and solid solutions of griseofulvin in PEG 4000, 6000, and 20,000

dissolve significantly more rapidly than the wetted micronized drug. In
the case of PEG 4000 and 20,000, this treatment provided supersaturated
solutions [23]. Subsequent studies with the PEG 6000 dispersion showed
that, in humans, the dispersed drug was more than twice as available as
from commercially available tablets containing the micronized drug [24].

In the majority of cases, efforts to alter solubilities of drugs are undertaken to improve the solubility. Occasionally, however, a less soluble form
is desired. Thus, in the case of clindamycin, the less soluble pamoate
salt is preferred over the soluble hydrochloride hydrate to circumvent the
problem of the unpleasant taste of the drug [25]. Likewise, when a drug
is inactivated by the acidity of gastric fluids, a less soluble form is preferred.

Knowledge of solubility of a drug substance not only helps in making
some judgment concerning its bioavailability but also is useful in the development of appropriate media for dissolution testing or for development of
an injectable dosage form for certain pharmacological and comparative bioavailability studies. In the investigation of dissolution of drugs insoluble
in a purely aqueous medium, a cosolvent may be used to provide sink conditions. In these situations, knowledge of solubility in water-miscible organic solvents such as lower molecular weight alcohols and glycols is useful. The latter data are also of use to a formulator in the development of
dosage forms of drugs that are administered in very small doses. Here
the drug is often dispersed among the excipients as a solution in an appropriate solvent. Solubility data are also useful to the formulator in
choosing the right solvent for the purposes of granulation and coating.
The use of a granulating solvent with a very high capacity to dissolve the
active ingredient can lead to a phenomenon known as *case hardening*. Here
the solute migrates and deposits on the periphery of granules during the
drying operation.

A good working knowledge of solubility is also essential at the preclini-
cal stage for the proper interpretation of biological data. These data are
invariably generated using extemporaneously prepared solutions/suspensions.
An inappropriate choice of solvent in these studies could show an active
drug to be inactive or a toxic one to be nontoxic because of inadequate
solubility and consequent incomplete absorption, and result in wrong selection of a compound for further development.

VI. DISSOLUTION

The absorption of solid drugs administered orally can be depicted by the
following flowchart:

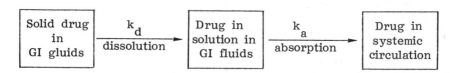

where k_d and k_a are rate constants for the dissolution and absorption
processes, respectively. When dissolution is the significantly slower of the
two processes (i.e., $k_d \ll k_a$) the absorption is described as *dissolution
rate-limited*. Since dissolution precedes absorption in the overall scheme,

any change in the process of dissolution would influence the absorption.
It is essential, therefore, to investigate the dissolution behavior of drug
substances, especially those with moderate and poor solubility.   Efforts
are then undertaken to alter this process if deemed necessary.   Also, a
knowledge of comparative dissolution rates of different chemical (salt, ester,
prodrug, etc.) and physical (polymorph, solvate, etc.) forms of a drug is
necessary in selecting the optimum form for further development.

A. Intrinsic Dissolution

The dissolution rate of a solid in its own solution is adequately described
by the Noyes–Nernst equation:

$$\frac{dC}{dt} = \frac{AD(C_s - C)}{hV} \tag{6}$$

where

dC/dt = dissolution rate

A = surface area of the dissolving solid

D = diffusion coefficient

C = solute concentration in the bulk medium

h = diffusion layer thickness

V = volume of the dissolution medium

C_s = solute concentration in the diffusion layer

During the early phase of dissolution, $C_s \gg C$ and is essentially equal to
saturation solubility S.   Surface area A and volume V can be held constant.
Under these conditions and at constant temperature and agitation, Equation
(6) reduces to

$$\frac{dC}{dt} = KS \tag{7}$$

where

$K = AD/hV$ = constant.

Dissolution rate as expressed in Equation (7) is termed the *intrinsic dissolution rate* and is characteristic of each solid compound in a given solvent under fixed hydrodynamic conditions.   The intrinsic dissolution rate
in a fixed volume of solvent is generally expressed as mg dissolved ×
(min^{-1} cm^{-2}).   Knowledge of this value helps the preformulation scientist
in predicting if absorption would be dissolution rate-limited.   Kaplan [26]
studied the dissolution of a number of compounds in 500 ml of medium
ranging in pH from 1 to 8, at 37°C, while stirring at 50 rpm.   His experience suggests that compounds with intrinsic dissolution rates greater
than 1 mg min^{-1} cm^{-2} are not likely to present dissolution rate-limited absorption problems.   Those with rates below 0.1 mg min^{-1} cm^{-2} are suspect

and usually exhibit dissolution rate-limited absorption. For compounds with rates between 0.1 and 1.0 mg min^{-1} cm^{-2}, usually more information is needed before making any prediction.

The determination of the intrinsic dissolution rate can be accomplished best using the rotating-disk method of Wood et al. [27]. A schematic diagram of the Wood apparatus is shown in Figure 4. This method allows for the determination of dissolution from a constant surface. A constant surface is obtained by compressing the solid in a tablet die against a flat surface using a hydraulic press. The punch used is cut down in length; the punch is left in the die and secured in position using a rubber gasket. The assembly is then attached to the shaft of a constant-speed rotor. To study dissolution, the rotor assembly is lowered in the dissolution medium to a preset position, and the rotor is activated. The progress of the dissolution is followed by periodically sampling and assaying the dissolution medium for the dissolved solute. Alternately, the dissolution medium may be circulated through the cell of a spectrophotometer for continuous recording. When the temperature, the pressure used to prepare the constant surface, and the hydrodynamics of the system are properly controlled, the method provides very reproducible results.

As expressed in Equation (7) dissolution rate of a compound is directly proportional to its solubility. However, solubilities of acidic and basic compounds, as mentioned earlier, are pH-dependent, and apparent deviations from the relationship expressed by Equation (7) have been reported for many ionizable drugs [28,29]. Thus, Serajuddin and Jarowski [17] noticed significantly different intrinsic dissolution behavior for phenazopyridine free base and its hydrochloride salt under apparently identical conditions. Their data are presented in Figures 5 and 6 and Table 7. It can be seen here that the rates of dissolution of the free base and its salt

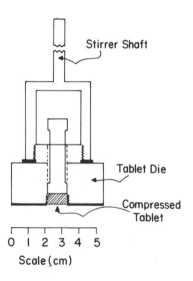

Figure 4   Schematic diagram of constant-surface assembly for the determination of intrinsic dissolution rates. [From Wood, J. H., Syarto, J. E., and Letterman, H., *J. Pharm. Sci.*, 54:1068 (1965). Reproduced with the permission of the copyright owner.]

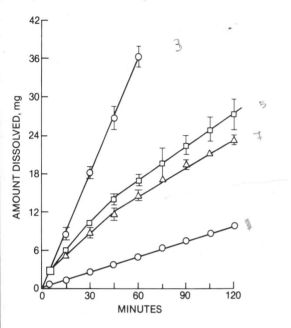

Figure 5 Dissolution profiles of phenzopyridine hydrochloride from a surface area of 0.95 cm^2 at 37°C under pH-stat conditions. Key: (○) pH 1.10: (○) pH 3.05: (□) pH 5.0: (△) pH 7.0. Each point represents the mean ± SD of three experimental values.

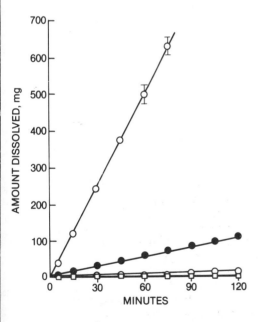

Figure 6 Dissolution profiles of phenazopyridine at 37°C from a surface area of 0.95 cm^2 under pH-stat conditions. Key: (○) pH 1.10: (●) 2.05: (○) pH 3.05: (□) pH 5.0. Each point represents the mean ± SD of three experimental values. Data are expressed as hydrochloride salt equivalents.

Table 7   Intrinsic Dissolution Rates (J/A) and
Solubilities in Bulk Media (C_s) of Phenazopyridine
and Its Hydrochloric Salt at 37°C

pH of medium	J/A, mg cm^{-2} min^{-1}[a]		C_s, mg/ml
	Salt	Base	Salt or base[a]
1.10	0.084	8.89	0.680
2.05	–	0.94	3.200
3.05	0.640	0.103	4.320
5.0	0.638	0.013	0.090
7.0	0.645	–	0.037

[a]Expressed as hydrochloride salt equivalents.
Source: Modified from Serajuddin, A. T. M.,
and Jarowski, C. I., *J. Pharm. Sci.*, 74:142
(1985). Reproduced with the permission of
copyright owner.

form are not directly proportional to their equilibrium solubilities. Also, the
rates of dissolution for the two forms under identical medium pH conditions
differ widely despite the constancy of equilibrium solubility. Such deviations
from Equation (7) are explained on the basis of self-buffering action of dissolving species in the diffusion layer. The pH at the dissolving surface in
these cases is different from the pH of the bulk medium. Under these conditions for the calculation of dissolution rate, one should use equilibrium
solubility value at the pH of the dissolving surface. A good approximation
of pH at the dissolving surface can be obtained by independently measuring
pH of a suspension in the medium.

B. Particulate Dissolution

Particulate dissolution is another method of studying the dissolution of solids.
Here no effort is made to maintain the surface area constant. A weighed
amount of powder sample from a particular sieve fraction is introduced in the
dissolution medium. Agitation is usually provided by a constant-speed pro-
peller. Particulate dissolution is used to study the influence on dissolution
of particle size, surface area, and mixing with excipients. Finholt [30]
studied the dissolution of phenacetin granules prepared using different sieve
fractions of the drug powder (Fig. 7). As expected, the rate of dissolution
increased with a decrease in the particle size. Occasionally, however, one
encounters an inverse relationship of particle size to dissolution, where particle size reduction decreases—or fails to improve—the dissolution. This
may be explained on the basis of effective or available, rather than absolute,
surface area; and it is caused by incomplete wetting of the powder. In such
areas incorporation of a surfactant in the dissolution medium may provide the
expected relationship.

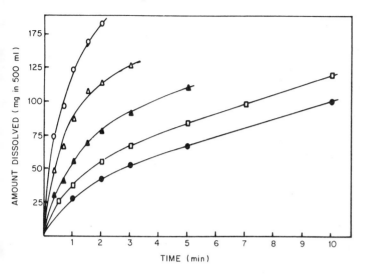

Figure 7 Effect of particle size of phenacetin on dissolution rate of the drug from granules. Key: ○ particle size 0.11−0.15 mm; △ particle size 0.15−0.21 mm; ▲ particle size 0.21−0.30 mm; □ particle size 0.30−50 mm; ● particle size 0.50−0.71 mm. (From Finholt, P., Influence of formulation on dissolution rate, *Dissolution Technology*, the Industrial Pharmaceutical Technology Section of the Academy of Pharmaceutical Sciences, Washington, D.C., 1974. Reproduced with the permission of the copyright owner.)

When dissolution is considered to be slow, a means of enhancing it may be sought. In the absence of a more soluble physical or chemical form of the drug, particle size reduction is the most commonly employed practice. Enhanced surface area, with a concomitant increase in the dissolution, can also be accomplished by adsorbing the drug on an inert excipient with a high surface area, such as fumed silicon dioxide [31]. Comelting, coprecipitating, or triturating a relatively insoluble drug with some excipients can also result in faster dissolution [32,33].

C. Prediction of Dissolution Rates

Since dissolution of solids is adequately described by the Noyes−Nernst equation, knowledge of different parameters in the equation should permit the calculation of theoretical rates. Hussain [34] used this approach to predict the dissolution rates of many slightly soluble drugs. He used a value of 9.0×10^{-6} cm^2 sec^{-1} for diffusion coefficient, a good approximation for most drugs, and a value of 50×10^{-3} cm for diffusion layer thickness when stirring at 50 rpm. The value of C_s [Eq. (6)] was approximated by saturation solubility. Surface areas were calculated using the mean particle diameter and assuming a spherical shape. The following example illustrates Hussain's method.

Sample Calculation

Consider the dissolution of 22 mg of 60- to 80-mesh hydrocortisone in 500 ml of water. The aqueous solubility of hydrocortisone is 0.28 mg cm^{-3}. The 60- to 80-mesh fraction (from sieve tables) corresponds to 212 μm or

2.12 × 10^{-2} cm in diameter. The density of hydrocortisone is 1.25 g cm^{-3}. The volume of s sphere is $4/3\pi r^3$. Assuming that all particles are spheres of the same diameter, 22 mg would correspond to

$$\frac{22 \times 10^{-3}}{1.25} \quad \frac{3}{4\pi \times (1.06)^3 \times 10^{-6}} = 3500 \text{ spherical particles}$$

The area of a sphere is given by $4\pi r^2$. Therefore, the area of 3500 particles of average radius 1.06 × 10^{-2} cm is

$$4\pi \times (1.06)^2 \times 10^{-4} \times 3500 = 4.94 \text{ cm}^2$$

The dissolution rate according to Equation (6) is

$$\frac{dC}{dt} = \frac{AD(C_s - C)}{hV}$$

where C_s can be approximated by the solubility, and C, the concentration during the early phase of dissolution, is essentially zero. Thus, for the sample of hydrocortisone,

$$\text{Initial dissolution rate} = \frac{4.94 \times 9.0 \times 10^{-6} \times 0.28}{5.0 \times 10^{-3} \times 500}$$

$$= 4.97 \times 10^{-6} \text{ mg cm}^{-2} \text{ sec}^{-1} \text{ ml}^{-1}$$

Hussain showed a good correlation between the calculated and the experimentally determined dissolution rates of hydrocortisone, benzoic acid, L-dopa, and griseofulvin. Hussain's method does not provide for the concept of effective surface area. It is nevertheless a useful approach, especially when the experimental determination of the dissolution cannot be accomplished.

VII.   PARAMETERS AFFECTING ABSORPTION

The absorption of drugs administered orally as solids consists of two consecutive processes: the process of dissolution, followed by the transport of the dissolved material across gastrointestinal membranes into the systemic circulation. As pointed out earlier for relatively insoluble compounds, the rate-determining step in the overall absorption process is generally the rate of dissolution. On the other hand, for relatively soluble compounds, the rate of permeation across biological membranes is the rate-determining step. In making a judgment concerning the absorption potential of a new drug entity, the preformulation scientist must undertake studies to delineate its dissolution as well as permeation behavior. The rate of dissolution can be altered via physical intervention. The rate of permeation, on the other hand, is dependent on size, relative aqueous and lipid solubilities, and ionic charge of the solute molecules. These properties can be altered, in the majority of cases, only through molecular modification. The characterization of the permeation behavior of a new drug must be performed at an early stage of drug development—primarily to help avoid mistaken efforts to improve its absorption by improving dissolution, when in reality the absorption is permeability-limited. Permeability studies are of even greater importance when analogs of the compound having similar pharmacological attributes are available. Permeability studies then would aid in the selection of the compound with the greatest absorption potential.

The significance of the solubility and the dissolution rate of a drug in the assessment of the absorption potential has already been discussed. Other physicochemical properties that are related to the process of absorption are the partition coefficient, which reflects the relative aqueous and lipid solubilities of a material, and the ionization behavior. Additionally, in vitro transport measurements using biological membranes are extremely useful. Together or singly, these three parameters help characterize the permeation behavior of a drug.

A. Partition Coefficient

Like biological membranes in general, the gastrointestinal membranes are largely lipoidal in character. Hence, the lipid solubility of a drug is an important factor in the assessment of its absorption potential. This point is well illustrated by the data reported by Kausch [35] for opium alkaloids. Comparing the absorption from the rat jejunum of structurally similar morphine, codeine, and thebaine, which contain two, one, and no hydroxyl groups, respectively, he found that the rate and extent of absorption decreased with the increasing polarity of molecules.

Lipids occurring in living membranes are complex and difficult to obtain in pure form. An indication of the relative lipid solubility, however, can be obtained by determining how a drug substance distributes itself between water and an immiscible organic solvent. When a solute is added to two immiscible liquids that are in contact with each other, it will distribute itself between the two phases in a fixed ratio. This ratio is known as the *partition coefficient* or the *distribution coefficient*, and is essentially independent of concentration of dilute solutions of a given solute species. Various organic solvents such as chloroform, ether, amyl acetate, isopropyl myristate, carbon tetrachloride, and n-octanol can be used in the determination of the partition coefficient, with the latter gaining increasing acceptance. The usefulness of partition coefficient data to assess the absorption potential of drugs is exemplified by the data of Schanker [36], shown in Table 8. These data show that for a series of barbituric acids with comparable ionization characteristics, there is a good rank-order correlation between the amounts absorbed from the rat colon and the chloroform/water partition coefficients of the un-ionized forms. However, the correlation of partition coefficient with absorption is not universal, underscoring that the actual body lipids are too complex to be simulated by an organic solvent and that the absorption process is more complex than the simple models used in the laboratory. The correlation can also depend on the choice of organic solvent used. This is illustrated by the data [37] shown in Figure 8. It can be seen here that for some barbiturates, the relationship between partition coefficients and absorption in vivo is very much dependent on the nature of the organic phase used. Nevertheless, in very many instances, the partition coefficient data are useful.

Table 8 Comparison Between Colonic Absorption and Lipid/
Water Partition of the Un-ionized Forms of Barbiturates

Barbiturate	Absorbed (%)	Chloroform/water partition coefficient
Barbital	12 ± 2	0.7
Aprobarbital	17 ± 2	4.0
Phenobarbital	20 ± 3	4.8
Allylbarbituric acid	23 ± 3	10.5
Butethal	24 ± 3	11.7
Cyclobarbital	24 ± 3	18.0
Pentobarbital	30 ± 2	23.0
Secobarbital	40 ± 3	50.7
Hexethal	44 ± 3	> 100.0

Source: From Schanker, L. S., *J. Pharmacol. Exp. Ther.*,
126:283 (1959). Reproduced with the permission of the
Williams & Wilkins Company, Baltimore.

Although the definition of partition coefficient refers to distribution
between two immiscible phases, in reality the lipid phase exhibits some
finite solubility in the aqueous phase and vice versa. For this reason, in
the determination of partition coeficient, both the aqueous and the organic
phases are presaturated with respect to each other. The drug is then
dissolved in either the aqueous or the organic phase, and the known volumes of the two phases are equilibrated by shaking. The phases are separated by standing or via centrifugation. For convenience, Leo et al. [38]
suggested the use of centrifuge bottles fitted with glass stoppers for
equilibration where centrifugation can be accomplished without further transfer of the liquid. The concentration of the solute is generally determined
in one of the phases and the concentration in the other is obtained by
difference. However, if there is a possibility that adsorption of the solute
to glass may occur, both phases must be analyzed. Leo et al. [38] also
caution against unnecessarily long shaking periods and vigorous shaking,
which tends to produce emulsions. Some emulsions may not break even
after centrifugation, thus giving incorrect partition coefficient values. The
presence of electrolytes in the aqueous phase could also affect the partition coefficients of many solutes. This should be carefully investigated
during preformulation study and must be taken into consideration while
comparing values generated by different laboratories.
    Another method applicable for estimation of partition coefficients of a
compound belonging to a family of structurally similar compounds utilizes
a reverse phase HPLC system [39–41]. Here, logarithmic value of partition
coefficient (log P) is correlated linearly with the logarithmic value of HPLC
capacity factor (log k) according to the following relationship:

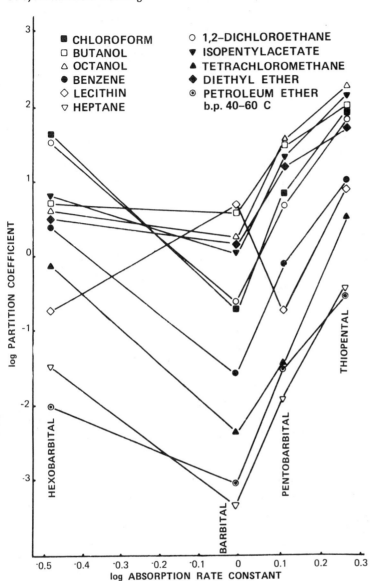

Figure 8 Influence of the nature of organic phase on relation between partition coefficient and rate of intestinal absorption of some barbiturates. The aqueous phase used was pH 5.5 buffer. (From Kurz, H., Principles of drug absorption, in *International Encyclopedia of Pharmacology and Therapeutics*, Section 39B, Vol. 1, Pergamon Press, 1975.)

$$\log P = a \log k + b$$

where a and b are constants. The capacity factor k is defined as

$$k = \frac{t_r - t_0}{t_0}$$

where t_0 is the column dead time and t_r is the retention time of the solute.

The advantages of the chromatographic method are that it (a) is fast, (b) uses micro samples, and (c) is suitable for substances containing impurities and for mixtures. However, this method requires a reference log P versus log k graph for structurally similar compounds.

B. Ionization Constant

Many drugs are either weakly acidic or basic compounds and, in solution, depending on the pH value, exist as ionized or un-ionized species. The un-ionized species are more lipid-soluble and hence more readily absorbed. The gastrointestinal absorption of weakly acidic or basic drugs is thus related to the fraction of the drug in solution that is un-ionized. The conditions that suppress ionization favor absorption. The factors that are important in the absorption of weakly acidic and basic compounds are the pH at the site of absorption, the ionization constant, and the lipid solubility of the un-ionized species. These factors together constitute the widely accepted pH partition theory [42−46].

The relative concentrations of un-ionized and ionized forms of a weakly acidic or basic drug in a solution at a given pH can be readily calculated using the Henderson−Hasselbalch equations:

$$pH = pK_a + \log \frac{[\text{un-ionized form}]}{[\text{ionized form}]} \quad \text{for bases} \tag{8}$$

$$pH = pK_a + \log \frac{[\text{ionized form}]}{[\text{un-ionized form}]} \quad \text{for acids} \tag{9}$$

Although Equations (8) and (9) tend to fail outside the pH limits of 4 to 10, or when the solutions are very dilute (where the hydronium ion concentration is about equal to or greater than 5% of the total solute concentration), a useful estimate can still be made. To use these equations, however, it is necessary to know the pK_a (the negative logarithm of the acidic ionization constant). The ionization constant refers to the following general reaction:

$$HB + H_2O \rightleftharpoons H_3O^+ + B^-$$

The most prevalent acid and conjugate base types are HB, B^- (e.g., acetic acid, acetate); HB^-, B^{2-} (e.g., bicarbonate, carbonate); and HB^+, B (e.g., glycinium, glycine), respectively.

Several methods are available for the determination of the ionization constant, and they are concisely described by Albert and Serjeant [47] and others [48]. For compounds with a reasonable solubility (about 0.01 M), acid-base potentiometric titrations can be performed on 100-ml portions using titrants of about 0.1 molarity. The procedure entails the measurement of the pH as a fucntion of the amount of titrant added. Automatic titrimeters are well suited to this purpose. Calculations of the dissociation constant can then be made from these data; and, often, an accurate value can be obtained by measuring the pH at the half-neutralization point where the pH equals the pK_a. If un-ionized and ionized forms of a drug in solution exhibit significantly different ultraviolet or visible absorption spectra, the absorbance data can be used for the determination of the ionization constant. Other methods for determining ionization constants include those based on the determination of solubility or partition coefficient as a function of pH of the aqueous phase and on conductimetric techniques.

It is apparent from the Henderson-Hasselbalch equations that for acidic compounds the relative concentration of the un-ionized form would increase with a decrease in the pH of a solution, whereas the converse would hold for basic compounds. This fact is graphically illustrated in Figure 9. The stomach contents are acidic, ranging in pH from 1 to 3, whereas the pH of intestinal fluids ranges from 5 to 8. Hence, weakly acidic but not basic drugs would be preferentially absorbed from the stomach, whereas the intestine is the primary site for the absorption of bases. The dependency of absorption of weakly acidic and basic drugs on the pH of intestinal solution is illustrated by the data of Hogben and coworkers [46], shown in Table 9. Schanker [36], who studied the absorption of a number of acidic and basic compounds from the rat colon, observed that weakly acidic compounds ($pK_a < 4.3$) were absorbed relatively rapidly; those with pK_a values ranging between 2.0 and 4.3 were absorbed more slowly; and strong acids ($pK_a > 2.4$) were hardly absorbed. For bases, those with pK_a values smaller than 8.5 were absorbed relatively rapidly; those with a pK_a between 9 and 12 were absorbed more slowly; and completely ionized quaternary ammonium compounds were not absorbed. Knowledge of the pK_a of a drug is thus very useful in determining the most likely site of absorption of acidic and basic drugs.

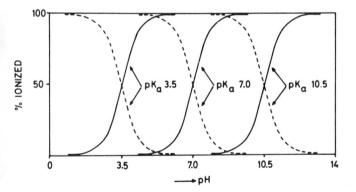

Figure 9 Correlation between pH, pK_a, and extent of ionization for acids (solid line) and conjugate acids of bases (dotted line) having pK_a values of 3.5, 7.0, and 10.5. (From Kurz, H., Principles of drug absorption, in *International Encyclopedia of Pharmacology and Therapeutics*, Section 39B, Vol. 1, Pergamon Press, 1975.)

Table 9 Intestinal Absorption of Drugs from Solutions of Various pH Values

Drug	pKa	Percent absorbed (pH range of intestinal solution)			
		3.6−4.3	4.7−5.0	7.2−7.1	6.0−7.8
Base					
Aniline	4.6	40 ± 7	48 ± 5	58 ± 5	61 ± 8
Aminopyrine	5.0	21 ± 1	35 ± 1	48 ± 2	52 ± 2
p-Toluidine	5.3	30 ± 3	42 ± 3	65 ± 4	64 ± 4
Quinine	8.4	9 ± 3	11 ± 2	41 ± 1	54 ± 5
Acids					
5-Nitrosalicylic	2.3	40 ± 0	27 ± 2	<2	<2
Salicylic	3.0	64 ± 4	35 ± 4	30 ± 4	10 ± 3
Acetylsalicylic	3.5	41 ± 3	27 ± 1	−	−
Benzoic	4.2	62 ± 4	36 ± 3	35 ± 4	5 ± 1
p-Hydroxypropiophenone	7.8	61 ± 5	52 ± 2	67 ± 6	60 ± 5

Source: Modified from Hogben, C. A. M., Tocco, D. J., Brodie, B. B., and Schanker, L. S., *J. Pharmacol. Exp. Ther.*, *125*:275 (1959). Reproduced with the permission of The Williams & Wilkins Company, Baltimore.

C. Permeation Across Biological Membranes

In the assessment of absorption potential of drugs, in addition to the determination of the physical parameters discussed above, in vitro experiments using biological membranes are gaining increasing acceptance among the preformulation scientists. These techniques measure the rate of permeation of drugs in solution across the intestine of mouse or rat and provide very useful information pertaining to the absorption characteristics of drugs. Many of these techniques are adequately reviewed by Bates and Gibaldi [49].

The method first described by Crane and Wilson [50] and modified by Kaplan and Cotler [51] is very simple and reproducible. The apparatus of Crane and Wilson is shown in Figure 10. The technique utilizes an isolated segment of intestine of laboratory animal such as a rat or a mouse. The animal is fasted overnight but is allowed access to drinking water. It is then anesthetized using ether or chloroform, and the small intestine is removed via a midline incision of the abdomen. The intestine is rinsed in cold normal saline. After discarding approximately a 10 to 15-cm section from the pyloric end, the entire intestine is everted, using a bluntheaded steel or glass rod. The everted gut is stretched under a weight of 10 g and cut into two 10-cm segments. A segment prepared in this manner is ligated at the distal end and attached at the proximal end to the

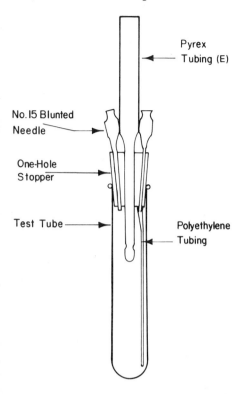

Figure 10   Test tube apparatus of Crane and Wilson.   [From Crane,
R. K., and Wilson, T. H., *J. Appl. Physiol.*, *12*:145 (1958).   Reproduced
with the permission of the copyright owner.]

canulated end of tube E (see Fig. 10).   A weight of 10 g is attached to the
ligated end to keep the sac in a vertical position.   The segment is suspended in about 80 ml of drug solution in a physiologically acceptable buffer,
such as Krebs bicarbonate buffer.   The drug-containing solution is preequilibrated at 37°C and is maintained at this temperature during the experiment.   The drug-containing solution is referred to as mucosal solution.
A 2-ml aliquot of drug-free buffer, also preequilibrated at 37°C and referred
to as the serosal solution, is introduced into the sac via tube E.   A 95:5
mixture of O_2/CO_2 is continuously bubbled through the mucosal solution at
a constant rate.   The serosal solution is withdrawn at predetermined intervals and replaced with fresh, drug-free buffer.   The concentration of the
drug in the serosal fluid samples is determined using a suitable assay.

Usually these experiments are carried out at different mucosal concentrations of drug.   Constancy of amount transferred per unit time per unit
concentration over a wide range of mucosal solution concentrations is indicative of passive transfer of drug.   Passive transfer refers to a free diffusion across a barrier composed of channels of various sizes; no biologically active or electrochemical processes are involved.   As the concentration
gradient across the barrier is increased, the flux across the barrier also
increases in direct proportion (Fick's first law).   Kaplan and Cotler [51]
studied a number of compounds using this technique and compared the

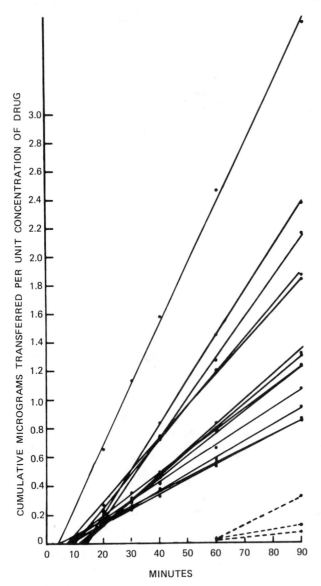

Figure 11   Cumulative amount of drug transferred per unit concentration of drug in the mucosal solution as a function of time.   [From Kaplan, S. A., and Cotler, S., *J. Pharm. Sci.*, *61*:1361 (1972).   Reproduced with the permission of the copyright owner.]

results to those obtained during in vivo **experiments** in dogs. Their results **are** shown in Figure 11. Of the 16 compounds studied, those that
exhibited lag times of 15 min or less, and clearance values between 0.01
and 0.04 ml min^{-1}, showed no permeability-related problem when tested
in vivo and administered in solution. Others with lag times of 50 to 60
min and essentially unmeasurable clearance values showed poor in vivo
absorption despite good dissolution characteristics. These data demonstrate the predictive value of the technique. The everted rat gut technique
is also useful in the investigation of site of absorption in the intestine and
in the determination of transport mechanisms [52].

Notwithstanding the usefulness of the everted rat gut technique, due
caution must be exerted in the interpretation of the data so derived. Thus,
Taylor and Grundy [53] report a very poor correlation between in vitro
clearance values and in vivo absorption in rat and man for practolol and
propranolol. The techniques based on use of isolated gut segments in
vitro also tend to underestimate absorption potential since such segments
lack a blood supply. In this regard, the in situ technique as described
by Doluisio and coworkers [54] is a more reliable method for the calculation
of absorption rates. In this technique an anesthetized male Sprague-Dawley
rat is surgically prepared such that the small intestine is exposed. Two
syringes are connected using L-shaped glass canulae and secured using
silk suture at the duodenol and ileal ends. After clearing the gut using
perfusion fluid, the drug solution is introduced into the intestine. Aliquots
of the lumen solution are then collected periodically at either the ileal or
duodenal end. Chow and coworkers [55] used this technique to assess absorption potential of a series of ACE inhibitor prodrugs. Their data [56]
presented in Table 10 showed good rank-order correlation between the first-
order absorption rate constant as determined in situ and percent of oral
dose absorbed in vivo.

Amidon [57] proposed calculation of a dimensionless parameter termed
intestinal permeability from the data obtained using in situ rat gut technique.
In this method, a solution of known concentration is perfused through a
segment of rat intestine. After the gut wall is equilibrated with the

Table 10   Relationship Between Absorption Rate Constants
for a Series of ACE Inhibitors as Determined in vitro Using
Doluisio Method and Their in vivo Absorption

Compound	% Absorption in vivo	Absorption rate constant k_a (hr^{-1})
A	74	0.58
B	39[a]	0.42
C	27	0.20
D	34	0.21
E	26	0.17
F	15	0.15

[a]Data from dog study; all other values obtained from rat.

solution, the perfusate is collected for an appropriate length of time. The
wall permeability is then calculated using the equation:

$$P^*_w = \frac{P^*_{eff}}{1 - P^*_{eff}/P^*_{aq}}$$ (10)

The terms P^*_{eff} and P^*_{aq} are calculated using the equations

$$P^*_{eff} = \frac{(1 - C_m/C_o)Q}{2\pi\, DL}$$

and

$$P^*_{aq} = A\left(\frac{\pi\, DL}{2Q}\right)^{1/3}$$

where C_m and C_0 are outlet and inlet perfusate concentrations, D the dif-
fusivity of solute in the perfusate, L the length of the intestinal segment,
Q the perfusate flow rate, and A a constant. For drugs that are transported by passive and nonpassive mechanisms, authors [58] have proposed
further modification of Equation (10). Amidon and coworkers [59] determined permeabilities for a number of drugs and correlated the same with
their reported bioavailabilities. Based on the correlation, incomplete absorption is suggested when calculated permeability ability is less than 1.
Using model compounds such as estrone, p-nitroanilide [60], higher alcohols,
and hydrocortisone [61], Amidon and coworkers have also shown the usefulness of permeability calculations in screening more soluble prodrugs with a
better potential for absorption in vivo.

VIII. CRYSTAL PROPERTIES AND POLYMORPHISM

Many drug substances can exist in more than one crystalline form with different space lattice arrangements. This property is known as polymorphism.
The different crystal forms are called polymorphs. Occasionally, a solid
crystallizes, entrapping solvent molecules in a specific lattice position and
in a fixed stoichiometry, resulting in a *solvate* or *pseudopolymorph*. Many
solids may be prepared in a particular polymorphic form via appropriate
manipulation of conditions of crystallization. These conditions include
nature of the solvent, temperature, rate of cooling, and other factors.
Many times a solute precipitates out of solution so that the molecules in
the resulting solid are not ordered in a regular array but in a more or
less random arrangement. This state is known as the amorphous form.
Usually shock cooling, a sudden change in the composition of the solvent
of crystallization, or lyophilization results in an amorphous form.
    Different polymorphic forms of a given solid differ from each other
with respect to many physical properties, such as solubility and dissolution,
true density, crystal shape, compaction behavior, flow properties, and solid-
state stability. It is essential, therefore, to define and monitor the solid
state of a drug substance. Occasionally, it may be deemed necessary to
actively search for a different polymorphic form to circumvent a stability,
bioavailability, or processing problem. The subject of polymorphism has

attracted considerable attention from preformulation scientists, and excellent reviews have appeared in the pharmaceutical literature [62–66].

A. Crystal Characteristics and Bioavailability

Differences in the dissolution rates and solubilities of different polymorphic forms of a given drug are well documented in the pharmaceutical literature [67,68]. When the absorption of a drug is dissolution rate-limited, a more soluble and faster dissolving form may be utilized to improve the rate and extent of bioavailability. The work of Aguiar and others [69,70] on polymorphs of chloramphenicol palmitate and that of Miyazaki et al. [71] on chlortetracycline hydrochloride illustrate this point.

Figure 12 shows comparative blood level data obtained in humans following oral administration of 1.5 g of pure A and pure B forms of chloramphenicol palmitate and their mixtures [69]. These data show that the pure, more soluble form B was most bioavailable, whereas the pure, less soluble form A was least bioavailable. The bioavailability of the mixtures fell between these two extremes and was directly proportional to the concentration of B.

Figure 13 shows intrinsic dissolution profiles for α and β forms of chlortetracycline hydrochloride. The in vivo data illustrated in Figure 14 show that the more soluble β form is also more bioavailable. As mentioned

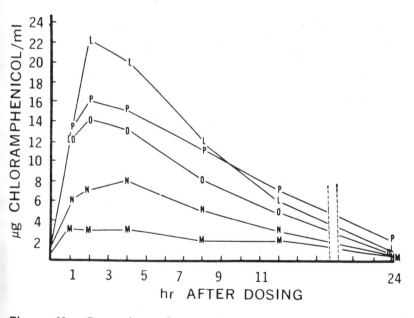

Figure 12   Comparison of mean blood serum levels obtained with chloramphenicol palmitate suspensions containing varying ratios of A and B polymorphs, following single oral dose equivalent to 1.5 g chloramphenicol. Percent polymorph B in the suspension: M, 0%; N, 25%; O, 50%; P, 75%; L, 100%. [From Aguiar, A. J., Krc, J., Kinkel, A. W., and Symyn, J. C., *J. Pharm. Sci.*, 56:847 (1967). Reproduced with the permission of the copyright owner.]

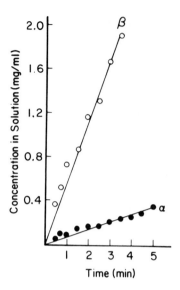

Figure 13   Dissolution curves of the α and β forms of chlortetracycline
hydrochloride from compressed disks in water at 37°C. [From Miyazaki, S.,
Arit, T., Hori, R., and Ito, K., *Chem. Pharm. Bull.*, *11*:638 (1974). Reproduced with the permission of the Pharmaceutical Society of Japan.]

earlier, the effect of polymorphism on bioavailability is mediated via enhanced dissolution. Hence, a deliberate attempt to uncover polymorphism
with the intention of improving bioavailability should be undertaken only
when there is reason to believe that the absorption is likely to be dissolution rate-limited. Obviously, for relatively soluble compounds this approach
may not be warranted.

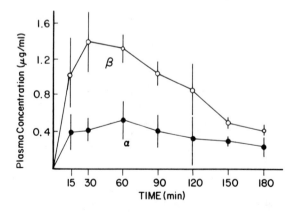

Figure 14   Plasma levels after intraduodenal administration of the α and β
forms of chlortetracycline hydrochloride to rabbits. [From Miyazaki, S.,
Arit, T., Hori, R., and Ito, K., *Chem. Pharm. Bull.*, *22*:638 (1974). Reproduced with the permission of the Pharmaceutical Society of Japan.]

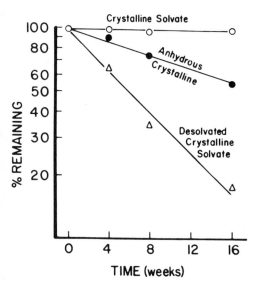

Figure 15 Solid-state decomposition of different polymorphic forms of an experimental compound.

B. Crystal Characteristics and Chemical Stability

For drugs prone to degradation in the solid state, the physical form of the drug influences the rate of degradation. For example, aztreonam, a monobactam antibiotic, exists in needlelike α- and dense spherical β-crystalline forms. In the presence of high humidity (37°C/75% RH), the α form undergoes β-lactam hydrolysis more readily with a half-life of about 6 months whereas the β form under identical conditions is stable for several years [72]. Inasmuch as two crystal forms of a labile drug could exhibit widely different solid-state stabilities, a preformuation scientist might consider changing the crystal form to alleviate and possibly eliminate a stability problem. This approach is demonstrated by the data presented in Figure 15 for an experimental drug. Under stress conditions, the anhydrous crystalline form of this experimental drug degraded rapidly with a half-life of about 18 weeks. A solvate form of the drug under the same conditions was essentially stable. Desolvation of the solvate caused by excessive heat resulted in a new crystal form distinct from the anhydrous and solvate forms. The desolvated form under the test conditions degraded most rapidly. This case history illustrates not only the possible use of a polymorphic form to solve a stability problem but also the importance of controlling processing variables so that the integrity of the selected form is maintained.

C. Crystal Characteristics and Tableting Behavior

In a typical tableting operation, flow and compaction behaviors of the powder mass to be tableted are important considerations. These properties, among others, are related to the morphology, tensile strength, and density of the powder bed. As mentioned earlier, two polymorphic forms of the same drug could differ significantly with respect to these properties. The morphology of a crystal also depends on crystal habit. The latter is a description of the outer appearance of a crystal. When the environment in which crystals grow changes the external shape of the crystals without altering their internal structure, then a different habit results. Crystal habit is influenced by the presence of an impurity, concentration, rate of crystallization, and hydrodynamics in the crystallizer.

Cole et al. [73] describe compaction processes as "packing of particles by diffusion into void spaces, elastic and plastic deformation, fracture and cold working and, finally, compression of the solid material." One or more of these subprocesses may be affected by crystal form and habit. Some investigation of polymorphism and crystal habit of a drug substance as it relates to pharmaceutical processing is desirable during its preformulation evaluation, especially when the active ingredient is expected to constitute the bulk of the tablet mass. Shell [74] studied the crystal habit and the tableting behavior of nine different lots of an experimental drug. Using single-crystal X-ray data and X-ray powder diffraction patterns, he found that the ratio of intensities at diffraction angles of 12.09 and 8.72° correlated well with the tableting behavior of the nine lots as judged by an experienced operator. Summers et al. [75] showed that different polymorphs of sulfathiazole, barbitone, and asprin differed significantly in their compression characteristics. Likewise, Imaizumi and coworkers [76] observed that the crystalline form of indomethacin yielded tablets with better hardness characteristics than the amorphous form.

D. Crystal Characteristics and Physical Stability

Although a drug substance may exist in two or more polymorphic forms, only one form is thermodynamically stable at a given temperature and pressure. The other forms would convert to the stable form with time. This transformation may be rapid or slow. When the transformation is not rapid, the thermodynamically unstable form is referred to as a metastable form. In general, the stable polymorph exhibits the highest melting point, the lowest solubility, and the maximum chemical stability. A metastable form nevertheless may exhibit sufficient chemical and physical stability under shelf conditions to justify its use for reasons of better dissolution or ease of tableting. When use of a metastable form is recommended, for whatever reason, a preformulation scientist must assure its integrity under a variety of processing conditions so that appropriate handling conditions may be defined.

Polymorphic transformations can occur during grinding, granulating, drying, and compressing operations. Digoxin, spironolactone, and estradiol are reported to undergo polymorphic transformations during the comminution process [77]. Phenylbutazone undergoes polymorphic transformation as a result of grinding and compression [78]. Granulation, since it entails the use of a solvent, can lead to a solvate formation. On the other hand, if the molecule is initially a solvate, the drying step in the process may cause transformation to an anhydrous crystalline or amorphous form [79].

Good knowledge of polymorphism and polymorphic stability is also needed to predict long-term physical stability of dosage forms. Yamaoka et al. [80] observed cappinglike cracking in tablets of anydrous crystalline carbochromen hydrochloride upon storage under high-humidity conditions. This was determined to be due to transformation of the anhydrous form into a dihydrate.

Even when the stable form is the form of choice, it is advisable to monitor the crystal form of each lot of raw material. In the case of calcium pantothenate, the preferred form is the crystalline form. In the preparation of multivitamin tablets, calcium pantothenate is granulated with a few other vitamins and appropriate excipients. An amorphous form of calcium pantothenate is known which readily reverts to the stable form when wetted with a variety of solvents used as granulating solvents. Use of the amorphous form in multivitamin tablets prepared by a granulation process is, however, not desirable because the polymorphic transformation renders the granulating mass sticky, making further granulation virtually impossible.

E. Techniques for Studying Crystal Properties

Various techniques are available for the investigation of the solid state. These include microscopy (including hot-stage microscopy), infrared spectrophotometry, single-crystal X-ray and X-ray powder diffraction, thermal analysis, and dilatometry. *Single-crystal X-ray* provides the most complete information about the solid state. It is, however, tedious, time consuming, and, hence, unsuitable for routine use.

Powder X-ray diffraction is both rapid and relatively simple, and is the method of choice. The powder X-ray diffraction pattern is unique to each polymorphic form: amorphous materials do not show any patterns or show one or two broad peaks attributable to the presence of shortrange ordering. Powder X-ray diffraction does not always indicate if the crystalline material is a true polymorph or a solvate. In Figure 16 are shown typical powder X-ray diffraction patterns for anhydrous amorphous, anhydrous crystalline, and crystalline trihydrate forms of the antibiotic epicillin [81,82].

Differential thermal analysis and differential scanning calorimetry are particularly useful in the investigation of polymorphism and in obtaining pertinent thermodynamic data. Figure 17 shows differential thermal analysis patterns for two polymorphs and a dioxane solvate form of SQ 10,996 [83]. Curve (1) is the differential thermogram for form A of SQ 10,996. It shows a melting endotherm at approximately 195°C, followed by a decomposition endotherm at 250 to 300°C. Curve (2) represents the differential thermogram for form B. It shows a melting endotherm at 180°C, followed by a small exotherm characterizing transition to form A, which then melts and decomposes at 190°C and 250 to 300°C, respectively. Curve (3) is a thermogram for the dioxane solvate. It is similar to that of form B with the exception that it has an extra endotherm at 140°C. This is a desolvation endotherm; upon desolvation, form B is generated. Other events on the thermogram of the solvate are identical to those seen for form B.

Desolvation endotherms are not always as distinct as shown in this example. In these situations thermogravimetric analysis is very useful. The thermogravimetric analysis pattern for the dioxane solvate showed a loss in weight that began at 105°C and was complete at about 140°C. The loss represented 13% of the total weight, which corresponded to a 1:1 solvate.

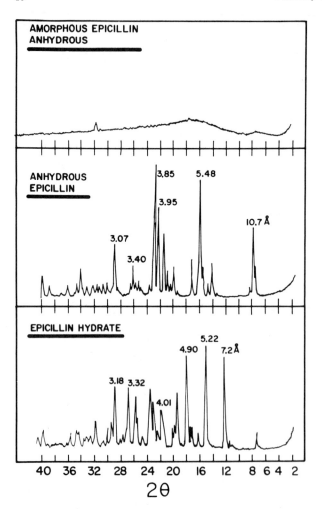

Figure 16   Powder X-ray diffraction patterns of amorphous, anhydrous
crystalline, and crystalline trihydrate forms of epicillin.

Presence of a solvate is best visualized by heating a sample of the suspected
solvate immersed in a high-boiling liquid in which it is soluble. In this
technique, desolvation is indicated by the appearance of bubbles. A hot-
stage microscope is very useful in the visualization. Another approach to
determine whether an observed endotherm is due to desolvation is suggested
in the work of Serajuddin [79]. His data for theophylline monohydrate are
presented in Figure 18. It can be seen here that the desolvation endotherm
shifted depending on manner of exposure of the sample. This difference
in the observed dehydration temperature was explained on the basis of the
partial pressure of water vapor prevalent over the sample under the different experimental conditions. On the other hand, the position of melting
endotherm is independent of the manner of sample presentation.

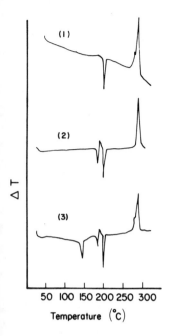

Figure 17 Differnetial thermograms of polymorphic forms of SQ 10,996. (1) Form A; (2) dioxane solvate; (3) form B. [From Gibbs, I., Heald, A., Jacobson, H., Wadke, D. A., and Weliky, I., *J. Pharm. Sci.*, *65*:1380 (1976). Reproduced with the permission of the copyright owner.]

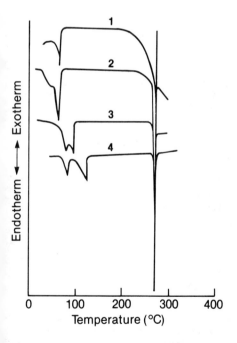

Figure 18 DSC thermograms of therophylline monohydrate recorded at a heating rate of 5°C min^{-1} by subjecting the samples to various atmospheric conditions. The atmospheric conditions were varied by placing the samples (1) on an open aluminium pan without purging of nitrogen (50 ml min^{-1}). (2) on an open pan with purging of nitrogen. (3) in a pan closed by crimping and (4) in a hermetically sealed pan.

IX. STABILITY

In designing a solid dosage form it is necessary to know the inherent stability of the drug substance; to have an idea of what excipients to use, as well as how best to put them together with the drug; and to know that no toxic substances are formed. Limits of acceptability and, therefore, compromises must be reasonably defined. Because the measurements of these aspects of stability as well as determination of the shelf life (or expiration date) for the final dosage form require long-term stability studies for confirmation, they can be expensive and time consuming. Consequently, the preformulation scientist must try to define those study designs and conditions that show the greatest probability of success [84]. The objective, therefore, of a preformulation stability program is to identify—and help avoid or control—situations where the stability of the active ingredient may be compromised. For a drug substance to be developed into a tablet dosage form, this objective may be achieved by investigating the stability of the drug under the following three categories: (1) solid-state stability of drug alone; (2) compatibility studies (stability in the presence of excipients); (3) solution phase stability (including stability in gastrointestinal fluids and granulating solvents).

The basic requisite for the execution of these studies is the availability of a reliable stability-indicating analytical method. For the most part, in the case of a new drug the preformulation scientist will not have a fully validated analytical method available. However, a reasonably reliable HPLC procedure can usually be developed very quickly. Also, and often as a precursor to adopting an HPLC method, TLC is very useful. TLC analysis can be quickly performed and several systems primarily using different solvents for development can easily be examined. The purpose of this type of approach is to increase the probability of the detection of degradation and/or impurities and to prevent being surprised later in the program, when such findings can have a devastating effect on schedules.

The preformulation scientist must also be aware of changes adopted in the synthesis of the drug substance. Although the molecule may be identical no matter what the synthetic route, its manner of presentation to the environment (as mediated by particle size, porosity, solvation, and/or crystalline form) can have profound effects on stability. This is not a rare occurrence.

Inasmuch as the tablet formulations are multicomponent systems, the physical state of excipients could influence the stability of the active. The state of hydration of excipient materials can have strong effects on an active. Using aspirin as a model drug, Patel et al. [85] showed how excipients that are either hydrated or contain adsorbed moisture can effect drug stability. In their study these researchers identified the ratio of drug to excipient content, equilibrium to ambient humidities, and the trapping of moisture in closed containers, thereby changing the internal environment of the package as the important factor affecting product stability.

A. Solid-State Stability

Solid-state stability refers to physical as well as chemical stability. In this section only chemical stability will be discussed. Physical changes caused by polymorphic transitions and hygroscopicity are discussed in Sections VIII and X, respectively.

In general, pharmaceutical solids degrade as a result of solvolysis, oxidation, photolysis, and pyrolysis. Any investigation of stability must begin with an examination of the chemical structure, which provides some indication of the chemical reactivity [86]. For example, esters, lactams, and, to a lesser extent, amides are susceptible to solvolytic breakdown. The presence of unsaturation or of electron-rich centers makes the molecule susceptible to free-radical-mediated or photocatalyzed oxidation. Strained rings are more prone to pyrolysis. With a number of possibilities suggested, it is possible to design the proper stress conditions to challenge the suspected weaknesses.

The physical properties of the drug, such as its solubility, pK_a, melting point, crystal form, and equilibrium moisture content, also influence its stability. As a rule, amorphous materials are less stable than their crystalline counterparts. For structurally related compounds, the melting point may indicate relative stabilities. For example, in a series of vitamin A esters, Guillory and Higuchi [87] observed that the zeroth-order rate constant for the degradation of the esters was inversely related to their fusion temperatures. The nature of thermal analysis curves may also help in a stability prognosis. Broad, shallow endotherms are suggestive of less stable, less homogeneous species. A relatively dense material may better withstand ambient stresses. For example, aminobenzylpenicillin trihydrate is denser [68] and more stable [88] than its anhydrous crystalline counterpart.

The mechanisms of solid-state degradation are complex and difficult to elucidate [89−92]. A knowledge of the exact mechanism, while always useful, is most often not the first objective. The stability study should be designed to identify the factos that cause degradation of the drug. As indicated earlier, the most common factors that cause solid-state reactions are heat, light, oxygen, and, most importantly, moisture. Clearly, there can be, and most often there is, considerable interplay among these factors. Heat and moisture can cause a material with a propensity to react with oxygen to do so more rapidly; conversely, the presence of moisture can render a substance more heat-labile. In the conduct of stability studies, where stability is influenced by more than one factor, it is advisable to study one factor at a time, holding others constant.

Solid-state reactions, in general, are slow, and it is customary to use stress conditions in the investigation of stability. The data obtained under stress conditions are then extrapolated to make a predicition of stability under appropriate storage conditions. This approach is not always straightforward, and due care must be exerted in the interpretation of the data. High temperatures can drive moisture out of a sample and render a material apparently stable that would otherwise be prone to hydrolysis. Degradative pathways observed at elevated temperatures may not be operant at lower temperatures. Some ergot alkaloids [93] degrade completely within a year when stored at temperatures above 45°C; however, the rate is less than 1% per year below 35°C. Above 65% relative humidity the β form of chlortetracycline hydrochloride transforms into the α form, the rate of transformation increasing with the increased aqueous tension. At or below 65% relative humidity, however, no transformation is observed [94]. Despite these shortcomings, accelerated stability studies are extremely useful in providing an early and a rapid prognosis of stability. Such studies are also used to force formation of degradants in amounts sufficient for isolation and characterization. This information can then be used not only in the understanding of reaction kinetics but, if necessary, to set limits on amounts of degradants.

Elevated Temperature Studies

The elevated temperatures most commonly used are 30, 40, 50, and 60°C —in conjunction with the ambient humidity. Occasionally, higher temperatures are used. The samples stored at the highest temperature should be examined for physical and chemical changes at frequent intervals, and any change, when compared to an appropriate control (usually a smaple stored at 5° or −20°C), should be noted. If a substantial change is seen, samples stored at lower temperatures are examined. If no change is seen after 30 days at 60°C, the stability prognosis is excellent. Corroborative evidence must be obtained by monitoring the samples stored at lower temperatures for longer durations. Samples stored at room temperature and at 5°C may be followed for as long as 6 months. The data obtained at elevated temperatures may be extrapolated using the Arrhenius treatment to determine the degradation rate at a lower temperature. Figure 19 shows the degradation of vitamin C at 50, 60, and 70°C [95].

Figure 20 shows the elevated-temperature degradation data plotted in the Arrhenius fashion, where the logarithm of the apparent rate constant is plotted as a function of the reciprocal of absolute temperature. The plot is linear and can be extrapolated to obtain the rate constant at other temperatures. Most solid-state reactions are not amenable to the Arrhenius treatment. Their heterogeneous nature makes elucidation of the kinetic order and prediction difficult. Long-term lower temperature studies are, therefore, an essential part of a good stability program. As indicated by Woolfe and Worthington [93], even a small loss seen at lower temperatures has greater predictive value when the assay variation is less than 2% and the experimental design includes adequate replication. These authors suggest a 3- to 6-month study at 33°C with three replications.

Stability Under High-Humidity Conditions

In the presence of moisture, many drug substances hydrolyze, react with other excipients, or oxidize. These reactions can be accelerated by exposing the solid drug to different relative humidity conditions. Controlled humidity environments can be readily obtained using laboratory desiccators containing saturated solutions of various salts [96]. The closed desiccators

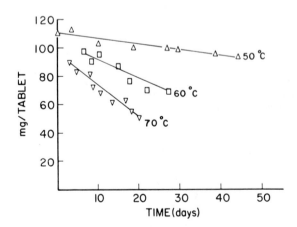

Figure 19 Degradation of vitamin C in a tablet formulation. [From Tardif, R., *J. Pharm. Sci.*, 54:281 (1965). Reproduced with the permission of the copyright owner.]

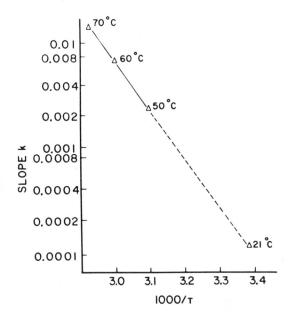

Figure 20   Arrhenius plot of the data shown in Fig. 19. [From Tardif, R., *J. Pharm. Sci.*, 54:281 (1965). Reproduced with the permission of the copyright owner.]

in turn are placed in an oven to provide a constant temperature. The data of Kornblum and Sciarrone [97] for the decarboxylation of p-aminosalicylic acid show a dependence on the ambient moisture (Fig. 21). These data reveal that the zeroth-order rate constant as well as the lag time depend on the aqueous tension. Preformulation data of this nature are useful in determining if the material should be protected and stored in a controlled low-humidity environment, or if the use of an aqueous-based granulation system should be avoided. They may also caution against the use of excipients that absorb moisture significantly.

Photolytic Stability

Many drug substances fade or darken on exposure to light. Usually the extent of degradation is small and limited to the exposed surface area. However, it presents an aesthetic problem—which can be readily controlled by using amber glass or an opaque container, or by incorporating a dye in the product to mask the discoloration. Obviously, the dye used for this purpose whould be sufficiently photostable. Exposure of the drug substance to 400 and 900 footcandles (fc) of illumination for 4- and 2-week periods, respectively, is adequate to provide some idea of photosensitivity. Over these periods, the samples should be examined frequently for change in appearance and for chemical loss, and they should be compared to samples stored under the same conditions but protected from light. The change in appearance may be recorded visually or quantitated by instruments specially designed for comparing colors or by diffuse reflectance spectroscopy. For example, a sample of cicloprofen became intensely yellow after 5 days under 900 fc of light. The progress of discoloration could be readily

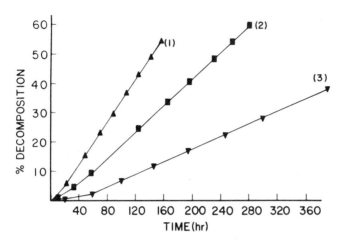

Figure 21   Percent decomposition-time curves for the decarboxylation of
p-aminosalicylic acid at 70°C under different aqueous tensions: (1) 144.0,
(2) 118.4, and (3) 52.3 mmHg. [From Kornblum, S. S., and Sciarrone,
G. J., *J. Pharm. Sci.*, *53*:935 (1964). Reproduced with the permission
of the copyright owner.]

followed using diffuse reflectance spectroscopy. Analysis of the exposed
sample showed less than 2% loss in cicloprofen. The degradation products
were determined to be safe. Discoloration in this instance was an aesthetic
problem only.

Stability to Oxidation

The sensitivity of each new drug entity to atmospheric oxygen must be
evaluated to establish if the final product should be packaged under inert
atmospheric conditions and if it should contain an antioxidant. Sensitivity
to oxidation of a solid drug can be ascertained by investigating its stability
in an atmosphere of high oxygen tension. Usually a 40% oxygen atmosphere
allows for a rapid evaluation. Some consideration should be given as to
how the sample is exposed to this atmosphere. As shallow a powder bed
as is reasonable should be used with an adequate volume of head space to
ensure that the system is not oxygen-limited. Results should be compared
against those obtained under inert or ambient atmospheres. Desiccators
equipped with three-way stopcocks are useful for these studies. Samples
are placed in a desiccator that is alternately evacuated and flooded with
the desired atmosphere. The process is repeated three to four times to
assure essentially 100% of the desired atmosphere. The procedure is somewhat tedious in that it must be repeated following each sample withdrawal.
While flooding the evacuated desiccator, the gas mixture should be brought
in essentially at the atmospheric pressure. This study can often be combined with an elevated temperature study, in that the samples under a 40%
oxygen atmosphere can also be heated.

B. Compatibility Studies: Stability in the Presence of Excipients

In the tablet dosage form the drug is in intimate contact with one or more excipients; the latter could affect the stability of the drug. Knowledge of drug—excipient interactions is therefore very useful to the formulator in selecting appropriate excipients. This information may already be in exist- ence for known drugs. For new drugs or new excipents, the preformula- tion scientist must generate the needed information.

A typical tablet contains binders, disintegrants, lubricants, and fillers. Compatibility screening for a new drug must consider two or more excipients from each class. The ratio of drug to excipient used in these tests is very much subject to the discretion of the preformulation scientist. It should be consistent with the ratio most likely to be encountered in the final tab- let, and will depend on the nature of the excipient and the size and poten- cy of the tablet. Table 11 shows ratios suggested by Akers [98]. Carstensen et al. [99] recommended drug/excipient ratios of 20:1 and 1:5 by weight for lubricants and other excipients, respectively. Often the interaction is accentuated for easier detection by compressing or granulat- ing the drug—excipient mixture with water or another solvent.

An illustration of importance of drug/excipient ratio on the drug stabil- ity is presented in Figure 22 [100]. These data show that the stability of captopril—a drug prone to oxidative degradation—in mixtures with lactose monohydrate was inversely proportional to its concentration. Similar obser- vations were made for stability in mixtures with microcrystalline celluslose and starch [101].

The three techniques commonly employed in drug—excipient compatibility screening are chromatographic techniques using either HPLC or TLC, dif- ferential thermal analysis, and diffuse reflectance spectroscopy.

Chromatography in Drug—Excipient Interaction Studies

This involves storage of drug—excipient mixture both "as is" and granulated with water or solvents at elevated temperatures. The granulation may be carried out so that the mixture contains fixed amounts (e.g., 5—20%) of mois- ture. The mixtures can be sealed in ampules or vials to prevent any escape of moisture at elevated temperatures. If desired, the type of gas in the headspace can be controlled using either air, nitrogen, or oxygen. The samples are examined periodically for appearance and analyzed for any decomposition using HPLC or TLC. Unstressed samples are used as con- trols. Any change in the chromatograph, such as the appearance of a new spot or a change in the R_f values or retention times of the components, is indicative of an interaction. HPLC may be quantitated if deemed neces- sary. If significant interaction is noticed at elevated temperatures, cor- roborative evidence must be obtained by examining mixtures stored at low- er temperatures for longer durations. If no interaction is observed at 50 to 60°C, especially in the presence of moisure and air, none can be expected at lower temperatures. Among the advantages of HPLC or TLC in this ap- plication are the following:

Evidence of degradation is unequivocal.
Spots or peaks corresponding to degradation products can be isolated
    for possible identification.
The technique can be quantitated to obtain kinetic data.

Differential Thermal Analysis in Drug—Excipient
Interaction Studies

Thermal analysis is useful in the investigation of solid-state interactions. Its main advantage is its rapidity. It is also useful in the detection of eutectics and other phase formations. Thermograms are generated for the pure components and their 1:3, 1:1, and 3:1 physical mixtures. In the absence of any interaction, the thermograms of mixtures show patterns corresponding to those of the individual components. In the event that interaction occurs, this is indicated in the thermogram of a mixture by the appearance of one or more new peaks or the disappearance of one or more peaks corresponding to those of the components. Figure 23 [102] shows separate thermograms of cephradine, a broad-spectrum antibiotic, and four excipients, namely, N-methylglucamine, tromethamine, anhydrous sodium

Table 11   Suggested Excipient/Drug Ratio in Compatibility Studies

Excipient	Weight excipient per unit weight drug (anticipated drug dose, mg)				
	1	5—10	25—50	75—150	>150
Alginic acid	24	24	9	9	9
Avicel	24	9	9	9	4
Cornstarch	24	9	4	2	2
Dicalcium phosphate dihydrate	24	24	9	9	9
Lactose	24	9	4	2	1
Magnesium carbonate	24	24	9	9	4
Magnesium stearate	1	1	1	1	1
Mannitol	24	9	4	2	1
Methocel	2	2	2	2	1
PEG 4000	9	9	4	4	2
PVP	4	4	2	1	1
Starch 1500	1	1	1	1	1
Stearic acid	1	1	1	1	1
Talc	1	1	1	1	1

Source: Modified from Akers, M. J., *Can. J. Pharm. Sci.*, *11*:1 (1976).
Reproduced with the permission of the Canadian Pharmaceutical Association.

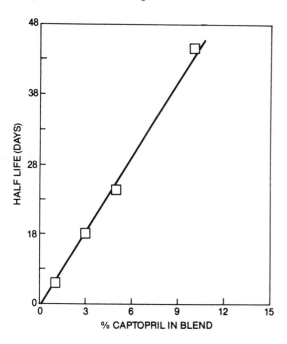

Figure 22   Degradation of captopril in presence of lactose Fast-Flo at 70°C and 75% RH.

carbonate, and trisodium phosphate dodecahydrate. Figure 24 shows the thermograms for the corresponding four mixtures. Only the thermogram for the mixture with anhydrous sodium carbonate retains the significant cephradine exotherm at about 200°C. An investigation of the stability at 50°C of cephradine in the presence of these excipients showed that all the excipients, with the exception of anhydrous sodium carbonate, had deleterious effects on stability.

Interpretation of thermal data is not always straightforward. When two substances are mixed, the purity of each is obliterated. Impure materials generally have lower melting points and exhibit less well-defined peaks in thermograms. In the absence of an interaction, this effect is usually small. By using the ratios for the mixtures suggested above, an insight can usually be obtained as to whether an interaction has occurred. The temperature causing thermal events to occur can be high, depending on the materials. If too high, the condition may be too stressful—forcing a reaction that might not occur at lower temperatures. Finally, if an interaction is indicated, it is not necessarily deleterious. The formation of eutectics, if not occuring at so low a temperature as to physically compromise the final product, is acceptable. The same may be true for compound or complex formation and solid solution or glass formation. Because thermal analysis involves heating, often it may be difficult to interpret the loss of features in the presence of, for example, polyvinylpyrrolidone. The latter melts at a relatively low temperature and, once liquid, may dissolve the drug.

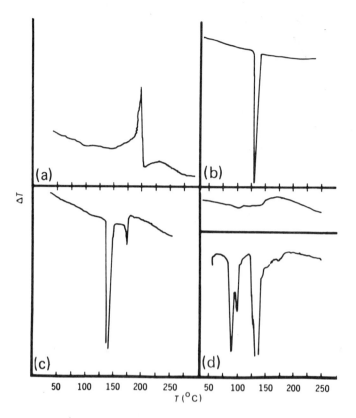

Figure 23   Thermograms of pure materials: (a) cephradine; (b) N-methyl-glucamine; (c) tromethamine; (d) anhydrous sodium carbonate; (e) tri-sodium phosphate dodecahydrate.   [From Jacobson, H., and Gibbs, I. S., *J. Pharm. Sci.*, *62*:1543 (1973).   Reproduced with the permission of the copyright owner.]

Diffuse Reflectance Spectroscopy in Drug—Excipient Interaction Studies

Diffuse reflectance spectrophotometry is a tool that can detect and monitor drug-excipient interactions [103].   In this technique solid drugs, excipients, and their physical mixtures are exposed to incident radiation.   A portion of the incident radiation is partly absorbed and partly reflected in a dif-fuse manner.   The diffuse reflectance depends on the packing density of the solid, its particle size, and its crystal form, among other factors. When these factors are adequately controlled, diffuse reflectance spectro-scopy can be used to investigate physical and chemical changes occurring on solid surfaces.   A shift in the diffuse reflectance spectrum of the drug due to the presence of the excipient indicates physical adsorption, whereas the appearance of a new peak indicates chemisorption or formation of de-gradation product.   The method of preparation of the drug—excipient mix-ture is very critical.   Equilibration of samples prepared by dissolving the drug and the excipient in a suitable solvent, followed by removal of the solvent by evaporattion, provides samples that are more apt to show small

changes in the spectrum. The dried solid mixture must be sieved to provide controlled particle size. When a suitable solvent in which both the
drug and excipient are soluble is not available, sample equilibration may be
effected using suspensions. Changes in the diffuse reflectance spectra may
be apparent in freshly prepared sample mixtures, indicating potential incompatibilities. In other instances, they may become apparent when samples
are stressed. In the latter case, diffuse reflectance spectroscopy can be
used to obtain kinetic information. Thus, Lach and coworkers [104] used
the technique to follow interactions of isoniazid with magnesium oxide and
with lactose in the solid state at elevated temperatures [104]. The data
were used to approximate the time needed for the reactions to be percept-
ible when samples are sotred at 25°C. In a like manner, Blaug and Huang
[105] studied ethanol-mediated interaction between dextroamphetamine sulfate and spray-dried lactose in solid mixtures.

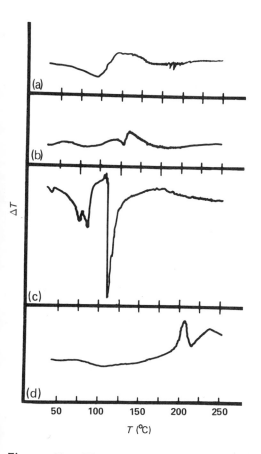

Figure 24   Thermograms of mixtures of cephradine with (a) N-methyl-
glucamine; (b) tromethamine; (c) trisodium phosphate dodecahydrate; (d)
anhydrous sodium carbonate. [From Jacobson, H., and Gibbs, I., *J. Pharm.
Sci.*, *62*:1543 (1973). Reproduced with the permission of the copyright
owner.]

C. Solution Phase Stability

Even for a drug substance intended to be formulated into a solid dosage form such as a tablet, a limited solution phase stability study must be undertaken. Among other reasons, these studies are necessary to assure that the drug substance does not degrade intolerably when exposed to gastrointestinal fluids. Also, for labile drugs, the information is useful in selection of granulation solvent and drying conditions. Thus, the stability of the dissolved drug in buffers ranging from pH 1 to 8 should be investigated. If the drug is observed to degrade rapidly in acidic solutions, a less soluble or less susceptible chemical form may show increased relative bioavailability. Alternately, an enteric dosage form may be recommended for such a compound. Erythromycin is rapidly inactivated in the acidic environment of the stomach. Stevens et al. [106] recommend the use of

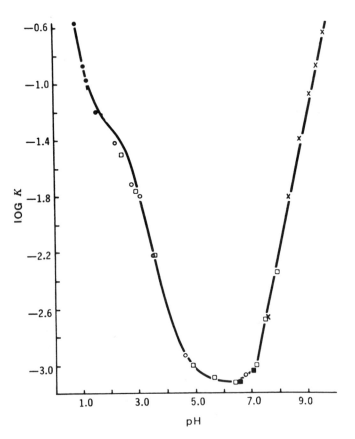

Figure 25   pH-Rate profile for the degradation of ampicillin in solution at 35°C. Apparent rate constants in buffers: $\bullet$, HCl-KCl; $\square$, citric acid-phosphate; $\times$, H_2BO_3-NaOH. Rate constants at zero buffer concentration: $\circ$, citric acid-potassium citrate; $\blacksquare$, NaH_2PO_4-Na_2HPO_4; $\square$, citric acid-phosphate buffer. [Modified from Hou, J. P., and Poole, J. W., *J. Pharm. Sci.* 54: 447 (1969). Reproduced with the permission of the copyright owner.]

relatively insoluble propionyl erythromycin lauryl sulfate (erythromycin estolate) to circumvent this problem. The work of Boggiano and Gleeson [107]
shows that other salts, such as stearates and salts of carboxylic acids, are
less satisfactory because hydrochloric acid of the gastric juice readily dis-
places the relatively weakly acidic anions and dissolves the antibiotic as the
soluble hydrochloride salt. The estolate, being a salt of a very strong
acid, lauryl sulfuric acid, is not affected by the hydrochloric acid. It remains undissolved and potent even after prolonged exposure to gastric acid.
    The availability of pH-rate profile data is sometimes useful in predicting
the solid-state stability of salt forms or the stability of a drug in the presence of acidic and basic excipients. The pH-rate profile for ampicillin, a
broad-spectrum β-lactam antibiotic (Fig. 25), shows that the antibiotic is
significantly less stable in both acidic and basic solutions [108]. Indeed,
both the hydrochloride and the sodium salt of ampicillin are significantly
less stable as solids, compared to free ampicillin, when exposed to moisture.
Compounds containing sulfhydryl groups are susceptible to oxidation in the
presence of moisture. These compounds are more stable under acidic conditions [109]. If a drug substance is judged to be physically or chemically
unstable when exposed to moisture, a direct-compression or nonaqueous
solvent granulation procedure is to be recommended for the preparation of
tablets. Before using a nonaqueous solvent for this purpose, stability of
the drug in the solvent must be ascertained—since many reactions that
occur in aqueous solutions may take place in organic solvents. Reactions
in solution proceed considerably more rapidly than the corresponding solid-
state reactions. Degradation in solution thus offers a rapid method for the
generation of degradation products. The latter are often needed for the
purposes of identification and synthesis (to study their toxicity where appropriate) and the development of analytical methods.

X. MISCELLANEOUS PROPERTIES

In addition to the physicochemical parameters described heretofore, information pertaining to certain other properties, such as density, hygroscopicity,
flowability, compactibility, compressibility, and wettability, is useful to the
formulator. These properties influence the process of manufacture and are
important considerations when the active drug constitutes the major portion
of the final dosage form.

A. Density

Knowledge of the absolute and bulk densities of the drug substance is very
useful in forming some idea as to the size of the final dosage form. Obviously, this parameter is very critical for drugs of low potency, which
may constitute the bulk of the final granulation of the tablet. The density
of solids also affects their flow properties. In the case of a physical mixture of powders, significant difference in the absolute densities of the components could lead to segregation.

B. Hygroscopicity

Many drug substances exhibit a tendency to adsorb moisture. The amount
of moisture adsorbed by a fixed weight of anhydrous sample in equilibrium

with the mosture in the air at a given temperature is referred to as *equilib-rium moisture content*. The significance of adsorbed moisture to the stabil-ity of the solids has already been discussed. Additionally, the equilibrium moisture content may influence the flow and compression characteristics of powders and the hardness of final tablets and granulations. The knowledge of the rate and extent of moisture pickup of new drug substances permits the formulator to take appropriate corrective steps when problems are antici-pated. In general, hygroscopic compounds should be stored in a well-closed container, preferably with a desiccant.

The sorption isotherms showing the equilibrium moisture contents of a drug substance and excipients as a function of a relative vapor pressure may be determined by placing samples in desiccators having different humid-ity conditions. Zografi and his coworkers [110,111] designed specialized equipments for more precise determination of the rate and extent of mois-ture sorption. Proper processing and storage conditions of drugs may be selected on the basis of sorption isotherms. A solid deliquesces or dis-solves in the adsorbed layer of water when the relative humidity of atmos-phere exceeds that of its saturated soltuion [112]. The latter condition is called critical relative humidity, or RH_0. The dissolution of a crystalline solid into adsorbed water (surface dissolution) would not be expected to occur below RH_0. However, Kontny et al. [111] recently showed that me-chanical processing of solids such as grinding, milling, micronization, com-paction, etc., can induce changes in their reactivity toward water vapor. As a result, the surface dissolution of drug may occur at a lower humidity, which may lead to chemical and physical instability problems during sub-sequent storage. Thus, whenever possible, preformulation study should be conducted with the form of material to be used in the final formulation.

The moisture contents of excipients can also influence the physicochemi-cal properties of solid dosage forms. The analysis of sorption isotherms of excipients such as cellulose and starch derivatives indicates that water may exist in at least two forms, "bound" ("solidlike") and "free" [113]. These two types of water may be differentiated by measuring heat of sorp-tion and by DSC and nuclear magnetic resonance studies. It has been sug-gested that serious stability problems may be avoided by minimizing free water in the excipients. On the other hand, it has been observed that the removal of unbound water reduces the ability of microcrystalline cel-lulose [114] and compressible sugar [113] to act as direct-compaction ma-terials. This is because free water is needed to provide plasticity to these systems. Free water on the external surface of powders can also affect powder flow [115].

C. Flowability

The flow properties of powders are critical for an efficient tableting opera-tion. A good flow of the powder or granulation to be compressed is neces-sary to assure efficient mixing and acceptable weight uniformity for the compressed tablets. If a drug is identified at the preformulation stage to be "poorly flowable," the problem can be solved by selecting appropriate excipients. In some cases, drug powders may have to be precompressed or granulated to improve their flow properties. During the preformulation evaluation of the drug substance, therefore, its flowability characteristic should be studied, especially when the anticipated dose of the drug is large.

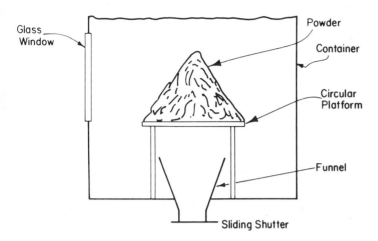

Figure 26 Schematic diagram of the apparatus for measuring angle of repose. [From Pilpel, N., Chem. *Process Eng.*, *46*:167 (1965). Reproduced with the permission of the publisher, Morgan-Grampian, London.]

Amidon and Houghton [116] discussed various methods of testing powder flow. Some of these methods are angle of repose, flow through an orifice, compressibility index, shear cell, etc. No single method, however, can assess all parameters affecting the flow.

When a heap of powder is allowed to stand with only the gravitational force acting on it, the angle between the free surface of the static heap and the horizontal plane can achieve a certain maximum value for a given powder. This angle is defined as the *static angle of repose* and is a common way of expressing flow characteristics of powders and granulations. For most pharmaceutical powders, the angle-of-repose values range from 25 to 45°, with lower values indicating better flow characteristics.

There are a number of ways to determine the angle of repose. The exact value of the measured angle depends on the method used. The value of the angle of repose determined from methods where the powder is poured to form a heap is often distorted by the impact of the falling particles. The method described by Pilpel [117] is particularly free of this distortion. The apparatus used by Pilpel is shown in Figure 26. It consists of a container with a built-in platform. The container is first filled with the powder, which is then drained out from the bottom, leaving a cone on the platform. The angle of repose is then measured using a cathetometer.

The angle-of-repose measurement has some drawbacks as a predictor of powder flow in that it lacks sensitivity. For example, in a study reported by Amidon et al. [116], sodium chloride, spray-dried lactose, and Fast-Flo lactose showed similar angles of repose, but their rates of flow through a 6-mm orifice were quite different. Therefore, the use of more than one method may be necessary for the adequate characterization of powder flow.

In general, acicular crystals (because of cross-bridging), materials with low density, and materials with a static charge exhibit poor flow. Grinding of acicular crystals generally results in an improvement in the flow. For other powders and granulations, incorporation of a lubricant

or glidant helps alleviate the problem. For powders with poor flow, usually
a granulation step is suggested.

D. Compactibility/Compressibility

Tablet formulations are multicomponent systems. The ability of such a mixture to form a good compact is dictated by compressibility and compactibility characteristics of each component.

Lueuenberger and Rohera [118] defined "compressibility" of a powder
as the ability to decrease in volume under pressure, and "compactibility"
as the ability of the powdered material to be compressed into a tablet of
specified tensile strength. Some indication of the compressibility and compactibility characteristics of a new drug substance alone and in combination
with some of the common excipients should therefore be obtained as part
of the preformulation evaluation. Use of a hydraulic press offers one of
the simplest ways to generate such data. Powders that form hard compacts
under applied pressure without exhibiting any tendency to cap or chip can
be considered as readily compactible.

The compactibility of pharmaceutical powders can be characterized by
studying tensile strength, indentation hardness, etc., of compacts prepared
under various pressures [118,119]. Hiestand and Smith [119] used tensile
strength and indentation hardness to determine three dimensionless parameters—
strain index, bonding index, and brittle fracture index—to characterize tableting performance of individual components and mixtures. For the determination of tensile strength, compacts are placed radially [120] or axially [121] between two platens, and forces required to fracture the compacts are measured.
Values of tensile strength calculated from the forces required radially and axially are called, respectively, radial and axial tensile strengths. Jarosz and
Parrott [122] suggested that a comparison of radial and axial tensile strengths
of compacts may indicate bonding strengths of compacts in two directions and
may be related to their tendency toward capping. They also used tensile
strength to evaluate the type and concentration of binders necessary to improve the compactibility of powders.

Hardness is defined as the resistance of a solid to deformation and is
primarily related to its plasticity. It is commonly measured by the static
impression method (Brinell test). The schematics of Brinell test apparatus
are shown in Figure 27. In this method [118], a hard, spherical indenter
of diameter D is pressed under a fixed normal load F onto the mooth surface of a compact. The resulting indentation diameter d is measured or
calculated using the depth h. The Brinell hardness number (BHN) is then
calculated by using the following equation:

$$\text{BHN} = \frac{2F}{\pi D(D - \sqrt{D^2 - d^2}}$$

Compressibility of powders is characterized from the density—compression pressure relationship according to the Heckel plot [123,124]. The
relevant equation is given below:

$$\log \frac{1}{1 - \rho_{rel}} = \frac{KP}{2.303} + A$$

where ρ_{rel} is the relative density, P is the compressional pressure, and K
and A are constants. Information about the extent of compression, the

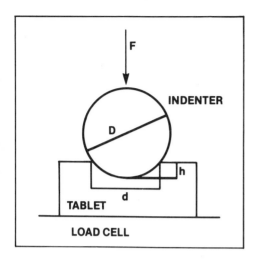

Figure 27   Schematics of apparatus for Brinell test.   [From Leuenberger, H., and Rohera, B. D., *Pharm. Res.*, 3:12 (1986).   Reproduced with the permission of The copyright owner.]

yield value or the minimum pressure required to cause deformation of solid, and the nature of deformation (plastic deformation, brittle fracture), etc., may be obtained from the Heckel plot.

E. Wettability

Wettability of a solid is an important property with regard to formulation of a solid dosage form [125]. It may influence granulation of solids, penetration of dissolution fluids into tablets and granules, and adhesion of coating materials to tablets. Wettability is often described in terms of a contact angle that can be measured by placing drops of liquids on compacts of materials. The more hydrophobic a material is, the higher is the contact angle, and a value above 90° (using water) implies little or no spontaneous wetting. Crystal structures can also influence the contact angle. For example, α and β forms of chloramphenicol palmitate have contact angles of 122 and 108°, respectively. Changes in surface characteristics may also occur on milling. A second method of determining wettability uses the Washburn equation [126]. In this method, the distance a liquid penetrates into a bed of powder or a compact is measured [127,128]. Problems associated with wettability of powders, namely, poor dissolution rate, low adhesion of film coating, and the like, may be solved by intimate mixing with hydrophilic excipients or by incorporating a surfactant in the formulation.

XI.   EXAMPLES OF PREFORMULATION STUDIES

As indicated earlier, selectivity is very important to the success of any preformulation program. To achieve this it is suggested that the data as they become available be analyzed to decide which areas warrant further scrutiny. The following examples of preformulation studies where certain parameters

were not studied will illustrate this approach. These examples also illustrate one format for organizing and presenting the data.

A. Preformulation Example A

  I. Background
      1. Compound: SQ 10,996
      2. Chemical name: 7-Chloro-5,11-dihydrodibenz(b,e)[1,4]oxazepine-
          5-carboxamide
      3. Chemical structure

$C_{14}H_{11}ClN_2O_2$ Molecular wt: 272.71

      4. Lot numbers: RR001RB and NN006NB
      5. Solvents of recrystallization: Lot RR001RB was crystallized from
          chloroform. Lot NN006NB was crystallized from a mixed solvent
          system consisting of ethyl acetate and ethyl alcohol.
      6. Purity: Lots RR001RB and NN006NB were 99.5 and 99.4% pure
          as determined by thin-layer chromatography. Lot RR001RB con-
          tained one impurity whereas NN006NB contained two impurities.
      7. Therapeutic category: Anticonvulsant, antidepressant
      8. Anticipated dose: About 400 mg single dose

 II. Organoleptic properties: SQ 10,996 is a white, odorless, and almost
      tasteless powder.

III. Microscopic examination: Microscopic examination of the "as is" powder
      revealed that the material was anisotropic and birefringent. Crystals
      in lot RR001RB were highly faceted with no specific shape predominating.
      Crystals in lot NN006NB were essentially rectangular and not as highly
      faceted as in lot RR001RB. The crystals in both lots ranged in diameter
      from 20 to 40 µm. On micronization, crystals in both lots were reduced
      to less than 10 µm in diameter.

IV. Physical characteristics
      1. Density: Densities of the two lots are shown in Table 12.
      2. Particle size
          a. Lot RR001RB "as is" was examined using a light-scattering
              technique. The data are presented in Table 13.

    b. Particle size distribution of lot RR001RB, micronized, was measured by the Coulter Counter. The data are shown in Table 14.

3. Surface area: Surface area of lot RR001RB "as is" increased from 0.5 to 2.7 m^2 g^{-1} on micronization.

4. Static charge: Neither lot exhibited any apparent static charge.

Table 12 Example A: Densities of Two Lots of SQ 10,996

	Density (g cm^{-3})	
Method	RR001RB	NN006NB
Fluff	0.34	0.45
Tap	0.58	0.55

Table 13 Example A: Particle Size Distribution of SQ 10,996, Lot RR01RB "As Is"

Size	Percentage
3—10 µm	63.25
Less than 20 µm	93.13
Less than 40 µm	99.77
Over 40 µm	0.25

Table 14 Example A: Particle Size Distribution of Micronized SQ 10,996

Size	Percentage
Less than 2.58 µm	2.5
Less than 4.09 µm	17.8
Less than 5.15 µm	36.8
Less than 10.3 µm	93.8
Less than 16.4 µm	98.8
Less than 20.6 µm	100.0

Micronization (RR001RB) resulted in the development of a surface static which was considered as manageable.

5. Flow properties: Both lots of SQ 10,996 exhibited good flow characteristics. An angle of repose measurement was not made.

6. Compressibility: SQ 10,996 compressed well into a hard disk which displayed some tendency to chip. Tableting of SQ 10,996 may need the incorporation of some granulating agent.

7. Hygroscopicity: SQ 10,996 powder (RR001RB) previously determined to be anhydrous by thermogravimetric analysis was found to pick up no moisture over a period of 8 weeks when exposed at room temperature to relative humidities of up to 90%.

8. Polymorphism: Because of the drug's low aqueous solubility a possible bioavailability problem existed. To circumvent this possibility, an intensive search to uncover a more soluble form of SQ 10,996 was made. These studies showed that lyophilization of a solution of SQ 10,996 in p-dioxane resulted in the formation of a dioxane solvate. Exhaustive drying eliminated the dioxane, leaving a polymorphic form (clearly demonstrable by powder X-ray diffraction and thermal analysis) and referred to as form II. The solubility of form II in aqueous solvent systems at room temperature was found to be twice that of for I. Under a variety of temperature and humidity conditions form II was found to be physically and chemically stable.

V. Solution properties

1. pH of 1% Suspension: Approximately 7

2. pK_a: Not determined

3. Solubility: The solubility data for the two lots of SQ 10,996 are presented in Table 15.

4. Effect of solubilizing agents: Because solubility in the aqueous systems was considered as very low, attempts were made to solubilize SQ 10,996 (RR001RB) using different surfactants. The data in Table 16 illustrate the influence of different surfactants on the solubility of SQ 10,996.

5. Partition coefficient: The n-octanol/water partition coefficient was very much in favor of the organic phase. The exact value was not determined.

6. Dissolution rates

   a. Intrinsic: In 1 L of distilled water with stirring at 100 rpm and at 37°C, the intrinsic dissolution rate of lot RR001RB was considerably lower than 0.1 mg min^{-1} cm^{-2}.

   b. Paritculate: Particulate dissolution studies were performed on loosely filled capsules containing 50 mg of SQ 10,996 (RR001RB). Because the dissolution of SQ 10,996 was considered as too slow, attempts to improve the dissolution rate were made. These included physically admixing with a surfactant, coprecipitating with a surfactant, micronizing, and granulating with sodium lauryl sulfate. In these instances mixtures containing the equivalent of 50 mg of SQ 10,996 were encapsulated and the dissolution investigated. The dissolution medium was 500 ml of 0.1 N HCl at 37°C, and it

Table 15 Example A: Solubilities in Various Solvents of SQ 10,996

	Solubility at 25°C (mg ml^{-1})	
Solvent	RR001RB	NN006NB
Water[a]	0.04	0.04
pH 7.2 Phosphate buffer[a]	0.04	—
0.1 N HCl[a]	0.04	—
Isopropyl alcohol[b]	3.10	3.00
Methyl alcohol[b]	15.30	15.70
Acetone[b]	34.40	34.30
Ethyl alcohol[b]	6.90	—

[a]Concentration of the saturated solutions determined spectrophotometrically by determining the absorbance at 290 nm.

[b]Determined gravimetrically by evaporating a known volume of the filtered saturated solution and determining the weight of the residue.

Table 16 Example A: Solubilities in Water of SQ 10,996 in the Presence of Various Surfactants

	Solubility (mg ml^{-1}) at 25°C in the presence of			
Surfactant/drug ratio (w/w)	Sodium lauryl sulfate	Tween 80	Sodium dihydrocholate	Dioctyl sodium sulfosuccinate
4/100	0.06	—	—	—
8/100	0.08	0.06	0.06	0.05
1/10	0.14	0.07	0.09	0.06
1/5	0.24	0.08	0.10	0.10

Note: All determinations were made using the spectrophotometric method.

was stirred at 50 rpm using the rotating basket. The concentration of the dissolved drug was determined spectrophotometrically. Because of the limited aqueous solubility of SQ 10,996, the dissolution was performed under nonsink conditions. The data are shown in Table 17.

VI. Stability (solid)
1. Heat: SQ 10,996 (RR001RB) was stable after 4 weeks at 60°C when assayed by thin-layer chromatography.
2. Humidity: SQ 10,996 (RR001RB) was stable after 8 weeks of exposure to 50% relative humidity at 60°C when assayed by thin-layer chromatography.
3. Light: SQ 10,996 (NN006NB) after 2 weeks of exposure to 900 fc of illumination at 33°C and ambient humidity did not show any visible discoloration or degradation when assayed by the thin-layer chromatography.

VII. Drug—excipient compatibility studies: Potential drug—excipient interactions were investigated using differential thermal analysis. Thermograms were obtained for the drug alone and for its 1:3, 1:1, and 3:1 physical mixtures and aqueous granulations with magnesium stearate, Sta-Rx 1500 starch, lactose, dicalcium phosphate dihydrate, talc, Avicel, cornstarch, PEG 6000, Plasdone C, and stearic acid. These studies failed to provide any evidence of potential drug—excipient interaction.

VIII. Solution stability: Because of excellent solid-state stability and very poor aqueous solubility, the solution phase stability of SQ 10,996 was not investigated.

IX. Recommendations: The major potential problem associated with SQ 10,996 is its poor aqueous solubility and consequent slow dissolution. This may result in incomplete and slow absorption. Use of the more soluble form II may alleviate this problem. The good solid-state physical stability of form II favors its usage. The method used in the present study for the preparation of form II is cumbersome, and an easier method which can be used in the manufacture of the bulk formulation should be developed. In the absence of the latter, the micronization of SQ 10,996 followed by granulation with an aqueous solution of sodium lauryl sulfate appears as a promising alternative. An in vivo study comparing the different alternatives must be undertaken at the earliest apportunity to select the right form of SQ 10,996. The stability prognosis for SQ 10,996 tablet dosage form is excellent.

B. Preformulation Example B
I. Background
1. Compound: SQ 20,009
2. Chemical name: 1-Ethyl-4[(1-methylethylidene)hydrazinol)-^{1}H-pyrazolo[3,4-b]pyridine-5-carboxylic acid, ethyl ester, hydrochloride (1:1)
3. Chemical structure

Table 17   Example A: Dissolution of SQ 10,996, Various Treatments

Time (min)	SQ 10,996 form I	1:1 Physical mixture with PEG 6000	1:1 Co-ppt with PEG 6000	1:1 Physical mixture with PVP	1:1 Co-ppt with PVP	Micronized SQ 10,996 granulated with sodium lauryl SO_4	1:1 Co-ppt with plusonic F-127
			Amount dissolved (mg ml^{-1})				
10	0.001	0.001	0.002	0.002	0.006	–	–
20	0.001	0.010	0.010	0.012	0.015	0.032	0.020
30	0.004	0.016	0.013	0.018	0.015	–	–
40	0.007	0.018	0.016	0.019	0.020	0.035	0.040
50	–	0.020	0.017	0.021	0.021	–	–
60	0.007	0.022	0.019	0.022	0.024	0.038	0.070

$$C_{14}H_{20}ClN_5O_2 \qquad \text{Molecular wt } 325.80$$

4. Lot number: RR004RA
5. Solvent of recrystallization: Acetone and aqueous hydrochloric acid.
6. Purity: Batch RR004RA contained 0.15% impurities as determined by paper chromatography
7. Therapeutic category: Psychotropic
8. Anticipated dose: 25 to 50 mg single dose

II. Organoleptic properties: SQ 20,009 is a white powder with a characteristic aromatic odor and a bitter taste.

III. Microscopic examination: The crystals of SQ 20,009 are needlelike.

IV. Physical characteristics

1. Density: Fluff and tap densities of SQ 20,009 were determined to be 3.0 and 3.5 g cm^{-3}, respectively.
2. Particle size (microscopic): The needlelike crystals of SQ 20,009 ranged in width from 2 to 10 μm. On grinding in a small ball-mill the average length was reduced to about 30 μm from about 80 μm.
3. Surface area: Not determined
4. Static change: SQ 20,009 "as is" material exhibited some static change. Grinding of SQ 20,009 did not significantly alter this property.
5. Flow properties: As would be expected with materials having needlelike crystals, SQ 20,009 was not very free flowing. Grinding of SQ 20,009 significantly improved its flow.
6. Compressibility: SQ 20,009 compressed well into a hard disk which did not show any tendency to cap or chip.
7. Hygroscopicity: When exposed to 80% relative humidity at room temperature, SQ 20,009 did not pick up any moisture over a 24-hr period.
8. Polymorphism: The potential problem associated with SQ 20,009 is its instability in solutions. For this reason a less soluble material is desirable. However, high solubility of the material makes it very unlikely that a sufficiently less soluble form can be discovered. For this reason investigation of polymorphism of SQ 20,009 was not undertaken. The free base of SQ 20,009 is an oily liquid and is not considered suitable for development into a development into a solid dosage form.

V. Solution properties
1. pH of 1% Solution: 1.9
2. pK$_a$: 2.04

3. Solubility: SQ 20,009 is exceedingly soluble in water and lower alcohols. In aqueous systems it dissolved in excess of 400 mg ml^{-1}, and in lower alcohols it dissolved in excess of 100 mg ml^{-1}. Because of the very high solubility, an exact solubility determination was not attempted.
4. Partition coefficient: Not determined
5. Dissolution (particulate): Capsules containing 50 mg of SQ 20,009 showed 100% dissolution in 15 min. The dissolution was studied in 1 L of water at 37°C at a stirring rate of 100 rpm using the rotating basket.

VI. Stability (solid)
1. Heat: SQ 20,009 was found to be stable after 12 months at 50°C and ambient humidity.
2. Humidity: Exposure of SQ 20,009 to a high humidity of 80% relative humidity showed a visible discoloration after 8 weeks. The samples were not assayed.
3. Light: Upon exposure to 900 fc of illumination at 33°C and ambient humidity, SQ 20,009 showed signs of yellowing after 2 weeks.

VII. Drug—excipient compatibility studies
1. Differential thermal analysis: Using weight ratios of 1:3, 1:1, and 3:1, mixtures of magnesium stearate, stearic acid, lactose, and Avicel with drug showed an interaction only with magnesium stearate.
2. Thin-layer chromatography: Mixtures of SQ 20,009 and magnesium stearate, lactose, stearic acid, and Sta-Rx 1500 starch were stable after 8 months at 50°C and 12 months at room temperature.

VIII. Solution stability: Aqueous solutions of SQ 20,009 showed rapid time-dependent changes in the ultraviolet spectrum. Analysis of the data and the degraded samples showed that the Schiff base moiety of SQ 20,009 underwent reversible hydrolysis to the corresponding hydrazine compound and acetone. The hydrolysis was pH-dependent. The half-lives for hydrolysis at 37°C in media of different pH are shown in Table 18. The ester function in SQ 20,009 is also susceptible to hydrolysis. Studies with a structural analog 1-ethyl-4-butylamino-^{1}H-pyrazolo[3,4-b]pyridine-5-carboxylic acid, ethyl ester showed that the ester function underwent significant hydrolysis only under alkaline conditions.

IX. Recommendations: Under acidic conditions SQ 20,009 hydrolyzes rapidly. To prevent the inactivation of SQ 20,009 by gastric acidity, use of the less soluble pamoate salt should be considered. The use of a less soluble form should also be considered for overcoming the problem of bitter taste. Because of the hydrolytic susceptibility of SQ 20,009, the use of aqueous-based granulating agent should be avoided. Because of the relatively low dose of SQ 20,009 it poor flowability is not likely to present any significant problems. Nevertheless SQ 20,009 should be ground, to improve its flow and allow for better homogeneity.

Table 18 Example B: Half-Lives for the Hydrolysis of SQ 20,009 under Various pH Conditions at 37°C

pH Condition	$T_{1/2}$(min)
0.1 N HCl	5
0.01 N HCl	50
pH 3.0	70
pH 4.0	150

C. Performulation Example C

    I. Background

        1. Compound: Cicloprofen (SQ 20,824)

        2. Chemical name: α-Methyl-^{9}H-fluorene-2-acetic acid

        3. Chemical structure

$C_{16}H_{14}O_2$ Molecular wt 238.29

        4. Lot numbers: EE003EA

                       EE007EA

                       EE009EC

        5. Solvents of recrystallization: Lots EE003EA and EE007EA were recrystallized out of acetone-water. Lot EE009EC was precipitated from aqueous ammoniacal solution with acetic acid.

        6. Purity: Lots EE003EA, EE007EA, and EE009EC contained 3.4, 4.0, and 0.7% impurities, respectively, when assayed by thin-layer chromatography.

        7. Therapeutic category: Nonsteroidal anti-inflammatory

        8. Anticipated dose: 100 to 250 mg

    II. Organoleptic properties: Cicloprofen is a pale cream-colored powder. It is practically odorless and tasteless.

   III. Microscopic examination: Microscopic examination of the three lots of cicloprofen showed that the powders were anisotropic and bire-

fringent. The crystals were platy and ranged in diameter form
1 to 50 μm.

IV. Physical characteristics
1. Density: Fluff, tap, and true densities of lot EE007EA were
determined to be 0.22, 0.33, and 1.28 g cm^{-3}, respectively.
2. Particle size: The particle size range of unmilled lot EE007EA
was 1 to 50 μm. About 30% of the particles counted were below 10 μm, with those below 5 μm accounting for about 50%
of the particles.
3. Surface area: Surface area of lot EE007EA was determined to
to be 1.05 m^2 g^{-1}. On milling the surface area increased to
3.50 m^2 g^{-1}.
4. Static charge: All three lots of cicloprofen exhibited significant
static charge. The problem of static charge was accentuated
on milling. Milling after mixing with an excipient such as lactose helped significantly in reducing the charge.
5. Flow properties: All three lots of cicloprofen exhibited poor
flow characteristics. On milling the material balled up in aggregates and had extremely poor flow. Granulating the milled and
unmilled materials with water significantly improved the flow behavior.
6. Compressibility: Cicloprofen compressed well into hard shiny
disks which showed no tendency to cap or chip.
7. Hygroscopicity: Cicloprofen adsorbed less than 0.1% moisture
after storage in an atmosphere of 88% relative humidity at 22°C
for 24 hr.
8. Polymorphism: Cicloprofen was recrystallized from 23 different
single solvents and 13 solvent-water mixtures, and from super-
cooled melts. No conclusive evidence of the existence of polymorphism was obtained.

V. Solution properties
1. pH of 1% suspension: 5.3
2. pK$_a$: A value of 4.1 was obtained using the solubility and the
spectrophotometric methods.
3. Solbility: The solubility data for cicloprofen are presented in
Table 19.
4. Partition coefficient: Partition coefficient (oil/water) of cicloprofen between amyl acetate and pH 7.3 McIlvaine citrate-phos-
phate buffer at 37°C was determined to be 17.0.
5. Dissolution rates
a. Intrinsic: In 1 L of pH 7.2, 0.05 M phosphate buffer at
37°C and at 50 rpm, the intrinsic dissolution rate of lot
EE007EA was 2.1 × 10^{-3} mg min^{-1} cm^{-2}.
b. Particulate: Dissolution studies were performed on loose-
filled capsules containing 200 mg unmilled and milled cicloprofen (EE007EA) and 400 mg of aqueous granulations of
1:1 mixtures of milled and unmilled cicloprofen with anhydrous lactose. The dissolution medium was 1 L of pH 7.2,
0.05 M phosphate buffer at 37°C, stirred at 50 rpm. Under
these conditions the 1:1 granulations dissolved the fastest
within 30 min. The DT50% (the time needed for 50% dissolu-

Table 19   Example C: Solubility
of Cicloprofen in Various Solvents
at 25°C

Solvent	Solubility (mg ml^{-1})
Water	0.06
0.1 N HCl	0.01
pH 7.0 buffer	1.10
Isopropyl alcohol	∿50
Methyl alcohol	∿80
Ethyl alcohol	∿75
Methylene chloride	>100

tion) values for the milled and unmilled cicloprofen were 50
and 40 min, respectively. The slower dissolution of the
milled material is believed to be due to powder agglomeration,
resulting in the reduction of effective surface area.

VI.   Stability (solid)
1.   Heat: After 6 months of storage at 50°C and ambient humidity,
cicloprofen (all three lots) showed approximately 4% degradation
when examined by thin-layer chromatography.
2.   Humidity: After 1 month at 40°C and 75% relative humidity, cicloprofen (all three lots) showed no detectable degradation.
3.   Light: On exposure to light cicloprofen became yellow. Samples
of cicloprofen exposed to 900 fc of illumination were intensely
yellow after 5 days. The exposed samples contained as many as
five degradation products when assayed by thin-layer chromatography and accounted for less than 2% of degradation of cicloprofen.

VII.   Drug–excipient compatibility studies: Mixtures in the ratios 1:1,
1:3, and 3:1 of cicloprofen (EE007EA) with alginic acid, microcrystalline cellulose, calcium phosphate, gelatin, lactose, magnesium stearate,
polyvinylpyrrolidone, sodium lauryl sulfate, cornstarch, stearic acid,
and talc were examined using differential thermal analysis. This
study failed to provide any evidence of potential interaction. Storage of these mixtures for 1 week at 70°C at 75% relative humidity
and up to 8 weeks at 40°C at 75% relative humidity, followed by
their examination by thin-layer chromatography, failed to provide
any evidence of degradation.

VIII.   Recommendations: The major potential problem areas associated with
cicloprofen are its low solubility, poor dissolution, poor flow, and

poor photolytic stability. Attempts to find a more soluble polymorph were not successful. Granulation of the powder is needed to improve both its flow and its dissolution. Any shearing of cicloprofen should be avoided to contain the problem of the static charge. Because of its photolytic instability cicloprofen should be protected from light as much as possible. Consideration also should be given to incorporation of a yellow dye in the tablets to mask any light-catalyzed discoloration.

REFERENCES

1. *Pharmacopeial Forum, 13*:2505 (1987).
2. *Pharmacopeial Forum, 13*:2683 (1987).
3. L. F. Prescott, R. F. Steel, and W. R. Ferrier, *Clin. Pharmacol. Ther., 11*:496 (1970).
4. R. M. Atkinson, C. Bedford, K. J. Child, and E. G., Tomich, *Nature, 193*:588 (1962).
5. J. Piccolo and A. Sakr, *Pharm. Ind., 46*:1277 (1984).
6. H. Weng and E. L. Parrott, *J. Pharm. Sci., 73*:1059 (1984).
7. E. L. Parrott, *Pharm. Mfg., 4*:31 (1985).
8. A. N. Martin, J. Swarbrick, and A. Cammarata, *Physical Pharmacy*, Lea & Febiger, Philadelphia, 1969.
9. C. Orr, Jr. and J. M. Dalla Valle, *Fine Particle Measurement*, MacMillan, New York, 1959.
10. S. J. Gregg and K. S. W. Sing, *Adsorption, Surface Area, and Porosity*, Academic Press, New York, 1967.
11. S. F. Kramer and G. L. Flynn, *J. Pharm. Sci., 61*:1896 (1972).
12. S Miyazaki, M. Oshiba, and T. Nadai, *Int. J. Pharm., 6*:77 (1980).
13. C. D. Herzfeldt and R. Kimmel, *Drug. Dev. Ind. Pharm., 9*:967 (1983).
14. Z. T. Chowhan, *J. Pharm. Sci., 67*:1257 (1978).
15. A. T. M. Serajuddin and D. Mufson, *Pharm. Res., 2*:65 (1985).
16. W. H. Streng and H. G. H. Tan, *Int. J. Pharm., 25*:135 (1985).
17. A. T. M. Serajuddin and C. I. Jarowski, *J. Pharm. Sci., 74*:142 (1985).
18. T. Higuchi, F. L. Shih, T. Kimura, and J. H. Rytting, *J. Pharm. Sci., 68*:1267 (1979).
19. R. Ohnishi and K. Tanabe, *Bull. Chem. Soc. Jap., 41*:2647 (1971).
20. G. Milosovich, *J. Pharm. Sci., 53*:484 (1964).
21. D. E. Guttman and M. Athalye, *J. Am. Pharm. Assoc. [Sci. Ed.], 49*:687 (1960).
22. D. A. Wadke and D. E. Guttman, *J. Pharm. Sci., 54*:1293 (1965).
23. W. L. Chiou and S. Riegelman, *J. Pharm. Sci., 58*:1505 (1969).
24. W. L. Chiou and S. Riegelman, *J. Pharm. Sci., 60*:1377 (1971).
25. A. A. Sinkula, W. Morozowich, and E. L. Rowe, *J. Pharm. Sci., 62*:1106 (1973).
26. S. A. Kaplan, *Drug Metab. Rev., 1*:15 (1972).
27. J. H. Wood, J. E. Syarto, and H. Letterman, *J. Pharm. Sci., 54*:1068 (1965).

28. K. G. Mooney, M. A. Mintun, K. J. Himmelstein, and V. A. Stella, *J. Pharm. Sci.*, *70*:22 (1981).

29. V. K. Prasad, R. S. Rapaka, P. W. Knight, and B. E. Cabana, *Int. J. Pharm.*, *11*:81 (1982).

30. P. Finholt, Influence of formulation on dissolution rate, in Dissolution Technology, Industrial Pharmaceutical Technology Section, Acad. Pharm Sci., Washington, D.C., 1974, p. 109.

31. D. C. Monkhouse and J. L. Lach, *J. Pharm. Sci.*, *61*:1431 (1972).

32. J. W. McGinity, D. D. Manes, and G. J. Yakatan, *Drug Dev. Commun.* *1*:396 (1974–75).

33. N. Shah, R. Pytelewski, H. Eisen, and C. Jorowski, *J. Pharm. Sci.*, *63*:1339 (1974).

34. A. Hussain, *J. Pharm. Sci.*, *61*:811 (1972).

35. O. Kausch, Vergleichende Untersuchungen der intestinalen Resorption von Opium. Alkoloiden mit Einem Beitrag zur Beantwortung der Frage nach der Abhangigkeit der Resorption von der chemischen Konstitution: Dissertation, Universitat des Saarlndes, Germany, 1968. Cited in Ref. 37.

36. L. S. Schanker, *J. Pharmacol. Exp. Ther.*, *126*:283 (1959).

37. H. Kurz, Principles of drug absorption, in International Encyclopedia of Pharmacology and Therapeutics, Vol. 1, Sec. 39B, Pharmacology of Intestinal Absorption-Gastro-Intestinal Absorption of Drugs, Pergamon Press, Elmsford, NY, 1975.

38. A. Leo, C. Hansch, and D. Elkins, *Chem. Rev.*, *71*:525 (1971).

39. R. Kaliszan, *Chromatography*, 1987, p. 19.

40. F. Gaspari and M. Bonati, *J. Pharm. Pharmacol.*, *39*:252 (1987).

41. T. Braumann, G. Weber, and L. J. Grimme, *J. Chromatography*, *261*: 329 (1983).

42. P. A. Shore, B. B. Brodie, and C. A. M. Hogben, *J. Pharmacol. Exp. Ther.*, *119*:361 (1957).

43. L. S. Schanker, P. A. Shore, B. B. Brodie, and C. A. M. Hogben, *J. Pharmacol. Exp. Ther.*, *120*:528 (1957).

44. L. S. Schanker, D. J. Tocco, B. B. Brodie, and C. A. M. Hogben, *J. Pharmacol. Exp. Ther.*, *123*:81 (1958).

45. C. A. M. Hogben, L. S. Schanker, D. J. Tocco, and B. B. Brodie, *J. Pharmacol. Exp. Ther.*, *120*:540 (1957).

46. C. A. M. Hogben, D. J. Tocco, B. B. Brodie, and L. S. Schanker, *J. Pharmacol. Exp. Ther.*, *125*:275 (1959).

47. A. Albert and E. P. Serjeant, The Determination of Ionization Constamts. Chapman & Hall, London, 1971.

48. I. M. Kolthoff, S. Bruckenstein, and R. G. Bates, Acids and Bases in Analytical Chemistry, Interscience, New York, 1966.

49. T. Bates, and M. Gibaldi, Gastro-intestinal absorption of drugs, Current Concepts in Pharmaceutical Sciences: Biopharmaceutics, Lea and Febiger, Philadelphia, 1970, p. 57.

50. R. K. Crane and T. H. Wilson, *J. Appl. Physiol.*, *12*:145 (1958).

51. S. A. Kaplan and S. Cotler, *J. Pharm. Sci.*, *61*:1361 (1972).

52. S. C. Penzotti and J. W. Poole, *J. Pharm. Sci.*, *63*:1803 (1974).

53. D. C. Taylor and R. U. Grundy, *J. Pharm. Pharmacol.*, *27* [Suppl.] (1975).

54. J. T. Doluisio, N. F. Billups, L. W. Dittert, E. T. Sugita, and J. V. Swintosky, *J. Pharm. Sci.*, *58*:1196 (1967).

55. W. S. Chow, S. A. Ranadive, S. A. Varia, and K. J. Kripalani, *Abstr. Acad. Pharm. Sci.*, *14*:109 (1984).
56. S. A. Ranadive, Private communication, 1987.
57. G. L. Amidon, Determination of intestinal wall permeabilities, in *Animal Models for Oral Delivery in Man: In Situ and In Vivo Approaches.* Am. Pharm. Assn., Acad. Pharm. Sci., Washington, D.C., 1983, p. 1.
58. G. L. Amidon, M. Chang, D. Fleisher, and R. Allen, *J. Pharm. Sci.*, *71*:1138 (1982).
59. G. L. Amidon and P. J. Sinko, *Proc. In. Symp. Control. Rel. Bioact. Mater.*, *14*:20 (1987).
60. G. L. Amidon, G. D. Leesman, and R. L. Elliot, *J. Pharm. Sci.*, *69*: 1362 (1980).
61. G. L. Amidon, B. H. Stewart, and S. Pognar, *J. Controlled Rel.*, *2*: 13 (1985).
62. J. Haleblian and W. McCrone, *J. Pharm. Sci.*, *58*:911 (1969).
63. S. Rosenstein and P. Lamy, *Am. J. Hosp. Pharm.*, *26*:598 (1969).
64. G. S. Mewada, D. R. Parikh, and S. Somsekhara, *Sci. Cult.*, *39*: 378 (1973).
65. J. Haleblian, *J. Pharm. Sci.*, *64*:1269 (1975).
66. S. R. Byrn, *Solid State Chemistry of Drugs*, Academic Press, New York, 1982.
67. E. Shefter and T. Higuchi, *J. Pharm. Sci.*, *52*:781 (1963).
68. D. A. Wadke and G. E. Reier, *J. Pharm. Sci.*, *61*:868 (1972).
69. A. J. Aguiar, J. Krc, A. W. Kinkel, and J. C. Symyn. *J. Pharm. Sci.*, *56*:847 (1967).
70. A. J. Aguiar and J. E. Zelmer, *J. Pharm. Sci.*, *58*:983 (1969).
71. S. Miyazaki, T. Arita, R. Hori, and K. Ito, *Chem. Pharm. Bull.*, *22*: 638 (1974).
72. D. M. Floyd, O. R. Kocy, D. C. Monkhouse, and J. D. Pipkin, U.S. Patent 282636 (1981).
73. E. T. Cole, J. E. Rees, and J. A. Hersey, *Pharm. Acta Helv.*, *50*: 28 (1975).
74. J. W. Shell, *J. Pharm. Sci.*, *52*:100 (1963).
75. M. P. Summers, R. P. Enever, and J. E. Carless, *J. Pharm. Pharmacol.*, *28*:89 (1976).
76. H. Imaizumi, N. Nambu, and T. Nagai, *Chem. Pharm. Bull.*, *28*:2565 (1980).
77. A. T. Florence and E. G. Salole, *J. Pharm. Pharmacol. 28*:637 (1976).
78. H. G. Ibrahim, F. Pisano, and A. J. Bruno, *J. Pharm. Sci.*, *66*: 669 (1977).
79. A. T. M. Serajuddin, *J. Pharm. Pharmacol. 38*:93 (1986).
80. T. Yamaoka, H. Nakamerchi, and K. Miyata, *Chem. Pharm. Bull.*, *30*:3695 (1982).
81. J. P. Hou and A. Restivo, *J. Pharm. Sci.*, *64*:710 (1975).
82. J. P. Hou, Private communication, 1976.
83. I. Gibbs, A. Heald, H. Jacobson, D. A. Wadke, and I. Weliky, *J. Pharm. Sci.*, *65*:1380 (1976).
84. D. C. Monkhouse, *Drug Dev. Ind. Pharm.*, *10*:1373 (1984).
85. N. K. Patel, S. J. Patel, A. J. Cutie, D. A. Wadke, D. C. Monkhouse, and G. E. Reier, *Drug Dev. Ind. Pharm.*, *14*:77 (1988).

86. C. Runti, *Farmaco* [*Prat.*], *28*:451 (1973).
87. K. Guillory and T. Higuchi, *J. Pharm. Sci.*, *51*:104 (1962).
88. D. A. Johnson and G. A. Hardcastle, U.S. Patent 3,157,640 (1963).
89. J. T. Carstensen, *Theory of Pharmaceutical Systems, Vol. 2: Heterogeneous Systems*, Academic Press, New York, 1973, p. 294.
90. J. T. Carstensen, *J. Pharm. Sci.*, *63*:1 (1974).
91. S. R. Byrn, *J. Pharm. Sci.*, *65*:1 (1976).
92. D. C. Monkhouse and L. Van Campen, *Drug. Dev. Ind. Pharm.*, *10*:1276 (1984).
93. A. J. Woolfe and H. E. C. Worthington, *Drug Dev. Commun.*, *1*:185 (1974).
94. S. Miyazaki, M. Nakano, and T. Arita, *Chem. Pharm. Bull.*, *24*:1832 (1976).
95. R. Tardif, *Pharm. Sci.*, *54*:281 (1965).
96. L. Mertes (ed.), *Handbook of Analytical Chemistry*, McGraw-Hill, New York, 1963, p. 3-29.
97. S. S. Kornblum and G. J. Sciarrone, *J. Pharm. Sci.*, *53*:935 (1964).
98. M. J. Akers, *Can. J. Pharm. Sci.*, *11*:1 (1976).
99. J. Carstensen, J. Johnson, W. Valentine, and J. Vance, *J. Pharm. Sci.*, *53*:1050 (1964).
100. N. B. Jain, Private communication, 1987.
101. N. B. Jain, K. W. Garren, and M. R. Patel, *Abstr. Acad. Pharm. Sci.*, *12*:146 (1982).
102. H. Jacobson and I. Gibbs, *J. Pharm. Sci.*, *62*:1543 (1973).
103. D. G. Pope and J. L. Lach, *Pharm. Acta Helv.*, *50*:165 (1975).
104. W. Wu, T. Chin, and J. L. Lach, *J. Pharm. Sci.*, *59*:1234 (1970).
105. S. M. Blaug and W. T. Huang, *J. Pharm. Sci.*, *61*:1770 (1972).
106. J. W. Stevens, J. W. Conine, and H. W. Murphy, *J. Am. Pharm. Assoc.* [*Sci. Ed.*], *48*:620 (1959).
107. B. G. Boggiano and M. Gleeson, *J. Pharm. Sci.*, *65*:497 (1976).
108. J. P. Hou and J. W. Poole, *J. Pharm. Sci.*, *58*:447 (1969).
109. W. E. Godwin, The Oxidation of Cysteine and Cystine. Ph.D. thesis, Oklahoma State University, 1962.
110. L. Van Campen, G. Zografi, and J. T. Carstensen, *Int. J. Pharm.*, *5*:1 (1980).
111. M. J. Kontny, G. P. Grandolfi, and G. Zografi, *Pharm. Res.*, *4*:104 (1987).
112. L. Van Campen, G. L. Amidon, and G. Zografi, *J. Pharm. Sci.*, *72*:1381 (1983).
113. G. Zografi and M. J. Kontny, *Pharm. Res.*, *3*:187 (1986).
114. R. Huettenrauch and J. Jacob, *Die Pharmazie*, *32*:241 (1977).
115. N. A. Armstrong and R. V. Griffiths, *Pharm. Acta. Helv.*, *45*:692 (1970).
116. G. E. Amidon and M. E. Houghton, *Pharm. Mfg.*, July 1985, p. 21.
117. N. Pilpel, *Chem. Process Eng.*, *46*:167 (1965).
118. H. Leuenberger and B. D. Rohera, *Pharm. Res.*, *3*:12 (1986).
119. E. N. Hiestand and D. P. Smith, *Powder Technol.*, *38*:145 (1984).
120. J. T. Fell and J. M. Newton, *J. Pharm. Sci.*, *59*:688 (1970).
121. S. T. David and L. L. Augsburger, *J. Pharm. Sci.*, *63*:933 (1974).
122. P. J. Jarosz and E. L. Parrott, *J. Pharm. Sci.*, *71*:607 (1982).
123. R. W. Heckel, *Trans. Metall. Soc. AIME*, *221*,671 (1961).
124. R. W. Heckel, *ibid.*, *221*,10001 (1961).

125. P. York, *Int. J. Pharm.*, *14*:1 (1983).
126. E. D. Washburn, *Phys. Rev.*, *17*:374 (1921).
127. D. T. Hansford, D. J. W. Grant, and J. M. Newton, *Powder Technol.*, *26*:119 (1980).
128. G. Buckton and J. M. Newton, *J. Pharm. Pharmacol.*, *38*:329 (1986).

2

Tablet Formulation and Design

Garnet E. Peck

*Purdue University
West Lafayette,
Indiana*

George J. Baley and
Vincent E. McCurdy

*The Upjohn Company
Kalamazoo, Michigan*

Gilbert S. Banker

*University of Minnesota
Health Sciences Center
Minneapolis, Minnesota*

I. INTRODUCTION

The formulation of solid oral dosage forms, and tablets in particular, has undergone rapid change and development over the last several decades with the emergence of precompression, induced die feeding, high-speed and now ultrahigh-speed presses, automated weight-control systems, the availability of many new direct compression materials, and the microprocessor control of precompression, compression, ejection forces, as well as upper punch tightness on tablet presses. Some of the newer tablet presses have tablet rejection systems that are operated by a computer. Computer-controlled tablet presses only require an operator to set up the press at the proper tablet weight and thickness (or pressure). The computer can then assume complete control of the run. Still other tablet presses only require the operator to provide a product identification code to make tablets within specifications previously established and stored in the computer memory.

Most recently, new concepts and federal regulations bearing on bioavailability and bioequivalence, and on validation, are impacting on tablet formulation, design, and manufacture.

Once, lavish gold-plated pills were manufactured and marketed with little knowledge of their pharmacological activity. Appearance and later stability of the dosage form were the prime requirements of pharmaceutical preparations. The introduction of the *friable pill* denoted in part the realization that solid medicinals must—in some fashion—disintegrate within the body for the patient to benefit from the drug. We now realize that disintegration and dissolution alone do not insure therapeutic activity. As only one example of this point, Meyer et al [1] presented information on 14 nitrofurantoin products, which were evaluated both in vitro and in vivo. All products tested met USP XVIII specifications for drug content, disintegration time, and dissolution rate; however, statistically significant differences in bioavailability were observed.

The design of a tablet usually involves a series of compromises on the part of the formulator, since producing the desired properties (e.g., resistance to mechanical abrasion or friability, rapid disintegration and dissolution) frequently involves competing objectives. The correct selection and balance of excipient materials for each active ingredient or ingredient combination in a tablet formulation to achieve the desired response (i.e., production of a safe, effective, and highly reliable product) is not in practice a simple goal to achieve. Add to this fact the need today to develop tablet formulations and processing methods which may be (and must in the future be) validated, and the complexity of tablet product design is further increased in contemporary pharmaceutical development. Increased competition among manufacturers (brand versus generic, generic versus generic, and brand versus brand) has necessitated that products and processes be cost-efficient. Thus cost of a raw material or a particular processing step must be considered before a final tablet formulation or manufacturing process is selected.

Tablet formulation and design may be described as the process whereby the formulator insures that the correct *amount* of drug in the right *form* is delivered at or over the proper *time* at the proper *rate* and in the desired *location*, while having its chemical *integrity* protected to that point. Theoretically, a validated tablet formulation and production process is one in which the range in the variation of the component specifications and physical properties of the tablet product quality properties is known from a cause and effect basis. It is further known that raw materials specifications, at their limits, and when considered as interaction effects of the worst possible combinations, cannot produce a product that is out of specification from any standpoint. Likewise a validated tablet-manufacturing process is one which, when all the operating variables are considered, at any extremes which could ever be encountered in practice, and under the worst possible set of circumstances, will produce products that are within specifications. Total validation of a tablet product includes all combination effects involving formulation, raw materials variables, and processing variables, as well as their interaction effects, to assure that any system produced will be within total product specifications.

The amount or quantity of a drug which is sufficient to elicit the required or desired therapeutic response can be affected by several factors. In the case of compendial or official drugs, the dosage levels have been predetermined. With certain drugs (e.g., griseofulvin), the efficiency of absorption has been shown to depend on the particle size and specific surface area of the drug. By reducing the particle size of such drugs, the dosage level may be reduced by one-half or more and still produce the same biological response.

The form in which the drug is absorbed can affect its activity. Most drugs are normally absorbed in solution from the gut. Since the absorption process for most orally administered drugs is rapid, the rate of solution of the drug will be the rate-limiting step from the point of view of blood level and activity.

Thus, we must consider the contribution and influence of the active components and nonactive components—both separately and together—to measure their impact on the pharmacological response of any tablet system. The timing of administration may affect when and how a drug will act (and to a certain extent where it acts) as will be discussed further in Section

IV.A. Also, the timing of administration may be crucial in order to reduce gastric irritation (uncoated strong electrolytes are often given following food); to reduce drug interactions with food (formation of insoluble complexes between the calcium of milk and several antibiotics), reducing their bioavailability; or to enhance the solubility and bioavailability of certain drugs in foods (notably fats) by their administration with foods (e.g., griseofulvin). Depending on such timing factors plus the relationship and rationale of fast, intermediate, or slow drug release as well as other release considerations, a particular design and tablet formulation strategy is often indicated.

Many excellent review articles have been written on tablet technology, including various formulation aspects. Cooper [2] presented a review monograph on the contributions from 1964 to 1968 in the areas of tablet formulation, processing, quality standards, and biopharmaceutics. Later, Cooper and Rees [3] continued the review and included similar topics covering the period 1969 to 1971. Recent book chapters on tablets include those by Banker [4] and Sadik [5].

The present chapter will detail the general considerations of tablet product design; will describe a systematic approach to tablet design, including the practical use of preformulation data; will describe the commonly used tablet excipients with particular emphasis on their advantages and limitations or disadvantages; and will present some general tablet formulation approaches. Extensive references to the literature should provide the reader with directed reading on topics where additional information may be obtained. While it is impossible to exhaustively cover as broad a topic as tablet formulation and design in one chapter of a book, it is the goal of this chapter to cover the major concepts and approaches, including the most recent thought bearing on validation, optimization, and programmatic methods related to the formulation, design, and processing of compressed tablets.

II. PREFORMULATION STUDIES

The first step in any tablet design or formulation activity is careful consideration of the preformulation data. It is important that the formulator have a complete physicochemical profile of the active ingredients available, prior to initiating a formulation development activity. Compilation of this information is known as preformulation. It is usually the responsibility of the pharmaceutical chemistry research area to provide the data shown below on the drug substances.

1. *Stability (solid state)*: light, temperature, humidity
2. *Stability (solution)*: excipient-drug stability (differential thermal analysis or other accelerated methods)
3. *Physicomechanical properties*: particle size, bulk and tap density, crystalline form, compressibility, photomicrographs, melting point, taste, color, appearance, odor
4. Physicochemical properties: solubility and pH profile of solution/dispersion (water, other solvents)
5. *In vitro dissolution*: pure drug, pure drug pellet, dialysis of pure drug, absorbability, effect of excipients and surfactants

The basic purposes of the preformulation activity are to provide a rational basis for the formulation approaches, to maximize the chances of success in formulating an acceptable product, and to ultimately provide a basis for optimizing drug product quality and performance. From a tablet formulator's perspective, the most important preformulation information is the drug-excipient stability study. The question then, for a new drug, or a drug with which the formulator lacks experience, is to select excipient materials that will be both chemically and physically compatible with the drug.

The question is compounded by the fact that tablets are compacts; and while powder mixtures may be adequately stable, the closer physical contact of particles of potentially reactive materials may lead to instability. The typical preformulation profile of a new drug is usually of limited value to the formulator in assuring him or her that particular drug-excipient combinations will produce adequate stability in tablet form. An added problem is that the formulator would like to identify the most compatible excipient candidates within days of beginning work to develop a new drug into a tablet dosage form rather than to produce a series of compacts, place them on stability, and then wait weeks or months for this information.

Simon [6], in reporting on the development of preformulation systems, suggested an accelerated approach, utilizing thermal analysis, to identify possibly compatible or incompatible drug-excipient combinations. In his procedure, mixtures are made of the drug and respective excipient materials in a 1:1 ratio and subjected to differential thermal analysis. A 1:1 ratio is used, even though this is not the ratio anticipated for the final dosage form, in order to maximize the probability of detecting a physical or chemical reaction, should one occur. The analyses are made in visual cells, and physical observations accompany the thermal analysis. The thermograms obtained with the drug-excipient mixtures are compared to thermograms for the drug alone and the excipient alone. Changes in the termograms of the mixture, such as unexpected shifts, depressions, and additions to or losses from peaks are considered to be significant. Simon [6] has given an example of the type of information which may be obtained from such a study by the data shown in Figure 1. The thermal peak due to the drug alone was lost when the thermal analysis was run on the drug in combination with the commonly used lubricant, magnesium stearate. This was strong evidence for an interaction between these materials. It was subsequently confirmed by other elevated-temperature studies that the drug did decompose rapidly in the presence of magnesium stearate and other basic compounds. Simon has concluded the differential thermal analysis can aid immensely in the evaluation of new compounds and in their screening for compatibility with various solid dosage form excipients. The combination of visual and physical data resulting from differential thermal analysis of drugs with excipients is suggested as a programmatic approach to the very rapid screening of the drug-excipient combinations for compatibility.

Following receipt of the preformulation information, the formulator may prepare a general summary statement concerning the drug and its properties relative to tablet formulation. This statement must often also take into account general or special needs or concerns of the medical and marketing groups for that drug. A typical statement might be as follows.

Compound X is a white crystalline solid with a pyridine odor and bitter taste, which may require a protective coating (film or sugar). It displays excellent compressing properties and has not been observed to possess any

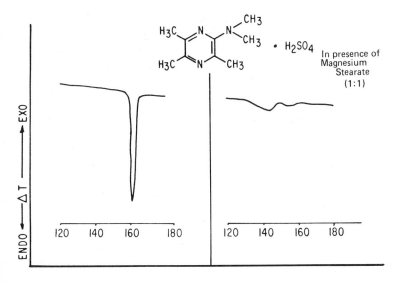

Figure 1   Thermograms showing the melting endotherm of triampyzine sulfate and loss of the endotherm in the presence of magnesium stearate.

polymorphs. It is nonhygroscopic, has low solubility in water, and in moderately volatile. It is an acidic moiety with a pK_a of 3.1 and a projected
dose of 50 to 100 mg. The compound is soluble in organic solvents and
aqueous media at pH 7.5. Below pH 5 it is sparingly soluble. In the dry
state it is physically and chemically stable. This product, while requiring
coating protection, must be designed for rapid drug dissolution release
(the drug is an acidic moiety, presumably best absorbed high in the gut).
No severe chemical stability problems are foreseen. The volatility of the
tableted form must be checked, and special packaging may be required.

III. A SYSTEMATIC AND MODERN APPROACH TO
TABLET PRODUCT DESIGN

Tablet product design requires two major activities. First, formulation activities begin by identifying the excipients most suited for a prototype formulation of the drug. Second, the levels of those excipients in the prototype
formula must be optimally selected to satisfy all process/product quality constraints.

A. Factors Affecting the Type of Excipient Used in a
Tablet Formula

The type of excipient used may vary depending on a number of preformulation, medical, marketing, economic, and process/product quality factors,
as discussed in the following sections.

Preformulation

Only those excipients found to be physically and chemically compatible with
the drug should be incorporated into a tablet formula. Preformulation

studies should also provide information on the flow and bonding properties
of the bulk drug. Excipients that tend to improve on flow (glidants) and
bond (binders) should be evaluated for use with poor-flowing and poor-
bonding compounds, respectively.

At the conclusion of a preformulation study, it may be known which
tableting process [direct-compression or granulation (wet/dry)] will be appropriate for the drug. If it is not known for certain which tableting
process is most appropriate after preformulation, then initial formulation
efforts should concentrate on a direct-compression method since it is most
advantageous. Direct compression is the preferred method of tablet manufacture for the following four major reasons: (a) It is the cheapest approach
since it is a basic two-step process (if components are of the proper particle size), involving only mixing and compressing, and it avoids the most
costly process of unit operating, drying. (b) It is the fastest, most direct
method of tablet production. (c) It has fewer steps in manufacture and
fewer formulation variables (in simple formulations). (d) It has the potential
to lead to the most bioavailable product (which may be critical if bioavailability is a problem).

Medical

The desired release profile for the tablet should be known early in tablet
development. Immediate, controlled, and combinations of immediate and
controlled release profiles require totally different approaches to formulation
development. Immediate release tablets usually require high levels of disintegrants or the use of superdisintegrants. Controlled release are usually
formulations of polymers or wax matrices.

In many instances, the rate-limiting factor to absorption of a drug is
dissolution. It may be necessary for the formulator to select excipients
which may increase drug dissolution and enhance absorption. Solvang
and Finholt [7] studied the effect of binder and the particle size of the
drug on the dissolution rate of several drugs in human gastric juice. Surface active agents such as sodium lauryl sulfate may be needed to promote
wetting of the drug. Alternatively, the use of disintegrants or superdisintegrants may improve dissolution. Hydrophobic lubricants may be used only
at low levels or not at all.

The targeting of drug delivery to various sites in the gastrointestinal
tract is sometimes required to maximize drug stability, safety, or efficacy.
This subject is discussed in detail in Section IV.A.2. Drugs that are acid-
labile or cause stomach irritation should not be released in the stomach.
The use of enteric coatings on tablets is the most common method of targeting the release of a drug in the small intestine. Tablets which are to be
coated should be formulated to withstand the rigors of a coating process
and to be compatible with the coating material. The use of alkaline excipients in the tablet may prove to weaken the integrity of the enteric coated
tablet.

Marketing

The appearance of a tablet dosage form is usually not thought to have a
large impact on the commercial success of a particular product. However,
all tablets must meet a minimal elegance criteria. The appearance of a
tablet can be evaluated by its color, texture, shape, size, and coating
(when present), and any embossing information.

Tablet appearance can be affected by the color and texture each excipient brings to a tablet formulation. Lactose, starch, and microcrystalline cellulose appear white to off-white when compressed. The inorganic diluents such as calcium sulfate, calcium phosphate, and talc produce more of a gray color in the tablet. Drugs will impact on the overall color and appearance of the tablet. Drug—excipient interactions may change the appearance of the tablet with time. The use of dyes may be required to improve the appearance of certain tablets. Relatively large amounts of stearates and high molecular weight polyethylene glycols produce glossy tablets.

The tableting properties (flow and compressibility) of tablet formulations containing a low percentage of active (<100 mg) are primarily dictated by the tableting properties of the excipients in the formulation. The formulator will frequently have numerous excipients to choose from because the drug does not dominate the behavior of the formulation during processing. However, if the tablet formula contains a large percentage of active, the formulator may be somewhat restricted in the choice of excipients. In order to be easily swallowed and remain elegant, tablet size and weight is limited in these formulations. Tablet formulas with a higher percentage of active can contain only minimal quantities of excipients. These excipients must therefore perform their functions at relatively low levels. The use of a more effective binder such as microcrystalline cellulose may be required to produce these tablets. Tablets with a high percentage of actives frequently require granulation methods of manufacture simply because excipients will not perform their desired function at low levels in a direct-compression method.

Marketing may request a coated tablet product. The quality of a coating on a tablet can be greatly affected by the tablet formulation onto which it is applied. Tablets with low resistance to abrasion (high friability) will result in coatings that appear rough and irregular. Coating adhesion can be greatly affected by the tablet excipients. Hydrophilic excipients can promote greater contact with the coating and result in superior adhesion. Hygroscopic excipients or drugs will cause swelling of a coated tablet and result in rupture of the film with time.

Embossing of compressed tablets is becoming increasingly popular. Embossing permits the tablet to have identifying information without requiring coating and printing operations. Embossing does exacerbate any picking or sticking problems usually observed during compression. This may necessitate higher levels of lubricants and glidant to alleviate these problems. Extreme care should be taken in designing tooling for embossed and scored tablets. It may take several design attempts to select a tooling design that will consistently produce acceptable embossed or scored tablets. Embossed tablets that are to be film-coated present additional coating problems such as bridging of the coat across a depression in a tablet.

Economics

One factor often overlooked in the development of a tablet formula is the cost of the raw materials and the process of manufacture. Direct compression is usually the most economical method of tablet production as previously discussed. In spite of the more expensive excipients used in direct compression, the cost (labor, energy, and time) of granulating is usually greater. Franz et al. [8] showed that a thorough analysis of cost versus time relationships can be performed using simulations before selecting a tableting process. Some companies have preferred manufacturing processes and raw materials. These general manufacturing processes and materials are considered the first choice when developing a new product. If it is demonstrated that the preferred manufacturing process or materials are not suitable for a new product, then alternative processes or materials are used. The use of preferred processes and materials helps keep the types of equipment needed to manufacture and materials in inventory at a minimum, thus reducing capital expenditures and material costs. Preferred manufacturing process and materials also makes it easier to automate a production facility for multiproduct use.

Process/Product Quality

Excipients should be selected that will enable the production of a tablet that will meet or exceed standard in-house quality tablet specifications. A formulator should be involved in the establishment of tablet specifications and be able to provide sound rationale for the critical specifications. Typical tests performed on tablets are as follows:

    Weight variation
    Hardness
    Friability
    Disintegration time
    Dissolution
    Water content
    Potency
    Content uniformity

Product quality is most often addressed at the tablet development stage. However, it is also important to monitor the processing quality of a formulation during development. Two reasons for monitoring processing quality during development are (a) to optimize the process as well as the product, and (b) to establish in-process quality control tests for routine production. It is more difficult to quantify the processing quality of a formulation than it is to meausre the product quality. Some measurements that could be performed on the process include

    Ejection force
    Capping
    Sticking
    Take-off force
    Flow of lubricated mixture
    Press speed (maximum)
    Frequency of weight control adjustments
    Sensitivity of formula to different presses
    Tooling wear
    Effect of consolidation load (batch size)
    Hopper angle for acceptable flow
    Hopper orifice diameter for acceptable flow
    Compressional forces
    Environmental conditions (temperature, humidity, and dust)

Each of the above processing parameters can become a source of trouble in scale-up or routine production. By monitoring these parameters in development, it may be possible to adjust the formula or process early enough to alleviate the source of trouble.

The expected production output (numbers of tablets) per unit time will determine what speed tablet press will be required for a particular tablet product. If the anticipated unit output for a tablet product is expected to be large, a high-speed press will be required. Attempts should be made in formulation development to design a tablet formula that will perform well on a high-speed press. A formula to run on a high-speed press should have excellent flow to maintain uniform die fill during compressing. It should have good bonding characteristics so that it can compress with a minimal dwell time.

B. Experimental Approach to Developing a Prototype Tablet Formula

After conducting an excipient compatibility study, a formulator may still have a wide choice of excipients available to use in the final tablet formula. The formulator must select a few excipients from a list of chemically compatible excipients. The formulator may later eliminate many drug-compatible excipients by selecting only those excipients known to provide a much needed function in the tablet formula as dictated by medical, marketing, economic, or process/product quality concerns. The objective in screening excipients for a prototype tablet formula is to choose a combination of excipients that most completely achieves desirable tableting characteristics. Tablets made at this stage of experimentation can be made on a Carver, single-punch, or rotary press depending on the amount of drug available. Obviously, no evaluation of the flow properties of a mixture can be made on a Carver or single-punch press. The following is a list of several experimental techniques that may be used to assist the formulator to develop a prototype formula.

> Analysis of variance (ANOVA)
> Statistical screening designs (first-order designs)
>> Plackett Burman
>> Extreme vertices

Analysis of Variance (ANOVA)

The ANOVA approach involves making statistical comparisons of different tablet formulas. Each formula represents a different combination of excipients. The selection of a prototype formula is done by running an ANOVA on the results of all the tests performed. The formula that is significantly better than the others tested becomes the prototype formula.

Statistical Screening Designs (First-Order Designs)

Plackett Burman Designs

A statistical screening involves setting lower and upper limits on the levels of each excipient considered for use in a tablet formula. Usually no more than 10 excipients are being considered for use in the tablet at this point. An experimental design is chosen that will enable a statistical test for the effect of each excipient on each process/product quality

Table 1   Twelve-Run Plackett-Burman Design

Trial	×1	×2	×3	×4	×5	×6	×7	×8	×9	×10	×11
1	+	+	−	+	+	+	−	−	−	+	−
2	+	−	+	+	+	−	−	−	+	−	+
3	−	+	+	+	−	−	−	+	−	+	+
4	+	+	+	−	−	−	+	−	+	+	−
5	+	+	−	−	−	+	−	+	+	−	+
6	+	−	−	−	+	−	+	+	−	+	+
7	−	−	−	+	−	+	+	−	+	+	+
8	−	−	+	−	+	+	−	+	+	+	−
9	−	+	−	+	+	−	+	+	+	−	−
10	+	−	+	+	−	+	+	+	−	−	−
11	−	+	+	−	+	+	+	−	−	−	+
12	−	−	−	−	−	−	−	−	−	−	−

characteristic (weight variation, hardness, friability, disintegration, dissolution, etc.).

This type of study requires at least n + 1 (n = number of excipients) trials to enable a statistical test. The type of statistical design employed in a screening study is referred to as a Plackett-Burman [9] design. Table 1 shows a 12-run Plackett–Burman design. Using this design, as many as 11 excipients could be screened for use in a tablet formula. Each column represents a different excipient. If seven excipients were to be screened, columns X1 to X7 would define the experimental design. Each row (tablet formula) in Table 1 represents combinations of high (+1) and low (−1) levels of each excipient (Xi) to be screened. The levels specified in each row are used to produce a tablet formula containing a fixed quantity of drug. Tablet formulas containing these mixtures of excipients are compressed and evaluated. A first-order regression model is fit to data collected during the tablet evaluation. Statistical tests can be performed to determine whether each excipient affected the tablet quality in a significantly positive or negative manner. Excipients that did not provide a significant "positive" effect on tablet quality may be either retested in a second screening study at different levels of eliminated from durtehr consideration for inclusion into the tablet formula. A second statistical screen may be performed on excipients to refine excipient ranges to more appropriate levels. Once acceptable excipients and excipient ranges have been established, formulation optimization can proceed.

Extreme Vertices

The extreme vertices design [10] is usually used as an optimization technique. However, it can be used as a screening study if at least n + 1 trials are run. The extreme vertices design is recommended when the number of components (excipients) is six or more. A first-order model is fit to the data to test for significant excipients as was done in the Plackett-Burman design. The disadvantage of using the extreme vertices design in tablet development is that tablet weight must be kept constant throughout the screening process.

C. Experimental Approach to Optimizing a Prototype Tablet Formula

A tablet formulation optimization study should be performed using an appropriately statistically designed experiment. Numerous experimental design texts [11,12] are available that can assist a formulator in selecting the appropriate experimental design. The extreme vertices design is not recommended in most tablet optimization studies unless tablet weight is to be held constant. It can be beneficial to have a statistician experienced in experimental designs select an appropriate design based on the established excipients and excipient ranges. All excipients should be varied in the optimization study to truly optimize the formulation. Excipients levels are usually the only factors or variables in a formulation optimization study. To reduce the number of factors in a study, a ratio of two excipients can be used. However, the total quantity of those two excipients must be fixed in the formula. When using excipient ratios as factors, include a factor for tablet weight. Tablet weight can then be varied as a factor. If a formulator suspects an interaction between an excipient and a particular process variable, the process variable should be considered for inclusion in the formulation optimization study. For example, in a sustained release direct-compression tablet, compression force may impact on the release rate of the drug from the tablet. In this example, compression force should be included as a factor in a formulation optimization study. Usually, all other process variables are maintained constant. Process variables that cannot be held constant but are *not* expected to impact on the tablet characteristics should be "blocked" appropriately in the design. For instance, different lots of raw materials or bulk drug may be used in an optimization study. The different lots should be treated as blocks in the experimental design. This will allow for a statistical test for block (lot) effect at the data analysis stage of the experiment. In this example, blocks serve as a flag to signal the formulator that the quality of the raw materials is not well controlled. Since the use of blocks do not "cost" the formulator any additional trials, blocks should be used wherever possible. Statisticians experienced in experimental design frequently state that you cannot lose by blocking!

It is important that all trails are performed in a randomized manner. After all the tablets have been manufactured, data analysis begins. A standard quadratic model is most often used to fit second-order experimental design data. Commercially available software (XSTAT, STATGRAPHICS, PCSAS, ECHIP) may be used to generate the coefficients and statistical tests on the raw data collected. This software will also provide a statistical analysis of the regression models produced. The analysis of the regression model provides the scientist information on how well the model explained the data variation. If a particular regression model does not satisfactorily explain the data variation, transformations of the raw data can be tried to improve the fit of the model. For a regression model to be acceptable, the $R_2 > 0.75$ the lack of fit should not be significant, and the residuals should have no more than a few outliers. Once acceptable models have been established for each tablet characteristic, the scientist should examine the models to determine which main effects, interactions, or quadratic terms are significant. The formulator should then generate response surface plots of significant interactions as a function of the tablet characteristic. Response surface plots of significant main effects and quadratic terms will also help the formulator to understand the critical relationships between tablet characteristics and the formulation factors.

Optimization of the final formulation can be performed using commercially available software (XSTAT, ECHIP, and PCSAS). Optimization invariably requires that constraints be placed on some or all of the critical response parameters. Constraints may also be placed on some or all of the factors as well. One critical tablet characteristic must be selected to optimize (minimize or maximize) while the other tablet characteristics and formulation factors are left constrained or unconstrained. For example, tablet friability could be constrained below 0.3% while dissolution rate is maximized. The mathematical algorithm used in specific optimization routines (software) varies. Optimization algorithms used in software routines are usually based on a simple method or a grid search method. The final formula determined to be optimal should be experimentally verified by manufacture and testing. Model predicted values for tablet characteristics should "agree" with actual experimental data collected on the optimal formula.

D. Establishment of Excipient and Preliminary Process Ranges

In light of the present interest in validating the product as well as the process of manufacture, it is to the formulator's advantage to establish excipient and process variable ranges. Having excipient and process ranges also allows production to make appropriate excipient or process changes without prior notification of the regulatory agencies.

If it can be demonstrated that the excipient ranges used for conducting the optimization study produced acceptable tablets (i.e., all tablets produced were acceptable, then the excipient ranges used in the study should be used as final product ranges. However, if the excipient ranges used in the optimization study were not always acceptable, the ranges should be narrowed to acceptable limits. This can be done by performing constrained optimization of the critical response variables using registration specifications on the response variables as the constraining limits.

E. Bioavailability Studies

In vivo test procedures appropriate for tablets and other solid dosage forms are also the subject of Chapter 6 in Volume II of this series. In some cases in vivo testing of tablet formulations involves studies in animals prior to studies in humans: in other cases the tablet formulations are studied directly in humans.

When in vivo studies in humans are undertaken, it may be desirable or even essential to conduct such studies with more than one formulation. This is particularly true if a goal of product design is product optimization, and a primary objective is to maximize bioavailability or response versus time profile. A bioavailability study should eventually be run comparing

the optimized formulation, a formulation (within the excipient ranges) predicted to have the slowest dissolution, and a formulation (within the excipient ranges) predicted to have the fastest dissolution. The bioavailability
study results can be used to establish a correlation between the in vitro
dissolution test and the in vivo bioavailability parameters. If the three
formulations (optimal, slow, and fast-dissolving) turn out to be bioequivalent, the excipient ranges are valid from the in vivo performance viewpoint.
If the three formulations are not bioequivalent, then the excipient ranges
should be tightened using the in vitro/in vivo correlation. The specifications for the dissolution of the tablet should be set based on this correlation.

F. Development of Stability Data for Tablet Formulations

Stability data should be collected on the bulk drug as well as the final
product stability. Stability on the bulk drug should be available in the
preformulation data. Based on the results of the bulk drug stability testing, recommendations should be made about the storage conditions and the
shelf life of the bulk drug.

The final tablet formulation should be placed up on stability as soon
as possible after its invention. Also, formulas that "cover" the proposed
excipient ranges may also be placed up on stability. Stability data should
be generated with the tablet in all the expected packaging configurations
(i.e., blisters, plastic and glass bottles, etc.). Ideally several lots of tablets should be put on stability using different lots of bulk drug. Having different lots of tablets containing different lots of bulk drug will give an indication of the lot-to-lot variability in product stability. Accelerated stability
testing (high temperature, humidity, or intense lighting) can be helpful in
judging the long-term stability of a tablet package system.

In addition to the stability data generated on the final formula, stability
data generated on *similar* formulations can sometimes be used as supportive
stability data. Usually there will be more supportive stability data available because the similar formulations were developed prior to the optimal
formula.

Based on the product stability data, a formulator must recommend
proper storage conditions, special labeling regarding storage, and an expiration date for each tablet package system.

G. Development of Validation Data for Tablet Formulations

As required under an NDA, process validation is the final step undertaken
after the process has been scaled up to full production batch size. Under
the concept of validation, an immense work load is placed on the pharmacy
development group, the pilot plant group, and possibly the production department to achieve the goals of validation as previously defined. Because
of the immense work load, some companies have created a group dedicated
to assist formulators in validating their manufacturing processes. As a
rule of thumb, the less complex the manufacturing process, the better defined the drug and excipient specifications, the easier the validation process.
The need to validate tablet products provides a great impetus to the use of
optimization techniques in tablet product design. The data base required
for product validation will often be adequate when development has

proceeded using optimization techniques. The validation of a new or re-
formulated tablet product requires two phases. In phase I the development
team formulates the product and general process of manufacture. In phase
II, emphasis is placed on the process validation of production scale batches.
Phase II is usually accomplished at the production startup of a new or re-
formulated product.

The objectives in phase I include:

1. Producing an optimal formula and process.
2. Identifying the most critical tablet characteristics and establishing
   specifications for the tablet.
3. Quantifying relationships between the critical tablet characteristics
   and process/formulation variables.
4. Establishing specifications for process/formulation variables to ensure that tablet specifications will be met.
5. Proposing in-process tests for critical process variables and raw
   materials specifications for critical formulation variables when appropriate.
6. Documenting above information.

The objectives in phase II include

1. Demonstrating that all manufacturing equipment and related systems (SOPs, equipment calibration, cleaning procedures, assays,
   packaging, and personnel training) have been qualified for use in
   the manufacture and testing of this product.
2. Drafting a process validation protocol before manufacture of first
   production lots that specifies the procedures to be validated. This
   protocol should be written to challenge the proposed limits on the
   critical process/formulation variables.
3. Running production/validation lots; collecting and analyzing data.
4. Demonstrating that all product specifications have been met in spite
   of the challenges presented to the process.
5. Documenting above information.

Usually several production lots are required to complete phase II validation. The more process/formulation variables, the more production lots
will have to used. If the production scale validation lots pass all the required specifications for that tablet product, the lots may be used for commercial sale.

IV. TABLET COMPONENTS AND ADDITIVES

A. Active Ingredients

General Considerations

Broadly speaking, two classes of drugs are administered orally in tablet
dosage form. These are (1) insoluble drugs intended to exert a local effect
in the gastrointestinal tract (such as antacids and absorbents) and (2)
soluble drugs intended to exert a systemic drug effect following their dissolution in the gut and subsequent absorption. With each class of drugs
very careful attention must be given to product formulation and design as
well as to manufacturing methods in order to produce an efficacious and

reliable product. The goal in designing tablet dosage forms for these two classes of drugs is different. When working with insoluble drugs whose action is usually strongly affected by surface phenomena (such as antacids and absorbents) it is critical that a product be designed that will readily redisperse the produce a fine particle size and large surface area. Accordingly the effect of formulation, granulation, and tableting on the surface properties of the material and the ability to regenerate a material in the gut with optimum surface properties are critical.

In the case of drug products intended to exert a systemic effect, the design of a dosage form which rapidly disintegrates and dissolves may or may not be critical, depending on whether the drug is absorbed in the upper gastrointestinal tract or more generally throughout the intestinal tract, and also based on the solubility properties of the drug at or above its absorption site. Dosage forms must, however, be designed which do disintegrate or dissolve to release the drug in an available form at or above the region of absorption in the gut.

The developmental pharmacist usually does not have a great deal of input into selecting the chemical form of an active ingredient. Drug-screening programs may not offer several salt or ester forms of the drug as candidates for a particular therapeutic claim. Instead the formulator, provided with small quantities of an active ingredient in a particular form to evaluate in the preformulation studies, is faced with the task of developing a tablet— which may be capable of handling only drugs of the same physical and chemical properties as the small sample. When large batches become available, often months later, they frequently differ in physical properties, making formulation and processing modification necessary. Given the opportunity, the preformulation scientist may suggest a particular salt or crystal form of the drug that is more stable, more suitable for tableting, or more bioavailable. As an example, ethanol-recrystallized (ethyl) ibuprofen is the form of drug initially developed to produce ibuprofen tablets. The ethyl drug is poorly compressible and usually must be tableted using wet granulation processing. Tablets made with the ethyl drug have a tendency to pick, stick, and laminate during compression. Methanol-recrystallized "methyl' ibuprofen [10] was subsequently developed. Methyl drug was capable of being tableted in a direct-compression formulation with no picking, sticking, or lamination problems. The difference between the crystal habits of the two drugs resulted in dramatically different tableting properties.

It is imperative that the physical properties of the active ingredient be thoroughly understood prior to the time of finalizing the formula. Indeed, these properties may provide a rational basis for a particular tablet design, such as rapid dissolution for a drug likely to be absorbed high in the upper gut, or the need for enteric or other forms of gastric protection for an acid-labile drug.

Although almost all tablets will require the addition of nonactive components or excipients—to produce satisfactory drug release, to achieve acceptable physical and mechanical properties, and to facilitate their manufacture—the formulator should not be anxious to begin adding excipients until the properties of the drug are thoroughly understood. If a substance possesses the proper crystalline structure, it can be compressed directly into a tablet without further treatment. Relatively few such materials (active or excipient) exist, and their number diminishes further if one considers only materials with therapeutic activity. Jaffe and Foss [13] confirmed that generally drugs of cubic crystalline structure are compressible directly, since upon compression the crystals are fractured, and the fragments form a close-packed arrangement which readily consolidates on compression. In a cube, the structure is the same along each axis; thus, no alignment is necessary in order for ionic or van der Waals bonding to occur between the individual particles. Sodium choride has a cubic structure and is an example of a directly compressible material.

In crystals which are not cubic, some realignment is necessary, which results in a reduced probability of bonding. Employing potassium chloride as a model, Lazarus and Lachman [14] found that the compaction of these crystals depended on many factors, such as particle size distribution, crystal shape, bulk density, and moisture content. If the drug to be formulated happens to possess a crystalline structure allowing for direct compaction, the formulator's task will be lessened. Rankell and Higuchi [15] have presented a theoretical discussion on the physical process which may be responsible for interparticulate bonding during compression. While the tableting aspects will be straightforward, the other requirements, such as acceptable friability, hardness, appearance, disintegration, and dissolution, must be met.

It is extremely rare to find a drug system which does not involve the use of excipients. The contribution of excipients will be discussed in Section IV.B. The treatment of processing which the active ingredient receives (alone or in combination with the excipients) will depend upon the dosage level, the physical and chemical properties of the active drug substance and the excipients used, the nature of the drug, its use, any absorption or bioavailability problems, and the granulation and tableting method employed. When potent drugs of limited solubility are involved, their particle size and uniform distribution throughout the tablet can dramatically affect the rapidity of their dissolution and absorption as well as content uniformity. However, if large dosage regimens of a soluble drug are considered, the effect of particle size is important—more from a processing standpoint than because of dissolution or absorption considerations. The relationship of various particle size factors to therapeutic effectiveness of drugs was discussed by Rieckmann [16]. He pointed out that one must be cautious in equating micronization, dissolution, and adsorption, especially with drugs such as nitrofurantoin, chloramphenicol, and spironolactone.

The role of the active ingredient can then be considered in two broad systems: first, when the drug—excipient interactions are considered primarily from a pharmacological (dissolution and absorption) viewpoint; and second, where in addition to the concerns in the first area, significant processing questions must be answered.

Bioavailability Considerations

Before drugs can effectively pass through the gastrointestinal wall they must be in solution. Drugs which are only sparingly soluble in the gastrointestinal contents at or above the absorption site can have, as the controlling process affecting their absorption, the rate of drug solution in these fluids. In this type of system, the drug goes into solution at a slow rate; absorption occurs almost immediately and is not, therefore, the rate-limiting step. In one study, Nelson [17] correlated the blood level concentration of various theophylline salts with their dissolution rates.

As noted earlier in this chapter and throughout this volume, drugs which exert a systemic effect must dissolve as a prerequisite to effective drug absorption. The various processes of tablet making, including the aggregation of drug into granular particles, the use of binders, and the compaction of the system into a dense compact, are all factors which miti- gate against a rapid drug dissolution and absorption in the gastrointestinal tract. In considering in a general manner the availability of drugs from various classes of dosage forms, drugs administered in solution will usually produce the most available drug product—assuming the drug does not pre- cipitate in the stomach or is not deactivated there.

The second most available form of a therapeutic agent would be drug dispersed in a fine suspension, followed by micronized drug in capsule form, followed by uncoated tablets, with coated tablets being the least bio- available drug product in general. In formulating and designing drug products as well as in considering methods of manufacture, the fact that the tablet dosage form is one of the least bioavailable forms (all other fac- tors being equal) should be kept in mind.

Many factors can affect drug dissolution rates from tablets, hence possibly drug bioavailability—including the crystal size of the drug; tablet disintegration mechanisms and rates; the method of granulation; type and amount of granulating agent employed; type, amount, and method of incorp- oration of disintegrants and lubricants; and other formulation and process- ing factors.

Levy et al. [18] showed the effects of granule size on the dissolution rate of salicylic acid. Salicylic acid of two mesh ranges, containing 300 mg of aspirin and 60 mg of starch, were compressed at 715 kg cm^{-2}. The data are shown in Figure 2.

Lachman et al. [19] studied the effect of crystal size and granule size on a delayed action matrix using tripelennamine hydrochloride. He noted that while granule and crystal size both affected release rate, in this in- stance the crystal size played a greater role than granule size in dissolu- tion rate.

Paul et al. [20] showed that with nitrofurantoin there was an optimal average crystal size of about 150 mesh, which resulted in adequate drug excretion (hence absorption and efficacy) but minimized emesis. This ex- emplifies a situation in which too rapid drug dissolution in the stomach may produce nausea and emesis; an intermediate release rate reduces this effect while achieving adequate bioavailability.

Numerous accounts of the effect of particle size on the dissolution rate of steroids have been reported. In one study Campagna et al. [21] showed that, in spite of good disintegration, therapeutic inefficacy of prednisone tablets could occur.

B. Nonactive Ingredients

The selection and testing of nonactive ingredients or excipients in tablet formulas present to the formulator the challenge of predictive foresight. While the ability to solve problems when they occur is a valuable attribute, the ability to prevent the problem through adequate experimental design is a virtue, leads to more reliable and expeditious product development, and, when coupled with optimization methods, enables the formulator to tell how close a particular formula is to optimum conditions.

It will become obvious to the formulator, on reviewing the literature, that the total number of significant excipients currently in use is probably less than 25. These 25 materials fulfill the needs of the six major excipient

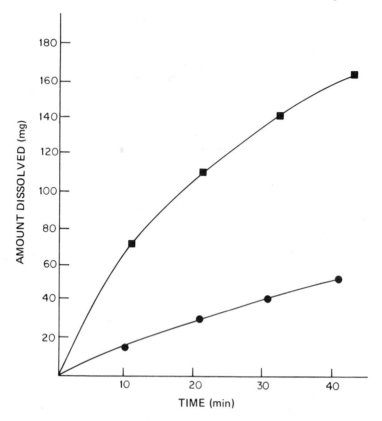

Figure 2 Effect of granule size on the dissolution rate of salicylic acid contained in compressed tablets. Key: ● 40- to 60-mesh granules; ■ 60- to 80-mesh granules.

categories: diluents, binders, lubricants, disintegrants, colors, and sweeteners (flavors excluded). The *United States Pharmacopeia* (USP XIX) recognized the important role excipients play in dosage form design by initiating a new section entitled "Pharmaceutic Ingredients." In time, official monographs may be developed for all the major or commonly used excipients. In 1974 the Swiss pharmaceutical companies, Ciba-Geigy, Hoffman-LaRoche, and Sandoz, joined together to publish in the German language an *excipient catalog (Katalog Pharmazeutischer Hilfsstoffe)*, covering almost 100 official and nonofficial excipients. The book contains general information, suppliers, tests, and specifications obtained from the literature or measured in the laboratories of the above companies. The development of an excipient codex was a major project of the Academy of Pharmaceutical Sciences of the American Pharmaceutical Association [22].

It will become apparent later in this section that many times the 25 or so excipients have been repeatedly evaluated over the past 50 years, and yet these same materials continue to stand the test of time. Rather than belabor the point we must simply be reminded that the tried and tested materials, by their longevity, deserve careful consideration. The formulator should not, however, be fearful of change or of evaluating new ingredients. Some formulators tend to "lock-in" on particular formulation types of approaches which have been successful in the past; the danger here is that one becomes dated. At the other extreme is the formulator who takes a quick look at a new disintegrant or binder, which then ends up in the formula months before sufficient data are available to make possible a sound judgment of total acceptability. Thus the best formulator is an individual who is constantly searching for new and better methods and systems, who avoids becoming sterotyped, and who is cautious and thoroughly analyzes new approaches without developing an undue proprietary or vested interest in them.

Additives are usually classified according to some primary function they perform in the tablet. Many additives will also often have secondary functions, which may or may not be of a beneficial nature in good, solid design of oral dosage forms. Some fillers or diluents may facilitate tablet dissolution, which is beneficial, while others may impair dissolution. The most effective lubricants are water repellent by their nature, which may retard both disintegration and dissolution.

Bavitz and Schwartz [23] concluded, in a paper evaluating common tablet diluents, that their proper choice becomes more critical when formulating water-insoluble drugs as opposed to water-soluble drugs. They showed that "inert ingredients" can profoundly affect the properties of the final dosage form. A knowledge of the properties of additives and how they affect the properties of the total formulation is necessary to provide guidelines in their selection. This is particularly true when the drug concentration is small. The drug plays a more significant role in determining the physical characteristics of the tablet as the drug concentration increases.

Two major classifications of additives by function include those which affect the compressional characteristics of the tablet:

Diluents
Binders and adhesives
Lubricants, antiadherents, and glidants

and those which affect the biopharmaceutics, chemical and physical stability, and marketing considerations of the tablet:

Disintegrants
Colors
Flavors and sweeteners
Miscellaneous components (e.g., buffers and adsorbents)

Diluents

Although diluents are normally thought of as inert ingredients, they can significantly affect the biopharmaceutic, chemical, and physical properties of the final tablet. The classic example of calcium salts interfering with the absorption of tetracycline from the gastrointestinal tract was presented by Bolger and Gavin [24]. The interaction of amine bases or salts with lactose in the presence of alkaline lubricants, and subsequent discoloration (as discussed by Costello and Mattocks [25] and Duvall et al. [26]), emphasized that excipient "inertness" may often not exist in the design of drug dosage form.

Keller [27] reviewed the properties of various excipients while Kornblum [28,29] proposed preformulation methods of screening materials for use as

diluents. Simon [6] described rapid thermal analytical methods of screening
for possible drug—excipient interactions. In another study Ehrhardt and
Sucker [30] discussed rapid methods to identify a number of excipients
used in tablet formulations.

Usually tablets are designed so that the smallest tablet size which can
be conveniently compressed is formed. Thus, where small dosage level
drugs are involved, a high level of diluent or filler is necessary. If, however, the dosage level is large, little or no diluent will be required, and
the addition of other excipients may need to be kept to a minimum to avoid
producing a tablet that is larger than is acceptable. In such large drug
dosage situations, nevertheless, excipient materials must often be added
to produce a granulation or direct-compression mixture which may be compressed into acceptable tablets.

Where moisture is a problem affecting drug stability, the initial moisture
level, as well as the tendency of the material to retain or pick up moisture,
must be considered. The hygroscopic nature of excipients, as described
by Daoust and Lynch [31], is an important consideration in formulation
studies for the following reasons:

1. Water sorption or desorption by drugs and excipients is not always
    reversible. Absorbed moisture may not be easily removed during
    drying.
2. Moisture can affect the way in which a system accepts aqueous
    granulating solutions.
3. The moisture content and rate of moisture uptake are functions of
    temperature and humidity and should be considered.
4. Moisture content in a granulation affects the tableting characteris-
    tics of the granulation.
5. Hygroscopicity data can aid in the design of tablet-manufacturing
    areas.
6. Moisture-sensitive drugs should not be combined with hygroscopic
    excipients.
7. Packaging materials should be chosen to suit the product.

Sangekar et al. [32] reported on the percent moisture uptake of tablets
prepared from various direct compression excipients. Figure 3 indicates
that a range of 1.7 to 5.6% uptake is possible, depending on the excipient
used. Dicalcium phosphate, lactose anhydrous DTG, and lactose beadlets
absorbed the minimum amount of moisture, while sorbitol and sucrose absorbed the maximum. Mannitol, dextrose, and monocalcium phosphate were
shown to be intermediate.

In selecting diluents, the materials will be found to contain two types
of moisture, bound and unbound. The manner in which a diluent holds its
moisture may be more important than the affinity of the material for moisture or the amount of moisture present. Calcium sulfate dihydrate, for
example, contains 12% moisture on a mole-for-mole basis. The water is
present, however, as bound moisture (as water of crystallization). Furthermore the tightly bound water is not liberated until a temperature of about
80°C is reached (well above normal product exposure temperatures). Since
calcium sulfate dihydrate is thermodynamically satisfied as to water content
and moisture demand, it is not hygroscopic and absorbs little moisture.
Since the bound water is generally unavailable for chemical reaction,
$CaSO_4 \cdot 2H_2O$ has been widely used in vitamin tablets and other systems

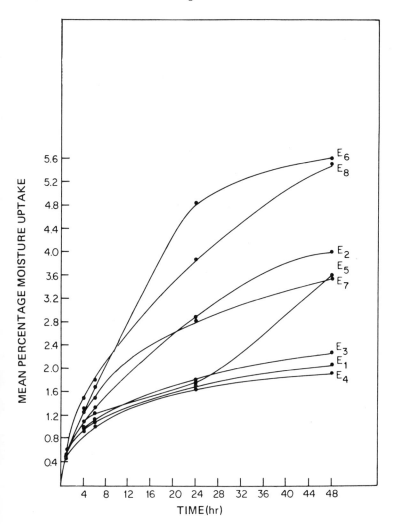

Figure 3   Direct-compression tablets with different excipients (E_1 to E_8), common binder (microcrystalline cellulose), and common disintegrant (alginic acid).   Mean percent moisture uptake across humidity levels of 43, 65, 75, and 100% relative humidity at 25°C.   Key: E_1, dibasic calcium phosphate dihydrate (unmilled); E_2, monobasic calcium phosphate monohydrate; E_3, lactose anhydrous DTG; E_4, lactose hydrous beadlets; E_5, mannitol granular; E_6, sorbitol crystalline, tablet type; E_7, dextrose; E_8, sucrose.

which are moisture-sensitive. Such a system, containing tightly bound water but with a low remaining moisture demand, may be vastly superior to an anhydrous diluent (or other excipient) which has a high moisture demand. When using a hydrate or excipient containing water of crystallization or other bound water, careful attention must be paid to the conditions under which this water is released.

The degree of cohesiveness which a diluent imparts to various drug substances when compacted into tablets becomes increasingly important when tablet size is a factor. Where size is not a factor, the ratio of the cohesiveness imparted by a diluent to its cost per kilogram should be considered. For example, if size is not a factor, a diluent that costs $3.08 per kilogram and is effective at a 10% concentration might be replaced by a diluent that must be present at a 25% concentration, that costs $0.66 per kilogram. Kanig [33] reviewed the ideal properties of a direct compaction diluent material, many of which hold true of any diluent.

In special tablets, such as chewable tablets, taste and mouth-feel become paramount in diluent selection. In these specialized tablets a consideration of unique aging effects, such as increased hardness and reduced "chewability," must be carefully examined.

The sensitivity of diluents to physicochemical changes caused by processing or manufacturing, both of which influence final tablet quality, should be considered in diluent selection. This is illustrated in Figures 4 and 5 [34] by a comparative evaluation of excipients for direct-compression formulas. These figures indicate the variety of disintegration and hardness

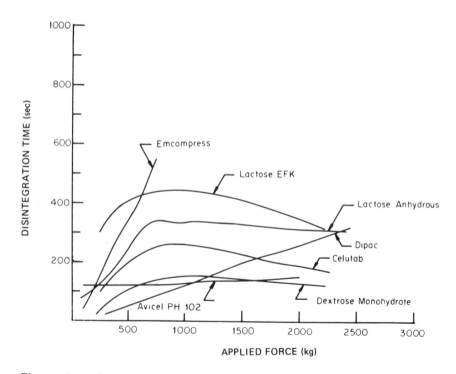

Figure 4   Disintegration time versus applied force for compacts of various materials.

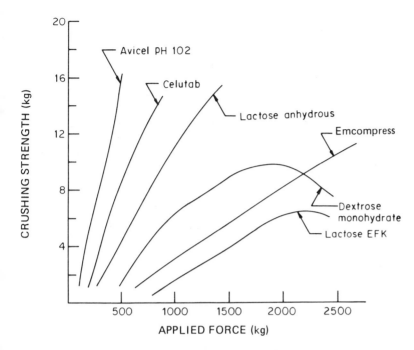

Figure 5 Crushing strength versus applied force for compacts of various materials.

profiles possible. Combinations of two or more excipients generally provide a final disintegration-hardness spectrum which lies between the values for each material when used separately. The figures also show the sensitivity of various agents to alterations in properties (disintegration time and crushing strength) with changes in compressive load. Emcompress, for example, was very sensitive to a change in compressive load in this study whereas Celutab and dextrose monohydrate are almost totally insensitive. Ideally, the diluent selected will not be sensitive to processing variables, such that the quality of the final tablet features can degrade appreciably under the processing variables encountered in production. This is an important consideration in the validation of a product and its method of manufacturing: identifying the range of product quality features produced by the expected limits of the processing variables encountered in production, and designing product formulation and processes so as to minimize such variability.

Lactose USP is the most widely used diluent in tablet formulation. It displays good stability in combination with most drugs whether used in the hydrous or the anhydrous form. Hydrous lactose contains approximately 5% water of crystallization. The hydrous form is commonly used in systems that are granulated and dried. Several suppliers offer various grades of hydrous and anhydrous lactose. The various grades have been produced by different crystallization and drying processes. It is most important not to assume that one form of lactose will perform in a similar manner as another form. Lactose is available in a wide range of particle size distributions. Nyqvist and Nicklasson [35] studied the flow properties of directly compressible lactose in the presence of drugs. While lactose is freely (but slowly) soluble in water, the particle size of the lactose employed can affect the release rate of the medicinal. Recent studies indicate the $T_{50\%}$ (time required for 50% of the drug to dissolve) was decreased by a factor of 8 when micronized lactose (2 to 5 mg^2 g^{-1}) was used rather than unmicronized lactose (0.5 m^2 g^{-1} surface area).

Lactose formulations usually show good drug release rates, are easy to dry (both in thrays and fluidized bed dryers), and are not sensitive to moderate variation in tablet hardness upon compression. They find exceptional application in tablets employing small levels of active ingredients (e.g., steroids). The cost of lactose is low relative to many other diluents. As noted previously, lactose may discolor in the presence of amine drug bases or salts and alkaline lubricants.

Lactose USP, anhydrous offers most of the advantages of lactose USP, hydrous, without the reactivity of the Maillard reaction, which leads to browning. Tablets generally show fast disintegration, good friability, and low weight variation, with an absence of sticking, binding, and capping. The applications of the anhydrous form have recently been evaluated by a number of investigators [36–39]. Mendell [40] has reported on the relative sensitivity of lactose to moisture pickup at elevated humidities. Blister packages should be tested at elevated temperatures and humidity to establish their acceptability with lactose-based formulas.

Lactose USP, spray-dried has improved flow and bond properties over the regular lactose due to the general spherical form of the aggiomerates. This shape can be affected by high-shear milling. The effect of particle diameter on particle and powder density, and angle of friction and repose, and the effect of orifice diameter on the flow rate have been studied by Alpar et al. [41] and Mendell [40]. Even when granulated, spray-dried lactose displays its flow and bond properties. It is commonly combined with microcrystalline cellulose and used as a direct-compaction vehicle. Alone, it usually must be used at a minimum concentration of 40 to 50% of the tablet weight for its direct-compaction properties to be of value. It has the capacity of holding 20 to 25% of active ingredients. Care must be exercised upon storage since loss of the usual 3% moisture content can adversely affect compressional properties.

Brownley and Lachman [42] reported that, as with lactose USP, care must be taken in using spray-dried lactose since it tends to become brown due to the presence of 5-(hydroxymethyl)-2-furaldehyde, when combined with moisture, amines, phosphates, lactates, and acetates. Similar findings were reported by Duvall et al. [26] even in systems not containing amines. The employment of neutral or acid lubricants such as stearic acid appears to retard the discoloration, while alkaline lubricants (e.g., magnesium stearate) accelerate the darkening. Bases as well as drugs which release radicals (e.g., amino salts) can bring about this browning, known as the Maillard reaction. Richman [43] reviewed the lubrication of spray-dried lactose in direct-compaction formulas and reported that this lactose form may affect the mechanism of action of lubricants.

The cost of spray-dried lactose is moderate; however, the fact that it is not available from a large number of suppliers could limit its widespread use. Tablets made with spray-dried lactose generally show better physical stability (hardness and friability) than regular lactose, but tend to darken more rapidly.

It was reported by Henderson and Bruno [39] that the tableting characteristics of spray-dried lactose were inferior to those of lactose beadlets. However, the physical stability of the resulting products was similar.

Starch USP may come from corn, wheat, or potatoes and finds application as a diluent, binder, and disintegrant. Tablets containing high concentrations of starch are often soft and may be difficult to dry, especially when a fluidized bed dryer is used. Commercially available starch USP may vary in moisture content between 11 and 14%. Certain specially dried types of starch are available at moisture levels of 2 to 4% at a premium price. Where the starch is used in a wet (aqueous) granulated system, the use of specially dried starch is wasteful since normal drying techniques will result in a moisture level of 6 to 8%. Recent studies indicate that, in some drug systems, starch—initially at a moisture level of 10% or greater—may perform differently with respect to dissolution than starch at a 5 to 7% level, even though the final equilibrium moisture levels of the tablet are the same.

There are also indications that, although starch reaches a moisture plateau of 11 to 14%, it often serves as a local desiccant to help stabilize moisture-sensitive drugs. This attribute can act in a negative fashion, however, as in steroid tablets, where the localization of moisture may result in reduced dissolution rates.

In a study on the effect of granule size, compression force, and starch concentration on the dissolution rate of salicylic acid, Levy [44] showed an increase in dissolution rate with decreasing granule size, increasing pre-compression force, and increasing starch content.

The effect of starch on the disintegration time of tolbutamide tablets was studied by Commons et al. [45]. They showed a critical starch concentration for different granule sizes of tolbutamide; however, disintegration times did not decrease with increasing starch levels.

Schwartz et al. [46] evaluated the incorporation of starch USP versus a modified cornstarch in various formulations. The modified starch generally exhibited improved processing characteristics and improved tablet properties, compared to starch USP.

Directly compressible starch, marketed commercially as Starch 1500, is physically cornstarch. Chemically, compressible starch does not differ from starch USP. It is a free-flowing, directly compressible excipient, which may be used as a diluent, binder, and disintegrating agent. When compressed alone, it is self-lubricating and self-disintegrating, but when combined with as little as 5 to 10% of an ingredient that is not self-lubricating, it requires additional lubricant and usually a glidant, such as colloidal silicone dioxide, at 0.25%.

Starch 1500 contains about 10% moisture and is susceptible to softening when combined with excessive amounts (greater than 0.5%) of magnesium stearate. Direct compaction starches have been reported [47] to not affect the stability of aspirin where moisture may be a concern. Most of the formulas evaluated also contained microcrystalline cellulose.

Underwood and Cadwallader [48] studied the effect of various starches on the dissolution rate of salicylic acid from tablets. They showed that the dissolution of the drug was most rapid from tablets containing a compressible starch (Fig. 6).

Mannitol USP finds increasing application in the formulation of chewable tablets where mouth-feel and palatability are important considerations. Its mouth-feel is related to its negative heat of solution and its slow solubility, which is experienced by the user as a cool sensation during dissolution of the sugar. It has been reported to be about 72% as sweet as sucrose. One gram dissolves in 5.5 ml of water. Chewable vitamins and antacids are the primary application for this material, although certain regular chewable

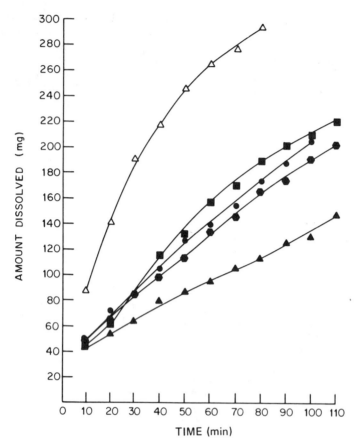

Figure 6 Dissolution rates of salicylic acid from tablets containing various starches, using the USP-NF method type 1 (basket, 100 rpm) at 37°C. Key: ● cornstarch; ■ potato starch; ▲ rice starch; ⬢ arrowroot starch; △ compressible starch.

tablets intended for swallowing do incorporate mannitol because of its non-hygroscopicity.

Mannitol formulations, because of their poor flow properties, usually require higher lubricant levels (3 to 6 times as great) and higher glidant levels for satisfactory compression than other diluents. Kanig [49] has reported on studies to overcome these shortcomings by spray-congealing fused mannitol alone with sucrose or lactose. A wide range of tablet hardness can be obtained with mannitol-based tablets. Staniforth et al. [50] crystallized mannitol to produce an excipient with an optimal particle size and surface coarseness for a direct-compression excipient. Mannitol is a relatively expensive diluent, and attempts are usually made to reduce its quantity per tablet. A granular form of mannitol is now available as a direct-compression excipient. Mannitol has been shown to be chemically compatible with moisture-sensitive compounds. It picks up less than 1.0% moisture at relative humidities as high as 90%.

Sorbitol is an optical isomer of *mannitol* but differs dramatically from it in that sorbitol is hygroscopic at humidities above 65% and is more water-soluble than mannitol. It may be combined with an equal weight of dicalcium phosphate to form a direct compaction carrier. Mannitol and sorbitol are noncariogenic sugars and are of low nutritional and caloric content.

Microcrystalline cellulose N.F., often referred to as Avicel, has found wide application in the formulation of direct-compaction products. Tablets prepared from the more widely used tablet grades PH 101 (powder) and 102 (granular) show good hardness and friability. The flow properties of microcrystalline cellulose have been described by Mendell [40] as poor, by Fox et al. [51] as good, and by Livingstone [52] as very good, once again indicating that each additive must be evaluated in the formulator's own system.

Numerous other investigators [53–58] have reviewed the applications of microcrystalline cellulose in tablet formulations. The capillarity of Avicel explains the penetration of water into a tablet, thereby destroying the cohesive bonds between particles. The hardness of the compressed tablet can significantly affect the disintegration time by breaking down the structure of the intermolecular spaces and destroying the capillary properties.

Avicel is a relatively expensive diluent when compared with lactose USP or starch USP. Usually it is not used in tablets alone as the primary diluent unless the formulation has a specific need for the bonding properties of Avicel. It is capable of holding in excess of 50% active ingredients and has certain unique advantages in direct compression which may more than offset its higher cost. As a diluent, Avicel offers many interesting possibilities to control drug release rates when combined with lactose, starch, and dibasic calcium phosphate. Bavitz and Schwartz [23,37] have reported on various combinations for use with water-soluble and water-insoluble drugs. Avicel possesses the ability to function both as a binder and disintegrant in some tablet formulas, which may make it very useful in tablets which require improvement in cohesive strength, but which cannot tolerate lengthened disintegration times.

Tablets containing high Avicel levels may be senstive to exposure to elevated humidities and may tend to soften when so exposed.

Dibasic calcium phosphate dihydrate NF, unmilled, is commonly used as a tablet diluent. A commercially available free-flowing form is marketed as Emcompress and has been described for use in tablet making by Mendell [40]. It is used primarily as a diluent and binder in direct-compaction formulas where the active ingredient occupies less than 40 to 50% of the final tablet weight. Emcompress is composed of 40- to 200-mesh material, is nonhygroscopic, and contains about 0.5% moisture. In direct-compaction formulas, 0.5 to 0.75% magnesium stearate is required as a lubricant. It shows no apparent hygroscopicity with increasing relative humidities (40 to 80%).

Bavitz and Schwartz [23] showed the negative effect on dissolution of increasing the ratio of dibasic calcium phosphate to microcrystalline cellulose in a system containing an "insoluble" drug, indomethacin USP (Fig. 7). Formula IV (50:50) released 66% of the drug in 30 min. The amount released decreased to 18% and 10% in 30 min as the ratio of dibasic calcium phosphate to microcrystalline cellulose increased to 70:30 (formula V) and 84:16 (formula VI), respectively. The study highlights the importance of carriers when insoluble drugs are employed.

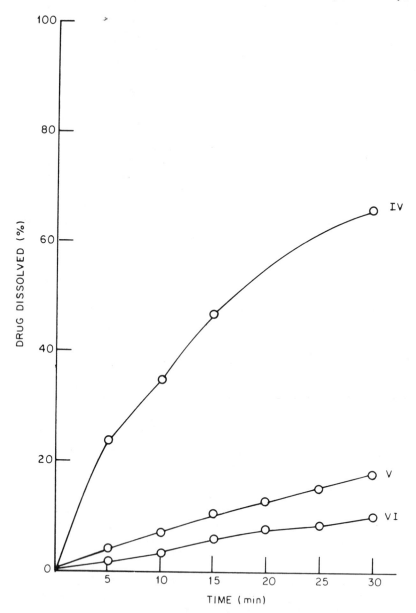

Figure 7   Drug release of an insoluble drug from direct-compression diluents diluents (see text).   IV = microcrystalline cellulose N.F./dibasic calcium phosphate N.F., 50:50.   V = microcrystalline cellulose N.F./dibasic calcium phosphate N.F., 30:70.   VI = microcrystalline cellulose N.F./dibasic calcium phosphate N.F., 16:84.

Khan and Rhodes [59] reviewed the disintegration properties of dibasic calcium phosphate dihydrate tablets employing insoluble and soluble disintegrating agents. The insoluble disintegrants showed a greater effect when compressional forces were varied than did the soluble disintegrants.

The use of a medium coarse dicalcium phosphate dihydrate has been reported [60, 61]. It has interesting applications in vitamin-mineral formulations as both a direct-compaction vehicle and as a source of calcium and phosphorus.

Sucrose-based tablet diluent-binders are available under a number of trade names which include Sugartab (90 to 93% sucrose plus 7 to 10% invert sugar), Di-Pac (97% sucrose plus 3% modified dextrins), NuTab (95% sucrose, 4% invert sugar, and 0.1 to 0.2% each of cornstarch and magnesium stearate).

All of the above sucrose-based diluent-binders find application in direct compaction tablet formulas for chewable as well as conventional tablets. All three demonstrate good palatability and mouth-feel when used in chewable tablets and can minimize or negate the need for artificial sweeteners. Due to their high sucrose level, they may exhibit a tendency to undergo moisture uptake. The initial moisture content is usually less than 1% on an "as-received" basis.

NuTab is available to two grades, medium (40 to 60 mesh) and coarse (20 to 40 mesh), in white only. Mendes et al. [62] reported on the use of NuTab as a chewable direct compression carrier for a variety of products. The medium grade of NuTab, in moisture uptake studies, initially took on moisture more rapidly than the coarse; however, both reached the same equilibrium uptake of 3.3 to 3.5% after 2 weeks at 80% relative humidity.

Di-Pac is available in one grade (40 to 100 mesh), the white and six colors, while Sugartab comes in one grade (20 to 80 mesh), the white only.

Tablets made with these sucrose-based diluents at high levels do not disintegrate in the classical sense but rather dissolve.

Confectioner's sugar N.F. may serve as a diluent in both chewable and nonchewable tablets, but does require granulation to impart bonding if present at significant levels. Powdered sugar is not pure sucrose; it contains starch.

Calcium sulfate dihydrate N.F. has been suggested as a diluent for granulated tablet systems where up to 20 to 30% of active ingredients are added to a stock calcium sulfate granulation. It is inexpensive, and has been reported to show good stability with many drugs. The recent lack of availability of an N.F. grade of material makes its choice as a diluent questionable. Two N.F. grades are marketed in the United States.

Bavitz and Schwartz [23] showed the effect on dissolution rate of a calcium sulfate and microcrystalline cellulose based vehicle (product no. 2834-125) when used with a water-soluble versus a water-insoluble drug. The water-soluble drugs showed a rapid release pattern while the water-insoluble drug was released slowly (Fig. 8).

Calcium lactate trihydrate granular N.F. has been used as diluent and binder in direct-compaction formulas with reasonable success. Its long-term availability should be reviewed before extensive studies are undertaken.

Emdex and Celutab are hydrolyzed starches containing 90 to 92% dextrose, 3 to 5% maltose, and the remainder higher glucose saccharides. They are free-flowing powders composed of spray-crystallized maltose-dextrose spheres. Hydrolyzed starches are often used as mannitol substitutes in chewable tablets because of their sweet taste and smooth

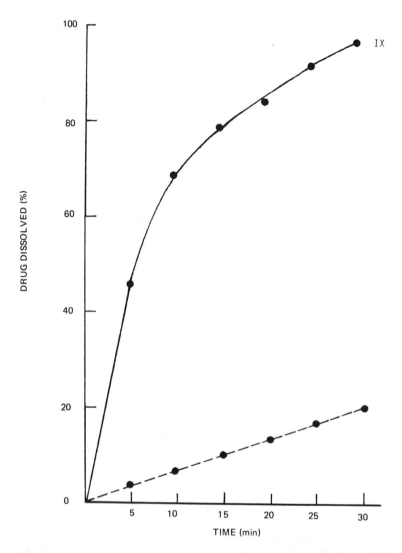

Figure 8   Release of a soluble (——, amitriptyline hydrochloride USP) compared to an insoluble (– – –, hydrochlorothiazide USP) drug from direct
compression diluents (see text).

mouth-feel. They show good stability with most drugs, but may react with drugs having active primary amino groups, when stored at high temperature and humidity. Tablets compressed using Emdex show an increase in hardness from 2 to 10 kg during the first few hours after compression. These materials contain 8.5 to 10.5% moisture, which must be considered when combining them with hydrolytically unstable drugs.

Dextrose, commercially available as *Cerelose*, can be used as filler, carrier, and extender where a sweet material is desired, as in chewable tablets. It is available as a hydrate (Cerelose 2001) and in an anhydrous form (Cerelose 2401) where low moisture is needed. It can be used to partly replace spray-dried lactose in direct-compaction formulas. It requires higher lubricant levels than spray-dried lactose and has been shown to have a lesser tendency to turn brown than spray-dried lactose. A comparison of dextrose and spray-dried lactose has been presented by Duvall et al. [26].

Inositol has been used as a replacement diluent for chewable tablets employing mannitol, lactose, and a sucrose-lactose mixture.

Hydrolyzed cereal solids such as the *Maltrons* and *Mor-Rex* have been suggested as lactose replacements. Except for economic considerations, their advantages are limited.

Amylose, a derivative of glucose, possesses interesting direct-compaction properties and has been described for use in tablets [63]. Since amylose contains 10 to 12% water, its use with drugs subject to hydrolytic decomposition should be avoided.

A list of *miscellaneous tablet diluents* would be extensive. Some additional materials used include *Rexcel* (food-grade natural source of α- and amorphous cellulose); *Elcema* (microfine cellulose, principally an α-cellulose) available in powder, fibrous, and granular forms; calcium carbonate; glycine; bentonite; and polyvinylpyrrolidone.

Binders and Adhesives

Binders or adhesives are added to tablet formulations to add cohesiveness to powders, thereby providing the necessary bonding to form granules, which under compaction form a cohesive mass or compact referred to as a tablet. The location of the binder within the granule can affect the quality of the granulation produced [64]. Granule strength is maximized when granulations are prepared by roller compaction followed by wet massing and spray drying [65]. The formation of granules aids in the conversion of powders of widely varying particle sizes to granules, which may more uniformly flow from the hopper to the feed system, and uniformly fill the die cavity.

Granules also tend to entrap less air than powders used in a direct-compression formulation. Table 2 summarizes some common granulating systems.

The primary criterion when choosing a binder is its compatibility with the other tablet components. Secondarily, it must impart sufficient cohesion to the powders to allow for normal processing (sizing, lubrication, compression, and packaging), yet allow the tablet to disintegrate and the drug to dissolve upon ingestion, releasing the active ingredients for absorption. Binder strength as a function of moisture has been reported by Healey et al. [66].

In a study [67] of a comparision of common tablet binder ingredients, the materials compressed were, in descending order of adhesive strength:

Table 2   Examples of Typical Granulating Systems

Material	System normally used (% of granulating)	Concentration used (% of formula)
Acacia	10—25	2—5
Cellulose derivatives	5—10	1—5
Gelatin	10—20	1—5
Gelatin-acacia	10—20	2—5
Glucose	25—50	2—25
Polymethacrylates	5—15	5—20
Polyvinylpyrrolidone	3—15	2—5
Starch paste	5—10	1—5
Sucrose	50—75	2—25
Sorbitol	10—25	2—10
Pregelatinized starch	2—5	1—10
Tragacanth	3—10	1—4
Sodium alginate	3—5	2—5

glucose, acacia, gelatin, simple syrup, and starch. Although starch has the least adhesive strength of the materials in the list, it also has the least deleterious effect on general tablet disintegration rates of the materials listed. Different binders can significantly affect the drying rate and required drying time of a granulation mass, and the equilibrium moisture level of the granulation.

Acacia, a natural gum, has been used for many years as a granulating solution for tablets. In solutions ranging from 10 to 25%, it forms tablets of moderate hardness. The availability of acacia has been uncertain over the past few years, and it should be avoided for that reason in new formulations. In addition to shortages, contamination by extraneous material and bacteria makes its use questionable.

Tragacanth, like acacia, is a natural gum which presents similar problems to those of acacia. Mucilage is difficult to prepare and use. Thus, adding it dry and activating it through the addition of water works best. Such wet granulation masses should be quickly dried to reduce the opportunity for microbial proliferation.

Sucrose, used as a syrup in concentration between 50 and 75%, demonstrates good bonding properties. Tablets prepared using syrup alone as a binder are moderately strong, but may be brittle and hard. The quantity of syrup used and its rate of addition must be carefully followed, especially in systems where overwetting occurs quickly.

Gelatin is a good binder. It forms tablets as hard as acacia or tragacanth, but is easier to prepare and handle. Solutions of gelatin must be used warm to prevent gelling. Alcoholic solutions of gelatin have been used but without great success. Jacob and Plein [68] and Sakr et al. [69]

have shown that increasing the gelatin content of tablets causes increases in their hardness, disintegration, and dissolution times.

Glucose as a 50% solution can be used in many of the same applications as sucrose.

Starch as a paste forms tablets which are generally soft and brittle. It requires heat to facilitate manufacture. Depending on the amount of heat employed, starch undergoes hydrolysis to dextrin and then to glucose. Thus, care in preparation of starch paste is necessary to produce a correct and consistent ratio of starch and its hydrolysis products, as well as to prevent charring.

Cellulose materials such as methylcellulose and sodium carboxymethylcellulose (CMC) form tough tablets of moderate hardness. They may be used as viscous solutions or added dry and activated with water, which results in less effective granule formation. They are available in a wide variety of molecular weights which affect the viscosity of the solution as well as their swelling properties.

Miscellaneous water-soluble or dispersible binders include alginic acid and salts of alginic acid, magnesium aluminum silicate, Tylose, polyethylene glycol, guar gum, polysaccharide acids, bentonites, and others.

Combinations of the previously discussed binding agents often impart the desirable properties of each. Some typical combinations include:

Gelatin + acacia
Starch paste + sucrose (as a syrup)
Starch + sucrose (as a syrup) + sorbitol
Starch + sorbitol

Some binders are soluble in nonaqueous systems, which may offer advantages with moisture-sensitive drugs. Most nonaqueous vehicle binders have as their main disadvantages the possible need for explosion-proof drying facilities and solvent recovery systems. A number of oven explosions have occurred in the pharmaceutical industry—related to the use of alcohol in wet granulation. Some manufacturers have used the approach of partially air-drying such granulations and then employing high air flow rates in their dryers to stay below the explosive limit of alcohol in air. While this approach may work for many years without incident, if a power failure occurs at the wrong time, alcohol vapor can build to the explosive limit, triggering an explosion when the power is turned back on. Great care should be taken in drying any granulation employing flammable solvents or in designing an oven system for such use.

Polyvinylpyrrolidone (PVP) is an alcohol-soluble material which is used in concentrations between 3 and 15%. Granulations using a PVP—alcohol system process (granulate) well, dry rapidly, and compress extremely well. PVP finds particular application in multivitamin chewable formulations where moisture sensitivity can be a problem.

Polymethacrylates (Eugragit NE30D, RS30D) can be used as binders in wet granulations. It is supplied as a 30% aqueous dispersion. Dilution with water prior to use is recommended.

Hydroxypropylmethylcellulose (HPMC) and hydroxypropylcellulose (Klucel) are soluble in various organic solvents or cosolvent systems, as well as water. L-HPC is a low molecular weight, crosslinked form of Klucel. It functions not only as a tablet binder but also a tablet disintegrant. Unlike Klucel, it is not soluble in water. It has tremendous swelling capability

which accounts for its disintegration property. L-HPC may be used in both
direct-compression as well as wet granulation tablet formulas. Various
grades of L-HPC may be used depending on whether the tablet is to be
wet-granulated or directly compressed.

Ethylcellulose (Ethocel) is used as alcohol solutions of 0.5 to 2.0% and
affords moisture-sensitive components a protective coating. Vitamin A and
D mixtures, which are usually sensitive to moisture, may be coated with
ethylcellulose solution, dried, and granulated with conventional aqueous
systems. Ethylcellulose may have a serious retardant effect on tablet disintegration and drug dissolution release.

Pregelatinized starch (National 1551 and Starch 1500) can be blended
dry with the various components of a tablet formula and activated with
water at the desired time of granulation. In a direct-compression formulation, no more than 0.5% magnesium stearate should be used to prevent
softening of the tablets.

Disintegrants

The purpose of a disintegrant is to facilitate the breakup of a tablet after
admisinistration. Disintegrating agents may be added prior to granulation
or during the lubrication step prior to compression or at both processing
steps. The effectiveness of many disintegrants is affected by their position within the tablet. Six basic categories of disintegrants have been described: starches, clays, celluloses, algins, gums, and miscellaneous. It
should be noted that many disintegrants have also been shown to possess
binder or adhesive properties. Since disintegration is the opposite operation to granulation (agglomeration) and the subsequent formation of strong
compacts, one must carefully weigh these two phenomena when designing
a tablet. Khan and Rhodes [70] reviewed the water sorption properties of
four tablet disintegrants: starch, sodium CMC, sodium starch glycolate,
and a cation exchange resin. The different disintegration properties were
related to the differing mechanisms by which the disintegrants affect tablet
rupture. Intergranular and extragranular disintegrating agents were reviewed by Shotton and Leonard [71]. The extragranular formulations disintegrated more rapidly than the intragranular ones, but the latter resulted
in a much finer dispersion of particles. A combination of the two types of
agents was suggested. Since the most effective lubricants are hydrophobic,
water-repellent, and function by granule coating, it is not surprising that
such materials may impede tablet wetting, disintegration, and dissolution.
To overcome this problem, disintegrants such as starch are often combined
with the lubricant to provide extragranular disintegration and to facilitate
tablet wetting. Such combinations of lubricant and disintegrant which are
added to tablet granulations prior to compression are termed *running
powders.*

Starches are the most common disintegrating agents (Table 3) in use
today. Ingram and Lowenthal [72] have attributed their activity as disintegrants to intermolecular hydrogen bonding which is formed during compression and is suddenly released in the presence of excess moisture. In
a later study, Lowenthal [73] evaluated the effects of pressure on starch
granules and showed that they do not regain their original shape when
moistened with water.

Lowenthal and Wood [74] showed that the rupture of the surface of a
tablet employing starch as a disintegrant occurred where starch agglomerates
were found. The conditions best suited for rapid tablet disintegration are

Table 3   Starch Disintegrants

Material	Usual range (%)
Natural starch (corn, potato)	1–20
Sodium starch glycollate (Primogel, Explotab)	1–20 (4% optimum)
Pregelatinized starch (National 1551)	5–10
Pregelatinized starch (Amijel)	5–10
Modified cornstarch (Starch 1500)	3–8

a sufficient number of starch agglomerates, low compressive pressure, and the presence of water.

Starches show a great affinity for water through capillary action, resulting in the expansion and subsequent disintegration of the compressed tablet. Formerly accepted swelling theories of the mechanism of action of starches as disintegrants have been generally discounted. In general, higher levels of starch result in more rapid disintegration times. However, high starch levels often result in a loss of bonding, cohesion, and hardness in tablets. It has been suggested [45] that an optimum starch level exists for many drugs such as tolutamide.

It is important to dry starch at 80 to 90°C to remove absorbed water. Equally important is starch storage while awaiting use, since starches will quickly equilibrate to 11 to 13% moisture by picking up atmospheric moisture.

Sodium starch glycolate modified starches with dramatic disintegrating properties are available as Primogel and Explotab, which are low-substituted carboxymethyl starches. While natural predried starches swell in water to the extent of 10 to 25%, these modified starches increase in volume by 200 to 300% in water. One benefit of using this modified starch is that disintegration time may be independent of compression force. However, high-temperature and humidity conditions can increase disintegration time, slowing dissolution of tablets containing this starch.

Clays such as Veegum HV (magnesium aluminum silicate) have been used as disintegrants at levels ranging from 2 to 10%. The use of clays in white tablets is limited because of the tendency for the tablets to be slightly discolored. In general clays, like the gums, offer few advantages over the other more common, often more effective, and no more expensive disintegrants such as the starches (including derivatives), celluloses, and alginates.

Celluloses, such as purified cellulose, methylcellulose, sodium carboxymethylcellulose, and carboxymethylcellulose, have been evaluated as disintegrants but have not found widespread acceptance. A crosslinked form of sodium carboxymethylcellulose (Ac-Di-Sol) has been well accepted as a tablet disintegrant. Unlike sodium carboxymethylcellulose, Ac-Di-Sol is essentially water-insoluble. It has a high affinity for water which results in rapid tablet disintegration. Ac-Di-Sol has been classifed as a "super-disintegrant."

Microcrystalline cellulose (Avicel) exhibits very good disintegrant properties when present at a level as low as 10%. It functions by allowing water

water to enter the tablet matrix by means of capillary pores, which breaks the hydrogen bonding between adjacent bundles of cellulose microcrystals. Excessively high levels of microcrystalline cellulose can result in tablets which have a tendency to stick to the tongue, due to the rapid capillary absorption, dehydrating the moist surface and causing adhesion.

Alginates are hydrophilic colloidal substances extracted from certain species of kelp. Chemically they are available as alginic acid or salts of alginic acid (with the sodium salt being the most common). They demonstrate a great affinity for water, which may even exceed that of cornstarch. Alginic acid is commonly used at levels of 1 to 5% while sodium alginate is used between 2.5 and 10%. Unlike starch, microcrystalline cellulose, and alginic acid, sodium alginates do not retard flow.*

National 1551 and Starch 1500 are *pregelatinized corn starches* with cold water swelling properties. They swell rapidly in water and display good disintegrant properties when added dry at the lubrication step. When incorporated into the wet granulation process, pregelatinized starch loses some of its disintegrating power.

Gums have been used as disintegrants because of their tendency to swell in water. Similar to the pregelatinized starches in function, they can display good binding characteristics (1 to 10% of tablet weight) when wet. This property can oppose the desired property of assisting disintegration, and the amount of gum must be carefully titrated to determine the optimum level for the tablet. Common gums used as disintegrants include agar, guar, locust bean, Karaya, pectin, and tragacanth. Available as natural and synthetic gums, this category has not found wide acceptance because of its inherent binding capabilities.

Miscellaneous disintegrants include surfactants, natural sponge, resins, effervescent mixtures, and hydrous aluminum silicate. Kornblum and Stoopak [75] evaluated cross-linked PVP (Povidone-XL) as a tablet disintegrant in comparison with starch USP and alginic acid. The new material demonstrated superiority over the other two disintegrants tested in most of the experimental tablet formulations made as direct compaction or wet granulation systems. Povidone-XL also falls under the classification of superdisintegrant.

Lubricants, Antiadherents, and Glidants

The primary function of tablet lubricants is to reduce the friction arising at the interface of tablet and die wall during compression and ejection. The lubricants may also possess antiadherent or glidant properties. Strickland [76] has described:

Lubricants: Reduce friction between the granulation and die wall during compression and ejection

Antiadherents: Prevent sticking to the punch and, to a lesser extent, the die wall

Glidants: Improve flow characteristics of the granulation

---

*A wide variety of grades are available from the Algin Corporation of America.

Lubricants

Lubrication is considered to occur by two mechanisms. The first is termed fluid (or hydrodynamic) lubrication because the two moving surfaces are viewed as being separated by a finite and continuous layer of fluid lubricant. A hydrocarbon such as mineral oil, although a poor lubricant, is an example of a fluid-type lubricant. Hydrocarbon oils do not readily lend themselves to application to tablet granulations and, unless atomized or applied as a fine dispersion, will produce tablets with oil spots. The second mechanism, that of boundary lubrication, results from the adherence of the polar portions of molecules with long carbon chains to the metal surfaces of the die wall. Magnesium stearate is an example of a boundary lubricant. Boundary-type lubricants are better than fluid-type lubricants since the adherence of a boundary lubricant to the die wall is greater than that of the fluid type. This is expected since the polar end of the boundary lubricant should adhere more tenaciously to the oxide metal surface than the nonpolar fluid type.

The type and level of lubricant used in a tablet formulation is greatly affected by the tooling used to compress the tablets. Mohn [77] reviewed the design and manufacture of tablet tooling. Proper inspection of tablet tooling is critical to ensure that tooling continues to perform up to expectations. Capping of tablet is more often formulation-related; however, it can be caused by improper tooling. Compressing tablets at pressures greater than what the tooling was designed to handle can result in damage to punch heads. The use of cryogenic material treatments can increase tooling life. Vemuri [78] discussed the selection of the proper tooling for high speed tablet presses.

Recommendations have been made to standardize tablet-tooling specifications by the IPT Section of the Academy of Pharmaceutical Sciences [79].

Mechtersheimer and Sucker [80] determined that die wall pressure is considerably greater when curve-faced punches are used to compress tablets instead of fat-faced punches. Additional lubricant is often needed in tablet formulations that are to be compressed with curved-face punches.

Lubricants tend to equalize the pressure distribution in a compressed tablet and also increase the density of the particle bed prior to compression. When lubricants are added to a granulation, they form a coat around the individual particles (granules) which remains more or less intact during compression. This coating effect may also extend to the tablet surface. Since the best lubricants are hydrophobic, the presence of the lubricant coating may cause an increase in the disintegration time and a decrease in the drug dissolution rate. Since the strength of a tablet depends on the area of contact between the particles, the presence of a lubricant may also interfere with the particle-to-particle bond and result in a less cohesive and mechanically weaker tablet. Matsuda et al. [81] reviewed the effect on hardness and ejection force of two methods of applying the lubricant (stearic acid, magnesium stearate, calcium stearate, and talc) to statically compressed tablets prepared from a lactose granulation. In one method of addition the lubricant was incorporated into the granulation during preparation, while in the other it was added to (mixed with) the final granules. The mixing method gave better results for ease of ejection and tablet hardness than the incorporation method.

As the particle size of the granulation decreases, formulas generally require a greater percent of lubricant. Danish and Parrott [82] examined the effect of concentration and particle size of various lubricants on the flow rate of granules. For each lubricant there was an optimum concentration, not exceeding 1%, which produced a maximum flow rate. For a constant concentration of lubricant, the flow rate increased to a maximum rate as the size of the lubricant particles was decreased to 0.0213 cm. A further reduction hindered the flow rate. Usually as the concentration of lubricant increases, the disintegration time increases and the dissolution rate decreases, as the ability of water to penetrate the tablet is reduced.

The primary function of a lubricant is to reduce the friction between the die wall and the tablet edge as the tablet is being ejected. Lack of adequate lubrication produces *binding*, which results in tablet machine strain and can lead to damage of lower punch heads, the lower cam track, and even the die seats and the tooling itself. Such binding on ejection is usually due to a lack of lubrication. Such tablets will have vertically scratched edges, will lack smoothness or gloss, and are often fractured at the top edges. With excessive binding the tablets may be cracked and fragmented by ejection. Ejection force can be monitored as an indicator of adhesion problems during compressing studies [83]. A film forms on the die wall, and ejection of the tablet is difficult.

Sticking is indicated by tablet faces which are dull. Earlier stages of sticking are often referred to as *filming* of the punch faces and may result when punches are improperly cleaned or polished or when tablets are compressed in a high humidity, as well as when lubrication is inadequate. Advanced states of sticking are called *picking*, which occurs when portions of the tablet faces are lifted or picked out and adhere to the punch face. Picking usually results from improperly dried granulations, from punches with incorrectly designed logos, and from inadequate glidant use, especially when oily or sticky ingredients are compressed.

Capping and *laminating*, while normally associated with poor bonding, may also occur in systems which are overlubricated with a lubricant such as a stearate. Attempts have been made to measure the tendency of a powder to cap and stick when compressed based on theoretical calculations [83]. Rue et al. [84] correlated acoustic emissions during tableting of acetaminophen with lamination and capping events. Acoustic emission analysis demonstrated that capping occurs within the die wall during the decompression phase and not during ejection. Capping or lamination observed with curve-face punches can often be eliminated by switching to flat-faced punches.

Lubricants may be further classified according to their water solubility (a (as water-soluble or water-insoluble). The choice of a lubricant may depend in part on the mode of administration and the type of tablet being produced, the disintegration and dissolution properties desired, the lubrication and flow problems and requirements of the formulation, various physical properties of the granulation or powder system being compressed, drug compatibility considerations, and cost.

Water-insoluble lubricants in general are more effective than water-soluble lubricants and are used at a lower concentration level. Table 4 summarizes some typical insoluble lubricants and their usual use levels.

In general lubricants, whether water-soluble or insoluble, should be 200 mesh or finer and are passed (bolted) through a 100-mesh screen (nylon cloth) before addition to the granulation. Since lubricants function by coating (as noted), their effectiveness is related to their surface area

Table 4   Water-Insoluble Lubricants

Material	Usual range (%)
Stearates (magnesium, calcium, sodium)	1/4−2
Stearic acid	1/4−2
Sterotex	1/4−2
Talc	1−5
Waxes	1−5
Stearowet	1−5

and the extent of particle size reduction. The specific lubricant, its surface area, the time (point) and procedure of addition, and the length of mixing can dramatically affect its effectiveness as a lubricant and the disintegration-dissolution characteristics of the final tablet.

Glyceryl behapate (Compritol 888) is a new addition to the list of tablet lubricants. It has the unique classification of being both a lubricant and a binder. Therefore, it should alleviate both sticking and capping problems. When used with magnesium stearate in a tablet formula, its level should be reduced. The stability of aspirin has been extensively studied in conjunction with various lubricants. In combination with talc, the rate of decomposition has been related to the calcium content and loss on ignition of the talc source. Alkaline materials such as alkaline stearate lubricants may be expected to have a deleterious effect on the stability of aspirin-containing products. For those formulations that are not sufficiently lubricated with stearates, the addition of talc may be beneficial. Mechtersheimer and Sucker [80] also found that talc should be added prior to the lubrication step to optimize the tableting properties. When added together, talc and magnesium stearate provided acceptable lubrication. Magnesium lauryl sulfate has been compared to magnesium stearate as a tablet lubricant [83]. Higher levels of magnesium lauryl sulfate were required to provide an equivalent lubricantion as measured by tablet ejection force. However, harder and more compressible blends can be prepared with magnesium lauryl sulfate than with magnesium stearate at the same ejection force.

Boron-coated tablet tooling has permitted the use of a lower lubricant level in some tablet formulations [85].

Water-soluble lubricants are in general used only when a tablet must be completely water-soluble (e.g., effervescent tablets) or when unique disintegration or, more commonly, dissolution characteristics are desired. Possible choices of water-soluble lubricants are shown in Table 5. Boric acid is a questionable member of the list due to the recognized toxicity of boron. A review of some newer water-soluble lubricants combined with talc and calcium stearate has been reported [86]. Polyethylene glycols and 20 low melting point surfactants have been suggested as water-soluble lubricants [87].

Table 5   Water-Soluble Lubricants

Material	Usual range (%)
Boric acid	1
Sodium benzoate + sodium acetate	1—5
Sodium chloride	5
DL-Leucine	1—5
Carbowax 4000	1—5
Carbowax 6000	1—5
Sodium oleate	5
Sodium benzoate	5
Sodium acetate	5
Sodium lauryl sulfate	1—5
Magnesium lauryl sulfate	1—2

Methods of Addition.   Lubricants are generally added dry at a point where the other components are in a homogeneous state. Thus, the lubricant is added and mixed for a period of only 2 to 5 minutes rather than the 10 to 30 minutes necessary for thorough mixing of a granulation. Overmixing may lead to diminished disintegration-dissolution characteristics and loss of bonding in the tablet matrix.

Lubricants have also been added to granulations as alcoholic solutions (e.g., Carbowaxes) and as suspensions and emulsions of the lubricant material. In one study [88] various lubricants were added, without significant loss of lubricating properties, to the initial powder mixture prior to wet granulation. However, as a rule, powdered lubricants should not be added prior to wet granulation since they will then be distributed throughout the granulation particles rather than concentrated on the granule surface where they operate. In addition, powder lubricants added in this manner will reduce granulating agent and binder efficiency.

Antiadherents

Antiadherents are useful in formulas which have a tendency to pick easily. Multivitamin products containing high vitamin E levels often display extensive picking, which can be minimized through the use of a colloidal silica such as Syloid. Studies have indicated that Cab-O-Sil, although similar chemically, does not perform satisfactorily, probably because of its lesser surface area.

Talc, magnesium stearate, and cornstarch display excellent punch-face or antiadherent properties. An extremely efficient yet water-soluble punch-face lubricant is DL-leucine. The use of silicone oil as an antiadherent has been suggested [89]. Table 6 summarizes the more common antiadherents.

Table 6 Antiadherents

Material	Usual range (%)
Talc	1–5
Cornstarch	3–10
Cab-O-Sil	0.1–0.5
Syloid	0.1–0.5
DL-Leucine	3–10
Sodium lauryl sulfate	<1
Metallic stearates	<1

Glidants

In general materials that are good glidants are poor lubricants. Table 7
lists a few of the common glidants. Glidants can improve the flow of granulations from hoppers into feed mechanisms and ultimately into the die cavity.
Glidants can minimize the degree of surging and "starvation" often exhibited
by direct-compaction formulas. They act to minimize the tendency of a granulation to separate or segregate due to excessive vibration. High-speed tablet presses require a smooth, even flow of material to the die cavities. When
flow properties are extremely poor, and glidants are ineffective, consideration
of forced-feed mechanisms may be necessary. The uniformity of tablet weights
directly depends on how uniformly the die cavity is filled.

Tablet Formulation and Design

A review by Augsburger and Shangraw [90] of a series of silica-type
glidants used decreased weight variation as a criterion of evaluation. The
use of starch as a glidant has been widely practiced in tablet and capsule
formulation. In general many materials commonly referred to as lubricants
possess only a minimal lubricating activity, and are better glidants or

Table 7 Glidants

Material	Usual range (%)
Talc	5
Cornstarch	5–10
Cab-O-Sil	0.1–0.5
Syloid	0.1–0.5
Aerosil	1–3

antiadherents. Thus, a blend of two or more materials may be necessary to obtain the three properties.

York [91] presented data indicating the relative efficiency of glidants for two powder systems and reported that the order of effectiveness was

Fine silica > magnesium stearate > purified talc

The mechanisms of action of glidants have been hypothesized by various investigators and include:

1. Dispersion of electrostatic charges on the surface of granulations [92, 93]
2. Distribution of glidant in the granulation [94]
3. Preferential adsorption of gases onto the glidant versus the granulation [94]
4. Minimization of van der Waals forces by separation of the granules [92]
5. Reduction of the friction between particles and surface roughness by the glidant's adhering to the surface of the granulation [92,93]

The most efficient means of measuring the effectiveness of a glidant in a powder blend is to compress the blend and determine weight variation. The use of shear cell and flowmeter data also gives some indication of the flow properties of a particular blend. A complete shear cell analysis of a powder blend can be performed to determine the appropriate hopper design (i.e. angle from vertical, orifice diameter, hopper diameter, and material of construction). Shear-cell analysis also provides information on the tendency of a blend to consolidate with time and under a load. Excessive consolidation can result in a good-flowing formulation turning into a poor-flowing formulation. Nyqvist [95] correlated the frequency of tablet machine adjustments with shear cell and flowmeter data. The moisture content of dried granulations was found to impact on the flowability of the granules.

The Running Powder. Since the best lubricants are not only water-insoluble but also water-repellent, and since lubricants function by coating the granulation to be compressed, it is not surprising that the lubricants used and the process of lubrication may have a deleterious effect on tablet disintegration and drug dissolution release. To overcome the tendency a second agent is often added to the lubricant powder to produce a less hydrophobic powder to be added as the lubricant system. The mixture of lubricant and a second, hydrophilic agent is called the *running powder*, since it is added to permit compression or running of the granulation on a tablet machine. The most common hydrophilic agent added to the lubricant is starch. The starch/lubricant ratio is typically in the range 1:1 to 1:4.

Colorants

Colors are incorporated into tablets generally for one or more of three purposes. First, colors may be used for identifying similar-looking products within a product line, or in cases where products of similar appearance exist in the lines of different manufacturers. This may be of particular importance when product identification (because of overdosing or poisoning and drug abuse) is a problem. Second, colors can help minimize the possiblity of mixups during manufacture. Third, and perhaps least important, is the addition of colorants to tablets for their aesthetic value or their marketing value.

The difficulties associated with the banning of FD&C Red No. 2 (amaranth), FD&C Red No. 4, and carbon black in 1976 should be a prime example of what may be the trend of the future. Other colors such as FD&C No. 40 and FD&C Yellow No. 5 have been questioned recently and will continue to be suspect for one reason or another. The pharmaceutical manufacturer can maximize the identification of his products through product shape and size, NDC number, and use of logos. One should not rely on color as a major means of eliminating in-house errors but should instead develop adequate general manufacturing practices to insure that mix-ups do not occur.

Today the formulator may choose a colorant from a decreasing list of colors designated as D&C and FD&C dyes and lakes, and a small number of acceptable natural and derived materials approved for use by the U.S. Food and Drug Administration. Historically, drug manufacturers have, for the most part, restricted their choice of dyes to the FD&C list. Table 8 summarizes the colors available at this time.

Dyes are water-soluble materials, whereas lakes are formed by the absorption of a water-soluble dye on a hydrous oxide (usually aluminum hydroxide), which results in an insoluble form of the dye.

The photosensitivity of lakes and dyes will be affected by the drug, excipients, and methods of manufacture and storage of each product. Ultraviolet-absorbing chemicals have been added to tablets to minimize their photosensitivity. Pastel shades generally show the least amount of mottling, especially in systems utilizing water-soluble dyes. Colors near the mid-range of the visible spectrum (yellow, green) will show less mottling than those at either extreme (blue, red).

Methods of Incorporation

Water-soluble dyes are usually dissolved in the granulating system for incorporation during the granulating process. This method assures uniform distribution through the granulation but can lead to mottling during the drying process. Colors may also be adsorbed onto carriers (starch, lactose, calcium sulfate, sugar) from aqueous or alcoholic solutions. The resultant color mixtures are dried and used as *stock* systems for many lots of a particular product. Water-soluble dyes may also be dry-blended with an excipient prior to the final mix.

Lakes are almost always blended with other dry excipients because of their insoluble nature. In general, direct-compression tablets are colored with lakes because no granulation step is used.

Flavors and Sweeteners

Flavors and sweeteners are commonly used to improve the taste of chewable tablets. Cook [96] reviewed the area of natural and synthetic sweeteners.

Flavors are incorporated as solids in the form of spray-dried beadlets and oils, usually at the lubrication step, because of the sensitivity of these materials to moisture and their tendency to volatilize when heated (e.g., during granulation drying). Aqueous (water-soluble) flavors have found little acceptance due to their lesser stability upon aging.

Since oxidation destroys the quality of a flavor, oils are usually emulsified with acacia and spray-dried. Dry flavors are easier to handle and are generally more stable than oils. Oils are usually diluted in alcohol and sprayed onto the granulation as it tumbles in a lubrication tub. Use of a P-K V-blender with an intensifier bar has also been used. Oils may also be adsorbed onto an excipient and added during the lubrication process. Usually, the maximum

Table 8   Status of Color Additives: Code of Federal Regulations (4-1-87)

FD&C Blue No. 1	May be used for coloring drugs in amounts consistent with current good manufacturing practice.
FD&C Blue No. 2	May be used for coloring drugs in amounts consistent with current good manufacturing practice.
D&C Blue No. 4	May be used in externally applied drugs in amounts consistent with current good manufacturing practice.
D&C Blue No. 9	May be used for coloring cotton and silk surgical sutures including sutures for ophthalmic use in amounts not to exceed 2.5% by weight of the suture.
FD&C Green No. 3	May be used for coloring drugs in amounts consistent with current good manufacturing practice.
D&C Green No. 5	May be used for coloring drugs in amounts consistent with current good manufacturing practice.
D&C Green No. 8	May be used in externally applied drugs in amounts not exceeding 0.01% by weight of the finished product.
D&C Orange No. 4	May be used for coloring externally applied drugs in amounts consistent with current good manufacturing practice.
D&C Orange No. 5	May be used for coloring mouthwashes and dentifrices and for externally applied drugs in amounts not to exceed 5 mg per daily dose of the drug.
D&C Orange No. 10	May be used for coloring externally applied drugs in amounts consistent with current good manufacturing practice.
D&C Orange No. 11	May be used for coloring externally applied drugs in amounts consistent with current good manufacturing practice.
D&C Orange No. 17	May be used for coloring externally applied drugs in amounts consistent with current good manufacturing practice.
FD&C Red No. 3	May be used for coloring ingested drugs in amounts consistent with current good manufacturing practice.
FD&C Red No. 4	May be used for externally applied drugs in amounts consistent with current good manufacturing practice.
D&C Red No. 6	May be used for coloring drugs such that the combined total of D&C Red No. 6 and D&C Red No. 7 does not exceed 5 mg per daily dose of the drug.
D&C Red No. 7	May be used for coloring drugs such that the combined total of D&C Red No. 6 and D&C Red No. 7 does not exceed 5 mg per daily dose of the drug.
D&C Red No. 8	May be used for coloring ingested drugs in amounts not exceeding 0.1% by weight of the finished product

Table 8 (Continued)

	and for externally applied drugs in amounts consistent with current good manufacturing practice.
D&C Red No. 9	May be used for externally applied drugs in amounts consistent with current good manufacturing practice.
D&C Red No. 17	May be used for externally applied products in amounts consistent with current good manufacturing practice.
D&C Red No. 19	May be used for externally applied products in amounts consistent with current good manufacturing practice.
D&C Red No. 21	May be used for coloring drug product in amounts consistent with current good manufacturing practice.
D&C Red No. 22	May be used for coloring drug product in amounts consistent with current good manufacturing practice.
D&C Red No. 27	May be used for coloring drug product in amounts consistent with current good manufacturing practice.
D&C Red No. 28	May be used for coloring drug product in amounts consistent with current good manufacturing practice.
D&C Red No. 30	May be used for coloring drug product in amounts consistent with current good manufacturing practice.
D&C Red No. 31	May be used for externally applied drugs in amounts consistent with current good manufacturing practice.
D&C Red No. 34	May be used for coloring externally applied in amounts consistent with current good manufacturing practice.
D&C Red No. 39	May be used for external germicidal solutions not to exceed 0.1% by weight of the finished drug product.
FD&C Red No. 40	May be used in coloring drugs subject to restrictions and in amounts consistent with current good manufacturing practice.
D&C Violet No. 2	May be used for coloring externally applied drugs in amounts consistent with current good manufacturing practice.
FD&C Yellow No. 5	In general products containing FD&C Yellow No. 5 (tartrazine) must be so labeled. The Code of Federal Regulations should be consulted for use restrictions that may be added.
FD&C Yellow No. 6	May be used for coloring drugs in amounts consistent with current good manufacturing practice.
D&C Yellow No. 7	May be used for externally applied drugs in amounts consistent with current good manufacturing practice.
D&C Yellow No. 10	May be used for coloring drugs in amounts consistent with current good manufacturing practice.

Table 8   (Continued)

D&C Yellow No. 11	May be used for externally applied drugs in amounts consistent with current good manufacturing practice.
D&C Lakes, Ext. D&C Lakes, FD&C Lakes	Consult the current regulations for status.

amount of oil that can be added to granulation without affecting the bond or flow properties is 0.75% (w/w).

Sweeteners are added primarily to chewable tablets when the commonly used carriers such as mannitol, lactose, sucrose, and dextrose do not sufficiently mask the taste of the components.

Saccharin, which is FDA-approved, is about 400 times sweeter than sucrose. The major disadvantage of saccharin is its bitter aftertaste, which can sometimes be minimized by incorporating a small quantity (1%) of sodium chloride. The saccharin aftertaste is highly discernible to about 20% of the population.

Aspartame, a nondrug approved artificial sweetener, is about 180 times sweeter than sucrose and is approved for use in beverages, desserts, and instant coffee and tea. It exhibits discoloration in the presence of ascorbic acid and tartaric acid, thus greatly limiting its use. Becuase of the possible carcinogenicity of the artificial sweeteners (cyclamates and saccharin), pharmaceutical formulators are increasingly attempting to design their tablet products without such agents. The following formulation represents such a system for a chewable antacid tablet.

Example 1:   Chewable Antacid Tablet, Aluminum Hydroxide, and Magnesium Carbonate Codried Gel (Direct Compression)

Ingredient	Quanity per tablet
Aluminum hydroxide and magnesium carbonate codried gel (Reheis F-MA 11)	325.0 mg
Mannitol, USP (granular)	675.0 mg
Microcrystalline cellulose	75.0 mg
Starch	30.0 mg
Calcium stearate	22.0 mg
Flavor	q.s.

Blend all ingredients and compress using a 5/9-in. flat-faced level edge punch to a hardness of 8 to 11 kg (Strong-Cobb-Arner tester).

Adsorbents

Adsorbents such as silicon dioxide (Syloid, Cab-O-Sil, Aerosil) are capable of retaining large quantities of liquids without becoming wet. This allows many oils, fluid extracts, and eutectic melts to be incorporated into tablets. Capable of holding up to 50% of its weight of water, silicon dioxide adsorbed systems often appear as free-flowing powders. This adsorbent characteristic explains why these materials function well in tablet formulations to alleviate picking, especially with high-level vitamin E tablets. Silicon dioxide also exhibits glidant properties and can play both a glidant and an adsorbent role in the formula.

Other potential adsorbents include clays like bentonite and kaolin, magnesium silicate, tricalcium phosphate, magnesium carbonate, and magnesium oxide. Usually the liquid to be adsorbed is first mixed with the adsorbent prior to incorporation into the formula. Starch also displays adsorbent properties.

V. REGULATORY REQUIREMENTS FOR EXCIPIENTS IN THE UNITED STATES

In 1974 the U.S. Congress received a report on *Drug Bioequivalence* from the Office of Technology Assessment which noted as a major conclusion the potential influence of excipients on the bioavailability of many drug products. A further major comment made in the report, which has been largely overlooked as readers focused on the bioavailability issue, was a strong criticism regarding the current standards for excipients in the compendia. Obviously, if test methods for excipients are nonspecific and incomplete, especially as these properties may relate to bioavailability of drug products, compendial and other government standards cannot provide good assurance of the bioequivalence of marketed drug products. The report went on to note that many commonly used excipients (including those used in tablets and other solid dosage forms) were not even included in the compendia.

The general notices of USP XX and NF XV contain broad, restrictive statements that require all excipients to be harmless in the amounts used, not to exceed the minimum amounts needed to produce the intended effect, not to impair the bioavailability or therapeutic effect of the drug(s) in the dosage form, and not to produce interference with any of the assays or tests required to determine adherence to compendial standards. Cooper [97] tabulated the various types of tests and standards applied to the 223 excipients listed in USP XIX and NF XIV. Each excipient has either a specific assay or an identity test, or both, together with various limit tests, which may include water content or loss on drying (for less than 80 excipients), tests for chloride, sulfate, arsenic, heavy metals, ash, residue on ignition, various specific or nonspecific impurities, tests for solubility or insolubility (23 excipients), and tests for other specified physicochemical properties (24 excipients).

A. Physicochemical Test Methods for Excipients

While it has been known for some time that many (if not most) pharmaceutical excipients were lacking in characterizing physicochemical tests, the Swiss drug companies were the first to take corrective steps, when they specified certain standard physical tests for excipients in their *Katalog Pharmazeutischer*

Hilfsstoffe (Catalog of Pharmaceutical Excipients). John Rees of the Department of Pharmacy, University of Aston, Birmingham, England, has translated these tests for German to English, as they are given in the Swiss catalog. Five of the standard tests are given there, since they relate to excipients for tablets, and since detailed tests for these properties are not given in the current compendia. Other tests in the catalog will not be detailed (for vapor density, flash point, fire point, ignition temperature, explosive limits, or maximum working conditions concentration).

The development of the *Handbook of Pharmaceutical Excipients* by the Academy of Pharmaceutical Sciences of the American Pharmaceutical Association in collaboration with the Pharmaceutical Society of Great Britain has produced a reference text with a comprehensive list of pharmaceutical excipients and suitable standards for each. This reference should prove to be invaluable to the formulator [22].

In selecting excipients for pharmaceutical dosage forms and drug products, the development pharmacist should be certain that standards exist and are available to assure the consistent quality and functioning of the excipient from lot to lot.

A major task of the committee that worked on the *Handbook of Pharmaceutical Excipients* was the development of standard test methods for important excipient properties. Standard methods to evaluate over 30 physical properties were developed.

The reader is urged to become familiar with the test methods, published in the *Handbook*, that allow comprehensive characterization of tablet excipient materials, especially the following:

Flow rate	Particle hardness	Shear rate
Gel strength (binders)	Particle size distribution:	Tensile strength
Lubricity (frictional)	(1) sieve analysis	Volume, bulk
Microbiological status	(2) air permeability	Water absorption
Moisture sorption	Porosity	Water adsorption
isotherm		

B. Tablet Formulation for International Markets

Many drug companies must consider regulatory requirements in many parts of the world when they undertake the formulation of new tablet products or reformulation of existing products. This is true not only for the largest drug companies with major international divisions, but is also the case for much smaller companies who market abroad through a separate foreign manufacturing or distributing company, or who hope (in the future) to license their product for foreign sale. Such formulations must take into account not only the acceptability of various excipients in the other countries and areas of the world of interest, but also the environmental restrictions of these countries which may impact on proposed manufacturing methods (e.g., the proposed solvents used, if any) and the worldwide availability of all excipient components in the required purity and specifications. While little information may be found in any literature compilation on this subject, Hess [98] presented a symposium paper in 1976 on the choice of excipients for international use; much of the following information has been drawn from this presentation.

Excipients that are in use in the pharmaceutical industry for tablets or other oral dosage forms generally fall into one of the following categories: (1) excipients permitted in foodstuffs; (2) excipients described in pharmacopoeias; (3) newer excipients with no official status, but registered with health authorities in various countries of the world, and approved for use in some of these countries.

Excipients permitted in foodstuffs are generally regarded as acceptable for like uses in drug products. Materials approved for excipient uses (e.g., fillers, surfactants, preservatives, binding agents) have usually been extensively tested in food and will be used in relatively low amounts as a tablet or pharmaceutical component compared to use as a food component. In general, an excipient listed in a major pharmacopoeia such as the United States, British, or European Pharmacopoeia can be used worldwide.

An exception to this rule should be noted for Japan, where only excipients named in one of the official Japanese compendia may be used. These compendia currently include: *Japan Pharmacopoeia VIII*, the *Japanese Standards of Food Additives III*, or the *Special Koseisho Regulations*. These compendia list some excipients not regularly used in the United States or Europe (e.g., calcium carboxymethylcellulose), while not listing such common ones as the free acid of saccharin (the sodium salt is listed) or diethyl phthalate (the dibutyl phthalate is listed). Polyvinylpyrrolidone, which was formerly acceptable, has now become restricted. Of the iron oxides only the red variety (Fe_2O_3) is permitted, while the use of the yellow (Fe_2O_3 monohydrate) and especially the black oxide ($FeO \cdot Fe_2O_3$) seems doubtful. Koseisho, the Japanese health authority, also restricts the use of excipients with a pharmacological effect (e.g., citric and ascorbic acid) to one-fifth of the minimum daily dose.

Pharmaceutical manufacturers must be careful to assure that excipients listed in pharmacopoeias, and made available by various suppliers around the world, do in fact comply with all the relevant pharmacopoeial specifications. In certain instances this may restrict the use of very similar, but not identical, compounds (e.g., cellulose ethers with different degrees of substitution).

The development of new materials for use as pharmaceutical excipients requires the demonstration of the absence of toxicity and freedom from adverse reactions. In most countries today it is very difficult to obtain approval by regulatory agencies for the use of new excipient agents. Reportedly, the only clear recommendations for the type of toxicological data currently required on a new excipient are provided in the German regulations (1971) and the European Economic Community Directives (EEC 75/318, dated May 20, 1975). These regulations and directives call for acute toxicity studies in three animal species, observed over 14 days. If possible, the LD_{50} by the parenteral route should also be established in one species. The combined acute and long-term studies may be summarized as follows:

Toxicological data on a new excipient: long-term oral administration
Acute toxicity: to standard international protocols
Repetitive administration: 6 months, 2 species (one nonrodent)
Carcinogenicity: 1 species (18 months, mouse or 2 years, rat)
Reproduction studies, segments 1, 11, and 111 (fertility, teratogenicity,
    effects on lactation): 1, 11, and 111 (rat); 11 (at least one other
    species nonrodent, e.g., rabbit)

In the FDA-oriented countries (Australia and Canada in addition to the United States), 2-year repetitive-dose studies in rats and 1-year studies in dogs may be expected to be required rather than the 6-month studies described above. It may also be necessary to conduct mutagenicity studies. For excipients with any potential for complexation or drug binding, drug bioavailability studies will be required for products in which the excipient is incorporated. If the excipient is absorbed its ADME and pharmacokinetic profile may need to be established. In the event that the agent can be clearly demonstrated to not be absorbed from the gut, these later studies may be simplified, shortened, or omitted. This would assume the excipient is also a well-characterized high-purity agent. Excipients that are clearly known to be components of the normal human diet, such as, for example, a form of pure cellulose, are much easier to clear with regulatory agencies than a compound not normal to the diet, or for which no prior knowledge of human exposure or exposure effects exists. The very high cost of obtaining the necessary toxicological data for a unique new excipient agent makes it obvious that few totally new excipient agents will make their appearance in the future.

Another consideration bearing on excipient use in international markets (that is expected to become increasingly important) is the subject of disclosure. Paragraph 10 of the 1976 Drug Law of the Federal Republic of Germany states that all active ingredients must be publicly declared. This requirement includes preservatives because of their antimicrobial activity. Whether dyestuffs with a weak allergenic potential should be included in this category is still debated. However, in countries such as Sweden, lists of drug preparations containing tartrazine and other azo dyestuffs have already been published. This obviously leads to a certain marketing disadvantage for these products. According to new regulations issued in November 1976, the azo dyestuffs tartrazine Sunset Yellow FCF, ponceau 4R, and amaranth were not to be permitted in foodstuffs in Sweden after 1979. Prohibitions or major restrictions against these, if not all, azo dyes may follow in the years ahead in other countries. Amaranth or FD&C Red No. 2 is currently prohibited in the United States, Taiwan, and Venezuela.

The choice of the excipients to be used in any drug product is usually a compromise. This is even more the case in selecting excipients for international use, since technical performance must be balanced against local restrictions in some countries as well as cost and availability in all countries where the product is to be produced.

Hess [98] has tabulated priorities of use for some common tablet and capsule excipients for international use. A number 1 indicates the highest priority for use based on all considerations (e.g., compatibility, availability, cost). His tabulations of priority of use for fillers and disintegrants and for binders, glidants, and lubricants are shown in Tables 9 and 10.

In the last few years some powerful new disintegrants for tablets have appeared. They are of great assistance where long disintegration times or slow dissolution rates are a problem. The compounds have been grouped below according to their acceptability; it appears that sodium carboxymethyl starch creates the least problem worldwide, even though it is not listed yet in any pharmacopoeia. The new disintegrants are:

Primogel, Scholten (NL): sodium carboxymethyl starch
Nymcel, ZSB-10 mod., Nyma (NL): sodium carboxymethylcellulose, low degree of substitution
Plasdone XL, GAF (USA): cross-linked polyvinylpyrrolidone
LHPC, Shinetsu (J): hydroxypropyl cellulose, low substitution

Table 9 Priority for Use: Fillers, Disintegrants

Substance	Comment	Rating
Cornstarch	OK (formaldehyde)	1
Lactose	OK (except primary amines)	1
Mannitol	OK (technical problems)	11
Sucrose	OK (hygroscopic point at 77.4% relative humidity)	11
Avicel	Somewhat less satisfactory than starch	1
Primogel		11
Emcompress	May lose water	11
Tricalcium phosphate	May accelerate hydrolytic degradations	11

Source: Adapted from Hess [98].

Ac-Di-Sol, FMC Corp: internally crosslinked form of sodium carboxy-methylcellulose of USP purity

Starch is ranked as the most inert filler and disintegrant. It is also generally available worldwide in satisfactory quality at relatively low cost. Lactose, though not completely inert, is given a priority of 1, based on its

Table 10 Priority for Use: Binders, Glidants, Lubricants

Substance	Comment	Rating
Starch paste	OK	1
PVP	Frequently accelerates degradation	11
HPMC	Better than PVP	11
Gelatin	Rather worse than HPMC or starch	11
Colloidal silica	Quite reactive	1
Talc	Mostly OK	11
Magnesium stearate	Individual incompatibilities, no general rules	1
Calcium stearate		11
Stearic acid		
Neutral fats	Usually nonreactive	11

Source: Adapted from Hess [98].

Table 11   Legal Status of Carotenoid Food Colors (April 1987)

Country	β-Carotene	β-Apocarotenal	Canthaxanthin
European Economic Community Countries	X	X	X
South American Countries	X	X	X
Switzerland	X	X	X
United States	X	X	X
Philippines	X	X	–
Japan	X	–	–
New Zealand	X	–	–
South Korea	X	–	–
Turkey	X	–	–
USSR and Eastern European Countries	X	–	–

Source: Adapted from Hess [98].

worldwide availability and good technical properties. Mannitol, though inert, is ranked as second choice because of its less satisfactory technical
properties. Sucorse is also quite inert and has compression properties similar to those of lactose, but has a relatively low hygroscopicity point, is
cariogenic, and is not a desired intake material in some patients.

The preferred binder, for reasons cited previously, is starch paste.
Hydroxypropylmethylcellulose (HPMC) and gelatin are less inert; gelatin
promotes microbial growth, and polyvinylpyrrolidone is not acceptable worldwide. Colloidal silica, while being potentially reactive, has unique technical
properties of combined binding, disintegrating, and lubricant action. Talc,
though not reactive, is difficult to obtain in good and constant quality.
Magnesium stearate is rated priority 1, based on availability, while it is
recognized that different lubricants must be evaluated individually for compatibility in any particular application. See Table 10.

The use of coloring agents to increase the elegance of coated and uncoated tablets, or for purposes of product identification, has changed rapidly since 1975. The trend in international product development appears to
be to use iron oxides and titanium dioxide as tablet colorants and carotenoid
food colors in tablet coatings in place of FD&C dyes. The legal status of
the carotenoid food colors is expected to expand in worldwide markets in
the future. The status of these colors given in Table 11.

Defined chemical composition and physical properties and defined chemical and microbiological properties are essential prerequisites for excipients
in general, and for excipients for international use in particular. Excipients
should conform to the same stringent requirements in all these properties
as must active ingredients. The most common problems with excipients used
in international pharmaceutical manufacture are the presence of undesired
impurities and unacceptable variations in technological performance. The

Table 12 Microcrystalline Cellulose: Differences in Commercial Grades

Type	Molecular weight	Degree of polymerization	Crystallinity (%)
Native cellulose (cotton)	300,000–500,000	2000–3000	90–94
Microcrystalline cellulose	30,000–50,000	200–300	—
Avicel	—	—	81–37
Elcema (Rehocel)	—	—	12–24

Source: Huttenrauch and Keiner, *Pharmazie*, *31*:183 (1976).

careful choice and continual monitoring of suppliers of excipients in international markets is essential. Suppliers who concentrate on the pharmaceutical and food industries are usually more reliable and better qualified to provide the high-quality products required by the drug industry.

Drug companies engaged in international manufacture must be assured of reliable availability of the excipients they use. The quality and performance of excipients used at every manufacturing site must be consistent and reliable. Some of the most commonly employed newer classes of tablet excipients used internationally include microcrystalline cellulose, most of the new disintegrants, directly compressible excipients composed of lactose, various sugars, dicalcium phosphate, and special types of starches. In most cases when working with these specialized but very useful materials, one product cannot easily be replaced by another. For example, there are several brands of so-called microcrystalline cellulose available internationally. One type, known by the trade name of Avicel, is obtained by mechanical as well as acid treatment; another type (Elcema) is produced by mechanical treatment only. This leads to different degrees of crystallinity, which may be expected to have an influence on the effectiveness of each agent and on the properties of the dosage forms in which they are contained. The much higher level in the crystallinity of the Avicel product (Table 12) compared to the other microcrystalline forms accounts for its being a superior product as a disintegrant and directly compressible material.

According to Hess [98] companies operating in international markets will usually employ brand name or specialty excipients only if they lead to a better product, usually one with better controlled bioavailability or one with superior mechanical or analytical properties. This will justify their use, their possibly higher price, and problems which may be encountered in importing these substances (including high import duties). In some countries, such as Mexico and India, such imports may not be possible at all or may be possible only with great difficulty. There are many difficult decisions, potential problems, and pitfalls in choosing excipients in a company which operates worldwide. Additional research and development and closer cooperation among the industries, the universities, and the regulatory agencies— to define the properties, the scope, and the use of pharmaceutical excipients— will be needed during the immediate future. In addition, the development of a catalog with standards for all the major excipients used in tablet making—which are accepted by regulatory agencies around the world—will provide a giant step forward for the quality assurance and standardization of products made in international markets.

REFERENCES

1. M. C. Meyer, G. W. A. Slywka, R. E. Dann, and P. L. Whyatt, *J. Pharm. Sci.*, *63*:1693 (1974).
2. J. Cooper, *Advances in Pharmaceutical Sciences*, Vol. 3, Academic Press, London, 1971.
3. J. Cooper and J. Rees, *J. Pharm. Sci.*, *61*:1511 (1972).
4. G. S. Banker, Tablets and tablet product design, in *American Pharmacy*, 7th ed., Lippincott, Philadelphia, 1974, Chap. 11.
5. F. Sadik, Tablets, in *Dispensing of Medication*, 8th ed. (J. E. Hoover, ed.), Mack Publ., Easton, PA., 1976, Chap. 5.
6. T. H. Simon, Preformulation studies, physical and chemical properties evaluation—Paper 1 of a symposium entitled, *A New Drug Entity A Systematic Approach to Drug Development*, Am. Pharm. Assoc. Acad. Pharm. Sci., Washington, D.C., 1967.
7. S. Solvang and P. Finholt, *J. Pharm. Sci.*, *59*:49 (1970).
8. R. M. Franz, G. E. Peck, G. S. Banker, and J. R. Buck, *J. Pharm. Sci. 69*:621 (1980).
9. R. L. Plackett and J. P. Burman, *Biometrika*, *33*:305 (1946).
10. U.S. Patent 4,476,248, October 9, 1984.
11. V. L. Anderson and R. A. McLean, *Design of Experiments: A Realistic Approach*, Marcel Dekker, New York, 1974.
12. R. H. Myers, *Response Surface Methodology*, 1976.
13. J. Jaffe and N. E. Foss, *J. Am. Pharm. Assoc., Sci. Ed.*, *48*:26 (1959).
14. J. Lazarus and L. Lachman, *J. Pharm. Sci.*, *55*:1121 (1966).
15. A. S. Rankell and T. Higuchi, *J. Pharm. Sci.*, *57*:574 (1968).
16. P. Rieckmann, *Pharm. Z.*, *34*:1207 (1971).
17. E. Nelson, *J. Pharm. Sci.*, *46*:607 (1967)
18. G. Levy, J. M. Antkowiak, J. A. Procknal, and D. D. White, *J. Pharm. Sci.*, *52*:1047 (1963).
19. L. Lachman, *J. Pharm. Sci.*, *54*:1519 (1965).
20. H. E. Paul, K. J. Hayer, M. F. Paul, and A. R. Borgmann, *J. Pharm. Sci.*, *56*:882 (1967).
21. F. A. Campagna, G. Cureton, R. A. Mirigian, and E. Nelson, *J. Pharm. Sci.*, *52*:605 (1963).
22. American Pharmaceutical Association, *Handbook of Pharmaceutical Excipients*, Washington, D.C., and the Pharmaceutical Society of Great Britain, London, 1986.
23. J. F. Bavitz and J. B. Schwartz, *Drug Cosm. Ind.*, *60* (April 1976).
24. W. P. Bolger and J. J. Gavin, *N. Engl. J. Med.*, *261*:827 (1959).
25. R. Costello and A. Mattocks, *J. Pharm. Sci.*, *51*:106 (1962).
26. R. N. Duvall, K. T. Koshy, and R. E. Dashiell, *J. Pharm. Sci.*, *54*: 1196 (1965).
27. O. Keller, *Informationsdienst APV*, *16*:75 (1970).
28. S. S. Kornblum, *J. Pharm. Sci.*, *58*:125 (1969).
29. S. S. Kornblum, *Drug Cosm. Ind.*, *32*:92 (1970).
30. L. Ehrhardt and H. Sucker, *Pharm. Ind.*, *32*:92 (1970).
31. R. G. Daoust and M. J. Lynch, *Drug Cosm. Ind.*, *93*:26 (1963).
32. S. A. Sangekar, M. Sarli, and P. R. Sheth, *J. Pharm. Sci.*, *61*:939 (1972).
33. J. L. Kanig, Paper presented at the Emcompress Symposium, London, 1970.

34. C. F. Lerk, G. K. Bolhuis, and A. H. DeBoer, *Pharm. Weekblad*, *109*:945 (1974).
35. H. Nyqvist and M. Nicklasson, *Drug Dev. Ind. Pharm.*, *11*:745 (1985).
36. N. H. Butuyios, *J. Pharm. Sci.*, *55*:727 (1966).
37. J. F. Bavitz and J. B. Schwartz, *Drug Cosm. Ind.*, *114*:44 (1974).
38. C. F. Lerk and G. K. Bolhuis, *Pharm. Weekblad*, *108*:469 (1973).
39. N. L. Henderson and A. J. Bruno, *J. Pharm. Sci.*, *59*:1336 (1970).
40. E. J. Mendell, *Mfg. Chemist Aerosol News*, *43*:43 (1972).
41. O. Alpar, J. A. Hersey, and E. Shotton, *J. Pharm. Pharmacol.*, *22*: 1S-7S (1970).
42. C. Brownley and L. Lachman, *J. Pharm. Sci.*, *53*:452 (1964).
43. M. D. Richman, M.S. thesis, University of Maryland (1963).
44. G. Levy, *J. Pharm. Sci.*, *52*:1039 (1963).
45. K. C. Commons, A. Bergen, and G. C. Walker, *J. Pharm. Sci.*, *57*: 1253 (1968).
46. J. B. Schwartz, E. T. Martin, and E. J. Dehner, *J. Pharm. Sci.*, *64*:328 (1975).
47. K. S. Manudhane, A. M. Contractor, H. Y. Kim, and R. F. Shangraw, *J. Pharm. Sci.*, *58*:616 (1969).
48. T. W. Underwood and D. E. Cadwallader, *J. Pharm. Sci.*, *61*:239 (1972).
49. J. L. Kanig, *J. Pharm. Sci.*, *53*:186 (1964).
50. J. N. Stainiford, et al., *Drug Dev. Ind. Pharm.*, *7*:179–190 (1981).
51. C. D. Fox, M. D. Richman, G. E. Reier, and R. R. Shangraw, *Drug Cosm. Ind.*, *92*:161 (1963).
52. J. L. Livingstone, *Mfg. Chemist Aerosol News*, *42*:23 (1970).
53. O. A. Battista and P. A. Smith, *Ind. Eng. Chem.*, *54*:20 (1962).
54. F. Jaminet and H. Hess, *Pharm. Acta Helv.*, *41*:39 (1966).
55. G. M. Enezian, *Prod. Prob. Pharm.*, *23*:185 (1968).
56. M. A. Shah and R. G. Wilson, *J. Pharm. Sci.*, *57*:181 (1968).
57. M. D. Richman, C. D. Fox and R. F. Shangraw, *J. Pharm. Sci.*, *54*: 447 (1965)
58. G. E. Reier and R. F. Shangraw, *J. Pharm. Sci.*, *55*:510 (1966).
59. K. A. Khan and C. T. Rhodes, *J. Pharm. Sci.*, *64*:166 (1975).
60. J. Kalish, *Drug Cosm. Ind.*, *102*:140 (1968).
61. F. Jaminet, *Pharm. Acta Helv.*, *43*:129 (1968).
62. R. W. Mendes, M. R. Gupta, I. A. Katz, and J. A. O'Neil, *Drug Cosm. Ind.*, *42* (1974).
63. K. C. Kwan and A. Milosovich, *J. Pharm. Sci.*, *55*:340 (1966).
64. H. Seager, I. Burt, J. Ryder, P. Rue, S. Murray, et al., *Int. J. Pharm. Technol. Prod. Manuf.*, *1*:36 (1979).
65. P. J. Rue, H. Seager, J. Ryder, and I. Burt, *Int. J. Pharm. Technol. Prod. Manuf.*, *1*:2 (1980).
66. J. N. C. Healey, M. H. Rubinstein, and V. Walters, *J. Pharm. Pharmacol.* *26*:41P (1974).
67. G. I. Rubio, *An. Fac. Quim. Farm. Chile*, *9*:249 (1957).
68. J. T. Jacob and E. M. Plein, *J. Pharm. Sci.*, *52*:802 (1968).
69. A. M. Sakr, A. A. Kassem, S. A. A. Aziz, A. H. Shalaby, *Mfg. Chem. Aerosol News*, *43*:38 (1972).
70. K. A. Khan and C. T. Rhodes, *J. Pharm. Sci.*, *64*:447 (1975).
71. E. Shotton and G. S. Leonard, *J. Pharm. Sci.*, *65*:1170 (1976).
72. J. T. Ingram and W. Lowenthal, *J. Pharm. Sci.*, *55*:614 (1966).
73. W. Lowenthal, *J. Pharm. Sci.*, *61*:455 (1972).

74. W. Lowenthal and J. H. Wood, *J. Pharm. Sci.*, *62*:287 (1973).
75. S. S. Kornblum and S. B. Stoopak, *J. Pharm. Sci.*, *62*:43 (1973).
76. W. A. Strickland, Jr., *Drug Cosm. Ind.*, *85*:318 (1959).
77. B. Mohn, *Pharm. Manuf.*, *3*, 30, 1986.
78. S. Vemuri, *Pharm. Tech.*, *6*:98 (1982).
79. *Tableting Specification Manual*, Academy of Pharmaceutical Sciences, American Pharmaceutical Association, Revised, 1981.
80. B. Mechtersheimer and H. Sucker, *Pharm. Tech.*, *10*:38 (1986).
81. Y. Matsuda, Y. Minamida, and S. Hayashi, *J. Pharm. Sci.*, *65*:1155 (1976).
82. F. Q. Danish and E. L. Parrott, *J. Pharm. Sci.*, *60*:752 (1971).
83. A. W. Holzer and J. Sjogren, *Drug Dev. Ind. Pharm.*, *3*:23 (1977).
84. P. J. Rue, P. M. R. Varkworth, W. P. Ridgway, P. Rough, D. C. Sharland, et al., *Int. J. Pharm. Technol. Prod. Manuf.*, *1*:2 (1979).
85. T. B. Tsiftsoglou and R. W. Mendes, *Pharm. Tech.*, *6*:30 (1982).
86. J. Maly and A. Maros, *Pharm. Ind.*, *29*:494 (1967).
87. P. Fuchs, E. Schottky, and G. Schenck, *Pharm. Ind.*, *32*:390 (1970).
88. J. Cooper and D. Pasquale, *Pharm. J.*, *181*:397 (1958).
89. N. T. Vegan, *Medd, Norsk Farm. Selskap*, *23*:169 (1961).
90. L. L. Augsburger and R. F. Shangraw, *J. Pharm. Sci.*, *55*:418 (1966).
91. P. York, *J. Pharm. Sci.*, *64*:1217 (1975).
92. T. M. Jones, Symposium on Powders, Society of Cosmetic Chemists of Great Britain, Dublin, April 1969.
93. M. Paleg and C. H. Mannheim, *Powder Technol.*, *7*:45 (1972).
94. B. S. Neumann, *Advances in Pharmaceutical Sciences*, Vol. 2. Academic Press, London, 1967, pp. 194, 207.
95. H. Nyqvist, *Int. J. Pharm. Technol. Prod. Manuf.*, *5*:21 (1984).
96. M. K. Cook, *Drug Cosm. Ind.*, Sept. (1975).
97. J. Cooper, *Aust. J. Pharm. Sci.*, *7*:9 (1978).
98. H. K. Hess, Choice of excipients for international use. Paper presented to the Industrial Pharmaceutical Technology Section in a symposium entitled "The Development of Drugs for International Markets," Am. Pharm. Assoc. Acad. Pharm. Sci., 21st National Meeting, Orlando, FL, November 1976.

3
Compressed Tablets by Wet Granulation

Fred J. Bandelin

Schering-Plough Corporation and University of Tennessee, Memphis, Tennessee

Compressed tablets are the most widely used of all pharmaceutical dosage forms for a number of reasons. They are convenient, easy to use, portable, and less expensive than other oral dosage forms. They deliver a precise dose with a high degree of accuracy. Tablets can be made in a variety of shapes and sizes limited only by the ingenuity of the tool and die maker (i.e. round, oval, capsule-shaped, square, triangular, etc.).

Compressed tablets are defined as solid-unit dosage forms made by compaction of a formulation containing the drug and certain fillers or excipients selected to aid in the processing and properties of the drug product.

There are various types of tablets designed for specific uses or functions. These include tablets to be swallowed per se; chewable tablets formulated to be chewed rather than swallowed, such as some antacid and vitamin tablets; buccal tablets designed to dissolve slowly in the buccal pouch; and sublingual tablets for rapid dissolution under the tongue. Effervescent tablets are formulated to dissolve in water with effervescence caused by the reaction of citric acid with sodium bicarbonate or some other effervescent combination that produces effervescence in water. Suppositories can be made by compression of formulations using a specially designed die to produce the proper shape.

The function of tablets is determined by their design. Multilayer tablets are made by multiple compression. These are called layer tablets and usually consist of two and sometimes three layers. They serve several purposes: to separate incompatible ingredients by formulating them in separate layers, to make sustained or dual-release products, or merely for appearance where the layers are colored differently. Compression-coated tablets are made by compressing a tablet within a tablet so that the outer coat becomes the coating. As many as two coats can be compressed around a core tablet. As with layer tablets, this technique can also be used to separate incompatible ingredients and to make sustained or prolonged release tablets. Sugar-coated tablets are compressed tablets with a sugar coating. The coating may vary in thickness and color by the addition of dyes to the sugar coating. Film-coated tablets are compressed tablets with a thin film of an inert polymer applied in a suitable solvent and dried. Film coating is today the preferred method of making coated tablets. It is the most economical and involves minimum time, labor, expense, and exposure of the tablet to heat and solvent. Enteric-coated tablets are compressed tablets coated with an inert substance which resists solution in gastric fluid, but disintegrates and releases the medication in the intestines. Sustained or prolonged release tablets are compressed tablets especially designed to release the drug over a period of time.

Most drugs cannot be compressed directly into tablets because they lack the bonding properties necessary to form a tablet. The powdered drugs, therefore, require additives and treatment to confer bonding and free-flowing properties on them to facilitate compression by a tablet press.

This chapter describes and illustrates how this is accomplished by the versatile wet granulation method.

I. PROPERTIES OF TABLETS

Whatever method of manufacture is used, the resulting tablets must meet a number of physical and biological standards. The attributes of an acceptable tablet are as follows:

1. The tablet must be sufficiently strong and resistant to shock and abrasion to withstand handling during manufacture, packaging, shipping, and use. This property is measured by two tests, the hardness and friability tests.

2. Tablets must be uniform in weight and in drug content of the individual tablet. This is measured by the weight variation test and the content uniformity test.

3. The drug content of the tablet must be bioavailable. This property is also measured by two tests, the disintegration test and the dissolution test. However, bioavailability of a drug from a tablet, or other dosage form, is a very complex problem and the results of these two tests do not of themselves provide an index of bioavailability. This must be done by blood levels of the drug.

4. Tablets must be elegant in appearance and must have the characteristic shape, color, and other markings necessary to identify the product. Markings are usually the monogram or logo of the manufacturer. Tablets often have the National Drug Code number printed or embossed on the face of the tablet corresponding to the official listing of the product in the National Drug Code Compendium of the Food and Drug Administration. Another marking that may appear on the tablet is a score or crease across the face, which is intended to permit breaking the tablet into equal parts for the administration of half a tablet. However, it has been shown that substantial variation in drug dose can occur in the manually broken tablets.

5. Tablets must retain all of their functional attributes, which include drug stability and efficacy.

II. FORMULATION OF TABLETS

The size and, to some extent, the shape of the tablet are determined by the active ingredient(s). Drugs having very small doses in the microgram range (e.g., folic acid, digitoxin, reserpine, dexamethasone, etc.) require the addition of fillers also called excipients to be added to produce a mass or or volume of material that can be made into tablets of a size that is convenient for patients. A common and convenient size for such low-dosage drugs is a 1/4-in. round tablet or equivalent in some other shape. It is difficult for some patients to count and handle tablets smaller than this. Tablets of this size ordinarily weigh 150 mg or more depending on the density of the excipients used to make up the tablet mass.

As the dose increases, so does the size of the tablet. Drugs with a dose of 100 to 200 mg may require tablet weights of 150 to 300 mg and round die diameters of 1/4 to 7/16 in. in diameter depending on the density and compressibility of the powders used. As the dose of the active ingredient(s) increases, the amount of the excipients and the size of the tablet may vary considerably depending on requirements of each to produce an acceptable tablet. While the diameter of the tablet may in some cases be fixed, the thickness is variable thus allowing the formulator considerable latitude and flexibility in adjusting formulations.

As the dose, and therefore the size, of the tablet increases, the formulator uses his expertise and knowledge of excipients to keep the size of the tablet as small as possible without sacrificing its necessary attributes. Formulation of a tablet, then, requires the following considerations:

1. Size of dose or quantity of active ingredients
2. Stability of active ingredient(s)
3. Solubility of active ingredient(s)
4. Density of active ingredient(s)
5. Compressibility of active ingredient(s)
6. Selection of excipients
7. Method of granulation (preparation for compression)
8. Character of granulation
9. Tablet press, type, size, capacity
10. Environmental conditions (ambient or humidity control)
11. Stability of the final product
12. Bioavailability of the active drug content of the tablet

The selection of excipients is critical in the formulation of tablets. Once the formulator has become familiar with the physical and chemical properties of the drug, the process of selecting excipients is begun. The stability of the drug should be determined with each proposed excipient. This can be accomplished as follows: In the laboratory, prepare an intimate mixture of the drug with an excess of each individual excipient and hold at 60°C for 72 hr in a glass container. At the end of this period, analyze for the drug using a stability-indicating assay. The methods of accelerated testing of pharmaceutical products have been extensively reviewed by Lachman et al in *The Theory and Practice of Industrial Pharmacy*, 3rd Ed., Lea and Febiger (1986).

Table 1   Suggested Excipient/Drug Ratio in Compatibility Studies

Excipient	Weight excipient per unit weight drug (anticipated drug dose, mg)				
	1	5—10	25—50	75—150	150
Alginic acid	24	24	9	9	9
Avicel	24	9	9	9	4
Cornstarch	24	9	4	2	2
Dicalcium phosphate dihydrate	34	34	9	9	9
Lactose	34	9	4	2	1
Magnesium carbonate	24	24	9	9	4
Magnesium stearate	1	1	1	1	1
Mannitol	24	9	4	2	1
Methocel	2	2	2	2	1
PEG 4000	9	9	4	4	2
PVP	4	4	2	1	1
Sta-Rx[a]	1	1	1	1	1
Stearic acid	1	1	1	1	1
Talc	1	1	1	1	1

[a]Now called starch 1500.
Source: Modified from Akers, M. J., *Can. J. Pharm. Sci.*, *11*:1 (1976). Reproduced with permission of the Canadian Pharmaceutical Association.

The suggested ratio of excipient to drug is given in Table 1. Excipients are specified according to the function they perform in the tablet. They are classified as follows:

    Fillers (diluents)
    Binders
    Disintegrants
    Lubricants
    Glidants
    Antiadherents

These additives are discussed in detail later in this chapter.

III. TABLET MANUFACTURE

A. Tablet Presses

The basic unit of any tablet press is a set of tooling consisting of two
punches and a die (Fig. 1) which is called a station. The die determines
the diameter or shape of the tablet; the punches, upper and lower, come
together in the die that contains the tablet formulation to form a tablet.
There are two types of presses: single-punch and rotary punch. The
single-punch press has a single station of one die and two punches, and
is capable of producing from 40 to 120 tablets per minute depending on
the size of the tablet. It is largely used in the early stages of tablet formulation development. The rotary press has a multiplicity of stations arranged
on a rotating table (Fig. 2) in which the dies are fed the formulation producing tablets at production rates of from a few to many thousands per
minute. There are numerous models of presses, manufactured by a number
of companies, ranging in size, speed, and capacity.

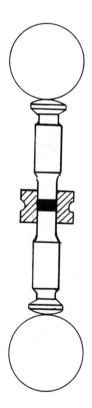

Figure 1   Two punches and die, comprises one station. (Courtesy of
Pennsalt Chemical Corporation, Warminster, Pennsylvania.)

Tablet presses consist of:

1. Hoppers, usually one or two, for storing and feeding the formulation to be pressed
2. Feed frame(s) for distributing the formulation to the dies
3. Dies for controlling the size and shape of the tablet
4. Punches for compacting the formulation into tablets
5. Cams (on rotary presses) that act as tracks to guide the moving punches

All other parts of the press are designed to control the operation of the above parts.

B. Unit Operations

There are three methods of preparing tablet granulations. These are (a) wet granulation, (b) dry granulation (also called "slugging"), and direct compression (Table 2). Each of these methods has its advantages and disadvantages.

The first two steps of milling and mixing of the ingredients of the formulation are identical, but thereafter the processes differ. Each individual operation of the process is known as a unit operation. The progress or flow of materials through the process is shown in the schematic drawing (Fig. 3).

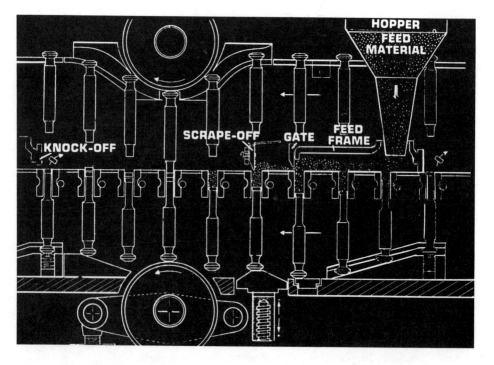

Figure 2   Punches and dies on rotary tablet press. (Courtesy of Pennwalt Chemical Corporation, Warminister, Pennsyovania.)

Table 2 Steps in Different Methods of Tablet Manufacture (Unit Operations)

Wet granulation	Dry granulation	Direct compression
1. Milling of drugs and excipients	1. Milling of drugs and excipients	1. Milling of drugs and excipients
2. Mixing of milled powders	2. Mixing of milled powders	2. Mixing of ingredients
3. Preparation of binder solution	3. Compression into large, hard tablets called slugs	3. Tablet compression
4. Mixing binder solution with powder mixture to form wet mass	4. Screening of slugs	
5. Coarse screening of wet mass using 6- to 12- mesh	5. Mixing with lubricant and disintegrating agent	
6. Drying moist granules	6. Tablet compression	
7. Screening dry granules with lubricant and disintegrant		
8. Mixing screened granules with lubricant and disintegrant		
9. Tablet compression		

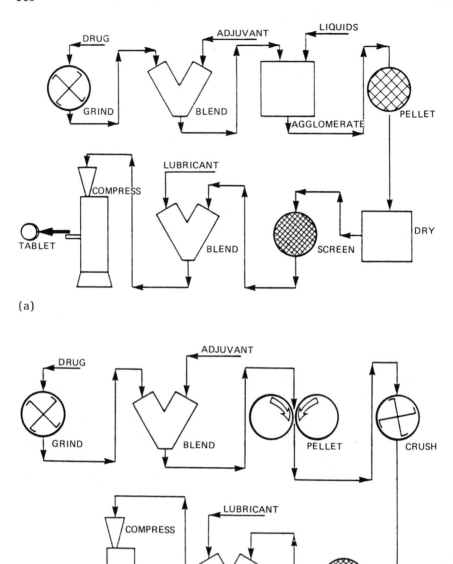

Figure 3 Unit operations in three methods of tablet manufacture: (a) wet granulation, (b) dry granulation, and (c) direct compression.

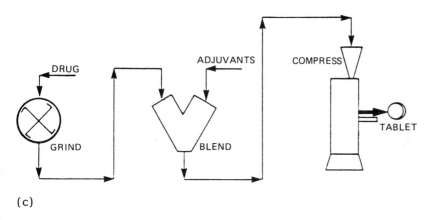

DRUG

GRIND

ADJUVANTS

BLEND

COMPRESS

TABLET

(c)

Figure 3   (Continued)

This chapter is devoted to the first of these processes—the wet granulation process.

The preliminary step of particle size reduction can be accomplished by a variety of mills or grinders such as shown in Figure 4. The next step is powder blending with a planetary mixer (Fig. 5) or a twin-shell blender (Fig. 6). The addition of the liquid binder to the powders to produce the wet mass requires equipment with a strong kneading action such as a sigma blade mixer (Fig. 7) or a planetary mixer mentioned above. The wet mass is formed into granules by forcing through a screen in an oscillating granulator (Fig. 8) or through a perforated steel plate in a Fitzmill (Fig. 9). The granules are then dried in an oven or a fluid bed dryer after which they are reduced in size for compressing by again screening in an oscillator or Fitzmill with a smaller orifice. The granulation is then transferred to a twin shell or other suitable mixer where the lubricant, disintegrant, and glidant are added and blended. The completed granulation is then ready for compression into tablets.

Fluid bed dryers have been adapted to function as wet granulators as depicted by the schematic drawings Figs. 10 and 11. In the latter, powders are agglomerated in the drying chamber by spraying the liquid binder onto the fluidized powder causing the formation of agglomerates while the hot-air flow simultaneously dries the agglomerates by vaporizing the liquid phase. This manner of wet granulation has the advantage of reducing handling and contamination by dust and offers savings in both process time and space [1-3]. It also lends itself to automation; however, by its nature it has the disadvantage of being limited to a batch-type operation. Unlike the wet-massing method, fluidized granulation is quite sensitive to small variations in binder and processing. Conversion of granule preparation from the wet massing to the fluid bed method is not feasible without extensive and time-consuming reformulation [4-8].

In one study it was noted that fluidized bed tablets were more friable than wet-massed tablets of the same tensile strength and attributes this to uneven distribution of the binder in the fluidized bed powders leading to drug-rich, friable areas on the surface and edges of the tablets causing breaking and chipping [9].

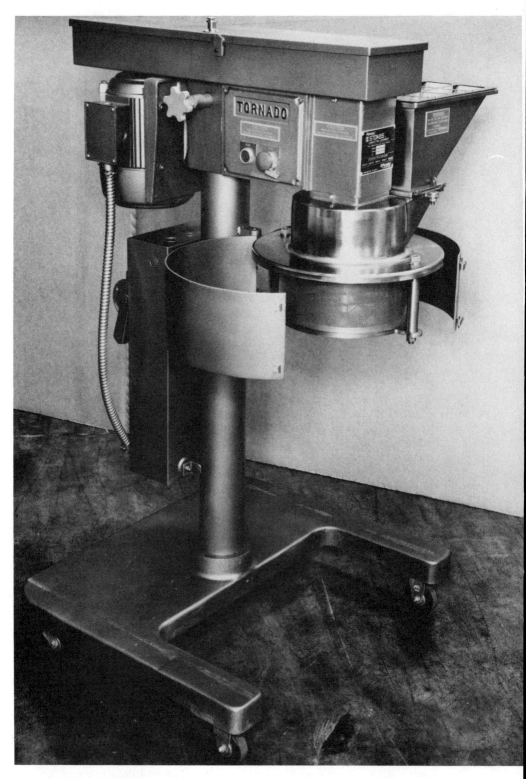

Figure 4   Tornado mill. (Courtesy of Pennwalt Chemical Corporation, Warminister, Pennsylvania.)

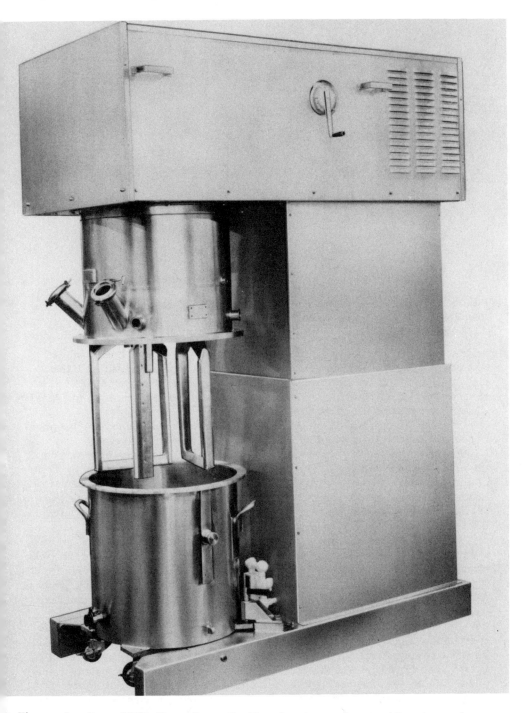

Figure 5 Ross HDM 40 sanitary double planetary mixer. (Courtesy of Charles Ross & Son Co., Happauge, New York.)

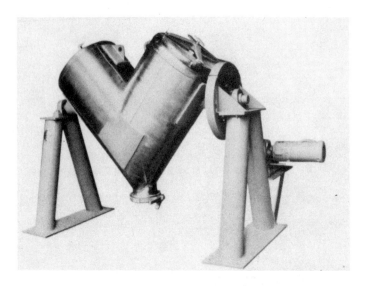

Figure 6   Twin-shell blender.   (Courtesy of Patterson-Kelley Company, East Strousberg, Pennsylvania.)

In the past few years considerable improvements have been made in equipment available for fluidized bed drying. These have reduced the risk of channeling by better design of the fluid bed, improved design from a Good Manufacturing Practices viewpoint, and by means of in-place washing together with automatic controls.

Several other methods of granulating not extensively used in the pharmaceutical industry but worthy of investigation are the following.

Pan granulating is achieved by spraying a liquid binder onto powders in a rotating pan such as that used in tablet coating. The tumbling action of the powders in the pan produces a fluidizing effect as the binder is impinged on the powder particles. The liquid (water or solvent) is evaporated in the heated pan by a current of hot air and the vapors are carried off by a vacuum hood over the upper edge of the pan opening.

Although pan granulation has found extensive application in other industries (e.g., agricultural chemicals), it has not found favor in the pharmaceutical industry. One reason may be the lack of acceptable design.

Spray drying can serve as a granulating process. The drying process changes the size, shape, and bulk density of the dried product and lends itself to large-scale production [10]. The spherical particles produced usually flow better than the same product dried by other means because the particles are more uniform in size and shape. Spray drying can also be used to dry materials sensitive to heat or oxidation without degrading them. The liquid feed is dispersed into droplets, which are dried in seconds, and the product is kept cool by the vaporization of the liquid. Seager and others describe a process for producing a variety of drug formulations by spray drying [11–13].

Extrusion, in which the wet mass is forced through holes in a steel plate by a spiral screw (similar to a meat grinder), is an excellent method of granulating and densifying powders. It lends itself to efficient,

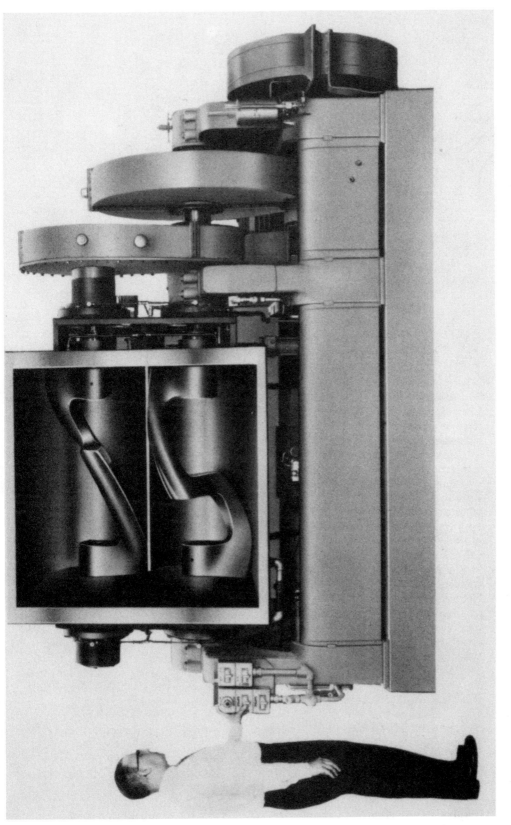

Figure 7   Sigma blade mixer.   (Courtesy of J. H. Day Company, Cincinnati, Ohio.)

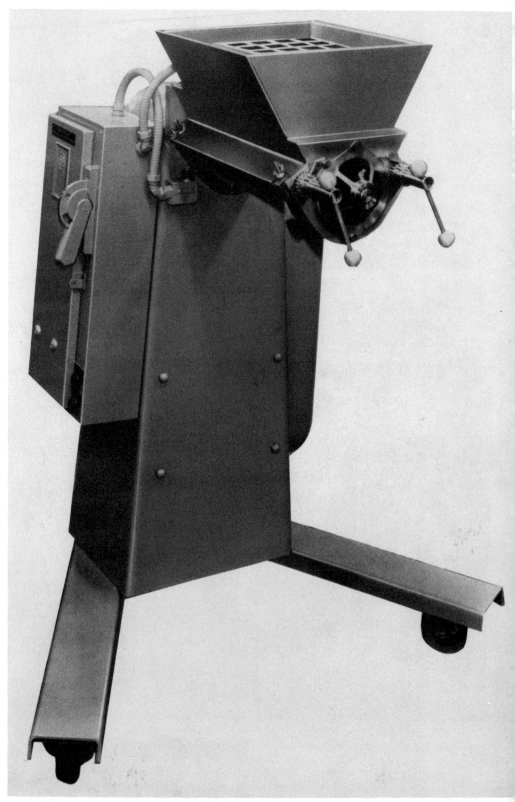

Figure 8 Oscillating granulator. (Courtesy of Pennsalt Chemical Corporation, Warminister, Ohio.)

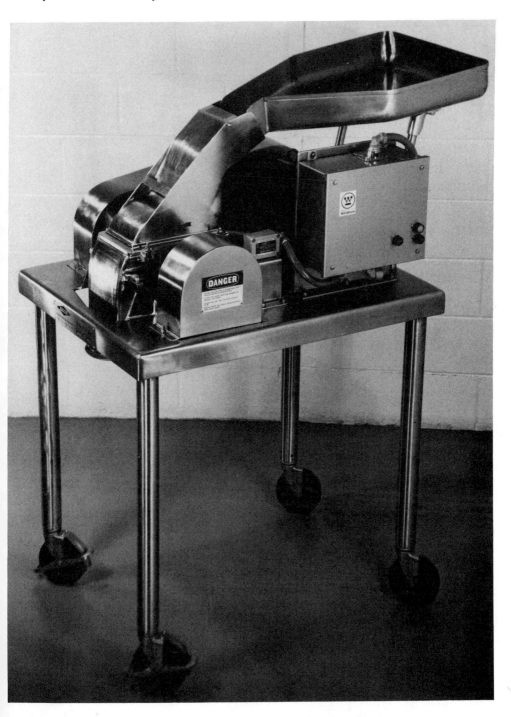

Figure 9   Fitzmill.   (Courtesy of The Fitzpatrick Company, Elmhurst, Illinois.)

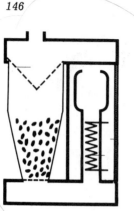

Figure 10   Fluid bed dryer.   (Courtesy of Aeromatic, Inc., South Somerville, New Jersey.)

large-scale production as part of an enclosed continuous wet-granulating system protected from airborne contamination.

The extruder can also act as a wet-massing mixer by providing a continuous flow of the binder into the screw chamber, allowing the spiral screw to act as the massing instrument as it moves the powder, infusing it with the liquid to form a wet mass that is then extruded to form granules. The extruder has the added advantage of being a small unit as compared with other mixers, and has a high production capacity for its size. It is easily cleaned and is versatile in its ability to produce granules of various size depending on the size of the plate openings used.

Pellets can be prepared by spheroidization of the wet mass after extrusion [14—16].

The transfer of wet granulation technology from lab batches to production equipment, generally known as "scale-up," is a critical step because

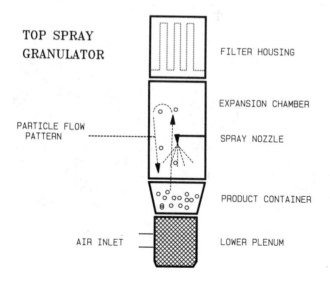

Figure 11   Spray granulator.   (Courtesy of Glatt Air Techniques, Inc., Ramsey, New Jersey.)

of the increased mass of the larger batches and different conditions in
larger equipment. To attempt to anticipate granulation variation due to
scale-up, intermediate pilot equipment facilitates the step-up to production
quantities. This permits the use of various types of equipment or unit
operations to determine which produces the best end result of the granulation process. Often, however, scale-up is limited to the available equipment, which limits, or locks in, the process. In this situation, it is in-
cumbent on the formulator to utilize his or her expertise and experience
in selecting excipients and binder which yield the best granulation and
tablets with the equipment available [17—19].

Attempts to apply experimental design to scaling up the wet granulation
process has not been rewarding so that, in practice, trial and error remains the most widely used procedure.

Wet granulation research has greatly increased and expanded in the
last decade because of the advent of new types of granulating equipment.
Notable among these are the Lodige, Diosna, Fielder, and Baker—Perkins
mixers. These are equipped with high-speed impellers or blades that rotate at speeds of 100 to 500 rpm. In addition to merely mixing the powders,
they produce rapid and efficient wetting and densification of the powders.
Most of these mixers are also equipped with a rotating chopper that operates at speeds of 1000 to 3000 rpm. This facilitates uniform wetting of the
powders in a matter of minutes. Granule formation can be achieved by the
controlled spraying or atomization of the binder solution onto the powders
while mixing [20]. While these highly efficient mixers serve to optimize the
wet granulation process, they also demand greater understanding of their
effects on the individual fillers and binders as processed by the mixers
[21].

Another mixer, blender, and granulator that has found application in
the pharmaceutical industry is the Patterson—Kelley twin-shell liquid-solids
Blender (Fig. 12). These twin-shell units are equipped with a jacket for

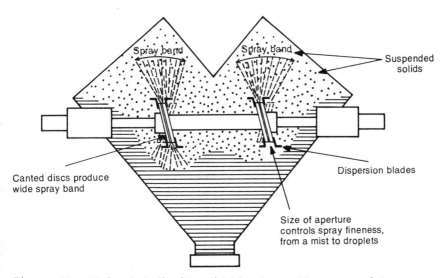

Figure 12   Twin-shell liquid-solid blender. (Courtesy of Patterson-
Kelley Company, East Stroudsburg, Pennsylvania.)

heating and cooling, a vacuum take-off, and a liquid dispersion bar through which a liquid binder can be added. As the blender rotates, liquid is sprayed into the powder charge through the rotating liquid dispersion bar, located concentric to the trunnion axis. The bar's dog-eared blades, rotating at 3300 rpm, aerates the powder to increase the speed and thoroughness of the blend. Granulation can be controlled by the rate of binder addition through the dispersion bar. After heating, the liquid of the binder is removed under reduced pressure. Mixing, granulating, heating, cooling, and removal of excess liquid are carried out in a continuous operation in an enclosed system, thereby protecting the contents from contamination and the adjacent area from contamination by the contents. Once the granulation process is completed, the remaining excipients can be added and blended by the simple rotating action of the blender. This unit is also known as a liquid-solids processor.

IV. GRANULATION

Most powders cannot be compressed directly into tablets because (a) they lack the proper characteristics of binding or bonding together into a compact entity and (b) they do not ordinarily possess the lubricating and disintegrating properties required for tableting. For these reasons, drugs must first be pretreated, either alone or in combination with a filler, to form granules that lend themselves to tableting. This process is known as granulation.

Granulation is any process of size enlargement whereby small particles are gathered together into larger, permanent aggregates [22] to render them into a free-flowing state similar to that of dry sand.

Size enlargement, also called agglomeration, is accomplished by some method of agitation in mixing equipment or by compaction, extrusions or globulation as described in the previous section on unit operations [4,23, 24].

The reasons for granulation as listed by Record [23] are to:

1. Render the material free flowing
2. Densify materials
3. Prepare uniform mixtures that do not separate
4. Improve the compression characteristics of the drug
5. Control the rate of drug release
6. Facilitate metering or volume dispensing
7. Reduce dust
8. Improve the appearance of the tablet

Because of the many possible approaches to granulation, selection of a method is of prime importance to the formulator.

A. Wet Granulation

Wet granulation is the process in which a liquid is added to a powder in a vessel equipped with any type of agitation that will produce agglomeration or granules. This process has been extensively reviewed by Record [23], Kristensen and Schaefer [26], and Capes [27].

It is the oldest and most conventional method of making tablets. Although it is the most labor-intensive and most expensive of the available methods, it persists because of its versatility. The possibility of moistening powders with a variety of liquids, which can also act as carriers for certain ingredients, thereby enhancing the granulation characteristics, has many advantages. Granulation by dry compaction has many limitations. It does not lend itself to all tablet formulations because it depends on the bonding properties of dry powders added as a carrier to the drug thereby increasing the size of the tablet. In wet granulation, the bonding properties of the liquid binders available is usually sufficient to produce bonding with a minimum of additives.

The phenomena of adhesion and cohesion may be defined as follows: adhesion is the bonding of unlike materials, while cohesion is that of like materials. Rumpf [28] identified mechanisms by which mechanical links are formed between particles. The following are involved in the bonding process:

1. Formation of crystalline bridges by binders during drying
2. Structures formed by the hardening of binders in drying
3. Crushing and bonding of particles during compaction

Wet granulation is a versatile process and its application in tablet formulation is unlimited.

B. Advantages of Wet Granulation

1. The cohesiveness and compressibility of powders is improved due to the added binder that coats the individual powder particles, causing them to adhere to each other so they can be formed into agglomerates called granules. By this method, properties of the formulation components are modified to overcome their tableting deficiencies. During the compaction process, granules are fractured exposing fresh powder surfaces, which also improves their compressibility. Lower pressures are therefore needed to compress tablets resulting in improvements in tooling life and decreased machine wear.
2. Drugs having a high dosage and poor flow and/or compressibility must be granulated by the wet method to obtain suitable flow and cohesion for compression. In this case, the proportion of the binder required to impart adequate compressibility and flow is much less than that of the dry binder needed to produce a tablet-by-direct compression.
3. Good distribution and uniform content for soluble, low-dosage drugs and color additives are obtained if these are dissolved in the binder solution. This represents a distinct advantage over direct compression where the content uniformity of drugs and uniform color dispersion can be a problem.
4. A wide variety of powders can be processed together in a single batch and in so doing, their individual physical characteristics are altered to facilitate tableting.
5. Bulky and dusty powders can be handled without producing a great deal of dust and airborne contamination.

6. Wet granulation prevents segregation of components of a homogeneous powder mixture during processing, transfering, and handling. In effect, the composition of each granule becomes fixed and remains the same as that of the powder mixture at the time of the wetting.

7. The dissolution rate of an insoluble drug may be improved by wet granulation with the proper choice of solvent and binder.

8. Controlled release dosage forms can be accomplished by the selection of a suitable binder and solvent.

C. Limitations of Wet Granulation

The greatest disadvantage of wet granulation is its cost because of the space, time, and equipment involved. The process is labor-intensive as indicated by the following.

1. Because of the large number of processing steps, it requires a large area with temperature and humidity control.

2. It requires a number of pieces of expensive equipment.

3. It is time consuming, especially the wetting and drying steps.

4. There is a possibility of material loss during processing due to the transfer of material from one unit operation to another.

5. There is a greater possibility of cross-contamination than with the direct-compression method.

6. It presents material transfer problems involving the processing of sticky masses.

7. It can slow the dissolution of drugs from inside granules after tablet disintegration if not properly formulated and processed.

A recent innovation in wet granulating, which reduces the time and energy requirements by eliminating the drying step, is the melt process. This method relies on the use of solids having a low softening or melting point which, when mixed with a powder formulation and heated, liquefy to act as binders [29,30]. Upon cooling, the mixture forms a solid mass in which the powders are bound together by the binder returning to the solid state. The mass is then broken and reduced to granules and compressed into tablets. Materials used as binders are polyethylene glycol 4000 and polyethylene glycol 6000 [31–33], stearic acid [30], and various waxes [34,35].

The amount of binder required is greater than for conventional liquid binders (i.e., 20 to 30% of the starting material).

Another advantage of the method is that the waxy materials also act as lubricants, although in some cases additional lubricant is required.

A new variation of the granulating process known as "moisture-activated dry granulation" [36] combines the efficiency of dry blending with the advantages of wet granulation. As little as 3% water produces agglomeration. The process requires no drying step because any free water is absorbed by the excipients used. After granulation, disintegrant and lubricant are added and the granulation is ready for compression.

The complex nature of wet granulation is still not well understood, which accounts for the continuing interest in research on the process. One significant problem is the degree of wetting or massing of the powders. Wetting plays an exceedingly important roll in the compression characteristics

of the granules, and also in the rate of drug release from the final tablet.
Some attempts at standardizing the wetting process have been made, particularly in the matter of overwetting [37−39]. Factors that affect wetting
are

1. Solubility of the powders
2. Relative size and shape of the powder particles
3. Degree of fineness
4. Viscosity of the liquid binder
5. Type of agitation

Conclusion

Although the wet granulation method is labor-intensive and time consuming, requiring a number of steps, it continues to find extensive application for a number of reasons. One reason is because of its universal
use in the past, the method persists with established products where,
for one reason or another, it cannot be replaced by direct compression.
Although a number of these products might lend themselves to the direct-
compression method, to do so would require a change in ingredients to
other excipients. A change of this nature would be considered a major
modification requiring a careful review to evaluate the need to carry out
additional studies or product stability, safety, efficacy, and bioavailability
as well as the impact of pertinent practical and regulatory considerations.
Since extensive data are likely to have been accumulated on the existing
product(s), there is understandable reluctance on the part of the drug industry to undertake such changes unless dictated by compelling reasons.
Another reason is that formulators prefer to use the wet granulation method
to assure content uniformity of tablets where small doses of drug(s) and/
or color additives are being dispersed by dissolving in the liquid binder.
This procedure affords better and more uniform distribution of the dissolved material. The method is also singular for use in the granulation of
drugs having a high dosage where direct compression, because of the necessity to add a considerable amount of filler to facilitate compaction, becomes
unfeasible because of the resulting increase in tablet size.

V. EXCIPIENTS AND FORMULATION

Excipients are inert substances used as diluents or vehicles for a drug. In
the pharmaceutical industry it is a catch-all term which includes various subgroups comprising diluents or fillers, binders or adhesives, disintegrants,
lubricants, glidants or flow promoters, colors, flavors, fragrances, and
sweeteners. All of these must meet certain criteria as follows:

1. They must be physiologically inert.
2. They must be acceptable to regulatory agencies.
3. They must be physically and chemically stable.
4. They must be free of any bacteria considered to be pathogenic or
   otherwise objectionable.
5. They must not interfere with the bioavailability of the drug.
6. They must be commercially available in form and purity commensurate
   to pharmaceutical standards.
7. For drug products that are classified as food, such as vitamins,
   other dietary aids, and so on, the excipients must be approved
   as food additives.

8. Cost must be relatively inexpensive.

9. They must conform to all current regulatory requirements.

Certain chemical incompatibilities have been reported in which the filler interfered with the bioavailability of the drug as in the case of calcium phosphate and tetracycline [40] and the reaction of certain amine bases with lactose in the presence of magnesium stearate [41,42].

To assure that no excipient interferes with the utilization of the drug, the formulator must carefully and critically evaluate combinations of the drug with each of the contemplated excipients and must ascertain compliance of each ingredient with existing standards and regulations.

Two comprehensive publications cataloging the various excipients used in the pharmaceutical industry are available. The first of these, published in German in 1974 by the combined Swiss Pharmaceutical firms of Ciba Geigy, Hoffman LaRoche, and Sandoz, and entitled *Katalog Pharmaceutischer Hillstoff* contains specifications, tests, and a listing of suppliers. More recently, the listing by the Academy of Pharmaceutical Science of the American Pharmaceutical Association entitled *Handbook of Pharmaceutical Excipients* was published.

The screening of drug—excipient and excipient—excipient interactions should be carried out routinely in preformulation studies. Determination of the optimum drug—excipient compatibility has been adequately presented in the literature [43—45].

A. Fillers (Diluents)

Tablet fillers or diluents comprise a heterogeneous group of substances that are listed in Table 3. Since they often comprise the bulk of the tablet, selection of a candidate from this group as a carrier for a drug is of prime importance. Since combinations are also a possibility, consideration should be given to possible mixtures.

Calcium sulfate, dihydrate, also known as terra alba or as snow-white filler, is an insoluble, nonhygroscopic, mildly abrasive powder. Better grades are white, others may be greyish white or yellowish white. It is the least expensive tablet filler and can be used for a wide variety of

Table 3   Tablet Fillers

Insoluble	Soluble
Calcium sulfate, dihydrate	Lactose
Calcium phosphate, dibasic	Sucrose
Calcium phosphate, tribasic	Dextrose
Calcium carbonate	Mannitol
Starch	Sorbitol
Modified starches (carboxymethyl starch, etc.)	
Microcrystalline cellulose	

acidic, neutral, and basic drugs. It has a high degree of absorptive capacity for oils and has few incompatibilities. Suggested binders are polymers such as PVP and methylcellulose, and also starch paste. See Example 1 for a typical formulation.

Determination of final tablet weight: Since the amount of starch added as starch paste in the massing procedure was not known, it is necessary to determine the amount added to find the tablet weight for pressing. One method of doing this is to weigh the completed granulation before pressing and determine the tablet weight as follows:

$$\frac{\text{Weight of completed granulation}}{\text{Theoretical number of tablets}} = \text{tablet weight}$$

Calcium phosphate, dibasic is insoluble in water, slightly soluble in dilute acids, and is a nonhygroscopic, neutral, mildly abrasive, fine white powder. It produces a hard tablet requiring a good disintegrant and an effective lubricant. Its properties are similar to those of calcium sulfate, but it is more expensive than calcium sulfate and is used to a limited extent in wet granulation. If inorganic acetate salts are present in the formulation, the tablets are likely to develop an acetic odor on aging. It can be used with salts of most organic bases, such as antihistamines, and with both water- and oil-soluble vitamines. Best binders are starch paste, PVP, methylcellulose, or microcrystalline cellulose. See Example 2.

Tricalcium phosphate Is an insoluble, slightly alkaline, nonhygroscopic, abrasive, fine white powder. It is used to a limited extent in wet granulation. It should not be used with strong acidic salts of weak organic bases or in the presence of acetate salts. It should not be used with the water-soluble B vitamines or with certain esters such as vitamin E or vitamin A acetate or palmitate.

Calcium carbonate is a dense, fine, white, insoluble powder. It is available in degrees of fineness. Precipitated calcium carbonate of a very fine particle size is used as a tablet filler. It is inexpensive, very white, nonhygroscopic, and inert. It cannot be used with acid salts or with acidic compounds. Its main drawback, when used as a filler, is that when granulated with aqueous solutions, care must be taken not to overwet by adding too much granulating liquid or overmixing because this produces a sticky, adhesive mass that is difficult to granulate, and tends to form hard granules that do not disintegrate readily. For this reason, it is best used in combination with another diluent such as starch or microcrystalline cellulose.

Calcium carbonate, in common with calcium phosphates, can serve as a dietary source of calcium. It also serves as an antacid in many products. A tablet with unique mouth-feel and a sweet, cooling sensation. See Example 3.

Microcrystalline cellulose (Avicel) is a white, insoluble, nonreactive, free-flowing, versatile filler. It produces hard tablets with low-pressure compression on the tablet press. It produces rapid, even wetting by its wicking action, thereby distributing the granulating fluid throughout the powder bed. It acts as an auxiliary wet binder promoting hard granules with less fines. It lessens screen blocking and promotes rapid, uniform drying. It promotes dye and drug distribution thus promoting uniform color dispersion without mottling. Microcrystalline cellulose also serves as a disintegrant, lubricant, and glidant. It has an extremely low coefficient

Example 1:   Phenylpropanolamine Hydrochloride Tablets

Ingredients	Quantity per tablet (mg)	Quantity per 10,000 tablets (g)
Phenylpropanolamine hydrochloride	60	600
Calcium sulfate, dihydrate	180	1800
10% Starch paste*	q.s.	q.s.
Starch 1500 (StaRx) (disintegrant)	12	120
Magnesium stearate (lubricant)	6	60

*Starch paste is made by mixing 10% starch with cold water and heating to boiling with constant stirring and until a thick, translucent white paste is formed.

Mix the phenylpropanolamine hydrochloride with the calcium sulfate in a sigma blade mixer for 15 min, then add sufficient starch paste to form a wet mass of suitable consistency.   Allow to mix for 30 min.   Pass the wet mass through a no. 14 screen and distribute on drying trays.   Dry in a forced-air oven at 120 to 130°F or in a fluid bed dryer.   When dry, screen through a no. 18 mesh screen, place in a twin-shell blender, add the starch 1500 starch and the magnesium stearate, blend for 6 to 8 min, and compress the completed granulation on a tablet press using 3/8-in. standard cup punches.

Example 2:   Diphenylhydramine (Benadryl) Tablets

Ingredients	Quantity per tablet (mg)	Quantity per 10,000 tablets (g)
Diphenhydramine hydrochloride	25	250
Calcium phosphate, dibasic	150	1500
Starch 1500 (StaRx)	20	200
10% PVP in 50% alcohol	q.s.	q.s.
Stearic acid, fine powder	75	75
Microcrystalline cellulose	25	250

Mix the diphenylhydramine hydrochloride, calcium phosphate, dibasic, and the starch in a planetary mixer.   Moisten the mixture with the poly-vinylpyrrolidone solution and granulate by passing through a 14-mesh screen.   Dry the resulting granules in an oven or fluid bed dryer at 120 to 130°F.   Reduce the size of the granules by passing through a

no. 20 mesh screen and dry. Add the stearic acid after passing
through a 30-mesh screen and the microcrystalline cellulose in a twin-
shell blender for 5 to 7 min. Compress to weight using 5/16-in. standard concave punches.

Important: In all formulations where an indeterminate amount of granulating agent is added, weigh the dried granulation *after* all other ingredients (e.g., lubricant, disintegrant, etc.), which were not part of
the wet granulation, and calculate the weight for compression of the
tablet as illustrated in Example 1.

Example 3: Calcium Carbonate-Glycine Tablets

Ingredients	Quantity per tablet (mg)	Quanity per 10,000 tablets (g)
Calcium carbonate, precipitated	400	4000
Glycine (aminoacetic acid)	200	2000
10% starch paste	q.s.	q.s.
Light mineral oil (50 to 60 SUS)	6.5	65

Mix the calcium carbonate and the glycine in a sigma blade or planetary
mixer for 10 min. Add the starch paste with constant mixing until sufficiently moistened to granulate.

Important: Powders are considered to be sufficiently moistened to granulate when a handful of the wet mass can be squeezed into a solid,
hand-formed mass that can be broken in half with a clean fracture
while the two halves retain their shape. (This method of determining
when powders are adequately moistened to granulate holds true for most
wet granulations.) Then force the wet mass through a no. 12 screen
and dry the resulting granulation in a forced-air oven at 130 to 140°F
or in a fluid bed dryer. Size the granules by passing thorugh a no.
12 mesh screen. Reduce the particle size by forcing through a no. 18
mesh screen. Using a 30-mesh screen, separate out all particles passing
through the screen. Finally, add the light mineral oil in a tumble
mixer. Mix for 8 min and compress to weight with 7/16-in. punches
and dies.

of friction, both static and dynamic, so that it has little lubricant requirement itself. However, when more than 20% of drug or other excipient is
added, lubrication is necessary. It can be advantageously combined with
other fillers such as lactose, mannitol, starch, or calcium sulfate. In
granulating, it makes the consistency of the wet mass less sensitive to
variations in water content and overworking. This is particularly useful
with materials which, when overwet or overmixed, become claylike, forming
a mass that clogs the screens during the granulating process. When dried,
these granules become hard and resistent to disintegration. Materials that

Example 4:   Calcium Carbonate and Water Only

Ingredient	Quantity
Calcium carbonate	1000 g
Water	300 ml

Example 5:   Calcium Carbonate Plus
Microcrystalline Cellulose and Water

Ingredient	Quantity
Calcium carbonate	1000 g
Avicel PH-101	100 g
Water	300 ml

cause this problem are clays such as kaolin and certain other materials
such as calcium carbonate.   This is illustrated by Examples 4 and 5.

The material of Example 4 produces a sticky mass, which is difficult to
granulate, whereas that of Example 5 produces a nonsticky mass, which
can be granulated through a no. 12 screen.

Microcrystalline cellulose added to a wet granulation improves bonding
on compression and reduces capping and friability of the tablet.

For drugs having a relatively small dose, microcrystalline cellulose used
as a filler acts also as an auxiliary binder, controls water-soluble drug
content uniformly, prevents migration of water-soluble dyes, and promotes
rapid and uniform evaporation of liquid from the wet granulation.

Although the usual method of making wet granulations is a two-step
procedure, Avicel granulations can be prepared by a one-step procedure.
In the two-step procedure, the drug and fillers are formed into granules
by wetting in the presence of a binder, drying the resulting moist mass,
and passing through a screen or mill to produce the desired granule size.
These granules are then blended with a disintegrant and lubricant, and,
if necessary, a glidant as in the following formulation (Example 6).

In the one-step method, the lubricant is included in the wet granulation contrary to what is usually taught concerning the necessity for small
particle size of these substances in order to coat the granules to obtain easy
die release.   Apparently, in the comminution of the granulation, sufficient lubricant becomes exposed to perform its intended function (Example 7).

The quantities used in the one-step formulations are the same as those
used in the two-step formulations.   This method eliminates the usual mixing
step for incorporating lubricants.   It is also a good idea to incorporate a
disintegrant in the wet granulation so that the granules will also disintegrate
readily when the tablet breaks up.   The practice is valid and can be widely used with modifications in one-step formulations.   The materials and

Example 6: Two-Step Avicel Granulation

Ingredients	Percent
Drug	q.s.
Avicel PH-101	q.s.
Confectioners sugar	2.5
Starch 1500	5.0
Starch paste, 10%	q.s.
Talc	3.0
Magnesium stearate	0.5
Sodium lauryl sulfate	1.0

Note: The amount of Avicel is replaced by the amount of the drug.
Blend the first four ingredients and pass through a no. 1 perforated plate (round hole) in a Fitzmill, hammers foreward. Add the starch paste to the powder to form a uniform wet mass. Dry at 140°F. Reduce the granule size by passing through a 20-mesh wire screen in a Fitzmill with knives foreward, medium speed. Transfer the dry granules to a twin-shell blender, add the last three ingredients, blend, and compress into tablets at the predetermined weight.

quantities used in the one-step method are essentially the same as those in the two-step method.

Example 7 illustrates the one-step method.

In the above formulation, if the amount of the drug is less than 10% of the total tablet weight, up to 30% of the Avicel may be replaced with calcium sulfate dihydrate.

Avicel PH-101 mixed with starch and cooked until the starch forms a thick paste makes an excellent wet granulating mixture. Using 60% Avicel and 40% starch as a 10% paste makes the wet mass easier to push through a screen, forms finer granulations and harder granules on drying with fewer fines than with starch paste alone.

Lactose, also known as milk sugar, is the oldest and traditionally the most widely used filler in the history of tablet making. In recent years, however, with new technology and new candidates, other materials have largely replaced it. Its solubility and sweetening power is somewhat less than that obtained with other sugars. It is obtained by crystallization from whey, a milk byproduct of cheese manufacture. Chemically, lactose exists in two isomeric forms, α and β. In solution, it tends to exist in equilibrium between the two forms. If it is crystallized at a temperature

Example 7:   One-Step Avicel Granulation

Ingredients	Percent
Drug	q.s
Avicel PH-101	q.s
Confectioners sugar	5.0
Starch 1500	6.0
Polyethylene glycol 6000	3.0
Talc	5.0
Magnesium lauryl sulfate	0.5
50% alcohol	q.s.

In a planetary mixer, blend all of the ingredients except the polyethylene glycol 6000 and the hydroalcoholic solution. Dissolve 1 part of polyethylene glycol 6000 in 1 part (w/v) of the 50% alcohol by heating to 50°C. Add this solution to the blended powders with constant mixing in a sigma blade mixer until uniformly moist. Spread the wet mass on trays and dry in an oven at 50°C. Pass the dry mass through a no. 2 perforated plate in a Fitzmill, knives foreward. Compress to predetermined size and weight. The use of alcohol is not essential, but it gives better control of wetting the powders and promotes more rapid drying.

over 93°C., β-lactose is produced that contains no water of crystallization (it is anhydrous). At lower temperatures, α-lactose monohydrate (hydrous) is obtained.

α-Lactose monohydrate is commercially available in a range of particle sizes from 200- to 450-mesh impalpable powder. The spray-dried form is used for the direct-compression method of producing tablets. Lactose is a reducing sugar and will react with amines to produce the typical Maillard browning reaction. It will also turn brown in the presence of highly alkaline compounds. Lactose is also incompatible with ascorbic acid, salicylamide, pyrilamine maleate, and phenylephrine hydrochloride [46]. Nevertheless, it has a place in tableting by the wet granulation method in the sense that on wetting some goes into solution thereby coating the drug and offering an amount of protection and slow release where rapid dissolution is not required.

Sucrose can be used as both a filler and as a binder in solution. It is commercially available in several forms: granular (table sugar), fine

Example 8:   Vitamin B$_{12}$ Tablets

Ingredient	Quantity per tablet	Quantity 10,000 per tablets
(1) Vitamin B$_{12}$ (Cyanocobalamin, USP)	55 µg*	0.55 g
(2) Lactose, anhydrous, fine powder	150 mg	1500 g
(3) 10% Gelatin solution	q.s.	q.s.
(4) Hydrogenated vegetable oil (Sterotex)	5 mg	50 g

*Includes 10% manufacturing overage.

Dissolve the vitamin B$_{12}$ in a portion of the gelatin solution. Slowly add
this to the lactose in a sigma blade mixer with constant mixing. Add sufficient additional gelatin solution to form a wet mass suitable to granulate.
Pass through a no. 14 mesh screen and dry in a suitable dryer. Reduce
the granule size by passing through a no. 20 mesh screen. Add the
Sterotex to the granules in a twin-shell blender and blend for 5 min. Compress using 1/2-in. punches and dies. This procedure forms hard tablets
that do not disintegrate readily but dissolve rather slowly.

granular, fine, superfine, and confectioners sugar. The latter is the most
commonly used in wet granulation formulations and contains 3% cornstarch
to prevent caking. It is very fine, 80% passing through a 325-mesh screen.
When used alone as a filler, sucrose forms hard granulations and tablets
tend to dissolve rather than disintegrate. For this reason, it is often used
in combination with various other insoluble fillers. It is used in chewable
tablets to impart sweetness and as a binder to impart hardness. In this
role it may be used dry or in solution. When used as a dry filler, it is
usually granulated with water only or with a hydroalcoholic binder. Various
tablet hardnesses can be obtained depending on the amount of binder used
to granulate. The more binder, the harder the granulation and the tablet.
If a mixture of water and alcohol is used, softer granules are produced.
      Sucrose has several disadvantages as a filler. Tablets made with a
major portion of it in the formulation tend to harden with time. It is not
a reducing sugar but with alkaline materials, it turns brown with time.
It is somewhat hygroscopic and tends to cake on standing.
      Dextrose has found some limited use in wet granulation as a filler and
binder. It can be used essentially in the same way as sucrose. Like sucrose, it tends to form hard tablets, especially if anhydrous dextrose is
used. It has the same disadvantages of both lactose and sucrose in that
it turns brown with alkaline materials and reacts with amines to discolor.
      Mannitol is a desirable filler in tablets when taste is a factor as in
chewable tablets. It is a white, odorless, pleasant-tasting crystalline powder that is essentially inert and nonhygroscopic. It is preferred as a
diluent in chewable tablets because of its pleasant, slightly sweet taste and
its smooth, cool, melt-down mouth-feel. Its negative heat of solution is

responsible for its cool taste sensation. Mannitol may be granulated with a
variety of granulating agents but requires more of the solution than either
sucrose or lactose and approximately the same as dextrose. The moisture
content of these granulations after overnight drying at 140 to 150°F for
sucrose, dextrose, and mannitol was less than 0.2%, except for dextrose
granulations made with 10% gelation and 50% glucose, in which case the
moisture content was 1.15 and 0.2%, respectively. In all lactose granulations,
the moisture content was between 4 and 5%. Mannitol and sucrose were the
lowest, having about the same moisture content. It was found, however,
that mannitol, although requiring more granulating solution, generally gave
a softer granulation than either sucrose or dextrose.

B.   Binders

Binders are the "glue" that holds powders together to form granules. They
are the adhesives that are added to tablet formulations to provide the cohesiveness required for the bonding together of the granules under compaction to form a tablet. The quantity used and the method of application
must be carefully regulated, since the tablet must remain intact until swallowed and must then release its medicament.

The appearance, elegance, and ease of compression of tablets are directly related to the granulation from which the tablets are compressed.
Granulations, in turn, are dependent on the materials used, processing
techniques, and equipment for the quality of the granulation produced. Of
these variables, none is more critical than the binder used to form the granulation, for it is largely the binder that is fundamental to the granulation
particle size uniformity, adequate hardness, ease of compression, and general quality of the tablet [47-50].

Binders are either sugars or polymeric materials. The latter fall into
two classes: (a) natural polymers such as starches or gums including
acacia, tragacanth, and gelatin, and (b) synthetic polymers such as polyvinylpyrrolidone, methyl- and ethylcellulose and hydroxypropylcellulose.
Binders of both types may be added to the powder mix and the mixture
wetted with water, alcohol-water mixtures, or a solvent, or the binder may
be put into solution in the water or solvent and added to the powder. The
latter method, using a solution of the binder, requires much less binding
material to achieve the same hardness than if added dry. In come cases,
it is not possible to get granules of sufficient hardness using the dry method.
In practice, solutions of binders are usually used in tablet production.
Reviews of binders and their effects are available [23,26,51,52]. A guide
to the amount of binder solution required by 3000 g of filler is presented
in Table 4.

A study on the addition of a plasticizer to the binder solution on the
tableting properties of dicalcium phosphate, lactose, and paracetamol
(acetaminophen) indicated that it improved the wet-massing properties of
the granulation. Including a placticizer in the binder increased the tensile
strength, raised the capping pressure, and reduced the friability of all
the tablets. The plasticizers used in this study were propylene glycol,
polyethylene glycol 400, glycerine, and hexylene glycol [53].

A list of commonly used binders is given in Table 5. These are treated
in detail as discussed in the following paragraphs.

Table 4   Granulating Solution Required by 3000 g of Filler

Volume of granulating solution required (ml)	Filler			
	Sucrose	Lactose	Dextrose	Mannitol
10% Gelatin	200	290	500	560
50% Glucose	300	325	500	585
2% Methylcellulose (400 cps)	290	400	835	570
Water	300	400	660	750
10% Acacia	220	400	685	675
10% Starch paste	285	460	660	810
50% Alcohol	460	700	1000	1000
10% PVP[a] in water	260[b]	340[b]	470[b]	525[b]
10% PVP[a] in alcohol	780[b]	650[b]	825[b]	900[b]
10% Sorbitol in water	280[b]	440[b]	750[b]	655[b]

[a]Polyvinylpyrrolidone.

[b]Derived by the author, not from source noted below.

Source: Taken in part from the *Technical Bulletin*, Atlas Mannitol, ICI Americas, Wilmington, Delaware, 1969.

Starch in the form of starch paste has historically been, and remains, one of the most used binders. Aqueous pastes usually employed range from 5 to 10% in concentration. Starch paste is made by suspending starch in 1 to 1-1/2 parts cold water, then adding 2 to 4 times as much boiling water with constant stirring. The starch swells to make a translucent paste that can then be diluted with cold water to the desired concentration. Starch paste may also be prepared by suspending the starch in cold water and heating to boiling in a steam-jacketed kettle with constant stirring. Starch paste is a versatile binder yielding tablets that disintegrate rapidly (see Example 9) and in which the granulation is made using starch as an internal binder and granulated with water only.

An example of granulation made by massing with starch paste as an internal binder rather than an external binder when wetted with water only as in Example 9 is given in Example 10.

Pregelatinized starch is starch that has been cooked and dried. It can be used in place of starch paste and offers the advantage of being soluble in warm water without boiling. It can also be used as a binder by adding it dry to the powder mix and wetting with water to granulate as indicated in Example 9.

Starch 1500 is a versatile, multipurpose starch that is used as a dry binder, a wet binder, and a disintegrant. It contains a 20% maximum cold water-soluble fraction which makes it useful for wet granulation. It can be

Table 5   Binders Commonly Used in Wet Granulation

Binder	Usual concentration
Cornstarch, USP	5–10% Aqueous paste
Pregelatinized cornstarch	5–10% Aqueous solution
Starch 1500	5–10% Aqueous paste
Gelatin (various types)	2–10% Aqueous solution
Sucrose	10–85% Aqueous solution
Acacia	5–20% Aqueous solution
Polyvinylpyrrolidone	5–20% Aqueous, alcoholic, or hydroalcoholic solution
Methylcellulose (various viscosity grades)	2–10% Aqueous solution
Sodium carboxymethylcellulose (low-viscosity grade)	2–10% Aqueous solution
Ethylcellulose (various viscosity grades)	2–15% Alcoholic solution
Polyvinyl alcohol (various viscosity grades)	2–10% Aqueous or hydroalcoholic solution
Polyethylenene glycol 6000	10–30% Aqueous, alcoholic, or hydroalcoholic solution

Example 9:   Aminophylline Tablets

Ingredients	Quantity per tablet (mg)	Quantity per 10,000 tablets (g)
Aminophylline	100	1.0
Tricalcium phosphate	50	0.5
Pregelatinized starch	15	0.15
Water	q.s.	q.s.
Talc	30	0.3
Mineral oil, light	2	0.02

Mix the aminophylline, tricalcium phosphate, and starch and moisten with water with constant mixing. Pass through a 12-mesh screen and dry at 110°F. Size the dry granulation through a 20-mesh screen; add the talc and mix in a suitable mixer for 8 min. Add the mineral oil, mix for 5 min, and compress with 5/16-in. standard concave punches.

Example 10: Pseudoephedrine Tablets

Ingredients	Quantity per tablet (mg)	Quantity per 10,000 tablets (kg)
Pseudoephedrine hydrochloride	60	0.6
Calcium sulfate, dihydrate	200	2.0
Citric acid, fine powder	5	0.05
Starch (as starch paste)	8	0.08
Sterotex (hydrogenated vegetable oil)	10	0.10
Alginic acid (disintegrant)	7	0.07
FD&C Yellow No. 6	0.005	(5 mg)

Mix the pseudoephedrine hydrochloride, citric acid, and calcium sulfate in an appropriate mixer for 15 min. Dissolve the FD&C Yellow No. 6 in the water used to make the starch paste, or dissolve the dye in a small quantity of water and add to the prepared paste. Add the starch paste sufficient to form a suitable wet mass and granulate through a 14-mesh screen. Dry at 120 to 130°F. Reduce the granules by passing through an 18-mesh screen, add the alginic acid, mix, and compress with 5/16-in. standard cup punches.

dry-blended with powder ingredients and granulated with ambient temperature water. The water-soluble fraction acts as an efficient binder, while the remaining fraction aids in the disintegration of the tablet. It also will not present overwetting problems as commonly experienced with pregelatinized starch.

Approximately 3 to 4 times as much starch is required to achieve the same tablet hardness as with starch paste.

Gelatin. If a still stronger binder is needed, a 2 to 10% gelatin solution may be used. Gelatin solutions should be made by first allowing the gelatin to hydrate in cold water for several hous or overnight, then heating the mixture to boiling. Gelatin solutions must be kept hot until they are used for they will gel on cooling. Although gelatin solutions have been extensively used in the past as a binder, they have been replaced to a large extent by various synthetic polymers, such as polyvinylpyrrolidone, methylcellulose, etc.

Gelatin solutions tend to produce hard tablets that require active disintegrants. The solutions are generally used for compounds that are difficult to bind. These solutions have another disadvantage in that they serve as culture media for bacteria and molds and, unless a preservative is added, they are quickly unfit to use.

Sucrose solutions are capable of forming hard granules. Some gradation of tablet hardness can be achieved by varying the concentration of sucrose from 20 to 85% depending on the strength of binding required.

In ferrous sulfate tablets, sucrose acts both as a binder and to protect the ferrous sulfate from oxidizing.

Example 11: Ferrous Sulfate Tablets

Ingredients	Quantity per tablet (mg)
Ferrous sulfate, dried	300
Corn starch	60
Sucrose as a 70% w/w syrup	q.s.
Explotab (sodium carboxymethyl starch)	45
Talc	30
Magnesium stearate	6

Mix the ferrous sulfate and the starch; moisten with the sugar solution to granulate through a 14-mesh screen. Dry in a tray oven overnight at 130 to 140°F. Size through an 18-mesh screen, add the Explotab, talc, and magnesium stearate, and compress to weight using 3/8-in. deep-cup punches. The reason for the deep-cup punches is that ferrous sulfate tablets need to be coated and tablets prepared with deep-cup punches lend themselves better to the coating process in that the edges at the perimeter are less obtuse than the standard punch tablets.

Sugar solutions are good carriers for soluble dyes, producing granulations and tablets of uniform color. Sugar syrups are used to granulate tribasic phosphate excipient, which usually requires a binder with greater cohesive properties than starch paste. Some other compounds for which sugar is indicated include aminophylline, acetophenetidin, acetaminophen, and meprobamate.

Acacia solutions have long been used in wet granulation, but now they have been largely replaced by more recently developed polymers such as polyvinylpyrrolidone and certain cellulose derivates. However, for drugs with a high dose and difficult to granulate, such as mephenesin, acacia is a suitable binder. It produces hard granules without an increase in hardness with time as is the case with gelatin. One disadvantage of acacia is that it is a natural product and is often highly contaminated with bacteria, making it objectionable for use in tablets. Tragacanth is another natural gum which, like acacia, has been used in 5 to 10% solutions as a binder. It does not produce granulations as hard as acacia solutions. Like acacia, it often has a high bacterial count. In the following formula, a soluble lubricant, polyethylene glycol 6000, is added to the acacia solution to assist both in tableting and in disintegration of the tablet (Example 12).

Polyvinylpyrrolidone has become a versatile polymeric binder. This compound, first developed as a plasma substitute in World War II, is inert and has the advantage of being soluble both in water and in alcohol. Although it is slightly hygroscopic, tablets prepared with it do not, as a rule, harden with age, which makes it a valuable binder for chewable tablets (Example

Example 12:   Mephenesin Tablets

Ingredients	Quantity per tablet (mg)
Mephenesin	400
Acacia, 10% aqueous solution with 1% polyethylene glycol 6000	q.s.
Talc	8
Starch	20

Add sufficient acacia-polyethylene glycol 6000 solution to the mephenesin in a planetary or other suitable mixer to granulate; pass the wet mass through
a 12-mesh screen and dry in an oven or other suitable dryer at 130 to 140°F. Force the dry granules
through a 16-mesh screen, add the talc and the
starch in a tumble mixer, mix for 10 to 15 min.
and compress using 1/2-in flat-face, bevel edge
punches.

13). Generally, it is better to granulate insoluble powders with aqueous or
hydroalcoholic solutions of PVP and to granulate soluble powders with PVP
in alcoholic solution. Effervescent tablets comprising a mixture of sodium
bicarbonate and citric acid can be made by wet granulation using solutions
of PVP in anhydrous ethanol since no acid-base reaction occurs in this
anhydrous medium. Anhydrous ethanol should always be used in this granulation and not anhyrous isopropanol, since the latter leaves a trace of its
odor in the tablets no matter how, or how long, the granulation has been
dried. A concentration of 5% PVP in anhydrous ethanol produces a granulation of good compressibility of fine powders of sodium bicarbonate and
citric acid, and makes the vigorous effervescence and rapid dissolution of
the resulting tablets. Polyvinylpyrrolidone is also an excellent binder for
chewable tablets, especially of the aluminum hydroxide—magnesium hydroxide
type (Example 12). The inclusion of 2 to 3% of glycerine (based on the
final weight of the tablet) tends to reduce hardening of these tablets with
age. It is a versatile and excellent all-purpose binder used in approximately the same concentration as starch, but considerably more expensive.

Methylcellulose in aqueous solutions of 1 to 5%, depending on the viscosity grade, may be used to granulate both soluble and insoluble powders.
A 5% solution produces granulations similar in hardness to 10% starch paste.
It has the advantage of producing granulations that compress readily, producing tablets that generally do not harden with age. Methylcellulose is
a better binder for soluble excipients such as lactose, mannitol, and other
sugars. It offers considerable latitude in binding strength because of the
range of viscosity grades available. Low-viscosity grades, 10 to 50 cps,
allow for higher working concentrations of granulating agent than higher
viscosity grades, such as the 1000 to 10,000 cps grades.

Example 13:   Chewable Antacid Tablets

Ingredients	Quantity per tablet (mg)
Aluminum hydroxide, dried gel	200
Magnesium hydroxide, fine powder	200
Sugar, confectioners 10X	20
Mannitol, fine powder	180
Polyvinylpyrrolidone, 10% solution in 50% alcohol solution	q.s.*
Magnesium stearate	12
Cab-O-Sil M-5	4
Glycerine	8
Oil of peppermint	0.2

Mix the first four ingredients in a suitable mixer. Add
the glycerine to the PVP solution and use to moisten
the powder mix. Granulate by passing through a 14-mesh
screen and dry at 140 to 150°F. Mix the oil of peppermint
with the Cab-O-Sil and the magnesium stearate, mix, and
size through a 20-mesh screen. Mix well and compress
using 1/2-in. flat-face, bevel edge punches.
*10 milligrams of dry PVP may be added to the powder mix
and granulated with 50% hydroalcoholic solution instead of
the PVP solution. This, however, is about 3 times as
much as is required when used in solution.

Sodium carboxymethylcellulose (sodium CMC) in concentrations of 5 to
15% may be used to granulate both soluble and insoluble powders. It produces softer granulations than PVP, and tablets have a greater tendency
to harden. It is incompatible with magnesium, calcium, and aluminum salts,
and this tends to limit its utility to some extent. Although producing
softer granulations, these generally compress well. However, tablets have
a relatively long disintegration time.

Ethylcellulose is insoluble in water and is used in alcohol solutions. Like
methylcellulose, it is available in a range of viscosities, depending on the
degree of substitution of the polymer. Low-viscosity grades are usually
used in concentrations of 2 to 10% in ethanol. It may be used to granulate
powders which do not readily form compressible granules, such as acete-
minophen, caffeine, meprobamate, and ferrous fumarate (Example 14), and
it offers a nonaqueous binder for medicaments that do not tolerate water
(Example 15).

Polyvinyl alcohols are water-soluble polymers available in a range of viscosities. As granulating agents they resemble acacia but have the advantage
of not being heavily laden with bacteria. They are film-formers and their
granulations are softer than those made with acacia, yielding tablets that

Example 14: Ferrous Fumarate Tablets

Ingredients	Quantity per tablet (mg)
Ferrous fumarate, fine powder	300
Ethylcellulose 50 cps, 5% in ethanol	q.s. (approx. 10 mg)
Avicel	30
Stearowet*	10
Cab-O-Sil	5

Slowly add the ethylcellulose solution to the ferrous fumarate in a double-S arm mixer with constant mixing until sufficiently moist to granulate. Force through a 16-mesh screen and dry in a suitable dryer. Transfer the dry granulation to a tumble mixer, add the Stearowet and the Cab-O-Sil, mix, and compress using 3/8-in. standard cup punches.
*Stearowet is a mixture of calcium stearate and sodium lauryl sulfate. This combination of hydrophobic and a hydrophilic lubricant tends to decrease the disintegration time of the tablets.

disintegrate more readily and generally do not harden with age. Viscosities lending themselves to tablet granulation range from 10 to 100 cps.

Polyethylene glycol 6000 may serve as an anhdrous granulating agent where water or alcohol cannot be used. Polyethylene glycol 6000 is a white to light yellow unctuous solid melting at 70 to 75°C and solidifying at 56 to 63°C.

Example 15: Ascorbic Acid Tablets

Ingredient	Quantity per tablet (mg)
Ascorbic acid, 20-mesh granules	250
Ethylcellulose 50 cps, 10% in ethanol	q.s. (approx. 4 mg)
Explotab (sodium carboxymethyl starch)	15
Calcium silicate	10

In a rotating drum or coating pan add the ethylcellulose solution slowly to the ascorbic acid with rapid rotation of the drum. Dry with warm air directed into the rotating drum or pan equipped with an exhaust system to remove alcohol vapor. When dry, transfer to a tumble mixer, add the Explotab and the calcium silicate, mix, and compress with 13/32-in. punches.

Example 16:   Polyethylene 6000 granulation

Ingredients	Quantity per tablet
Drug	q.s.
Filler, calcium sulfate dihydrate, or dicalcium phosphate, or lactose, or any other suitable filler	q.s.
Polyethylene glycol 6000 up to 30% of the above mixture*	
Explotab	q.s.
Magnesium stearate	q.s.
Aerosil 200	q.s.

Uniformly mix the drug with the filler and the polyethylene glycol 6000 and pass through a pulverizer using a no. 20 screen. Spread on trays and place in an oven at 75 to 80°C for 3 hr. Cool the heated mass to room temperature and screen through an 18-mesh screen, blend with the balance of the ingredients, and compress into tablets of proper weight.

*Because of variation of drug and filler, the amount of polyethylene glycol 6000 needs to be determined on an experimental basis for each formula.

A procedure for making tablets by this method has been given by Shah et al. [29] in which polyethylene glycol 6000 acts as the binding agent (Example 16).

Another method described by Rubenstein [32] carries out the granulation in a coating pan modified so that the pan contents can be heated to 60°C. The disintegrant is charged into the pan followed by 4% of polyethylene glycol 6000 in powder form. The heated pan is then rotated to melt the polyethylene glycol. The drug is then added and the whole mass is tumbled and heated for 5 min. The molten PEG 6000 acts as a binder covering the surface of the powders. After thoroughly mixing, the heat is discontinued and the mass allowed to cool to room temperature. During the cooling period, the PEG 6000 solidifies coating the powders to produce granules. The resulting granules are free flowing but require the addition of a glidant (0.2% Aerosil 200) for tableting. The granules are not self-lubricating and require the addition of a lubricant to permit tableting.

Sustained Release Applications

Binders as waterproofing agents having been used to obtain sustained or prolonged release dosage forms. By granulating or coating powders with relatively insoluble or slowly soluble binders (i.e. shellac, waxes, fatty acids and alcohols, esters and various synthetic polymers), tablets having delayed or prolonged release properties have been formulated. This application is discussed later in this chapter.

C. Lubricants

Lubricants are used in tablet formulations to ease the ejection of the tablet from the die, to prevent sticking of tablets to the punches, and to prevent excessive wear on punches and dies. They function by interposing a film of low shear strength at the interface between the tablet and the die wall and the punch face. Lubricants should be carefully selected for efficiency and for the properties of the tablet formulation.

Metal stearates because of their unctuouse nature and available small particle size, are probably the most efficient and commonly used lubricants. They are generally unreactive but are slightly alkaline (except zinc), and have the disadvantage of retarding tablet disintegration and dissolution because of their hydrophobic nature [59,63,64]. Of the metal stearates, magnesium is the most widely used. It also serves as a glidant and antiadherent. Butcher and Jones [59] showed that particle size, packing density, and frictional shear tests are necessary to evaluate the quality and suitability of commercially available stearates as lubricants.

Stearowet C, because of its surfactant component, is less likely to interfere with disintegration and dissolution. Sodium lauryl sulfate is an auxiliary lubricant as well as a surfactant.

In instances where lubrication is a problem, an internal and an external lubricant can be used in conjunction with each other as given in Example 17.

Allow the gelatin to soak in 70% of the water for several hous or overnight. Heat to 80°F, add the polyethylene glycol 6000, stir until dissolved, and cool slowly to 110 to 120°F. Add water, maintaining the temperature in the above range. The solution must be used at this temperature because it will gel on cooling.

Stearic acid is a less efficient lubricant than the metal stearates. It melts at 69 to 70°C, so that it does not melt under usual conditions of storage. It should not be used with alkaline salts of organic compounds such as sodium barbiturates, sodium saccharin, or sodium bicarbonate. With these compounds it has a tendency to form a gummy, sticky mass that causes sticking to the punches.

Numerous studies of lubricants indicate that there is no universal lubricant and that the formula, method of manufacture, and the formulators knowledge and experience determine the choice and amount used [56–60].

In selecting a lubricant, the following should be considered:

1. Lubricants markedly reduce the bonding properties of many excipients.
2. Overblending is one of the main causes of lubrication problems. Lubricants should be added last to the granulation and tumble-blended for not more than 10 min.
3. The optimum amount of lubricant must be determined for each formulation. Excess lubricant is no more effective but rather interferes with both disintegration and bioavailability by waterproofing the granules and tablet.
4. Lubricant efficiency is a function of particle size; therefore, the finest grade available should be used and screened through a 100 to 300-mesh screen before use.

Ragnarssen et al. [61] found that a short mixing time for magnesium stearate in excipient blends resulted in poor distribution of the lubricant but did not impair the lubricating efficiency in tablet compression.

Example 17:   Analgesic-Decongestant Tablets

Ingredients	mg per tablet
Acetaminophen	325
Pseudoephedrine hydrochloride	30
Chlorpheniramine maleate	2
Sucrose	20
10% gelatin—5% polyethylene glycol 6000 aqueous solution*	q.s.
Microcrystalline cellulose	30
Starch 1500	15
Stearowet C	15
Cab-O-Sil (silica aerogel)	0.2

Mix the acetaminophen, pseudoephedrine hydrochloride, chlorpheniramine maleate, and sucrose, and granulate with the gelatin —polyethylene 6000 solution, passing the wet mass through a 12-mesh screen. Dry at 130 to 140°F and size through an 18-mesh screen. Add the Cab-O-Sil, Starch 1500, and microcrystalline cellulose in order and blend for 15 min. Finally, add the Sterowet C and blend for 3 min. Compress using 7/16-in. standard cup punches.
*Preparation of gelatin-polyethylene glycol 6000 solution.

Another study [62] found that prolonged mixing time tends to limit or reduce lubricant effectiveness and that glidants should be added first and intimately blended after which the lubricant is added and blended for a relatively short time.

Insufficient lubrication causes straining of the tablet press as it labors to eject the tablet from the die. This may cause a characteristic screeching sound and straining of the press parts involved. Another indication of insufficient lubrication is the presence of striations or scratch marks on the edges of the tablets.

Lubricants fall into two classes: water-insoluble and water-soluble. A listing of the hydrophobic and the soluble lubricants is given in Table 6.

Hydrogenated vegetable oils, commercially available as Sterotex and Duratex, are bleached, refined, and deodorized hydrogenated vegatable oils of food grade. They are usually available in spray-congealed form. While the particle size is not as small as may be desirable, the establishment of appropriate blending times with specific granulations can aid in the distribution on the granules through attrition of the lubricant powder. These have special application where alkaline metal stearates cannot be used, or where their metallic taste may be objectional as in tablets or lozenges to be dissolved in the mouth. Example 18 illustrates this use.

Table 6 Lubricants: Typical Amounts Used

Lubricants	Amount used in granulations (% w/w)
Hydrophobic	
Metal stearates, calcium, magnesium, zinc	0.5–2
Stearowet C: a water-wettable mixture of calcium stearate and sodium lauryl sulfate	0.5–2
Stearic acid, fine powder	1.0–3.0
Hydrogenated vegetable oils (Sterotex, Duratex)	1–3
Talc	5–10
Starch	5–10
Light mineral oil	1–3
Water-Soluble	
Sodium benzoate	2–5
Sodium chloride	5–20
Sodium and magnesium lauryl sulfate	1–3
Polyethylene glycol 4000 and 6000 (Carbowax 4000 and 6000), fine powder	2–5

High-Melting Waxes. Numerous food grade waxes are available, and while these are not generally used as lubricants, they offer possibilities for investigation. Waxes of both mineral sources (ceresin) and vegetable sources (carauba) offer possibilities as lubricants.

Talc acts as both lubricant and glidant. It is less efficient than the previously mentioned products and larger quantities are required for adequate lubrication. It has the disadvantage of retarding disintegration. Smaller quantities can be used in conjunction with other lubricants. It is essential that talc used in tableting be asbestos-free and, to this end, each lot should be accompanied by a certification from the supplier to this effect.

Starch is derived from a number of sources: corn, potatoe, rice, and tapioca. It may exist as dry granules, powder, swollen granules, in solution, and may be used as a filler, binder, disintegrant and film-former. It is available both as hydrophilic and hydrophobic corn starch.

Pharmaceutically cornstarch is the item of commerce most commonly used. Although there are much more efficient lubricants, starch because of its multiple properties is often included in formulations as an auxiliary lubricant because of its many applications in tablet making by the wet granulation method.

Mineral oil. Light mineral oil having a Saybolt viscosity of 50 to 60 SUS (approximately 8 centistokes) is a liquid lubricant with universal application because it is unreactive, odorless, tasteless, and can be easily sprayed onto

Example 18:   Medicated Throat Lozenges

Ingredients	per tablet
Sucrose, fine powder (10X confectioners sugar	8.00
Acacia, fine powder	0.50
Citric acid, fine powder	15 mg
10% Gelatin solution	q.s.
Menthol	12 mg
Benzocaine	10 mg
Hexylresorcinol	2.4 mg
Hydrogenated vegetable oil (Sterotex, Duratex)	160 mg
Ethanol 95%	0.04 ml

Mix the sucrose, acacia, and citric acid and mass with the gelation solution. Granulate through an 8-mesh screen and dry at 130 to 140°F. Dissolve the methol, benzocaine, and the hexylresorcinol in the ethanol and distribute on the granulation in a twin-shell blender. Spread on trays in an oven and remove alcohol with forced air at ambient temperature. Transfer the granulation to a tumbel blender, add the hydrogenated vegetable oil, blend for 5 min, and compress with 3/4-in. flat-face, bevel edge punches.

granulations. It should be sprayed onto the formulation in a closed container, preferably in a twin-shell or double-cone blender equipped with a spray head or an intensifier bar. On compression, tablets lubricated with mineral oil often show mottling with oil spots on the surface of the tablet. This is more noticeable with colored tablets, especially dark colors. This mottling disappears after a day or two as the oil disperses in the tablet. One disadvantage of mineral oil as a lubricant is that the granulation, after the addition of the oil, must be compressed within 24 to 48 hr because the oil has a tendency to penetrate into the granules and thereby lose its effectiveness as a lubricant. Mineral oil is a largely neglected but excellent lubricant that greately reduces die wall friction and sticking to punches.

Sodium benzoate and sodium chloride have limited application in pharmaceuticals but find some use in household products. Sodium benzoate is essentially tasteless and can be used in tablets intended to be chewed or allowed to dissolve in the mouth.

Sodium and magnesium lauryl sulfate are water-soluble surfactants that can be used instead of the metal stearates to counteract their waterproofing properties as tablet lubricants. Studies indicate that granulations run on a rotary tablet press using both magnesium stearate and magnesium lauryl sulfate as lubricants, produced tablets having less variation in physical properties with the latter than with the former. It appears that magnesium lauryl sulfate is at least as efficient as magnesium stearate and has the advantage of reduced interference with dissolution [65,66].

Magnesium lauryl sulfate also has less taste than the sodium salt and is therefore better for chewable tablets.

Polyethylene glycol 4000 and 6000, also known as Carbowax 4000 and 5000, are water-soluble lubricants that find considerable use in tablet manufacture and in the formulation of chewable tablets. They are generally unreactive and can be used with sensitive ingredients such as aspirin, ascorbic acid, and other vitamins.

As with other lubricants, the smaller the particle size, the greater the distribution on granules, which makes for more efficient lubrication. Solid polyethylene glycols in very fine powder are not commercially available; however, they may be micronized if cooled to $-10°$ to $-20°C$.

Polyethylene glycol 6000 can be used in aqueous, alcoholic, or hydroalcoholic solution with various binders thereby obtaining a binder-lubricant combination that can be used in wet massing. Solutions may also be sprayed or atomized onto powders in a fluidized bed granulator or in a twin-shell or double-cone blender equipped with a vacuum takeoff to remove solvent thus applying both binder and lubricant.

Recently, two new additions to the field of lubricants have been proposed. These are sodium stearyl fumarate and glyceryl behenate [67]. Using magnesium stearate for comparison, these were added to granulations of lactose and salicylic acid and compressed with equivalent force on an instrumented tablet press. The new lubricants showed less effect on tablet strength and had a lesser effect on dissolution rate of the active ingredients than did magnesium stearate. Magnesium stearate and sodium stearyl fumarate were effective at 1 to 3% levels whereas glyceryl behenate required 3% for effective lubrication.

In tablet formulation, a lubricant often permits the resolution of several production problems that are related to compression. Lubrication facilitates glidancy of granules during material flow, eliminates binding in the die, and minimizes picking and sticking to punch-face surfaces on compression. Mixing time in the scale-up of tablet production is greatly influenced by the type of mixing equipment and by the batch size. Vigorous mixing shortens the time required for the distribution of the disintegrant and the batch size, due to the shear weight on the charge, influences the mixing time because of the increased flow of particles in tumble-, twin-shell, and double-cone-type mixers. The release characteristics and performance criteria of the final tablet (such as physical integrity and stability) depend on lubricant— excipient interaction and the manner in which these materials are affected by mixing.

D. Disintegrants

Disintegrant is the term applied to various agents added to tablet granulation for the purpose of causing the compressed tablet to break apart (disintegrate) when placed in an aqueous environment. Basically, the disintegrant's major function is to oppose the efficiency of the tablet binder and the physical forces that act under compression to form the tablet. The stronger the binder, the more effective must be the disintegrating agent in order for the tablet to release its medication. Ideally, it should cause the tablet to disrupt, not only into the granules from which it was compressed, but also into the powder particles from which the granulation was prepared [68–71].

There are two methods used for incorporating disintegrating agents into tablets. These methods are called *external addition* and *internal addition*.
In this, the disintegrant is added to the sized granulation with mixing just
prior to compression. In the internal addition method, the disintegrant is
mixed with other powders before wetting the powder mixture with the granulating solution. Thus, the disintegrant is incorporated within the granule.
When this method is used, part of the disintegrant can be added internally
and part externally. This provides immediate disruption of the tablet into
the previously compressed granules while the disintegrating agent within
the granules produces further erosion of the granules to the original powder particles. Although this latter is an attractive theory, it is only
partially effective in practice because any disintegrating agent bound within
the granules loses some of its disruptive force due to its encasement by the
binder. Nevertheless, the two-step method usually produces better and
more complete disintegration than the usual method of adding the disintegrant
to the granulation surface only.

Disintegrants constitute a group of materials that, on contact with water,
swell, hydrate, change in volume or form, or react chemically to produce a
disruptive change in the tablet. This group includes various forms of
starch, cellulose, algins, vegetable gums, clays, ion exchange reins, and
acid-base combinations. A list of commonly used tablet disintegrants and
the amounts usually used are given in Table 7.

Starch is the oldest and probably the most widely used disintegrant
used by the pharmaceutical industry. Regular cornstarch USP, however,
has certain limitations and has been replaced to some extent by modified
starches with specialized characteristics to serve specific functions. Starch
1500 is a physically modified cornstarch that meets all the specifications of
pregelatinized starch NF. It is somewhat unique in that it lends itself well

Table 7 Disintegrants: Typical Amounts Used

Disintegrant	Concentration in granulation (% w/w)
Starch USP	5–20
Starch 1500	5–15
Avicel PH 101, PH 102 (microcrystalline cellulose	
Solka floc (purified wood cellulose)	5–15
Alginic acid	5–10
Explotab (sodium starch glycolate)	2–8
Guar gum	2–8
Polyclar AT (polyvinylpyrrolidone, crosslinked PVP)	0.5–5
Amberlite IPR 88 (ion exchange resin)	0.5–5
Methylcellulose, sodium carboxymethylcellulose, hydroxy-propylmethylcellulose	5–10

to conventional manufacturing techniques, especially to wet granulation. There are many classical theories that attempt to explain the mode of action of disintegrants, especially starches. One theory is that the disintegrant forms pathways throughout the tablet matrix that enable water to be drawn into the structure by capillary action, thus leading to disruption of the tablet. An equally popular concept relates to the swelling of starch grains on exposure to water, a phenomenon that physically ruptures the particle–particle bonding in the tablet matrix. Neither of these mechanisms explains the dramatic explosion that often takes place when tablets containing starch are exposed to water. Unique work carried out by Hess [72] would seem to suggest that on compression there is a significant distortion of the starch grains. On exposure to water, these grains attempt to recover their original shape, and in so doing release a certain amount of stress which, in effect, is responsible for the destruction of interparticulate hydrogen bonds and causes the tablet to be literally blown apart. Starch thus functions as the classical disintegrant. Starch 1500, by virtue of its manufacturing process, retains the disintegrant qualities of the parent cornstarch. These qualities make it a versatile disintegrating agent as both an internal and external disintegrant in tablet formulations (Example 19).

Avicel (microcrystalline cellulose) is a highly effective disintegrant. It has a fast wicking rate for water, hence, it and starch make an excellent combination for effective and rapid disintegration in tablet formulations. One drawback to its use is its tendency to develop static charges with increased moisture content, sometimes causing striation or separation in the granulation. This can be partially overcome by drying the cellulose to remove the moisture. When wet-granulated, dried, and compressed, it does not disintegrate as readily as when unwetted. It can be used with almost all drugs except those that are moisture-sensitive (such as aspirin, penicillin, and vitamins) unless it is dried to a moisture content of less than 1% and then handled in a dehumidified area.

Solka floc (purified wood cellulose) is a white, fibrous, inert, neutral material that can be used alone or in combination with starch as a disintegrating agent for aspirin, penicillin, and other drugs that are pH- and moisture-sensitive. Its fibrous nature endows it with good wicking properties and is more effective when used in combination with clays such as kaolin, bentonite, or Veegum. This combination is especially effective in tablet formulations possibly having a high moisture content (such as ammonium chloride, sodium salicylate, and vitamins).

Alginic acid is a polymer derived from seaweed comprising D-mannuronic and L-glucuronic units. Its affinity for water and high sorption capacity make it an excellent disintegrant. It is insoluble in water, slightly acid in reaction, and should be used only in acidic or neutral granulations. It can be used with aspirin and other analgesic drugs. If used with alkaline salts or salts of organic acids, it tends to form soluble or insoluble alginates that have gelling properties and delay disintegration. It can be successfully used with ascorbic acid, multivitamin formulations, and acid salts of organic bases.

Explotab (sodium starch glycolate) is a partially substituted carboxymethyl starch consisting of granules that absorb water rapidly and swell. The machanism by which this action takes place involves accelerated absorption of water leading to an enormous increase in volume of granules. This results in rapid and uniform tablet disintegration. Explotab is official in the N.F. XVI.

Example 19: Multivitamin Tablets

Ingredients	Per tablet
Vitamin A (coated)	5000 USP units
Vitamin D (coated)	400 USP units
Vitamin C (ascorbic acid, coated)	60 mg
Vitamin B_1 (thiamine mononitrate)	2 mg
Vitamin B_2 (riboflavin)	1.5 mg
Vitamin B_6 (pyridoxine hydrochloride)	1 mg
Vitamin B_{12} (cyanocobalamin)	2 µg
Calcium pantothenate	3 mg
Niacinamide	10 mg
Sodium saccharin	0.3 mg
Mannitol NF (fine powder)	350 mg
Starch 1500 (internal disintegrant)	65 mg
Magnesium stearate	10 mg
Talc	12 mg
Starch 1500 (external disintegrant)	40 mg
Flavor	q.s.

Blend the mannitol, saccharin, and internal Starch 1500
with 10% of the riboflavin and all the other vitamins
except A, D, and C. Granulate this blend with water.
Dry at 120°F, pass through a 16-mesh screen, and add
the flavor. Mix the ascorbic acid with the magnesium
stearate; mix the vitamins A and D with the remainder of
the riboflavin. Add these and the talc and the external
Starch 1500 to the previous mixture and mix well. Compress using 7/16-in., flat-face, bevel edge punches.

Guar gum is a naturally occurring gum that is marketed under the
trade name Jaguar. It is a free-flowing, completely soluble, neutral polymer composed of sugar units and is approved for food use. It is available
in various particle sizes and finds general use as a tablet disintegrant. It
is not sensitive to pH, moisture content, or solubility of the tablet matrix.
Although an excellent disintegrant, it has several drawbacks. It is not
always pure white, and it sometimes varies in color from off-white to tan.
It also tends to discolor with time in alkaline tablet.

Polyclar AT (Polyplasdone XL and Polyplasdone XL10) are crosslinked,
insoluble homopolymers of vinylpyrrolidone. Polyplasdone XL ranges in
particle size from 0 to 400 + µm, and Polyplasdone XL10 has a narrower
range and smaller particle size (0 to 74 µm), which makes for better distribution and reduced mottling in tablet formulations. Tablet hardness

and abrasion resistance are less affected by the addition of Polyplasdone XL as compared to starches, cellulose, and pectin compounds [73]. A tendency toward tablet capping is reduced [74]. Polyplasdone XL disintegrants do not reduce tablet hardness and provide rapid disintegration and improved dissolution [75–77]. Polyplasdone, due to its high capillary activity, rapidly draws water into the tablet causing swelling which exceeds the tablet strength, reuslting in spontaneous tablet disintegration.

Amberlite IPR 88 (ion exchange resin) has the ability to swell in the presence of water thereby acting as a disintegrant. Care must be taken in the selection of a resin as a disintegrant since many resins have the ability to adsorb drugs upon them. Anionic and cationic resins have been used to absorb substances and release them when the charge changes.

Methyl cellulose, sodium carboxymethylcellulose, and hydroxypropyl-cellulose are disintegrants to some extent depending on their ability to swell on contact with water. Generally, these do not offer any advantage over more efficient products such as the starches and microcrystalline cellulose. However, in certain cases they may be of benefit when used in conjunction with the above.

E. Glidants

Glidants are materials that improve the flow characteristics of granulations by reducing interparticulate friction. They increase the flow of materials from larger to smaller apertures, from the hopper into the die cavities of the tablet press.

The effects produced by different glidants depend on (a) their chemical nature in relation to that of the powder or granule (i.e., the presence of unsaturated valences, ionic or hydrogen bonds on the respective surfaces that could interact chemically) and (b) the physical factors including particle size, shape, and distribution of the glidant and various other formulation components, moisture content, and temperature. In general, hydrophilic glidants tend to be more effective on hydrophilic powders, and the opposite is true for hydrophobic glidants. For any particular system there is usually an optimum concentration above which the glidant may start to act as a antiglidant [78]. This optimum depends, among other factors, on the moisture level in the granulation [79].

When fine particles of less than the optimum for flowability are added to a bulk powder of similar chemical constitution, there is often an improvement in the rate of flow through an orifice [80]. The improvement is dependent on the size and concentration of the fine particles; the smaller the particles, the lower the concentration required to produce an increased flow.

Some glidants commonly used and suggested concentrations for optimum glidant effect are shown in Table 8.

The silica-type glidants are the most efficient probably because of their small particle size. In one study [81], it was found that all silica-type glidants improved the flow properties of granulations as reflected in increased tablet weight and in decreased weight variation in the tablets. Chemically, the silica glidants are silicon dioxide. They are available as two types, both insoluble: (a) the pyrogenic silicas prepared by burning silicon tetrachloride in an atmosphere of oxygen and (b) the hydrogels, which are prepared by the precipitation of soluble silicates. The pyrogenic

Table 8   Commonly Used Glidants and
Usual Concentration Range

Glidant	Percent
Silica aerogels	
Cab-O-Sil M-5	0.1–0.5
Aerosil 200	0.1–0.5
QUSO F-22	0.1–0.5
Calcium stearate	0.5–2.0
Magnesium stearate	0.2–2.0
Stearowet C*	0.2–2.0
Zinc stearate	0.2–1.0
Calcium silicate	0.5–2.0
Starch, dry flow	1.0–10.0
Starch 1500	1.0–10.0
Magnesium lauryl sulfate	0.2–2.0
Magnesium carbonate, heavy	1.0–3.0
Magnesium oxide, heavy	1.0–3.0
Talc	1.0–5.0

silicas are generally composed of smaller particles that tend to be more spherical in shape.   Pyrogenic silicas are available in both hydrophilic and hydrophobic form [82].   The particle size of most commercially available silicas used as glidants range in size from 2 to 20 nm and have an enormous surface area averaging 200 to 300 m^2 g^{-1}.

There are no specific rules dictating the amount of any glidant required for a particular granulation.   Glidants differ not only in chemical properties but also in physical characteristics such as size, frictional properties, structure, and density.   For these reasons the amount of glidant varies with the material to which it is added.   Since it is the purpose of the glidant to confer fluidity on the granulation, this property may be measured by one of several methods [83].   One method is the determination of the angle of repose [84,85].   When powdered material is allowed to fall freely from an orifice onto a flat surface, the material deposited forms a cone. The base angle of the cone is referred to as the angle of repose.   By this method it has been found, for example, that the repose angle of a sulfathiazole granulation increases with decreasing particle size.   Talc added in small quantities reduces the angle of repose, indicating greater flow, but tends to increase the repose angle at higher concentrations, thus becoming an antiglidant.   The addition of fines causes a marked increase in the repose angle.

Another method of determining the effect of glidants on the flow properties of a granulation is that of allowing a given amount of granulation, with and without glidant, to flow through an orifice ranging in size from

3/8 to 1 in. in diameter depending on the size of the granules, and observing the efflux time. The glidant efficiency factor may then be determined as follows:

$$f = \frac{\text{rate of flow in presence of glidant}}{\text{rate of flow in absence of glidant}}$$

Since many materials used as glidants are also efficient lubricants, a reduction in interparticulate friction may also be encountered. This reduction can occur in two ways: (a) The fine material may adhere to the surface rugosity, minimizing the mechanical interlocking of the particles. (Rugosity refers to surface roughness or deviation of shape from spherical. The coefficient of rugosity is defined as the ratio of actual surface area, as determined by a suitable method, to the geometric surface area found by microscopy.) (b) Certain glidants, such as talc and silica aerogels, roll under shear stresses to produce a "ball bearing" effect or type of action, causing the granules to roll over one another.

Many powders acquire a static charge during handling, in mixing, or in an induced die feed. The addition of 1% or more of magnesium stearate or polyethylene glycol 4000 or 2% or more of talc effectively lowers the accumulated charge.

Magnesium oxide should be considered an auxiliary glidant to be used in combination with silica-type glidants, especially for granulations that tend to be hygroscopic or somewhat high in moisture content. Magnesium oxide binds water and keeps the granulation dry and free flowing.

That anomalies exist in the action of glidants has been pointed out [86] in some cases of the physical and mechanical properties of mixtures of lactose, paracetamol, and oxytetracycline when small amounts of silica glidants are added to them. Owing to the differing propensities to coat the particles of the host powders, the silica aerogels act as a glidant for lactose and paracetamol but as an antiglidant for oxytetracycline.

Selection of glidants must be determined by the formulator by trial and error since there is no way of predicting which will be effective in a specific granulation.

VI. MULTILAYER TABLETS

Multilayer tablets are tablets made by compressing several different granulations fed into a die in succession, one on top of another, in layers. Each layer comes from a separate feed frame with individual weight control. Rotary tablet presses can be set up for two or three layers. More are possible but the design becomes very special. Ideally, a slight compression of each layer and individual layer ejection permits weight checking for control purposes.

A. Advantages of Multilayer Tablets

1. Incompatible substances can be separated by formulating them in separate layers as a two-layer tablet or separating the two layers by a third layer of an inert substance as a barrier between the two.

2. Two layer tablets may be designed for sustained release—one
    layer for immediate release of the drug and the second layer for
    extended release, thus maintaining a prolonged blood level.
3. Layers may be colored differently to identify the product.

B. Layer Thickness

Layer thickness can be varied within reasonable proportions within the
limitations of the tablet press. Thinness is dependent on the fineness of
the granulation.

C. Sizes and Shapes

Size is limited by the capacity of the machine with the total thickness
being the same as for a single-layer tablet. Many shapes other than
round are possible and are limited only by the ingenuity of the die maker.
However, deep concavities can cause distortion of the layers. Therefore,
standard concave and flat-face beveled edge tooling make for the best appearance, especially when layers are of different colors.

D. Granulations

For good-quality tablets with sharp definition between the layers, special
care must be taken as follows:

1. Dusty fines must be limited. Fines smaller than 100 mesh should
    be kept at a minimum.
2. Maximum granule size should be less than 16 mesh for a smooth,
    uniform scrape-off at the die.
3. Materials that smear, chalk, or coat on the die table must be
    avoided to obtain clean scrape-off and uncontaminated layers.
4. Low moisture is essential if incompatibles are used.
5. Weak granules that break down easily must be avoided. Excessive
    amounts of lubrication, especially metallic stearates, should be
    avoided for better adhesion of the layers.
6. Formulation of multilayer tablets is more demanding than that of single-
    layer tablets. For this reason, selection of additives is critical.

E. Tablet Layer Press

A tablet multilayer press is simply a tablet press that has been modified
so that it has two die-filling and compression cycles for each revolution of
the press. In short, each punch compresses twice, once for the first
layer of a two-layer tablet and a second time for the second layer. Three-
layer presses are equipped with three such compression cycles.

There are two types of layer presses presently in use—one in which
each layer can be ejected from the press separately for the purpose of
weight checking, and the second in which the first layer is compressed so
hard that the second layer will not bond to it, or will bond so poorly
that upon ejection the layers are easily separated for weighing. Once the

proper weight adjustments have been made by adjusting the die fill, the pressure is adjusted to the proper tablet hardness and bonding of the layers.

One hazard of layer tablet production is the lack of proper bonding of the layers. This can result in a lot of 100,000 tablets ending up as 200,000 layers after several days if the layers are not sufficiently bonded.

In a two-layer tablet press, two hoppers above the rotary die table feed granulated material to two separate feed frames without intermixing. Continuous, gentle circulation of the materials through the hoppers and feed frames assures uniform filling without segregation of particle sizes that would otherwise carry over to the second layer and affect layer weight, tablet hardness, and, in the case of differently colored granulations, the appearance of the tablet. The same procedure is followed in the three-layer press with three hoppers for the three granulations instead of two.

Certain single-layer or unit tablet presses are equipped with two pre-compression stations prior to the final compaction. This provides high-speed production by increasing dwell time of the material under pressure making for harder, denser tablets.

VIII. PROLONGED RELEASE TABLETS

Prolonged or sustained release tablets can be made by the wet granulation method using slightly soluble or insoluble substances in solution as binding agents or low-melting solids in molten form in which the drug may be incorporated. These include certain natural and synthetic polymers, wax matrices, hydrogenated oils, fatty acids and alcohols, esters of fatty acids, metallic soaps, and other acceptable materials that can be used to granulate, coat, entrap, or otherwise limit the solubility of a drug to achieve a prolonged or sustained release product.

Freely soluble drugs are more difficult to sustain than slightly soluble drugs because the sustaining principle is largely a waterproofing effect.

Ideally, the ultimate criterion for a sustained release tablet is to achieve a blood level of the drug comparable to that of a liquid product administered every 4 hr. To this end, prolonged release dosage forms are designed to release the drug so as to provide a drug level within the therapeutic range for 8 to 12 hr with a single dose rather than a dose every 4 hr (Fig. 13). They are intended as a convenience so that the patient needs to take only one dose morning and evening and need not get up in the night.

Prolonged drug forms are not without disadvantages. Since gastrointestinal tracts are not all uniform, certain individuals may release too much drug too soon and experience toxic or exaggerated response to the drug, whereas others may liberate the drug more slowly and not receive the proper benefit or response anticipated. This is especially true of older people whose gastrointestinal tract is less active than that of the younger. Also, where liberation is slow, there is danger of accumulation of the drug after several days resulting in high blood levels and a delayed exaggerated response.

Prolonged release products may be divided into two classes:

1. Prolonged release
2. Repeat action

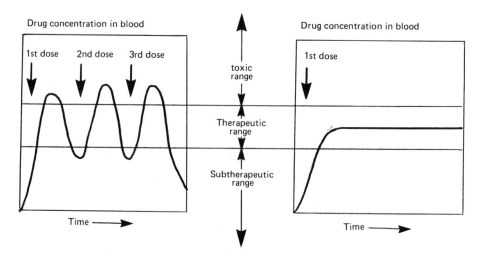

Figure 13 Conventional versus prolonged release dosage forms. (Left) repeated doses of conventional drug, and (right) single dose of ideal controlled release drug.

A prolonged (or sustained) release product is one in which the drug is initially made available to the body in an amount sufficient to produce the desired pharmacological response as rapidly as is consistent with the properties of the drug and which provides for the maintenance of activity at the initial level for a desired number of hours.

A repeat action preparation provides for a single usual dose of the drug and is so formulated to provide another single dose at some later time after administration. Repeat action, as defined here, is difficult to achieve and most products on the market today are of the sustained release type.

Many varied materials have been used in practice to achieve prolonged release dosage forms. The following example illustrates the ubiquitous nature shown in Example 20.

Prolonged release tablets must be tested for the rate of drug release by the prescribed in vitro laboratory method. Each product has an inherent release rate based on properly designed clinical trials of blood concentration and excretion in humans which is compared to the concentration and pharmacological activity resulting from the usual single-dose schedule of the drug administered in solution.

Once established, the in vitro testing based on the above is valuable for manufacturing control purposes to assure batch-to-batch uniformity of drug release.

Typical examples of release rates by laboratory tests are illustrated in Example 21.

Different drugs require different time release patterns depending on the half-life of the drug in the blood.

A prolonged release tablet containing two drugs in a single granulation has been patented in Example 22.

Some formulations are so constructed as to separate the ingredients into two formulations, one for immediate release and one for prolonged

Example 20:   Ferrous Sulfate Prolonged Release Tablets

Ingredients	mg per tablet
Ferrous sulfate, anhydrous, fine powder	325
Lactose, fine powder	70
Methocel E 15LV	100
Ethylcellulose, 50 cps, 15% in 95% ethanol	35
Magnesium stearate, fine powder	15
Cab-O-Sil	2

Mix the ferrous sulfate and the lactose and granulate
with the ethylcellulose solution and dry at 120 to 130°F.
(It will be necessary to granulate several times to achieve
25 mg per tablet of ethylcellulose. The batch must be
weighed after each addition until the proper weight is
attained.)
     In a twin-shell blender, add the Cab-O-Sil and blend
for 5 min, next add the magnesium stearate and blend
for 2 min. Compress with 13/32-in.-deep cup punches.
Coat the tablets with cellulose acetate phthalate solution
in alcohol and ethyl acetate.

release. The following formulation illustrates this by employing a two-layer
tablet for the formulations.
     Still another type is a tablet containing the prolonged release drug(s)
in the core tablet and the immediate release dose in the coating as is illustrated by Example 24.
     Prolonged release tablets have also been prepared by incorporating the
drug in a granulation for immediate release and in another granulation for
prolonged release, then mixing the two granulations and compressing as
given in Example 24.

Example 21:   Typical In Vitro Drug
Release Rates

Time increment (hr)	Percent cumulative release	
	Product A	Product B
1	28	36
2	26	44
4	54	58
6	71	74
8	82	86

Example 22:   Prolonged Release Hydrochlorothiazide
with Probenecid Tablets [87]

Ingredients	mg per tablet
Hydrochlorothiazide	12.5
Probenecid	250.0
Lactose	100.0
Starch	20.0
Cellulose acetate phthalate (5% solution in acetone)	7.5
Starch	30.0
Magnesium stearate	5.0

Mix the hydrochlorothiazide, probenecid with the
lactose and 20 mg of starch, granulate with the
cellulose acetate phthalate solution; pass the wet
mass through a 10-mesh screen.   Dry at 120 to
130°F.   Screen through a 20-mesh screen, incorporate the magnesium stearate and the remaining starch, and compress into tablets.

Example 23:   Prolonged and Immediate Release
Tablet Containing Pentaerythritol Tetranitrate
Two-Layer Tablets

Ingredients	mg per layer
Immediate Release Layer	
Pentaerythritol tetranitrate	20
Phenobarbital	10
Calcium sulfate, dihydrate	140
Starch	50
Starch paste, 10%	q.s.
Magnesium stearate	12
Prolonged Release Layer	
Penterythritol tetranitrate	60
Phenobarbital	35
Lactose	30
Beeswax	180

Example 23 (Continued)

Ingredients	mg per layer
Prolonged Release Layer	
Acacia, powdered	30
Cab-O-Sil M-5	15

Procedure for immediate release layer: Mix the first four ingredients and granulate with the starch paste through a 12-mesh screen. Dry at 130 to 140°F and size the dry granulation through a 20-mesh screen, add the magnesium stearate, and blend for 3 min. Hold for compressing on the following layer.

Procedure for prolonged release layer: Melt the beeswax and add all of the ingredients except the Cab-O-Sil with constant stirring and heating to maintain the molten state. Allow to cool and granulate by passing the mass through an 18-mesh screen; blend in the Cab-O-Sil.

Compression: On a two-layer tablet press, first compress the immediate release layer with 7/16-in. flat-face, bevel edge punches; then compress the prolonged release layer on top of it. Check the tablets for layer bonding.

Example 24: Antihistamine Decongestant Prolonged Release Tablet

Ingredients	mg in core tablet	mg in coating
Brompheniramine maleate	8	4
Phenylpropanolamine hydrochloride	10	5
Calcium sulfate, dihydrate	160	—
Kaolin	30	—
Zein granulating solution*	q.s.	—
Zinc stearate	10	—

*Zein granulating solution is prepared as follows:

Zein G-200[a]	100 g
Propylene glycol	10 g

Example 24   (Continued)

Stearic acid	10 g
Ethyl alcohol, 90%	200 ml

Dissolve the stearic acid in the alcohol at 35 to 40°F, next add the propylene glycol and then the zein with constant agitation until all is in solution.

[a]Zein G-200 is a protein derived from corn. It is resinlike and is acceptable for food use. Zein resists microbial decomposition. Granulating procedure for core tablet: Mix the three drugs with the calcium sulfate and the kaolin, and moisten with the zein granulating solution until evenly wetted. Granulate by passing through a 12-mesh screen and dry at 120 to 130°F. Pass the dry granulation through an 18-mesh screen, add the zinc stearate, and compress with 5/16-in.-deep cup punches.
Sugar coating: Dissolve the three drugs for immediate release in a solution of 810 g of sucrose, 80 g of acacia in 400 ml water, and apply as a sugar coating in a coating pan.

Example 25:   Chloroprophenpyridamine Tablets [88]

Ingredients	Pounds
Prolonged release granulation—A	
Chloroprophenpyridamine maleate, 50 mesh	5.0
Terra alba, 60 mesh	45.0
Sucrose, 75% w/v aqueous solution	15.0
Cetyl alcohol	10.0
Stearic acid	5.0
Glyceryl trilaurate	20.0

The cetyl alcohol, stearic acid, and glyceryl trilaurate are melted together. The chloroprophenpyridamine maleate and terra alba are added to the melted mixture with stirring. After mixing, the mixture is cooled until congealed to a hard mass. The mass is ground and sieved through a 30-mesh screen. The sucrose syrup is added to the powder obtained and thoroughly mixed to mass the powder. The resulting product is ground through a 14-mesh screen. The granules thus formed are dried at 37°C and sieved through aa 18-mesh screen.

Example 25   (Continued)

Ingredients	Pounds
Immediate release granulation—B	
Chloroprophenpyridamine maleate, 60 mesh	5.0
Terra alba, 60 mesh	65.0
Dextrose, 40 mesh	20.0
Lactose, 60 mesh	4.0
Starch, 80 mesh	5.0
Gelatin, 13% aqueous solution	1.0

Mix the chloroprophenpyridamine maleate, terra alba,
lactose, dextrose, and starch and mass with the gelatin
solution. Granulate through a 14-mesh screen and dry
at 40°C. Sieve the dried granules through an 18-mesh
screen.

Mix equal quantities of the prolonged release granulation—A and immediate release granulation—B and compress into 200-mg tablets.

Example 26:   Prednisolone Tablets [89]

Ingredients	mg per tablet
Prednisolone	5.0
Dicalcium phosphate	117.0
Aluminum hydroxide, dried gel	25.0
Sugar, as syrup	25.0
Magnesium stearate	3.4

Blend the first three ingredients and wet with
15 ml of syrup having a sugar concentration
0f 850 g/L. Screen through a 20-mesh screen
to form granules and dry at 60°C for 12 hr.
The dried material is then passed through
a 20-mesh screen to form final granules.
These granules are blended with the magnesium
stearate and compressed into tablets. This
formulation is claimed to have a disintegration
time of 12 hr.

Drugs may also be prepared in prolonged release form by adsorbing on acceptable materials such as ionic synthetic resins, aluminum hydroxide, and various clays. The following example presents the use of aluminum hydroxide and an aqueous granulating liquid (Example 26).

Prolonged action drug tablets have also been prepared with drugs bound to ion exchange resins that permit slow displacement of the drug from the drug-resin complex when it comes into contact with the gastrointestinal fluids. The displacement reaction of drug-resin complex may be described by the following equation:

$$(R-SO_3-H_3N-R') - (X-Y) \longrightarrow (R-SO_3-Z) - (H_3N-R'Y)$$

where X is H or some other cation and Y is Cl or some other anion. The opposite of this would occur if an acidic drug were bound to an anion exchange resin with Cl or other anion causing drug displacement.

Preparation of drug—ion exchange complexes are described in several patents [89—93]. Drug in solution in excess or less than the amount required by stoichiometric considerations is exposed to a suitable resin displacing the cation or anion, as the case may be, for the resin. After washing with water, the resin is dried and is then incorporated into a tablet granulation.

VIII. MANUFACTURING PROBLEMS

Although tablet presses have become more complex over the years as a result of numerous modifications, the compaction of material in a die between upper and lower punches remains essentially the same. The main differences that have been made are increase in speed, mechanical feeding of the material from the hopper into the die, and electronic monitoring of the press. Precompression stations allow for the elimination of air from the granulation by partially compressing the tablet material prior to final pressing of the tablet. This makes for harder, firmer tablets with less tendency toward capping and lower friability. The number of tablets a press can produce is determined by the number of tooling stations and the rotational speed of the press. Large presses can produce as many as 10,000 tablets per minute. All these advancements and innovations, however, have not decreased the problems often encountered in production, and in fact have increased the problems because of the complexities of the presses and the greater demands of quality.

The production of faulty or imperfect tablets creates problems that range from annoying to serious. These are time consuming and costly. Imperfections may arise from causes inherent in the granulation to improper machine adjustment and/or tooling.

A. Binding

Binding in the die or difficult ejection is usually due to insufficient lubrication. It is the resistance of the tablet to ejection from the die. This can cause the tablet press to labor and squeak producing tablets with rough edges and vertical score marks on the edges. This may be overcome by,

1. Increasing lubrication
2. Using a more efficient lubricant
3. Improving the distribution of the lubricant by screening through an 30-mesh screen and mixing with a portion of fines screened from the granulation
4. Reducing the size of the granules
5. Increasing the moisture content of the granulation
6. Using tapered dies
7. Compressing at a lower temperature and/or humidity.

B. Sticking, Picking, and Filming

Sticking is usually due to improperly dried or lubricated granulation causing the tablet surface to stick to the punch faces. Contributing to this are tablet faces that are dull, scratched, or pitted. This condition usually becomes progressively worse.

Picking is a form of sticking in which a small portion of granulation sticks to the punch face and grows with each revolution of the press, picking out a cavity on the tablet face.

Filming is a slow form of picking and is largely due to excess moisture in the granulation, high humidity, high temperature, or loss of highly polished punch faces due to wear. These may be overcome by

1. Decreasing the moisture content of the granulation
2. Changing or decreasing the lubricant
3. Adding an adsorbent (i.e., silica aerogel, aluminum hydroxide, microcrystalline cellulose)
4. Polishing the punch faces
5. Cleaning and coating the punch faces with light mineral oil, low-viscosity dimethylpolysiloxane

C. Capping and Laminating

Capping occurs when the upper segment of the tablet separates from the main portion of the tablet and comes off as a cap. It is usually due to air entrapped in the granulation that is compressed in the die during the compression stroke and then expands when the pressure is released. This may be due to a large amount of fines in the granulation and/or the lack of sufficient clearance between the punch and the die wall. It is often due to new punches and dies that are tight fitting. Other causes may be too much or too little lubricant or excessive moisture.

Lamination is due to the same causes as capping except that the tablet splits and comes apart at the sides and is ejected in two parts. If tablets laminate only at certain stations, the tooling is usually the cause. The following should be tried to overcome capping and laminating:

1. Changing the granulation procedure
2. Increasing the binder
3. Adding dry binder such as pregelatinized starch, gum acacia, powdered sorbitol, PVP, hydrophilic silica, or powdered sugar
4. Increasing or changeing lubrication

5. Decreasing or changing lubrication
6. Using tapered dies
7. Decreasing the upper punch diameter by 0.0005 in. to 0.002 in. depending on the size

D. Chipping and Cracking

Chipping refers to tablets having pieces broken out or chipped, usually around the edges. This may be due to damaged tooling or an improperly set takeoff station. These problems are similar to those of capping and laminating, and are annoying and time consuming. Cracked tablets are usually cracked in the center of the top due to expansion of the tablet, which is different from capping. It may occur along with chipping and laminating and/or it may be due to binding and sticking. It often occurs where deep concave punches are used. These problems may be overcome by one or more of the following:

1. Polishing punch faces
2. Reducing fines
3. Reducing granule size
4. Replacing nicked or chipped punches
5. Adding dry binder such as pregelatinized starch, gum acacia, PVP, spray-dried corn syrup, powdered sugar, or finely powdered gelatin

Solving many of the manufacturing problems requires an intimate knowledge of granulation processing and tablet presses, and is acquired only through long study and experience.

The foregoing are just a few of the problems of tablet manufacture that are encountered in production by the pharmaceutical scientist, and as new technologies develop, new problems arise.

For decades wet granulations have been processed on a purely empirical basis, often on a small scale. If tablet compression ran smoothly, reproducibility of the granulation was unimportant. Today, however, high-speed presses, demanding specifications, GMP regulations, and validation requirements have given rise to the need for more and greater effort to assure uniformity and reproducibility of the granulation. Experience indicates that formulation and process variables greatly influence the performance characteristics of the final product. Recent developments in techniques utilizing various high-shear mixers, granulating by extrusion, spray drying, pan granulating, and fluid bed agglomeration have presented new areas of investigation. Fast-running, automated processes demand greater control through instrumental and computer monitoring for satisfactory scale-up from laboratory to production scale. It is to this end that more research needs to be directed.

REFERENCES

1. D. E. Fonner, G. S. Banker, and J. Swarbrick, *J. Pharm. Sci.*, 55: 181–186 (1966).
2. P. J. Sherington and R. Oliver, *Granulation*, Heyden and Son Ltd., Philadelphia (1981).

3. T. Schaefer and O. Worts, *Arch. Pharm. Chem. Sci. Ed.*, 6:69–72 (1978).
4. T. Schaefer and O. Worts, *Arch. Pharm. Chim. Sci. Ed.*, 6:14–25 (1978).
5. M. E. Aulton and M. Banks, *Int. J. Pharm. Technol. Prod. Manufact.*, 2:24–28 (1981).
6. T. Schaefer and O. Worts, *Arch. Pharm. Chem., Sci. Ed.*, 6:5:178–193 (1977).
7. K. T. Jaiyeoba and M. S. Spring, *J. Pharm. Pharmacol.*, 33:5–11 (1981).
8. K. V. Sastry and D. W. Fuerstenau, in K. V. Sastry (ed.), *Agglomeration*, AIME, New York, 1977, p. 381.
9. M. J. Gamlen, H. Seager, and J. K. Warrach, *Int. J. Pharm. Tech. Prod. Manufact.*, 3:(4)108–114 (1982).
10. E. Nuernberg, *Acta Pharm. Technol.*, 26:39–42 (1980).
11. H. Seager and C. R. Trask, *Mfg. Chem. Aerosol News*, Dec. 10, 1976.
12. H. Seager, *Mfg. Chem. Aerosol News*, April 2, 1977.
13. D. M. Jones, *Pharm. Tech.*, 9:50 (1985).
14. H. J. Malinowski and W. E. Smith, *J. Pharm. Sci.*, 63:285–288 (1974).
15. H. J. Malinowski, *J. Pharm. Sci.*, 64:1688–1692 (1975).
16. R. C. Rowe, *Pharm. Ind.*, 46:119–125 (1985).
17. T. Schaefer et al., *Pharm. Ind.*, 48:1083–1095 (1986).
18. R. Kinget and R. Kemel, *Acta Pharm. Technol.*, 31:57–61 (1985).
19. H. Lewenberger, *Acta Pharm. Technol.*, 29:274–283 (1983).
20. P. Holm et al., *Pharm. Ind.*, 45:886–888 (1983).
21. T. Schaefer et al., *Arch. Pharm. Chem., Sci. Ed.*, 14:1–8 (1986).
22. *Chemical Engineer's Handbook*, 5th ed., McGraw-Hill, New York, 1975, pp. 53–58.
23. P. C. Record, *Int. J. Pharm. Prod. Dev.*, 1:32–39 (1980).
24. W. A. Knepper (ed.), *Agglomeration*, John Wiley and Sons, New York, 1962, pp. 365–383.
25. C. Orr, *Particulate Technology*, Macmillan, New York, 1966, pp. 400–432.
26. H. G. Kristensen and T. Schaefer, *Drug. Dev. Ind. Pharm.*, 13:(4 and 5),803–872 (1987).
27. C. E. Capes, *Particle size enlargement*, in Vol. 1, *Handbook of Powder Technology*, J. C. Williams and T. Allen (eds.), Elsevier, Amsterdam, 1980.
28. H. Rumpf, *Chem. Ind. Technol.* 46: (1974).
29. R. C. Shah, P. V. Raman, and P. L. Sheth, *J. Pharm. Sci.* 66:1554–1561 (1977).
30. M. H. Rubenstein and B. Musikabhumma, *Drug Dev. Ind. Pharm.*, 6:451–58 (1976).
31. K. Pataki et al., *Proc. Conf. Appl. Chem. Unit Oper. Processes*, 3(4):258–270 (1983).
32. M. H. Rubenstein, *J. Pharm. Pharmacol.*, 28: Suppl. 67P (1976).
33. J. L. Ford and M. H. Rubenstein, *Pharm. Helv. Acta*, 55:1–14 (1980).
34. P. Flanders et al, *Proc. Pharm. Tech. 5th Conf.*, 2:40 (1986).
35. J. C. McTaggert et al., *Int. J. Pharm.*, 19:139–145 (1984).
36. I. Ullah et al., *Pharm. Tech.*, 11:48–54 (1987).
37. J. T. Carstensen et al., *J. Pharm. Sci.*, 65:992–997 (1976).
38. M. A. Zoglio et al., *J. Pharm. Sci.*, 65:1205–1208 (1976).

39. A. Rogerson et al., *J Pharm. Pharmacol.*, *28*: Suppl. 63D (1976).
40. W. P. Bogar and J. J. Gavin, *N. Engl. J. Med.*, *261*:827 (1959).
41. R. Costello and A. J. Mattocks, *J. Pharm. Sci.*, *51*:106–110 (1962).
42. R. M. Duvall et al., *J. Pharm. Sci.*, *54*:607–611 (1965).
43. A. L. Jacobs, *Pharm. Mfg.* June; pp. 43–45 (1985).
44. M. J. Akers, *Can. J. Pharm. Sci.*, *11*:1–8 (1976).
45. L. Lachman and P. DeLuca, *Theory and Practice of Industrail Pharmacy*, 2nd Chap. 2, Lea and Febiger, Philadelphia, 1976.
46. S. A. Botha, A. P. Lötter, and J. L. dePreez, *Drug. Dev. Ind. Pharm.*, *13*:1197–1215 (1987).
47. M. T. Sclosserman and A. S. Feldman, *J. Soc. Cos. Chem.*, *24*:357–361 (1973).
48. E. Doelker and E. J. Shotton, *J. Pharm. Sci.*, *66*:193–196 (1977).
49. J. Carstensen et al., *J. Pharm. Sci.*, *65*:992–998 (1976).
50. A. A. Chalmers and P. H. Elsworthy, *J. Pharm. Pharmacol.*, *28*:228–230 (1976).
51. Z. T. Chowhan and Y. D. Chow, *Int. J. Pharm. Prod. Mfr.*, *2*:29–34 (1981).
52. J. L. Fabricans and J. Cicala, *J. Drug. Dev. Ind. Pharm.*, *13*:1217–1227 (1987).
53. J. I. Wells, D. A. Bhatt, and K. A. Khan, *J. Pharm. Pharmacol.*, *32*:55–59 (1980).
54. H. N. Wolkoff and G. Pinchuk, U.S. Patent 3,511,914 (1970).
55. Tablet Making, Tech. Bull. 14-100.500A, Pennwalt-Stokes, Warminster, PA.
56. Y. Matenda, V. Minamida, and Hayashi, *J. Pharm. Sci.*, *65*:1158–1162 (1976).
57. R. Appino, G. Banker, and G. DeKay, *Drug Stand.*, *27*:193–195 (1959).
58. A. C. Carman, *Soc. Chem. Ind.*, *London*, *57*:225–231 (1939).
59. A. E. Butcher and T. M. Jones, *J. Pharm. Pharmacol.*, *24*:163–166 (1972).
60. E. Nelson et al., *J. Am. Pharmaceut. Assn., Sci. Ed.*, *43*:596–601 (1954).
61. G. Ragnarssen, A. W. Höltzer, and S. Sjögren, *Int. J. Pharm.*, *3*:127–131 (1979).
62. G. K. Bolhuis and C. F. Lerk, *J. Pharm. Pharmacol.*, *33*:790 (1981).
63. P. J. Jarosz and E. L. Parrott, *Drug Dev. Ind. Pharm.*, *10*:259–273 (1984).
64. M. E. Johnsson and M. Nicklasson, *J. Pharm. Pharmacol.*, *38*:51–54 (1986).
65. M. I. Blake, *J. Am. Pharmaceut. Assn., New Series*, *11*:603 (1971).
66. A. C. Caldwell and W. J. Westlake, *J. Pharm. Sci.*, *61*:984–988 (1972).
67. N. H. Shah et al., *Drug. Dev. Ind. Pharm.*, *12*:329–246 (1986).
68. A. A. Khan and C. T. Rhodes, *J. Pharm. Sci.*, *64*:447–453 (1975).
69. K. A. Khan and D. J. Rooke, *J. Pharm. Pharmacol.*, *28*:6336 (1976).
70. L. A. Bergman and F. J. Bandelin, *J. Pharm. Sci.*, *54*:445–448 (1965).
71. E. Shotton and G. S. Leonard, *J. Pharm. Sci.*, *65*:1170–1176 (1976).
72. H. Hess, *Pharm. Tech.*, *2*:36–57 (1978).
73. R. Huttenrauch and I. Kleiner, *Pharmazie*, *28*:40–48 (1973).
74. A. H. Bronnsack, *Pharm. Ind.*, *38*:40–45 (1978).
75. D. Gessinger and A. Stamm, *Pharm. Ind.*, *42*:189–195 (1980).

76. H. Flasch, G. Asmussen, and N. Heinz, *Ar. Forsch.*, 28:1–12 (1978).
77. K. A. Kahn and D. J. Rooke, *J. Pharm. Pharmacol.*, 28:633 (1976).
78. H. G. Kristensen, *Dan. Tidsskr. Farm.*, 45:114–120 (1971).
79. N. Pilpel, in *Advances in Pharmaceutical Sciences*, Vol. 3, Chap. 3, H. S. Bean (ed.), Academic Press, London, 1971.
80. G. Gold et al., *J. Pharm. Sci.*, 57:667–671 (1968).
81. R. Tawashi, *Pharm. Ind.*, 26:682 (1964).
82. Tech. Bull. 49, *Aerosil in Pharmaceuticals and Cosmetics*, Degussa, New York.
83. Silanox Bull., Cabot Corp., Boston.
84. E. J. Nelson, *J. Am. Pharmaceut. Assn., Sci. Ed.*, 44:435–441 (1955).
85. T. M. Jones, *J. Soc. Cos. Chem.*, 21:483–489 (1970).
86. S. Varthalis and N. Pilpel, *J. Pharm. Pharmacol.*, 29:37 (1977).
87. J. E. Baer, Br. Patent 646,426 (1967).
88. E. V. Svedres, U.S. Patent 2,793,999 (1957).
89. E. Schuster, U.S. Patent 3,469,545 (1971).
90. S. P. Rety et al., Br. Patent 862,242 (1958).
91. E. L. Gustus, U.S. Patent 4,101,390 (1977).
92. C. R. Hamilton, U.S. Patent 4,473,957 (1982).
93. F. J. Keller, U.S. Patent 3,687,465 (1975).

4
Compressed Tablets by Direct Compression

Ralph F. Shangraw

The University of Maryland School of Pharmacy, Baltimore, Maryland

I. INTRODUCTION AND HISTORY

Until the late 1950s the vast majority of tablets produced in the world
were manufactured by a process requiring granulation of the powdered
constituents prior to tableting. The primary purpose of the granulation
step is to produce a free-flowing and compressible mixture of active ingredients and excipients. The availability of new excipients or new forms of old
excipients, particularly fillers and binders, and the invention of new (or the
modification of old) tablet machinery have allowed the production of tablets
by the much simpler procedure of direct compression. However, in spite
of its many obvious advantages, tableting by direct compression has not
been universally adopted even in those cases where it would seem to be
technically feasible and advantageous. The reasons for this can be understood only by reviewing the development of direct-compression technology
and the decision-making steps involved in selecting one manufacturing
process over another.

The term *direct compression* was long used to identify the compression
of a single crystalline compound (usually inorganic salts with cubic crystal
structures such as sodium chloride, sodium bromide, or potassium bromide)
into a compact without the addition of other substances. Few chemicals
possess the flow, cohesion, and lubricating properties under pressure to
make such compacts possible. If and when compacts are formed, disintegration usually must take place by means of dissolution—which can take a considerable length of time, delaying drug release and possibly causing physiological problems such as have occurred in potassium chloride tablets.

Note: A glossary of direct-compression excipients, trade names, and
supplies can be found on page 243.

Furthermore, the effective dose of most drugs is so small that this type of direct compression is not practical for most drug substances.

Pellets of potassium bromide are directly compressed for use in infrared spectrophotometry, and disks of pure drug have been directly compressed for the study of intrinsic dissolution rates of solids. However, there are few examples today of direct compression as classically defined in the literature. The term direct compression is now used to define the process by which tablets are compressed directly from powder blends of the active ingredient and suitable excipients (including fillers, disintegrants, and lubricants), which will flow uniformly into a die cavity and form into a firm compact. No pretreatment of the powder blends by wet or dry granulation procedures is necessary. Occasionally, potent drugs will be sprayed out of solution onto one of the excipients. However, if no granulation or agglomeration is involved, the final tableting process can still be correctly called direct compression. The first significant discussion of the concept of direct compression was presented by Milosovitch in 1962 [1].

Increasingly, there has been a trend toward integrating traditional wet granulation and direct-compression processes wherein triturations of potent drugs or preliminary minigranulations are added to direct-compression filler binders and then compressed. These techniques will be described later in the chapter.

The advent of direct compression was made possible by the commercial availability of directly compressible tablet vehicles that possess both fluidity and compressibility. The first such vehicle was spray-dried lactose, which, although it was subsequently shown to have shortcomings in terms of compressibility and color stability, initiated the "direct-compression revolution" [2]. Other direct-compression fillers were introduced commercially in the 1060s, including: Avicel (microcrystalline cellulose), the first effective dry binder/filler [2]; Starch 1500, a partially pregelatinized starch that possesses a higher degree of flowability and compressibility than plain starch while maintaining its disintegrant properties; Emcompress, a free-flowing compressible dicalcium phosphate; a number of direct-compression sugars such as Nutab, Di-Pac, and Emdex; and a variety of sorbitol and mannitol products. The relatively minimal compression properties of spray-dried lactose were improved by enhanced agglomeration of smaller crystals and the problems of browning due to impurities in the mother liquid were corrected. At the same time major advances were made in tablet compression machinery, such as improved positive die feeding and precompression stages that facilitate direct-compression tableting. By the beginning of the 1980s, the excipients and machinery had become available to make possible the direct compression of the vast majority of tablets being manufactured. It is important to understand why this has not occurred.

The simplicity of the direct-compression process is obvious. However, it is this apparent simplicity that has caused so many initial failures in changing formulations from wet granulation to direct compression. *Direct compression should not be conceived as a simplified modification of the granulation process for making tablets.* It requires a new and critical approach to the selection of raw materials, flow properties of powder blends, and effects of formulation variables on compressibility. During the wet granulation process the original properties of the raw materials are, to a great extent, completely modified. As a result, a new raw material, the granulation, is what is finally subjected to compression. Many inadequacies in the raw materials are covered up during the granulation step. This is not true in direct compression and therefore the properties of each and every raw material and the process by which these materials are blended become extremely critical to the compression stage of tableting. If direct compression is approached as a unique manufacturing process requiring new approaches to excipient selection, blending, and compressibility, then there are few drugs that cannot be directly compressed. If this is not done, failures are very likely to be encountered.

II. ADVANTAGES AND DISADVANTAGES OF THE WET GRANULATION PROCESS

The process of wet granulation is historically embedded in the pharmaceutical industry. It produces in a single process (although many steps may be involved) the two primary requisites for making a reproducible tablet compact (i.e., fluidity and compressibility). The various methods of granulation as well as the steps involved in the process of granulation and the materials used are reviewed in an article by Record [4] and described extensively in Chapter 3 of this book.

The advantages of the wet granulation process are well established and the advent of high-shear mixers and fluidized bed granulation and drying equipment has made wet granulation a more efficient process today than it was a quarter of a century ago. The advantages include the fact that it (a) permits mechanical handling of powders without loss of mix quality; (b) improves the flow of powders by increasing particle size and sphericity; (c) increases and improves the uniformity of powder density; (d) improves cohesion during and after compaction; (e) reduces air entrapment; (f) reduces the level of dust and cross-contamination; (g) allows for the addition of a liquid phase to powders (wet process only); and (h) makes hydrophobic surfaces hydrophilic.

On the other hand, the granulation process is subject to a great many problems. Each unit process gives rise to its own specific complications. The more unit processes, the more chance for problems to occur. Granulation essentially involves the production of a new physical entity, the granule. It is therefore necessary to control and validate all the steps involved in making a new material (the granulation) and to assure that this final material is in fact reproducible.

In addition to blending, problems include (a) type, concentration, rate of addition, distribution, and massing time of the binder solution; (b) effects of temperature, time, and rate of drying on drug stability and distribution during the drying process; and (c) granule size and segregation during the dry screening and subsequent final granulation blending. Each of these factors often involves a considerable effort in regard to both process and equipment validation.

When taken as an aggregate, these problems can be imposing, and it is easy to see why direct compression has both a scientific and economic appeal. However, it certainly offers no panacea for the unwary or unthinking formulator.

III. THE DIRECT-COMPRESSION PROCESS

A. Advantages

The direct-compression process assumes that all materials can be purchased or manufactured to specifications that allow for simple blending and tablet- ing.

The most obvious advantage of direct compression is economy. It is safe to say that there would be a relatively minor interest in the process of direct-compression tableting if economic savings were not possible. Savings can occur in a number of areas, including reduced processing time and thus reduced labor costs, fewer manufacturing steps and pieces of equipment, less process validation, and a lower consumption of power. Two unit processes are common to both wet granulation and direct-compression tableting: blending and compression. Prior micronization of the drug may be necessary in either process. Although a number of pieces of equipment, such as granulators and dryers, are not needed in preparing tablets by direct compression, there may be a need for greater sophistication in the blending and compression equipment. However, this is not always the case.

The most significant advantage in terms of tablet quality is that of processing without the need for moisture and heat which is inherent in most wet granulation procedures, and the avoidance of high compaction pressures involved in producing tablets by slugging or roll compaction. The unneces- sary exposure of any drug to moisture and heat can never be justified; it cannot be beneficial and may certainly be detrimental. In addition to the primary problem of stability of the active ingredient, the variabilities en- countered in the processing of a granulation can lead to innumerable tablet- ing problems. The viscosity of the granulating solution—which is depend- ent on its temperature, and sometimes on how long it has been prepared— can affect the properties of the granules formed, as can the rate of addi- tion. The granulating solution, the type and length of mixing, and the method and rate of wet and dry screening can change the density and par- ticle size of the resulting granules, which can have a major effect on fill weight and compaction qualities. The drying cycles can lead not only to critical changes in equilibrium moisture content but also to unblending as soluble active ingredients migrate to the surfaces of the drying granules. There is no question that, when more unit processes are incorporated in production, the chances of batch-to-batch variation are compounded.

Probably one of the least recognized advantages of direct compression is the optimization of tablet disintegration, in which each primary drug par- ticle is liberated from the tablet mass and is available for dissolution. The granulation process, wherein small drug particles with a large surface area are "glued" into larger agglomerates, is in direct opposition to the principle of increased surface area for rapid drug dissolution.

Disintegrating agents, such as starch, added prior to wet granulation are known to be less effective than those added just prior to compression. In direct compression all of the disintegrant is able to perform optimally, and when properly formulated, tablets made by direct compression should disintegrate rapidly to the primary particle state. However, it is important that sufficient disintegrant be used to separate each drug particle if ideal dissolution is to occur. One bioavailability advantage of making tablets by wet granulation has never been fully appreciated. The wetting of hydro- phobic drug surfaces during the granulation step and the resulting film of hydrophilic colloid that surrounds each drug particle can certainly speed up the dissolution process providing that each one of the primary drug particles can be liberated from the granule. Although this is not as likely to occur in a tablet made by direct compression as in one made by granulation, it is possible to add a wetting agent in the dry blend of powders to enhance dissolution rates. Prime particle disintegration in direct-compression tablets depends on the presence of sufficient disintegrating agent and its uniform distribution throughout the tablet matrix. High drug concentrations can lead to cohesive particle bonding during compression with no interjecting layer of binder or disintegrating agent.

Although it is not well documented in the literature, it would seem obvious that fewer chemical stability problems would be encountered in tablets prepared by direct compression as compared to those made by the wet granulation process. The primary cause of instability in tablets is moisture. Moisture plays a significant role not only in drug stability but in the compressibility characteristics of granulations. While some direct-compression excipients do contain apparently high levels of moisture, this moisture in most cases is tightly bound either as water of hydration (e.g., lactose monohydrate) or by hydrogen bonding (e.g., starch, microcrystalline cellulose) and is not available for chemical degradation. The role of moisture is discussed further under the description of individual excipients.

One other aspect of stability that warrants increasing attention is the effect of tablet aging on dissolution rates. Changes in dissolution profiles are less likely to occur in tablets made by direct compression than in those made from granulations. This is extremely important as the official compendium now requires dissolution specifications in most solid dosage form monographs.

B. Concerns

On the basis of the distinct advantages listed above, it is difficult to understand why more tablets are not made by the direct-compression process. To understand this fully, one must have an appreciation of not only the technology, but the economics and regulation of the pharmaceutical industry.

The technological limitations revolve mainly about the flow and bonding of particles to form a strong compact, and the speed at which this must be accomplished in an era of ever-increasing production rates.

With an increased emphasis on dissolution and bioavailability, many drugs are commonly micronized. Micronization invariably leads to increased interparticulate friction and decreased powder fluidity, and may also result in poor compressibility. Very often a decision has to be made as to whether to granulate a micronized powder—which may result in a longer dissolution time—or to directly compress a slightly larger particle size of the drug. In either case the decision should be based on in vivo blood studies as well as in vitro dissolution tests.

The choice of excipients is extremely critical in formulating direct-compression tablets. This is most true of the filler-binder, which often serves as the matrix around which revolves the success or failure of the formulation. Direct-compression filler-binders must possess both compressibility and fluidity. In most cases they are specialty items available from only one supplier and often cost more than comparable fillers used

in granulations. In addition, there is a need to set functionality specifications on properties such as compressibility and fluidity, as well as on
the more traditional physical and chemical properties. These specifications
must be rigidly adhered to in order to avoid lot-to-lot variations in raw
materials, which can seriously interfere with tableting qualities. This is
as true of the drug substance as it is of the excipients. The costs of
raw materials and raw material testing are thus higher in direct compression. However, this increased cost is often more than offset by the econo-
mies described earlier.

Many active ingredients are not compressible in either their crystalline
or their amorphous forms. Thus, in choosing a vehicle it is necessary to
consider the dilution potential of the major filler-binder (i.e., the proportion of active ingredient that can be compressed into an acceptable compact
utilizing that filler). Fillers-binders range from highly compressible materials such as microcrystalline cellulose to substances that have very low
dilution capacity such as spray-dried lactose. It is not possible to give
specific values for each filler because the dilution capacity depends on the
properties of the drug itself. In some cases it is necessary to employ
tablet presses with precompression capabilities in order to achieve an acceptable compact at a reasonable dilution ratio.

Outside of compressibility failures, the area of concern most often mentioned by formulators of direct-compression tablets is content uniformity.
The granulation process does lock active ingredients into place and, provided
the powders are intimately dispersed before granulation and no drying-
initiated unblending occurs after wetting, this can be advantageous. Direct-
compression blends are subject to unblending in postblending handling steps.
The lack of moisture in the blends may give rise to static charges that can
lead to unblending. Differences in particle size or density between drug
and excipient particles may also lead to unblending in the hopper or feed
frame of the tablet press.

The problems of unblending can be approached in either of two ways.
The traditional approach involves trying to keep particle sizes or densities
uniform. Ideally the vehicle itself (drug and/or filler binder) should incorporate a range of particle sizes corresponding as closely as possible to
the particle size of the active ingredients. This range should be relatively
narrow and should include a small percentage of both coarse and fine particles to ensure that voids between larger particles of drugs or filler excipients are filled by smaller sized particles. In such an approach, Avicel
or Starch 1500 could be used to fill voids between larger excipient particles
such as Emdex or Emcompress. The problem can also be solved by ordered
blending which is discussed in detail later in the chapter.

One other technical disadvantage of direct compression related to blending is the limitation in coloring tablets prepared in this manner. There is
no satisfactory method for obtaining tablets of a uniformly deep color.
However, it is possible through the use of highly micropulverized lakes
preblended or milled with fillers such as Starch 1500 or microcrystalline
cellulose to obtain a wide variety of pastel shade tablets.

Lubrication of direct-compression powder blends is, if anything, more
complicated than that of classical granulations. In general the problems
associated with lubricating direct-compression blends revolve around both
the type and amount needed to produce adequate lubrication and the softening effects that result from lubrication. It may be necessary to avoid

the alkaline stearate lubricants completely in some direct-compressi_{on} formulations.

The most common approach to overcome the softening as well phobic effects of alkaline stearate lubricants is to substantially limit the length of time of lubricant blending often to as little as 2 to 5 min. In fact, it is probably advisable in all direct-compression blending not to include the lubricant during the majority of the blending period. Lubricants should never be added to direct-compression powder blends in a high-shear mixer. In addition, the initial particle size of the lubricant should be carefully controlled. Another approach is to abandon the alkaline stearate lubricant and use hydrogenated vegetable oils such as Sterotex, Lubritab, and Compritol. In such cases, higher concentrations are necessary than would be used to lubricate granulations of similar filler/drug mixtures with magnesium stearate.

Outside of the limitations imposed by vehicle and formulation, there are economic and regulatory considerations necessary in making a decision to convert present products or to develop new products utilizing direct-compression technology.

It is interesting to note that, except for spray-dried lactose, all direct-compression excipients were developed after the 1962 Kefauver–Harris amendment to the Food, Drug and Cosmetic Act, which placed very strigent restrictions on dosage form as well as drug development. There is no question that this has led to a much more conservative approach to product development and formulation. Because of a 3- or 5-year or longer interval between formulation and marketing, many product development pharmacists hesitate to develop direct-compression formulations with unproven excipients. Of even greater uncertainty today is the physical specifications of the drug substance after its production has been scaled up to commercial proportions. In addition, there are increasing pressures to develop formulations that will be accepted internationally. In this respect, direct compression is much more widely used in the States than in Europe, although this situation is rapidly changing. Direct compression is more likely to be used by noninnovator companies because by the time patents have expired, the physical properties of the drug substance are more clearly defined.

Complicating this picture in the past was the sampling of experimental direct-compression excipients that were never marketed commercially or were subsequently withdrawn, leading to instability in the specialty excipient marketplace. Lot-to-lot variation in common direct-compression fillers commercially available today is rare. Of equal importance is the number of companies that have tried direct-compression formulations that failed when placed in full-scale production. In many cases this could be attributed to a failure to appreciate the complexities of the direct-compression technology, failure to set adequate specifications on raw materials, and failure of lot-to-lot reproducibility in the drug substances, particularly high-dose active ingredients.

In order to reduce the likelihood of raw material failure, it is advisable to set quality specifications on particle size, bulk density fluidity, and even compressibility. The latter can be easily done using a Carver press or single-punch machine under carefully prescribed conditions and determining the breaking strengths of resulting compacts.

The major advantages and concerns for the wet granulation and direct-compression processes are contrasted in Table 1.

Table 1   Comparison of Direct-Compression and Wet Granulation Processes for Making Tablets

Wet granulation	Direct Compression
Compressibility	
Harder tablets for poorly compressible substances	Potential problem for high-dose drugs
Fluidity	
Excellent in most cases	Many formulations may require a glidant
	Cannot micronize high-dose drugs
Particle Size	
Larger with greater range	Lower with narrower range
Content Uniformity	
Massing and drying induced	Segregation may occur in mass transport, hopper, and feed frame
Mixing	
High or low shear	Low shear with ordered blending
Lubricant	
Less sensitive to lubricant softening and overblending	Minimal blending with magnesium stearate
Disintegration	
Often problems with granules	Lower levels usually necessary
Dissolution	
1. Drug wetted during processing	1. No wetting, may need surface active agent
2. Drug dissolution from granules may be a problem	2. Dissolution may be slower if larger size drug crystals used
3. Generally slower than direct compression	3. Generally faster than wet granulation
Costs	
Increase in equipment, labor, time, process validation, energy	Increase in raw materials and their quality control

Table 1 (Continued)

Wet granulation	Direct compression
Flexibility of Formulation	
Granulation covers raw material flaws	Properties of raw materials must be carefully defined
Stability	
1. Problems with heat or moisture	1. No heat or moisture added
2. Dissolution rate may decrease with time	2. Dissolution rate rarely changes
Attitude of Equipment Suppliers	
Positive	Very negative
Tableting Speed	
May be faster	May require lower speed
Dust	
Less dusty	More dusty
Color	
Deep or pastel (dyes or lakes)	Pastel only (lakes only)

IV. DIRECT-COMPRESSION FILLER BINDERS

A. General Considerations

Direct-compression excipients, particularly filler-binders, are specialty excipients. In most cases they are common materials that have been modified in the chemical manufacturing process to impart to them greater fluidity and compressibility. The physical and chemical properties of these specialty products are extremely important if they are to perform optimally. It is most important for the direct-compression formulator to understand that there is no chance to cover up flaws in raw materials in direct compression as there is in the wet granulation process.

Many factors influence the choice of the optimum direct-compression filler to be used in a tablet formulation. These factors vary from primary properties of powders (particle size, shape, bulk density, solubility) to characteristics needed for making compacts (flowability and compressibility) to factors affecting stability (moisture), to cost, availability, and governmental acceptability. It is extremely important that raw material specifications be set up that reflect many of these properties if batch-to-batch

Table 2   Factors Influencing Choice of Direct-Compression Fillers

1. Compressibility[a]
   a. Alone
   b. Dilution factor or capacity
   c. Effect of lubricants, glidants, disintegrants
   d. Effect of reworking

2. Flowability[a]
   a. Alone
   b. In the finished formulation
   c. Need for glidant

3. Particle Size[a] and Distribution
   a. Effect on flowability
   b. Effect on compressibility
   c. Effect on blending
   d. Dust problems

4. Moisture Content and Type[a]
   a. Water of hydration (lactose, dextrose, dicalphosphate)
   b. Bound and free moisture
   c. Availability for chemical degradation
   d. Effect on compressibility
   e. Hydroscopicity

5. Bulk Density[a]
   a. Compression ratio $= \dfrac{\text{volume of tablet}}{\text{bulk volume of powder}}$
   b. Effect of handling and blending

6. Compatibility with Active Ingredient
   a. Moisture
   b. pH
   c. Effect on assay

7. Solubility (in GI Tract)
   a. Rate of dissolution
   b. Effect of pH

8. Stability of Finished Tablets
   a. Color
   b. Volume
   c. Hardness

9. Physiological Inertness
   a. Toxicity
   b. Reducing sugar
   c. Osmotic effect
   d. Taste and mouth-feel (if appropriate)

10. Cost and Availability

11. Governmental Acceptability
    a. United States and foreign countries
    b. Master File
    C. GRAS status
    d. Compendial standards (N.F.)

[a]Need to set purchase specifications for each lot of raw material.

manufacturing uniformity is to be assured. This is particularly true in the case of the filler-binders because they often make up the majority of the tablet weight and volume. However, this fact is still not fully appreciated by pharmaceutical formulators and production personnel. A list of factors involved in the choice of a filter-binder can be found in Table 2.

Most all of the classic tablet fillers have been modified in one way or another to provide fluidity and compressibility. In viewing the scanning electron photomicrographs of the various direct-compression filler-binders, one is taken with the fact that none of the products consist of individual crystals. Instead, all of them are actually minigranulations or agglomerations that have been formed in the manufacturing process by means of co-crystallization, spray drying, etc. The resulting material thus is able to deform plastically in much the same manner as the larger particle size granules formed during the traditional wet granulation process. The key to making any excipient or drug directly compressible thus becomes obvious and the possibility of making all tablets by direct compression appears to be within the scope of present technology.

B. Soluble Filler-Binders

Lactose

Spray-dried lactose is the earliest and still one of the most widely used direct-compression fillers. It is one of the few such excipients available from more than a single supplier. In spite of many early problems, this material revolutionized tableting technology.

Coarse and regular grade sieved crystalline fractions of α-lactose monohydrate have very good flow properties but lack compressibility. However spray drying produces an agglomerated product that is more fluid and compressible than regular lactose [1].

In the production of spray-dried lactose, lactose is first placed in an aqueous solution which is treated to remove impurities. Partial crystallization is then allowed to occur before spray-drying the slurry. As a result the final product contains a mixture of large α-monohydrate crystals and spherical aggregates of smaller crystals held together by glass or amorphous material. The fluidity of spray-dried lactose results from the large particle size and intermixing of spherical aggregates. The compressibility is due to the nature of the aggregates and the percentage of amorphous material present and the resulting plastic flow, which occurs under compaction pressure.

The problem of compressibility of spray-dried lactose is still real and troublesome. The compressibility of spray-dried lactose is borderline, and furthermore, it has relatively poor dilution potential. Spray-dried lactose is an effective direct-compression filler when it makes up the major portion of the tablet (more than 80%), but it is not effective in diluting high-dose drugs whose crystalline nature is, in and of itself, not compressible. Furthermore, spray-dried lactose does not lend itself to reworking because it loses compressibility upon initial compaction.

Spray-dried lactose has excellent fluidity, among the best for all direct-compression fillers. It contains approximately 5% moisture, but most of this consists of water of hydration. The free surface moisture is less than

0.5% and does not cause significant formulation problems. It is relatively nonhygroscopic.

Spray-dried lactose is available from a number of commercial sources in a number of forms [5]. Because the processing conditions used by different manufacturers may vary, all spray-dried lactoses do not necessarily have the same properties particularly in terms of degree of agglomeration, which influences both fluidity and compressibility. Alternative sources of supply should be validated, as is true of all direct-compression fillers.

When spray-dried lactose was first introduced, two major problems existed. The one that received the most attention was that of browning [2]. This browning was due to contaminants in the mother liquid, mainly 5-hydroxyfurfural, which was not removed before spraying. This browning reaction was accelerated in the presence of basic amine drugs and catalyzed by tartrate, citrate, and acetate ions [6]. Although the contaminants are now removed during the manufacturing process in most commercial products, the specter of browning still remains. However, at the present time, there appears to be no more danger of browning in spray-dried lactose than in any other form of lactose.

After many abortive attempts to improve on spray-dried lactose, a much more highly compressible product was introduced in the early 1970s [7]. This product, called Fast-Flo lactose, consists mainly of spherical aggregates of microcrystals. These microcrystals are lactose monohydrate, and they are held together by a higher concentration of glass than is present in regular spray-dried lactose. During the manufacturing process the microcrystals are never allowed to grow but are agglomerated into spheres by spray drying. Because it is much more compressible, it has replaced regular spray-direct lactose in many new direct-compression formulations.

Because of the spherical nature of the spray-dried aggregates, Fast-Flo lactose is highly fluid. It is nonhygroscopic and, as is the case with most spray-dried lactose, contaminants that could lead to browning are removed in the manufacturing process. Tablets made from Fast-Flo lactose are three to four times harder than those made from regular spray-dried lactose when compressed at the same compression force. An agglomerated form of lactose that is more compressible than spray-dried but less compressible than Fast-Flo lactose is marketed under the name Tabletose.

Anhydrous lactose is a free-flowing crystalline lactose with no water of hydration, first described in the literature in 1966 [8]. The most common form of anhydrous lactose is produced by crystallization above 93°C which produces the β form. This is carried out on steam-heated rollers, the resultant cake being dried, ground, and sieved to produce the desired size. It is available in a white crystalline form that has good flow properties and is directly compressible. Its compressibility profile (compression force versus hardness) is similar to that of Fast-Flo lactose. Anhydrous lactose can be reworked or milled with less loss of compactability than occurs with other forms of lactose. However, anhydrous lactose contains a relatively high amount of fines (15 to 50% passes through a 200-mesh screen), so that its fluidity is less than optimal. The use of a glidant such as Cab-O-Sil or Syloid is recommended if high concentrations are included in a formulation.

At high relative humidities anhydrous lactose will pick up moisture, forming the hydrated compound. This is often accompanied by an increase in the size of the tablets if the excipient makes up a large portion of the total tablet weight. At a temperature of 45°C and a relative humidity of 70%, plain anhydrous lactose tablets will increase in size by as much as 15% of their original volume. Much has been made of the fact that anhydrous lactose contains less moisture than regular lactose and thus is a better filler for moisture-sensitive drugs. In fact, the surface moisture of the anhydrous and hydrous forms is about the same (0.5%) and the water of hydration does not play a significant role in the decomposition of active ingredients. Anhydrous lactose possesses excellent dissolution properties, certainly as good as, if not better than, α-lactose monohydrate.

Anhydrous lactose possesses excellent dissolution properties which is due in part to the fact that it is predominantly β-lactose. The intrinsic dissolution rate is considerably faster than α-lactose monohydrate. Lactose N.F., anhydrous, direct tableting, is available in the United States from Sheffield products while both high-β- and high-α-content anhydrous lactose are produced by DMV in Europe. Dehydration of the hydrous form must occur above 130°C in order to obtain stable anhydrous crystals needed for pharmaceutical use. A number of excellent articles on the various types of lactose and their tableting properties have been published by Lerk, Bolhuis, and coworkers [9—14].

Sucrose

Sucrose has been extensively used in tablets both as a filler, usually in the form of confectioners sugar, and in the form of a solution (syrup), as a binder in wet granulations. Attempts to directly compress sucrose crystals have never been successful, but various modified sucroses have been introduced into the direct-compression marketplace. One of the first such products was Di-Pac, which is a cocrystallization of 97% sucrose and 3% highly modified dextrins [15]. Each Di-Pac granule consists of hundreds of small sucrose crystals "glued" together by the dextrin. Di-Pac has good flow properties and needs a glidant only when atmospheric moisture levels are high (greater than 50% relative humidity). It has excellent color stability on aging, probably the best of all the sugars.

Di-Pac is a product that points out the need for setting meaningful specifications in purchasing raw materials for direct compression. The concentration of moisture is extremely critical in terms of product compressibility. Compressibility increases rapidly in a moisture range of 0.3 to 0.4%, plateaus at a level of 0.4 to 0.5%, and rises again rapidly up to 0.8% when the product begins to cake and lose fluidity [16]. The moisture-compressibility profile of Di-Pac is closely related to the development of monomolecular and multimolecular layers of moisture on both the internal and external surfaces of the sucrose granules—a process that increases hydrogen bonding on compression. The dilution potential of Di-Pac and most other sucroses is only average, ranging from 20 to 35% active ingredients.

While a moisture concentration of 0.4% is probably optimal for most pharmaceuticals, material of high moisture content is extremely advantageous when making troches or candy tablets. Interestingly, as moisture levels increase, lubricant requirements decrease. Tablets containing high concentrations of Di-Pac tend to harden slightly (1- to 2-kg units) during the first hours after compression, or when aged at high humidities and then dried. This is typical of most direct-compression sucroses or dextroses. Like all direct-compression sucroses, the primary target products are chewable tablets, particularly where artificial sweeteners are to be avoided. Both the process for making cocrystallized sucrose products and their properties are described in an article by Rizzuto et al. [17].

Nutab is a directly compressible sugar consisting of processed sucrose, 4% invert sugar (equimolecular mixture of levulose and dextrose), and 0.1 to 0.2% each of cornstarch and magnesium stearate [18]. The latter ingredients are production adjuncts in the granulation process by which the product is made and are not intended to interject any disintegrant or lubricant activity in a final tablet formulation. NuTab has a relatively large particle size distribution which makes for good fluidity but could cause blending problems if cofillers and drugs are not carefully controlled relative to particle size and amounts. In formulations NuTab has poor color stability relative to other direct-compression sucroses and lactoses.

Dextrose

One of the most dramatic modifications of natural raw materials for improving tableting characteristics is directly compressible dextrose marketed under the name Emdex [19]. This product is spray-crystallized and consists of 90 to 92% dextrose, 3 to 5% maltose, and the remainder higher glucose polysaccharides. It is available as both an anhydrous and a hydrous product (9% moisture). Reports indicate that the anhydrous form is slightly more compressible than the monohydrate; but the compressibility of both is excellent, being second only to microcrystalline cellulose when not diluted with drugs or other excipients. The most widely used product is the monhydrate and the water of hydration does not appear to affect drug stability. At approximately 75% relative humidity both forms of Emdex become quite hygroscopic, particularly if they have been milled or sheared on the surface of a die table. Above 80% relative humidity both products liquefy. Tablets produced from Emdex show an increase in hardness of approximately 2 kg at all levels of initial hardness up to 10 kg. The increase occurs in the first few hours after compression with no further significant hardening on long-term storage under ambient conditions. However, hardness increases do not result in significant changes in rates of dissolution.

Emdex possesses the largest particle size of all the common direct-compression excipients. Blending problems can occur if blends of other smaller particle size excipients are not used to fill in voids. This filler lends itself to ordered blending, where the micronized drug is first blended with the large particle size Emdex, before other excipients are added to the blender. The micronized drug becomes lodged in the pores on the surfaces of the large spheres and are apparently held in place with sufficient attractive force to prevent dislodging during subsequent blending operations.

Sorbitol

Sorbitol is one of the most complex of all direct-compression fillers. It is available from a number of suppliers in various direct-compression forms. However, sorbitol exists in a number of polymorphic crystalline forms as well as an amorphous form. Failure of many suppliers to fully appreciate the ramifications of these crystalline forms on both compressibility and stability has caused major problems among users. The less stable (α and β) polymorphic forms of sorbitol will convert to the more stable form (γ), which often results in dendritic growth (small, hairlike crystals). This causes a caking of particles and is accentuated by the presence of moisture. More stable products such as Sorbitol 834 and NeoSorb 60, consisting almost solely of the γ form, are now available and overcome most of the stability problems. However, all γ-sorbitols are not crystallized in the same way and thus still have different compressibilities and lubricant requirements. At the present time interchange of one directly compressible form for another is not recommended without some validation of processing characteristics. The complexities of sorbitol and the modification of its crystalline structure to influence tableting properties are described by DuRoss [20], while an evaluation of ascorbic acid and gamma sorbitol tablets is presented by Guyot-Hermann and Leblanc [21].

Sorbitol is widely used as the sole ingredient in "sugar-free" mints and as a vehicle in chewable tablets. It forms a relatively hard compact, has a cool taste and good mouth-feel. However, it is hygroscopic and will clump in the feed frame and stick to the surfaces of the die table when tableted at humidities greater than 50%.

Lubricant requirements increase when the moisture content of the sorbitol drops below 0.5% or exceeds 2%.

Mannitol

Recently, there has been an increased interest in direct-compression mannitol. Mannitol does not make as hard a tablet as sorbitol but is less sensitive to humidity. Mannitol is widely used in the direct compression of reagent tablets in clinical test kits where rapid and complete solubility is required and can be lubricated sufficiently for this purpose using micronized polyethylene glycol 6000. One company has developed a highly specialized technique to produce beads of sensitive biological materials and mannitol or sorbitol for direct compression [22,23]. Its use as a filler in chewable tablets is limited by its cost, although its cool mouth feel is highly attractive. Mannitol also exists in a number of polymorphic forms and this phenomenon should be explored if a lot of mannitol behaves in a peculiar fashion. Debord et al. [24] tested four polymorphic forms of mannitol, two of which they obtained in pure state. Different forms were shown to have different compression characteristics.

Maltodextrin

A free-flowing agglomerated maltodextrin is available for direct-compression tableting under the name Maltrin. The product is highly compressible, completely soluble, and has very low hygroscopic characteristics.

C. Insoluble Filler-Binders

Starch

One of the most widely used tablet excipients starch, does not in its natural state possess the two properties necessary for making good compacts: compressibility and fluidity. There have been many attempts to modify starch to improve its binding and flow properties. The only modification of starch that has received widespread acceptance in direct compression is Starch 1500. Starch 1500 is more fluid than regular starch and meets the specifications for pregelatinized starch, N.F. Starch 1500 consists of intact starch grains and ruptured starch grains that have been partially hydrolyzed and subsequently agglomerated [25]. It has an extremely high moisture content (12 to 13%), but there is little indication that this moisture is readily available to accelerate the decomposition of moisture-sensitive drugs [26].

Although Starch 1500 will readily compress by itself, it does not form hard compacts. Its dilution potential is minimal, and it is not generally used as the filler-binder in direct compression, but as a direct-compression filler disintegrant. The major advantage of Starch 1500 is that it retains the disintegrant properties of starch without increasing the fluidity and compressibility of the total formulation, which is not the case with plain starch. Because Starch 1500, like all starches, deforms elastically when a compression force is applied, it imparts little strength to compacts. As few clean surfaces are formed during compaction, lubricants, particularly the alkaline stearate lubricants, tend to dramatically soften tablets containing high concentrations of Starch 1500, Lubricants such as stearic acid or hydrogenated vegetable oils are preferred in such formulations.

Cellulose

The first widespread use of cellulose in tableting occurred in the 1950s when a floc cellulose product, Solka-Floc, was introduced as a filler disintegrant. Solka-Floc consists of cellulose that has been separated from wood by digestion and formed into sheets that are mechanically processed to separate and break up individual fibers into small pieces. This converts the cellulose into a free-flowing powder. However, this material has poor fluidity and compressibility, and is not used as a direct-compression excipient.

The most important modification of cellulose for tableting was the isolation of the crystalline portions of the cellulose fiber chain. This product, microcrystalline cellulose (Avicel), was introduced as a direct-compression tableting agent in the early 1960s and stands today as the single most important tablet excipient developed in modern times [3]. Although it was developed with no though of tableting in mind, its properties are close to optimal. Microcrystalline cellulose is derived from a special grade of purified alpha wood cellulose by severe acid hydrolysis to remove the amorphous cellulose portions, yielding particles consisting of bundles of needlelike microcrystals. Microcrystalline cellulose for direct-compression tableting comes in a number of grades, the most widely used of which is PH 101, which was the original product, and PH 102, which is more agglomerated and possesses a larger particle size, resulting in slightly better fluidity but with no significant decrease in compressibility.

Microcrystalline cellulose is the most compressible of all the direct-compression fillers and has the highest dilution potential. This can be explained by the nature of the microcrystalline particles themselves, which are held together by hydrogen bonds in the same way that a paper sheet or an ice cube is bonded [27]. Hydrogen bonds between hydrogen groups on adjacent cellulose molecules account almost exclusively for the strength and cohesiveness of compacts. When compressed, the microcrystalline cellulose particles are deformed plastically due to the presence of slip planes and dislocations on a microscale, and the deformation of the spray-dried agglomerates on a macroscale. A strong compact is formed due to the extremely large number of clean surfaces brought in contact during the plastic deformation and the strength of the hydrogen bonds formed.

Other factors are important in the ability of a comparatively small amount of microcrystalline cellulose to bind other materials during compaction, the low bulk density of the microcrystalline cellulose, and the broad range of particle sizes. An excipient with a low bulk density will exhibit a high dilution potential on a weight basis, and the broad particle size range provides optimum packing density and coverage of other excipient materials.

Microcrystalline cellulose has an extremely low coefficient of friction (both static and dynamic) and therefore has no lubricant requirements itself. However, when more than 20% of drugs or other excipients are added, lubrication is necessary. Because it is so compressible, microcrystalline cellulose generally withstands lubricant addition without significant softening effects. However, when high concentrations (greater than 0.75%) of the alkaline stearate lubricants are used, and blending time is long, the hardness of tablets compressed at equivalent compression forces is lower.

Because of cost and density considerations, microcrystalline cellulose is generally not used as the only filler in a direct-compression tablet but is more often found in concentrations of 10 to 25% as a filler-binder-disintegrant. Although it is not as effective a disintegrant as starch in equivalent concentrations, it can be used as the only disintegrant at levels of 20% or higher and has an additive effect with starch at lower levels. Hard compacts of microcrystalline cellulose disintegrate rapidly due to the rapid passage of water into the compact and the instantaneous rupture of hydrogen bonds. The fluidity of microcrystalline cellulose is poor compared to that of most other direct-compression fillers because of its relatively small particle size. However, comparisons with other direct-compression fillers *based on a weight per unit time flow through an orifice are misleading due to its inherently low-bulk density* [28]. A comparison of the relative volumetric and gravimetric flow rates of typical direct-compression fillers can be seen in Table 3. Small amounts of glidant are recommended in many formulations containing high concentrations of microcrystalline cellulose.

Tablets made from higher concentrations of microcrystalline cellulose soften on exposure to high humidities due to moisture pickup and loosening of interparticulate hydrogen bonds. This softening is often reversible when tablets are removed from the humid environment. Cycling of temperature and moisture over a period of time can cause both increases or decreases of equilibrium hardness, depending on the total formulation.

Because microcrystalline cellulose is highly compressible, self-lubricating, and a disintegrant, attempts have been made to use it as the only filler-binder in tablets containing drugs with low doses. It has been found that formulations containing more than 80% microcrystalline cellulose may slow the dissolution rates of active ingredients having low water solubility. Apparently, the small particles get physically trapped between the deformed microcrystalline cellulose particles, which delays wetting and dissolution. This phenomenon can be easily overcome by adding portions of water-soluble direct-compression excipients such as Fast-Flo lactose.

During the middle 1980s, a number of cellulose products were introduced into the marketplace to compete with Avicel. These products represent a continuum from floc to crystalline celluloses, some of which meet N.F. specifications for microcrystalline cellulose (i.e., Emcocel). Personen and Paronen [29] compared the crystallinity, particle size, densities, flow, and binding properties of Emcocel and Avicel PH 101.

However, the most complete comparative evaluation of microcrystalline cellulose products was conducted by Doelker et al. [30]. They studied the tableting characteristics of N.F. grade microcrystalline celluloses produced by seven manufacturers. The powders were examined for moisture content, particle size, densities, flow, and tableting properties (on an instrumented press) by measuring diametral crushing force of the compacts.

Table 3   Volumetric and Gravimetric Comparative Flow Rates of Selected Direct-Compression Fillers

Filler-binder	Poured bulk density (g cm^{-3})	Gravimetric flow rate (kg min^{-1})	Volumetric flow rate based on poured bulk density (L in.$^{-1}$)
Microcrystalline cellulose[a]	0.314	1.300	4.140
Powdered cellulose[b]	0.531	1.499	2.823
Pregelatinized starch[c]	0.589	1.200	2.037
Hydrous lactose[d]	0.650	2.200	3.385
Compressible sugar[e]	0.694	3.747	5.399
Dibasic calcium phosphate[f]	0.933	4.300	4.609

[a]Avicel PH-102, FMC Corp. Philadelphia, Pennsylvania.

[b]Elcema G-250, Degussa Corp., Teterboro, New Jersey.

[c]Starch 1500, Colorcon, Inc., West Point, Pennsylvania.

[d]Fast-Flo, Foremost Whey Products, Barzboo, Wisconsin.

[e]Di-Pac, Amstar Corp., New York, New York.

[f]Di-Tab, Stauffer Chemical Co., Westport, Connecticut.
Source: From *Pharm. Tech.*, *7*(9), 94 (1983).

Great differences in packing and tableting properties and in sensitivity to the addition of a lubricant were generally observed between products from various manufacturers. In contrast, lot-to-lot variability was quite accept- able. Using an empirical scale, the authors rated the various products and found Avicel and Emcocel to overall outperform other products. How- ever, the functionality of microcrystalline cellulose depends as much on physical form as it does on crystalline content. Equivalence of microcrystal- line products varies with desired functionality and substitutions of one product for another must be validated. Often less compressible microcrystal- line cellulose can be substituted for Avicel with acceptable results because products may have been overly formulated with microcrystalline cellulose to begin with.

It should be remembered that the effectiveness of microcrystalline cel- lulose as a binder decreases as moisture is added to it in processing. Thus microcrystalline cellulose is effective as a binder in direct compression, slugging, roller compaction, or when added to a granulation in the free- flowing mix directly before compression. Its binding advantages in granu- lation decrease with an increase in water addition.

Another form of cellulose advocated for direct compression is microfine cellulose, (Elcema). This material is a mechanically produced cellulose powder which also comes in a granular grade (G-250), which is the only form that possesses sufficient fluidity to be used in direct compression. Microfine cellulose is a compressible, self-disintegrating, antiadherent form of cellulose that can be made into hard compacts. However, unlike microcrystalline cellulose, it possesses poor dilution potential, losing its compressibility rapidly in the presence of noncompressible drugs. It is not a particularly effective dry binder due to the large particle size of the G-250 granules and the resistance to fracture under compression. Microfine cellulose forms few fresh or clean surfaces during compression because of the lack of slip planes and dislocations in the cellulose granules. Thus little interparticulate binding occurs, and sufaces "contaminated" by lubricant during mixing show little inclination to form firm compacts.

Inorganic Calcium Salts

The most widely used inorganic direct-compression filler is unmilled dicalcium phosphate, which consists of free-flowing aggregates of small microcrystals that shatter upon compaction. This material is available in a tableting grade under the names Emcompress or DiTab. Dicalcium phosphate is relatively inexpensive and possesses a high degree of physical and chemical stability. It is nonhygroscopic at a relative humidity of up to 80%. Dicalcium phosphate in its directly compressible form exists as a dihydrate. Although this hydrate is stable at room and body temperature, it will begin to lose small amounts of moisture when exposed to temperatures of 40 to 60°C [31]. This loss is more likely to occur in a humid environment than a dry environment. This anomaly is theorized to occur because at low humidities and high temperatures, the outer surfaces of the particles lose water of hydration and become case-hardened, preventing further loss. In a humid environment the loss continues to occur. When combined with a highly hygroscopic filler like microcrystalline cellulose, the loss of moisture may be sufficient to cause a softening of the tablet matrix due to weakening of the interparticulate bonds and to accelerate decomposition of moisture-sensitive drugs like vitamin A.

The fluidity of dicalcium phosphate is good, and glidants are generally not necessary. While it is not as compressible as microcrystalline cellulose and some sugars (Fast-Flo lactose, Emdex), it is more compressible than spray-dried lactose and compressible starch. It apparently deforms by brittle fracture when compressed, forming clean bonding surfaces. Lubricants exert little softening effect on compacts.

Because it is relatively water-insoluble, tablets containing 50% or more of dicalcium phosphate disintegrate rapidly. Dicalcium phosphate does dissolve in an acidic medium, but it is practically insoluble in a neutral or alkaline medium. Therefore, it is not recommended for use in high concentrations in combination with drugs of low water solubility. This is of particular concern in formulating tablets that may be used in geriatric patients where the incidence of achlorhydria is significant.

Dicalcium phosphate dihydrate is slightly alkaline with a pH of 7.0 to 7.3, which precludes its use with active ingredients that are sensitive to even minimal amounts of alkalinity. Tricalcium phosphate (TriTab) is less compressible and less soluble than dicalcium phosphate but contains a higher ratio of calcium ions [32]. Calcium sulfate, dihydrate N.F., is also available in direct-compression forms [Delaflo, Compactrol].

Cel-O-Cal is the first significant direct-compression tablet filler specifically designed to combine the advantages of dissimilar materials by the method of coprocessing. It consists of 30 parts of microcrystalline cellulose and 70 parts of anhydrous calcium sulfate coprocessed in a spray dryer. It combines the compressibility and disintegrant advantages of microcrystalline cellulose with the cost advantages of calcium sulfate. The product is significantly more compressible than a physical mixture of its component parts and produces tablets of much lower friability. It is also less subject to lubricant softening effects due to its larger particle size. Because Cel-O-Cal is composed of two substances that are not water-soluble, care should be taken in using it in formulation of drugs with low water solubility particularly if the product is to be wet-granulated.

Calcium Carbonate

Calcium carbonate has been used in the past as a tablet filler even though it does have a significant pharmacological effect (antacid). It is available from a number of suppliers in directly compressible forms. There has been a renewed interest in calcium carbonate in the United States because of its use as a nutritional supplement in the prophylaxis of osteoporosis. Although its effectiveness for this condition has been questioned, numerous calcium supplements, including combinations with vitamin D and multivitamins are being marketed. Calcium carbonate is available in a number of forms including precipitated, ground oyster shells and mined limestone. There is no evidence that any one of these sources provides a nutritionally superior product and all have similar dissolution profiles. They do differ in terms of degree of whiteness, particle size, and impurities. Calcium carbonate has been coprocessed with various binders to make it directly compressible. The solubility of calcium carbonate does depend on pH. The effectiveness of calcium carbonate as a source of calcium in achlorhydric patients has been questioned.

On the other hand, calcium carbonate is much more soluble than either dicalcium phosphate, tricalcium phosphate, or calcium sulfate. The use of these other substances even in normal patients would appear to be even less justified.

A glossary of direct compression excipients, trade names, and suppliers can be found at the end of the chapter.

V. FACTORS IN FORMULATION DEVELOPMENT

More than in any other type of tablets, successful formulations of direct-compression tablets depend on careful consideration of excipient properties and optimization of the compressibility, fluidity, and lubricability of powder blends. The importance of standardizing the functional properties of the component raw materials and the blending parameters cannot be over-stressed. Preformulation studies are essential in direct-compression tableting even for what would appear to be a simple formulation.

A. Compressibility

Formulation should be directed at optimizing tablet hardness without applying excessive compression force while at the same time assuring rapid tablet disintegration and drug dissolution. In those cases where the drug makes up a relatively minor proportion of the tablet, this is usually no problem, and concern revolves around homogeneous drug distribution and content uniformity. Often much simpler excipient systems can be utilized, and factors such as relative excipient costs become more important. In those cases where the drug makes up the greater part of the final tablet weight, the functional properties of the active ingredient and the type and concentration of the excipient dominate the problem. Often the decision resolves about the question of what is the least amount of excipient necessary to form an acceptable and physically stable compact. In regard to the active ingredient it is important to determine the effect of particle size on compressibility as well as the effect of crystalline form (crystalline or amorphous) on compressibility. It may be necessary to granulate the active ingredient by slugging to improve compressibility and increase density.

The most effective dry binder is microcrystalline cellulose. It can add significant hardness to compacts at levels as low as 3 to 5%. It should always be considered first if the major problem in the formulation is tablet hardness or friability. It has been used at levels as high as 65% to bind active ingredients with extremely poor compressibility characteristics. No other direct-compression excipient acts as well as a dry binder in low concentrations. The compressibilities of varying fillers have been discussed as they relate to individual substances. Most disintegrating agents (such as starch) or glidants have negative effects on compressibility, although compressible starch is better than plain cornstarch.

A comparison of the relative compressibilities of various direct-compression fillers using magnesium stearate and stearic acid as lubricants is presented in Figures 1 and 2. As can be seen, microcrystalline cellulose is by far the most compressible of the substances tested. Magnesium stearate causes a softening of compacts to the point that Starch 1500 cannot be tableted. However, the relative compressibility of the fillers remains constant.

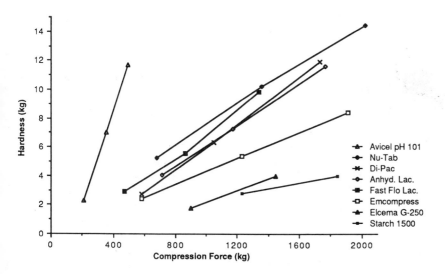

Figure 1   Excipient compressibility with 2% stearic acid as lubricant.

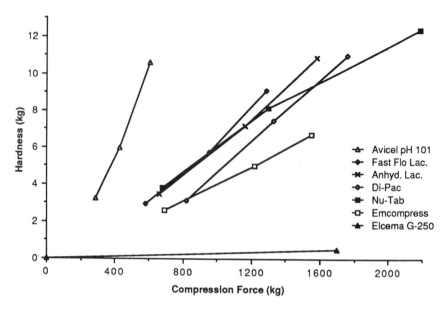

Figure 2   Excipient compressibility with 0.75% magnesium stearate as lubricant.

It is possible to compare the relative compressibility of a variety of direct-compression lactoses in a similar manner (Fig. 3). As can be seen, there can be as great as a twofold difference in the compressibility of two different forms at equivalent compression forces.

It might be expected that compressibility properties would be additive (i.e., that a mixture of microcrystalline cellulose and spray-dried lactose would have a compressibility profile of some proportionate value between those of the individual ingredients). For instance, Lerk et al. [33] showed an additive effect between most lactose fillers when they were combined with other lactoses or microcrystalline cellulose. However, an antagonistic behavior was demonstrated by blends of fast-dissolving vehicles such as dextrose or sucrose with cellulose or starch products. For instance, almost all combinations of microcrystalline cellulose and compressible dextrose gave poorer compressibility profiles and longer disintegration times than either ingredient alone. Bavitz and Schwartz [34] showed essentially additive effects in hardness when blending fillers, but their work did not include either sucrose or dextrose.

Almost all disintegrating agents retard compressibility as well as fluidity due to particle size. In order to have optimal disintegration into primary particles, it is desirable to have the particle size of the disintegrating agent as small as possible, preferably smaller than that of the active ingredient. This is not always possible.

One of the major advances in the development of direct-compression technology and its adoption by industry has been the introduction of the "superdisintegrants." These agents, which include Croscarmellose N.F. (AcDiSol), Crospovidone N.F. (Polyplasdone XL), and sodium starch glycolate N.F. (Explotab and Primogel), allow for faster disintegration of tablets, and lower use levels, therefore minimizing the softening effect and fluidity problems encountered when high levels of starch are used. Fortunately, direct-compression formulations generally do not require as high a disintegrant concentration as wet granulation because the problem of intragranular disintegration does not exist.

As direct-compression blends may not possess ideal compressibility, operational problems may be reduced by the use of one or two precompression stages or use of large compression rolls.

It is generally concluded that direct-compression formulations are less compressible than wet granulation formulations. Obviously, this depends to a great extent on the materials used. However, when direct-compression and wet-granulated formulations of norfloxacin were compared in a recent publication, it was found that the direct-compression formulation was superior not only in terms of disintegration and dissolution, but was also more compressible [35].

B. Fluidity

The fluidity of tablet blends is important not only from the direct effect on uniformity of die fill and thus uniformity of tablet weight, but also from the role it plays in blending and powder homogeneity. Because of the overall smaller particle size encountered in direct-compression blends, fluidity is a much more serious problem than in the case of granulations. A comparison of the bulk densities and particle size of some of the most common direct-compression fillers can be found in Table 4.

It is important that fluidity specifications be placed on all active ingredients and fillers that make up more than 5% of a final tablet formulation. Fluidity of active ingredients becomes a factor when the drug has been micronized to improve dissolution rate or provide more key particles of

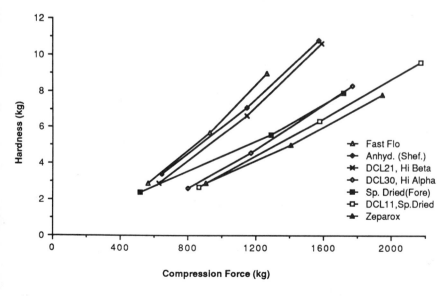

Figure 3 Compressibility profiles of different directly compressible lactoses.

Table 4   Physical Specifications of Direct-Compression Fillers

Filler	Moisture (%)	Bulk density (loose) (g ml^{-1})	Particle size[b]
Spray-dried lactose Foremost	5.0[a]	0.68	100% through 30 30–60% on 140 15–50% through 200
Fast-Flo lactose	5.0[a]	0.70	0.5–1.5% on 60 25–65% on 140 15–45% through 200
Anhydrous lactose	0.25–0.5	–	16% on 60 65% between 60–200 20% through 200
Emdex	7.8–9.2	0.64	1% on 20 20% max. through 100
Di-Pac	0.4–0.75	0.58	3% max. on 40 75% min. on 100 5% max. through 100
Nu-Tab	<1	0.70	50% min. on 60 10% max. through 120
Microcrystalline cellulose			
Avicel pH 101	<5	0.32	1% max. on 60 7% through 200
Avicel pH 102	<5	0.34	8% max. on 60 45% on 200
Starch 1500	12	0.62	0% on 8 0.5% max. on 40 90% through 100
Emcompress	0.5	0.91	5% max on 40 15 max through 200

[a]Contains 4.5% water of hydration.

[b]Mesh size of screen.

drug per tablet. If the amount of drug is small, this problem can be overcome by a proper choice of excipient fillers. However, when the drug
makes up higher proportions of the tablet weight, the use of glidants in
addition to careful selection of tablet fillers is necessary. The most effective glidants are the micronized silicas such as Cab-O-Sil and Syloid.
They are generally used in concentrations of 0.1 to 0.25%. At higher levels
the weight variation of tablets will often increase, and tablet hardness per
specific die volume fill becomes less [36]. However, higher concentrations
may be helpful as antiadherents, and may reduce filming and picking problems on punch faces.

Most direct-compression fillers are purposely designed to give good
flow properties. In most cases, fluidity in terms of *volume* (not weight)
flow per unit time is directly related to particle size (Table 3). The two
fillers with poorest flow appear to be microcrystalline cellulose and
compressible starch. However, flow of these materials is not as poor as
is often recorded when gravimetric flow and not volumetric flow data are
presented [28].

The trend toward higher tablet machine output has necessitated the
development of more sophisticated feeders because in older designs the dwell
time of the die cavity in contact with the feeder was not adequate to allow
uniform filling. This problem can become even more critical in direct compression because of the smaller mean particle size of direct-compression
powder. There are two basic approaches to increasing die-feeding efficiency: (a) to force material into the die cavity; (b) to improve flow properties of material directly above the die cavity so that the material will
naturally flow downward. The latter approach appears to be the more
realistic and serves as the basis for most tablet machine modifications for
improvement of die fill. One such system, designed by the Manesty Corporation, employs a rotary feeder with two horizontal paddles, which rotate
in opposite directions. The paddle speeds can be synchronized with the
main drive. It is possible that the use of such positive die-feeding equipment may be necessary if optimum fluidity cannot be obtained through
careful selection of ingredients and choice of their concentrations.

C. Content Uniformity

Highly fluid powder blends facilitate unblending. The narrower the particle size range of all components and the more alike the particle densities,
the less chance for unblending or segregation. It is important to note
that it is the particle density and not the bulk density that is important
in segregation. Cellulose and starch products tend to have lower true
densities than sugars or inorganic chemicals. However, the small and
angular particle shape of microcrystalline cellulose makes it difficult for
higher density particles to sift down through the spaces between the blend
of materials. Major problems with segregation can occur in spherically
shaped fillers, particularly if the particle is large and spherical, such as
is the case with compressible dextrose (Emdex). In such cases it is necessary to select other excipients to fill the empty spaces or to purposely pre-
blend a micronized active ingredient with the large-particle filler. This
approach is recommended by Ho and Crooks [37], who blended sulfaphenazole (mean particle diameter of 2 μm) with coarse direct-compression tablet
fillers, and then studied the blends, using a sampling method and electron
microscopy. After mixing with a 180- to 250 μm fraction of direct-compression

sucrose (DiPac) for 100 min, the standard deviation of 200-mg samples containing 4 mg of sulfaphenazole was equivalent to that predicted for a random mix. The mix did not appear to segregate during mixing or vibration. It is theorized that blending of the filler particles first (with lubricant, etc.) or simply blending all materials at once would have interfered with the surface attraction of drug particles to filler and resulted in decreased homogeneity. There are a number of other excellent articles on ordered blending that point out its importance to direct compression [38–40].

D. Lubrication

Lubrication has always been one of the most complicated and frustrating aspects of tablet formulation. The lubrication of direct-compression powder blends is, if anything, more complicated than that of classical granulations. In general, the problems associated with lubricating direct-compression blends can be divided into two categories: (a) type and amount needed to produce adequate lubrication; (b) the softening effects of lubrication.

Because the overall mean particle size of direct-compression blends is less than that for granulations, higher concentrations of lubricants are often needed. The recognized need for small particle size of lubricants in granulations is of even greater importance in direct compression.

Because there are already many more surfaces covered with lubricant in direct-compression blends, the softening effect upon compression is magnified. This is particularly true in direct-compression fillers that exhibit almost no fracture or plastic flow on compression. Even when all surfaces of a granulation are covered by a layer of lubricant, significant clean surfaces are formed during compression. In most instances standard blending times will result in complete coverage of these surfaces. The same blending times in direct-compression blends may or may not cover all primary surfaces. Thus length of blending becomes much more critical in direct compression than in lubrication of tablet granulations. If blended long enough, alkaline stearate lubricants will shear off and completely cover all exposed particle surfaces. It may be necessary to avoid the alkaline stearate lubricants completely in some direct-compression formulations. The influence of the duration of lubricant and excipient mixing on the processing characteristics of powders and on the properties of compacts prepared by direct compression was studied by Shah and Mlodozeniec [41]. They found that ejection force, hardness, disintegration, and dissolution of directly compressed tablets of lactose and microcrystalline cellulose were all significantly affected by blending times. The properties of directly compressed tablets can also be dramatically affected by the type of blender, which can be a major problem when scaling up from laboratory to production equipment [42]. When operated at the same rotation speed, the decrease in crushing strength of tablets was much faster for the large industrial mixers than for the laboratory blenders. Lubrication of direct-compression formulations is one of the more complex and difficult problems faced by a pharmaceutical formulator.

VI. MORPHOLOGY OF DIRECT-COMPRESSION FILLERS

The compressibility of direct-compression filler-binders can be more easily understood by viewing the morphology of individual particles. As was mentioned previously, most direct-compression fillers are minigranulations in which the raw material itself has in some way been agglomerated or granulated after being chemically or physically modified.

The scanning electron microscope has provided a unique tool to visualize such modifications while at the same time allowing for a qualitative assessment of product quality. The scanning electron microscope was dramatically used by Hess to depict the nature of pharmaceutical compacts and the effects of compression force and disintegrating agents on tablet morphology [43]. The use of scanning electron photomicrographs for the characterization of direct-compression excipients was first reported by Shangraw et al. [44,45] and updated in a later article that further reviewed the usefulness of scanning electron microscopy in studying excipient properties [46].

As can be seen in Figures 4 and 5, the spray drying of lactose can result in agglomerates consisting of small α-monohydrate crystals held together by amorphous glass. These agglomerates now have the prerequisite flow and deformation properties to make them compressible. The cocrystallization of sucrose with modified dextrins changes the poorly compressible sucrose crystals into a highly deformable dense aggregate of crystallites (Figs. 6 and 7).

It was not possible to utilize fibrous cellulose as a tableting agent until it was mechanically formed into a large-particle floc that improved flow characteristics but with little improvement in compressibility (Fig. 8). However, it was the acid hydrolysis of cellulose and the subsequent spray drying of the more crystalline portions of the fibers into a free-flowing powder that revolutionized direct-compression tableting. This product, microcrystalline cellulose (Fig. 9), not only forms extremely hard compacts, but has the ability to improve the compressibility of other substances when it is added in concentrations of 10 to 30%.

A scanning electron photomicrograph of unmilled dicalcium phosphate provides evidence of the aggregates of crystallites that shatter upon compaction to give tablet strength (Fig. 10). The agglomeration of starch

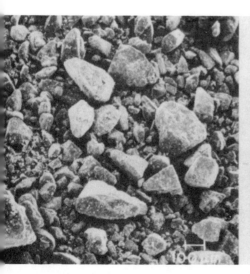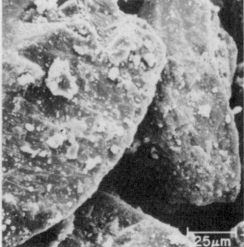

Figure 4   Crystalline lactose, N.F. (non-spray-dried).

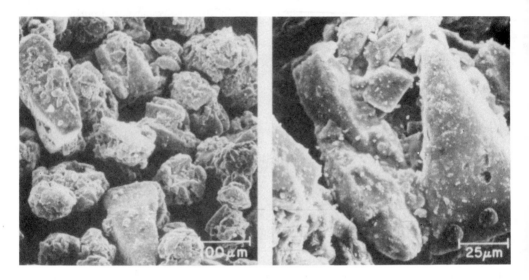

Figure 5   Lactose, N.F.   Spray-dried. (Fast-Flo).

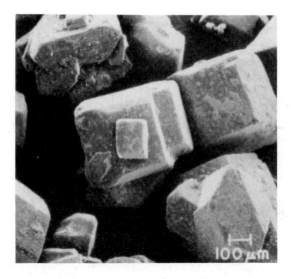

Figure 6   Sucrose, N.F. (crystalline).

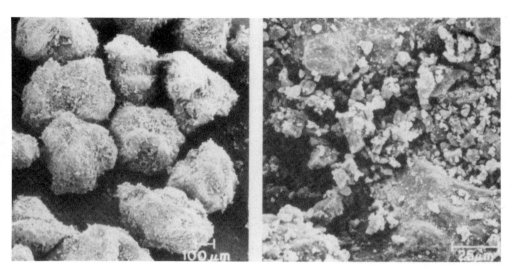

Figure 7   Compressible sugar, N.F. (Dipac).

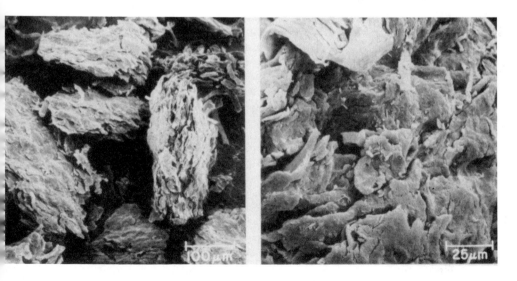

Figure 8   Powdered cellulose, N.F. (Elcema 250).

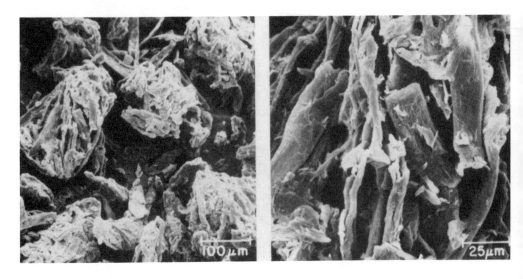

Figure 9   Microcystalline cellulose, N.F. (Avicel pH 102)

with partially hydrolyzed starch to form a free-flowing compressible granulation can be seen in Figure 11.

One of the most significant contributions to the literature of pharmaceutical excipients is *The Handbook of Pharmaceutical Excipients* [47].   Of
particular interest to those concerned with morphology and functionality
are the book's scanning electron photomicrographs of almost all tablet fillers and disintegrating agents.   A wide range of data is also presented
for products that have the same chemical composition yet different morphologies.   Such data include information about particle size, compressibility,
and moisture sorption.

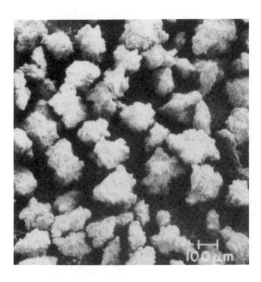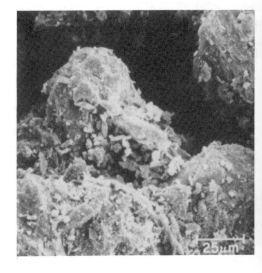

Figure 10   Dibasic calcium phosphate, USP unmilled (Di-Tab, Emcompress).

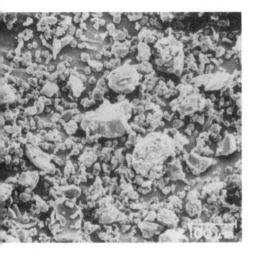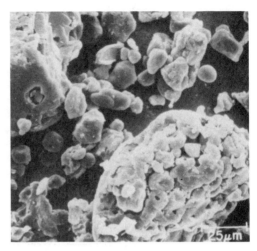

Figure 11   Pregelatinized starch N.F. compressible (Starch 1500).

VII. COPROCESSED ACTIVE INGREDIENTS

As it has become more and more apparent what makes chemical substances
compressible and also what enhances their dissolution rates, it has become
increasingly obvious that emphasis in tablet formulation has been misplaced.
There is nothing less compressible or less rapidly soluble than a perfectly
pure crystalline material.   Yet for a century there has been an emphasis
on producing the purest possible drug crystals.   It is then up to the pharmaceutical formulator to take those crystals and mask the inadequacies
of compressibility and dissolution inherent in them by means of external
excipients.   A more logical approach would be to supply the drug in an
impure form (with known quantities of known impurities) so that the crystals are actually flawed or in fact do not exist as large crystals but as
aggregates of microfine crystals.   Although this has not yet been done for
drug substances, pregranulations of some common drugs are available commercially.
     Ascorbic acid has long been available in a number of powder or granu-
lar forms.   Ascorbic acid is commonly crystallized in monoclinic, platelike
crystals.   The term granular simply means large crystals (similar to granular sugar), not a granulation in terms of aggregated powders.
     In the mid 1970s Roche marketed ascorbic acid C-90 in which micronized
ascorbic acid particles are granulated with starch paste.   The product appears to be extruded through a compactor and then ground.   Each large
particle is actually a granule of ascorbic acid and pasted starch, and is
much more compressible than the pure crystalline material.   However, the
product does have an extremely wide variation in particle size, and addition
of some filler-binder, such as microcrystalline cellulose, is recommended to
optimize compressibility.   More recently, Roch marketed a C-95 ascorbic acid
that contains only 5% excipients and utilizes methylcellulose rather than
starch as the binder.   Takeda Chemical Industries markets both a C-97
direct-compression ascorbic acid and SA-99, a direct-compression sodium
ascorbate.

Because of the increasing popularity of acetaminophen as an analgesic, it was only natural that a modification of this substance to improve compressibility would be attempted. Acetaminophen generally occurs as large monoclinic crystals, a crystal form which is not easily deformed and resists compaction. A direct-compression form of acetaminophen is available commercially from Mallinckrodt containing 90% acetaminophen and 10% of partially pregelatinized starch under the name COMPAP [48]. The spherical nature of the particles indicates that the material is prepared by spray drying; each particle is almost a perfect minigranule. Deformation can occur along any plane and multiple clean surfaces are formed during the compaction process. Moreover, each granule consists of hundreds of small crystals with wetted surfaces which optimize dissolution. Tablets with rapid dissolution can be easily formed by the addition of small concentrations of AcDiSol (2%) and lubricant (0.5% magnesium stearate). A self-lubricating version of this material is also available (COMPAP-L) as well as a combination of acetaminophen and codeine (Codacet-60).

Another direct-compression acetaminophen product is marketed by Monsanto under the name DC-90 [49]. This product is prepared by fluidized bed granulation instead of spray drying. It has a compressibility profile similar to that of COMPAP but is only available in the self-lubricating form. Both products exhibit rapid dissolution profiles when formulated with effective disintegrant systems. The compressibility of both materials can be enhanced by the addition of 10 to 20% microcrystalline cellulose. The different morphologies or these products is debicted in Figure 12a and b.

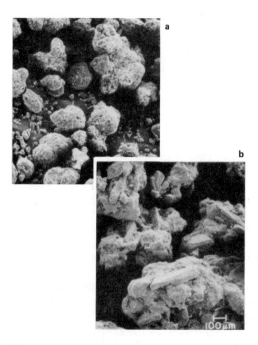

Figure 12   Direct-compression acetaminophen: (a) Compap (Mallinckrodt);
(b) DC 90 (Monsanto).

In 1982, Mallinckrodt introduced a directly compressible ibuprofen product under the name DCI. However, this product contains only 63% active ingredient and appears to be a classic granulation with little innovation.

In some respects the term direct-compression is a misnomer when applied to any of these products. However, it is apparent that these products will continue to multiply and provide convenient intermediate materials for manufacturing companies with limited processing equipment. In many ways, they resemble the slugged aspirin/starch (90/10) granulations that became popular in the post-World War II period and are still commercially available.

There is no reason to believe that it would not be possible to convert any active ingredient into a compressible form by crystal modification. The question remains as to whether or not this technique will be applied to drug substances or if pharmaceutical formulators will be forced to continue working with noncompressible, poorly soluble pure crystals.

VIII. MODIFICATION AND INTEGRATION OF DIRECT-COMPRESSION AND GRANULATION PROCESSES

It is in the area of dry granulation and mixed processing systems where the most recent impact of direct-compression technology has taken place.

When initially developed, direct compression was thought of as an all-or-nothing system. Gradually the integration of direct compression with various granulation processes has occurred. These include:

1. Use of direct-compression excipients in postgranulation running powders
2. Optimization of granulations prepared by roll compaction and Chilsonation
3. Semi- or pseudogranulations, mini- or microgranulations, preblending of triturations
4. Matrix for controlled relese granules or beads

The use of microcrystalline cellulose, which was originally thought of as a direct-compression binder-filler, in the postgranulation running powder for increasing tablet hardness has been a common practice almost since its introduction. Subsequently, microcrystalline cellulose has gained acceptability in mini- or microgranulations in which small quantities of wet binders are used but are more thoroughly distributed in loosely agglomerated powders [50]. This allows for the maximization of the effect of both the wet binder and the dry binder. However, care in the granulation step has to be taken because the overwetting of the granules tends to reduce the binding effectiveness of the microcrystalline cellulose.

A unique modification of this process was proposed by Ullah using a process called "moisture-activated dry granulation" (MADG) [51]. In this procedure, the binder (polyvinylpyrrolidone) is blended with the drug plus filler, a small amount of water is added, and the combination is then mixed thoroughly. Microcrystalline cellulose is subsequently added to sorb the small amount of moisture present. No traditional drying step is involved. The granulation tends to be nondense, with a relatively small particle size.

Direct compression has had a significant impact on the particle size originally thought necessary for tablet manufacture. Formulators have come to realize that with the use of glidants, much smaller mesh materials can be used as granulations and the particle size of granules can in fact approach the particle size of direct-compression fillers. In fact, as was stated earlier, most direct-compression fillers are nothing more than micro- or minigranulations.

The innovative use of compressible excipients for increasing the compressibility of a difficult material to tablets is illustrated by one approach to manufacturing 800-mg ibuprofen tablets [52]. Ibuprofen has a very low bulk density, low melting point, poor compaction properties, and tablets produced by wet granulations may age due to scintering. The patent for a stable high-dose high-bulk-density ibuprofen granulation describes the preparation of a dry granulation of croscarmellose and ibuprofen by roll compaction or chilsonation, and the subsequent blending of the granulation with additional croscarmellose and microcrystalline cellulose to produce a tablet. One might argue that this process is not direct compression, but the fact of the matter is that without the unique sorbent and disintegrating properties of croscarmellose and the unusual dry-binding properties of microcrystalline cellulose in the post blend powder, this product would not be possible.

A further modification of the direct-compression process is the use of premixed triturations of potent drug substances with one or more fillers and the subsequent addition of other fillers and binders before the final blend is directly compressed. This process is now being used successfully for making tablets of such potent drugs as clonidine with tablet strengths of 0.1, 0.2, and 0.3 mg. Preparation of tablets of this strength by direct compression would have been thought impossible 10 years ago.

More recently, two potassium supplements have been introduced into the marketplace that involve the compression of coated potassium chloride crystals into directly compressed tablet matrices. One product is made by coating KCl crystals with a solution/suspension of paraffin, acetyl tributyl citrate, ethylcellulose, and silicon dioxide in isopropanol. The coated crystals are then blended with microcrystalline cellulose, rice starch, magnesium stearate, and talc, and then compressed. The tablets are easily crushed and can be administered as a powder without changing the release characteristics of the KCl.

A similar potassium chloride tablet with a strength of 20 meq has also been marketed. The tablet is extremely hard but disintegrates into the primary coated KCl crystals very rapidly. Microcrystalline cellulose and crospovidone act both as compressible cushioning agents during compaction and disintegrating agents during the very rapid breakup that occurs on exposure to fluids, which allows the tablet contents to be administered as a suspension if so desired.

IX. FUTURE OF DIRECT-COMPRESSION TABLETING

In spite of the slow adoption of direct-compression tableting by the pharmaceutical industry, there is every indication that its acceptance will continue to grow. Its use in the manufacture of generic drug and nonprescription drug products, where innovation is easier to apply and just-ify economically, is now widespread. As was mentioned in the last section, there is an increasing inclination to integrate aspects of direct compression, dry granulation, and wet granulation in product manufacture. Co-processing of excipients and active ingredients to provide drum-to-hopper tableting of raw materials will no doubt also increase in volume. It is difficult to envision significant new filler-binders because the basic building materials that are both chemically and physiologically acceptable have already been modified. However, there will be a continuing search for dry binders that can mimic or exceed the properties of microcrystalline cellulose and to discover a lubricant with the functionality of magnesium stearate but without its hydrophobic properties.

X. FORMULATIONS FOR DIRECT COMPRESSION

As indicated above, the development of formulations for direct compression is both an art and a science. All formulations are highly dependent on the properties of the raw materials including the drug substance. It is not desirable to change sources of supply or grades of raw materials without validating effects on fluidity, compressibility, and solubility. This applies to the active ingredient also, particularly in a high-dose drug. Following is a collection of formulations taken from the literature (Examples 1 to 25) illustrating many of the points discussed in the chapter. These are guide formulations only and results may vary depending on the properties of the drug substance and the type of blender or tablet press used. A number of them have been taken or adapted from formularies available from FMC, Food and Pharmaceutical Products Division and Edward Mendell Co., Inc.

Example 1:   Aspirin Tablets USP (325 mg)

Ingredient	Composition (%)	Quantity per tablet (mg)
1. Aspirin, USP (40-mesh)	80.0	325.0
2. Avicel PH 102	12.0	48.0
3. Cornstarch, N.F.	8.0	32.0
	100.0	405.0

Note: Hardness of finished tablets can be improved by replacing corn starch with Starch 1500 with no resultant decrease in disintegration. Use of stearic acid is optional depending on aspirin type and concentration of Avicel. Blend all the ingredients for 20 min. Compress into tablets using 7/16-in. standard concave tooling.

Example 2:   Aspirin-Caffeine Tablets

Ingredient	Composition (%)	Quantity per tablet (mg)
1. Aspirin, USP (40-mesh crystal)	80.0	384.00
2. Caffeine, USP	3.30	15.84
3. Avicel PH 102	10.00	48.00
4. Cornstarch, N.F.	5.95	28.56
5. Stearic acid, N.F.	0.75	3.60
	100.0	480.00

Blend all ingredients in a P-K blender or equivalent for 20 min.   Compress into tablets using 7/16-in. standard concave tooling.

Example 3:   Acetaminophen Tablets USP (325 mg)

Ingredient	Composition (%)	Quantity per tablet (mg)
1. Acetaminophen, USP, granular	56.5	325.0
2. Solka Floc-BW 100	20.9	120.0
3. Emcocel	18.8	108.3
4. Cab-O-Sil M-5	0.5	3.0
5. Explotab	2.5	14.40
6. Magnesium stearate, N.F.	0.7	4.30
	100.0	575.0

Mix 1, 2, and 3 together for 10 min.   Add 4 and 5 and blend for 10 min.   Add 6 and blend for 5 min. and compress at maximum compression force.
Note: Harder tablets can be made by replacing additional portions of Solka Floc with Emcocel.

Example 4:   Acetaminophen Tablets USP (325 mg)

Ingredient	Composition (%)	Quantity per tablet (mg)
1. Acetaminophen USP	70.00	325.00
2. Avicel PH 101	29.65	138.35
3. Stearic acid, N.F. (fine powder)	0.35	1.65
	100.00	465.00

Note: If smaller crystalline size acetaminophen is desired to improve dissolution, it would be necessary to use a higher proportion of Avicel and to use PH 102 in place of PH 101, and to use a glidant.   All lubricants should be screened before adding to blender.
Blend 1 and 2 for 20 min.   Screen in 3 and blend for an additional 5 min.   Compress tablets using 7/16-in. standard concave or flat bevel tooling.

Example 5:   Analgesic Tablets

Ingredient	Composition (%)	Quantity per tablet (mg)
1. Asprin, USP	33.44	194.00
2. Salicylamide, USP	16.72	97.00
3. Acetaminophen, USP (large crystals or granular)	16.72	97.00
4. Caffeine, USP (granular)	5.60	32.50
5. Avicel PH 101	25.00	145.00
6. Stearic acid (powder), N.F.	2.00	11.50
7. Cab-O-Sil	0.52	3.00
	100.00	580.00

Blend all the ingredients except 5 for 20 min.   Screen in 5 and blend for an additional 5 min.   Compress into tablets using 7/16-in. standard concave tooling.

Example 6:   Propoxyphene Napsylate-Acetaminophen
(APAP) Tablets (100/650 mg)

Ingredient	Composition (%)	Quantity per tablet (mg)
1. 90% Pregranulated APAP	93.01	722.19
2. Propyoxyphene napsylate, USP	11.49	100.00
3. Avicel PH 102	4.00	34.77
4. Ac-Di-Sol	1.00	8.70
5. Cab-O-Sil	0.15	1.30
6. Magnesium stearate, N.F.	0.35	3.04
	100.00	870.00

Note: Pregranulated APAP is available from both
Mallinckrodt and Monsanto in directly compressible forms
containing 90% active ingredient.
Screen 2 and 6 through a 40-mesh sieve. Screen 5
through a 20-mesh sieve. Blend 1, 2, 3, 4, and 5 in
a twin-shell blender for 15 min. Add 6 and blend for 5
min. Compress using precompression force equal to
one-third the final compression force.

Example 7:   Chewable Ascorbic Acid Tablets (100 mg)

Ingredient	Composition (%)	Quantity per tablet (mg)
1. Ascorbic acid, USP (fine crystal)	12.26	27.60
2. Sodium ascorbate, USP	36.26	81.60
3. Avicel PH 101	17.12	38.50
4. Sodium saccharin (powder), N.F.	0.56	1.25
5. DiPac	29.30	66.00
6. Stearic acid, N.F.	2.50	5.60
7. Imitation orange juice flavor	1.00	2.25

Example 7: (Continued)

Ingredient	Composition (%)	Quantity per tablet (mg)
8. FD&C Yellow No. 6 dye	0.50	1.10
9. Cab-O-Sil	0.50	1.10
	100.00	225.00

Note: It is not possible to make chewable ascorbic acid tablets with over 50% active ingredient. Other direct-compression sugars such as Emdex could be used to replace DiPac. Magnesium stearate should be avoided in ascorbic acid formulations. Addition of a higher concentration of Avicel will not usually increase tablet hardness. Blend all ingredients, except 6, for 20 min. Screen in the stearic acid and blend for an additional 5 min. Compress into tablets using 7/16-in. standard concabe tooling.

Example 8: Ascorbic Acid Tablets, USP (250 mg)

Ingredient	Composition (%)	Quantity per tablet (mg)
1. Ascorbic acid, USP (fine crystal or granular)	60.0	250.0
2. Avicel PH 101	20.0	84.0
3. Starch 1500	17.5	75.5
4. Stearic acid, N.F. (powder) or Sterotex	2.0	8.5
5. Cab-O-Sil	0.5	2.0
	100.0	418.0

Note: It is important to use free-flowing types of ascorbic acid due to the high concentration in the formulation. Ascorbic acid concentration could be increased slightly by using more Avicel and less Starch 1500.
Stearic acid, Sterotex, Compritol 888, and Lubritab are interchangeable in most formulations.
Blend all the ingredients, except 4, for 25 min. Screen in 4 and blend for an additional 5 min. Compress into tablets using 7/16-in. standard concave tooling.

Example 9:   Thiamine Hydrochloride Tablets, USP (100 mg)

Ingredient	Composition (%)	Quantity per tablet (mg)
1. Thiamine hydro-chloride, USP	30.0	100.00
2. Avicel PH 102	25.0	83.35
3. Lactose, N.F. anhydrous	42.5	141.65
4. Magnesium stearate, N.F.	2.0	6.65
5. Cab-O-Sil	0.5	1.65
	100.0	333.30

Note: Anhydrous lactose could be replaced with Fast-Flo lactose with no loss in tablet quality. This would reduce (the need for a glidant (which is probably present in too high a concentration in many formulations). (Usually only 0.25% is necessary to optimize fluidity.) Blend all ingredients, except 4, for 25 min. Screen in 4 and blend for an additional 5 min. Compress using 13/32-in. standard concave tooling.

Example 10:   "Maintenance" Multivitamin Tablets

Ingredient	Composition (%)	Quantity per tablet (mg)
1. Vitamin A acetate (dry form 500 IU and 500 D_2 per mg)	5.5	11.0
2. Thiamine monoitrate, USP	0.8	1.65
3. Riboflavin, USP	1.1	2.20
4. Pyridoxine HCl, USP	1.0	2.10
5. 1% Cyanocobalamin (in gelatin)	0.1	0.22
6. D-Calcium pantothenate, USP	3.75	7.50
7. Ascorbic acid, USP (fine crystals)	33.25	66.50
8. Niacinamide	11.0	22.00

Example 10:   (Continued)

Ingredient	Composition (%)	Quantity per tablet (mg)
9. Emcompress of DiTab	13.1	26.23
10. Microcrystalline cellulose, N.F.	25.0	50.00
11. Talc USP	3.0	6.00
12. Stearic acid, N.F. (powder)	1.5	3.00
13. Magnesium stearate, N.F. (powder)	1.0	2.00
	100.00	200.00

Note: This formulation could be converted into a chewable tablet by adding 40 to 50% sugar filler (i.e., Di-Pac and a small quantity of saccharine or aspartame). Blend all ingredients in a suitable blender. Compress at a tablet weight of 200 mg using 3/8-in. standard concave tooling.

Example 11:   Geriatric Formula Vitamin Tablets

Ingredient	Composition (%)	Quantity per tablet (mg)
1. Ferrous sulfate, USP 95% Ethecal granulation	30.00	156.00
2. Thiamine mononitrate, USP	1.09	6.00
3. Riboflavin, USP	1.00	5.50
4. Niacinamide, USP	6.00	33.00
5. Ascorbic acid, C-90	17.45	96.00
6. Calcium pantothenate, USP	0.73	4.00
7. Pyridoxine HCl, USP	0.14	0.75
8. Cyanocobalamin, 0.1% spray-dried	0.82	4.50
9. AcDisol	2.00	11.00
10. Stearic acid N.F. (powder)	2.00	11.00

Example 11: (Continued)

Ingredient	Composition (%)	Quantity per tablet (mg)
11. Magnesium stearate N.F.	0.25	1.38
12. CeloCal	38.52	211.87
	100.00	550.00

Prepare a premix of items 2, 3, 6, 7. Mix in other ingredients except 10 and 11 and blend for 15 min. Add
10 and mix for 5 min. Add 11 and blend for an additional 5 min. Compress using oval punches (1 = 0.480-
in., w = 0.220 × cup = 0.040-in.). Sugar or film coat.

$$SD = \sqrt{\frac{\Sigma(x - \bar{x})^2}{N-1}}$$

Example 12: Pyridoxine HCl Tablets (10 mg)

Ingredient	Composition (%)	Quantity per tablet (mg)
1. Pyridoxine HCl, USP	5.0	10.00
2. Emcompress	92.5	185.00
3. Emcosoy	2.0	4.00
4. Magnesium stearate, N.F.	0.5	1.00
	100.0	200.00

Blend 1 and 2 together for 10 min in a twin-shell
blender. Add 3 and blend for an additional 10 min.
Add 4 and blend for 5 more min and compress.

Example 13: Sodium Fluoride Chewable Tablets (2.2 mg)

Ingredient	Composition (%)	Quantity per tablet (mg)
1. Sodium fluoride	2.0	2.200
2. Emdex	96.75	106.425
3. Artificial grape flavor S.S. (Crompton and Knowles)	0.25	0.275
4. Color, grape S3186 (Crompton and Knowles)	0.25	0.275
5. Magnesium stearate, N.F.	0.75	0.825
	100.00	110.000

Mix ingredient 1 and one-third of 2 for 10 min. Add remaining amount of 2 and 4 and mix thoroughly for 20 min. Add 3 and blend for 10 min. Add 5 and blend 5 additional min and compress.

Example 14: Chewable Antacid Tablets

Ingredient	Composition (%)	Quantity per tablet (mg)
1. FMA-11* (Reheis Chemical Co.)	25.2	400.00
2. Syloid 244	3.2	50.00
3. Emdex	69.3	1100.00
4. Pharmasweet powder (Crompton and Knowles)	1.3	20.00
5. Magnesium stearate, N.F.	1.0	16.00
	100.0	1586.00

Note: An appropriate flavor may be added.
*Aluminum hydroxide/magnesium carbonate co-dried gel.
Mix 1 and 2 together for 5 min. Screen through 30-mesh screen (if ingredients no already prescreened) and mix for 10 to 15 min. Add 3 and 4 and blend thouroughly for 10 to 15 min. Add 5, blend 5 min, and compress.

Example 15:   Calcium Lactate Tablets (10 gr)

Ingredient	Composition (%)	Quantity per tablet (mg)
1. Calcium lactate,* USP	71.25	470
2. AcDiSol	1.25	10
3. Avicel PH 101	10.00	80
4. Stearic acid, N.F. (powder)	2.50	20
5. Magnesium stearate, N.F.	0.50	4
6. CeloCal	14.50	116
	100.00	800

*Equivalent to calcium lactate pentahydrate 650 mg.
Mix ingredients 1, 2, 3, and 6 for 10 min. Add 5 and
blend for an additional 5 min. Compress on Stokes 551
using 1/2-in. standard concave upper bisect punches.

Example 16:   Pyrilamine Meleate Tablets, USP (25 mg)

Ingredient	Composition (%)	Quantity per tablet (mg)
1. Pyrilamine maleate, USP	12.50	25.00
2. Avicel PH 101	17.00	34.00
3. Lactose, N.F. anhydrous	68.40	136.80
4. AcDiSol	1.00	2.00
5. Cab-O-Sil	0.35	0.70
6. Stearic acid, N.F. (powder)	0.25	0.50
7. Magnesium stearate, N.F.	0.50	1.00
	100.00	200.00

Screen 1, 6, and 7 through 40-mesh sieve. Belnd 1 and
3 for 3 min in V blender. Add 2, 4, and 5 to step-2 and
blend for 17 min. Add 6 to step 3 and blend for 3 min.
Add 7 to step 4 and blend for 5 min. Tablet using
5/16-in standard concave punches to a hardness of
5.5 kg.

Example 17: Doxylamine Succinate Tablets USP

Ingredient	Composition (%)	Quantity per tablet (mg)
1. Doxylamine succinate, USP	6.4	25.13
2. Syloid 244	0.85	3.35
3. Solka Floc, BW100	4.05	16.70
4. Emcompress	83.95	331.82
5. Explotab	5.0	20.0
6. Magnesium stearate, N.F.	0.75	3.0
	100.00	400.0

Screen 6 through 30 mesh screen and blend with 2 for 10 to 15 min. Add 3 and one-third of 4 and mix for 10 min. Add remaining 4 and blend for 10 min. Add 5 and blend for 5 to 7 min. Add 6 and blend for 3 to 5 min.

Example 18: Amitriptyline HCl Tablets USP (25 mg)

Ingredient	Composition (%)	Quantity per tablet (mg)
1. Amitriptyline HCl, U.S.P.	22.73	25.0
2. Fast-Flo lactose	59.52	05.47
3. Avicel PH 102	15.00	16.50
4. Ac-Di-Sol	2.00	2.20
5. Cab-O-Sil	0.25	0.28
6. Magnesium stearate, N.F.	0.50	0.55
	100.00	110.0

Screen 1, 2, and 6 through a 40-mesh screen. Blend 1, 2, 3, 4, and 5 in a suitable twin-shell blender for 5 min using intensifier bar. Blend above mixture for an additional 5 min without the intensifier bar. Add 6 and blend for another 5 min. Compress.

Example 19:   Furosemide Tablets USP (40 mg)

Ingredient	Composition (%)	Quantity per tablet (mg)
1. Furosemide, USP	25.00	40.00
2. Avicel, PH-102	12.00	19.20
3. AcDiSol	1.50	2.40
4. Fast-Flo lactose	59.50	95.20
5. Cab-O-Sil	0.50	0.80
6. Stearic acid, N.F.	1.00	1.60
7. Magnesium stearate, N.F.	0.50	0.80
	100.00	160.00

Screen 5 through a 20-mesh sieve. Screen 6 and 7 through a 40-mesh sieve. Blend 1, 2, and 4 in twin-shell blender without intensifier bar for 1 min and then blend with aid of intensifier bar for 0.5 min and without intensifier bar for 1.5 min. Add 3 and 5 and blend for 3 min. Add 6 and blend for 3 min. Add 7 and blend for 5 min. Discharge blender and pass blend through 40-mesh sieve using oscillating granulator. Charge blender with sieved blend and blend for 5 min. Compress using 6/16-in. flat-faced, beveled edge punches. Compression force as needed to give a tablet of 6-kg hardness.

Example 20:   Allopurinol Tablets (300 mg)

Ingredient	Composition (%)	Quantity per tablet (mg)
1. Allopurinol, USP	55.74	300.00
2. Emcompress	37.2	200.00
3. Explotab	3.8	20.50
4. Talc	1.8	10.00
5. Cab-O-Sil	0.5	2.50
6. Magnesium stearate, N.F.	1.0	5.00
	100.0	538.00

Blend 1 and 2 for 10 min. Add 3 and blend for 10 more min. Add 4 and 5 and blend 3 to 5 min. Add 6 and blend 5 more min.

Example 21: Chlorpheniramine Maleate and
Pseudoephedrine HCl Tablets (4/60 mg)

Ingredient	Composition (%)	Quantity per tablet (mg)
1. Chlorpheniramine maleate, USP	1.82	4.0
2. Pseudoephedrine HCl, USP	27.27	60.0
3. Avicel PH-101	16.95	37.3
4. Fast-Flo lactose	51.36	113.0
5. AcDiSol	1.00	2.2
6. Cab-O-Sil	0.50	1.1
7. Stearic acid, N.F.	0.59	1.3
8. Magnesium stearate, N.F.	0.50	1.1
	100.00	220.00

Screen 2, 7, and 8 through 40-mesh sieve. Blend 1, 2,
and 3 in V blender for 3 min. Add 4, 5, and 6 to step
2 and blend for 17 min. Add 7 to step 3 and blend for
3 min. Add 8 to step 4 and blend for 5 min. Tablet
to a hardness of 5.3 kg using 5/16-in standard concave punches.

Example 22: Penicillin V Potassium Tablets USP
(250 mg; 400 IU)

Ingredient	Composition (%)	Quantity per tablet (mg)
1. Penicillin V potassium, USP	50.00	250.00
2. Avicel PH 102	24.25	121.25
3. Ditab or Emcompress (unmilled dicalcium phosphate)	22.00	110.00
4. Magnesium stearate, N.F.	3.75	18.75
	100.00	500.00

Blend 1, 2, and 3 for 25 min. Screen in 4 and blend
for an additional 5 min. Compress using 7/16-in.
standard concave tooling.

Example 23:   Quinidine Sulfate Tablets USP (200 mg)

Ingredient	Composition (%)	Quantity per tablet (mg)
1. Quinidine sulfate, USP	55.85	200.0
2. Avicel PH 102	40.25	144.0
3. Cab-O-Sil	0.50	1.8
4. Stearic acid, N.F. (powder)	2.50	9.0
5. Magnesium stearate, N.F.	0.90	3.2
	100.10	358.0

Blend 1, 2, and 3 for 25 min. Screen in 4 and 5 and blend for 5 min more. Compress using 3/8-in. standard concave tooling.

Example 24:   Chlorpromazine Tablets USP (100 mg)

Ingredient	Composition (%)	Quantity per tablet (mg)
1. Chorpromazine hydro-chloride, USP	28.0	100.00
2. Avicel PH 102	35.0	125.00
3. Ditab or Emcompress	35.0	125.00
4. Cab-O-Sil	0.5	1.74
5. Magnesium stearate, N.F.	1.5	5.25
	100.0	357.00

Blend all the ingredients, except 5, for 25 min.
Screen in 5 and blend for an additional 5 min. C
Compress into tablets using 11/32-in. tooling.

Example 25: Isosorbide Dinitrate Tablets (10 mg, oral)

Ingredient	Composition (%)	Quantity per tablet (mg)
1. Isosorbide dinitrate (25% in lactose)	20.00	40.00
2. Avicel PH 102	19.80	39.60
3. Fast-Flo lactose	59.45	118.90
4. Magnesium stearate, N.F.	0.75	1.50
	100.00	200.00

Blend 1, 2, and 3 in a P-K blender for 25 min. Blend
in 4 for 5 min. Compress into tablets using 5/16-in.
standard concave tooling.

Glossary of Trade Names and Manufacturers

Trade name	Chemical/description	Manufacturer
Ac-Di-Sol	Croscarmellose, N.F.	FMC Corporation, Philadelphia, PA 19103
Anhydrous lactose	Lactose N.F. (anhydrous direct tableting)	Sheffield Chemical, Union, NJ 07083
		DMV Corp., Veghel, The Netherlands
Avicel 101, 102	Microcrystalline cellulose, N.F	FMC Corp., Philadelphia, PA 19103
Compritol 88	Glyceryl behenate, N.F.	Gattefose Corp., Elansford, NY 10523
DCL-Lactose	Lactose, N.F. (various types)	DMV Corp., Veghel, Holland
Delaflo	Direct-compression calcium sulfate	J.W.S. Delavau Co., Philadelphia, PA 19122
Des-Tab	Compressible sugar, N.F.	Desmo Chemical Corp., St. Louis, MO 63144
Di-Pac	Compressible sugar, N.F.	American Sugar Co., New York, NY 10020
Di-Tab	Dibasic calcium phosphate, USP (unmilled)	Stauffer Chemical Co., Westport, CT 06880
Elcema G-250	Powdered cellulose, N.F.	Degussa, D-6000 Frankfurt (Main) Germany

Glossary of Trade Names and Manufacturers (Continued)

Trade name	Chemical/description	Manufacturer
Emcocel	Microcrystalline cellulose, N.F.	Edward Mendell Co., Carmel, NY 10512
Emcompress	Dibasic calcium phosphate, USP special size fraction	Edward Mendell Co., Carmel, NY 10512
Emdex	Dextrates, N.F. (dextr	Edward Mendell Co., Carmel, NY 10512
Explotab	Sodium starch glycolate, N.F.	Edward Mendell Co., Carmel, NY 10512
Fast-Flo Lactose	Lactose, N.F. (spray dried)	Foremost Whey Products Banaboo, Wi. 53913
Lubritab	Hydrogenated vegetable oil, N.F.	Edward Mendell Co., Carmel, NY 10512
Maltrin	Agglomerated maltrodextrin	Grain Processing Corp., Muscatine, IA 52761
Neosorb 60	Sorbitol, N.F. (direct-compression)	Roquette Corp., 645 5th Avenue New York, NY 10022
Nu-Tab	Compressible sugar, N.F.	Ingredient Technology, Inc., Pennsauken, NJ 08110
Polyplasdone XL	Crospovidone, N.F. (cross-linked polyvinylpyrrolidone)	GAF Corp., New York, NY 10020
Primojel	Sodium starch glycolate, N.F. (carboxymethyl starch)	Generichem Corp., Little Falls, NJ 07424
Solka Floc	Cellulose floc	Edward Mendell Co., Carmel, NY 10512
Sorbitol 834	Sorbitol, N.F. (crystalline for direct compression)	ICI United States, Wilmington, DE 19897
Spray-dried lactose	Lactose N.F. (spray-dried)	Foremost Whey Products, Baraboo, Wi. 53913
		DMV Corp., Vehgel, Holland
Sta-Rx 1500 (Starch 1500)	Pregelatinized starch, N.F. (compressible)	Colorcon, Inc., West Point, PA 19486
Sterotex	Hydrogenated Vegetable oil, N.F.	Capital City Products Co., Columbus, OH 43216

Glossary of Trade Names and Manufacturers (Continued)

Trade name	Chemical/description	Manufacturer
Tab-Fine	Trade name identifying a number of direct-compression sugars including sucrose, fructose, dextrose	Edward Mendell Co., Carmel, NY 10512
Tablettose	Lactose, N.F. hydrous (for direct compression)	Fallek Chemical Co., New York, NY 10022 (Product of Meggle Milchindustrie—GMBM & Co., KG
TriTab	Tricalcium phosphate anhydrous direct compression	Stauffer Chemical Co., Westport, CT 06881
Vitacel	Coprocessed product containing 30% calcium carbonate and 70% microcrystalline cellulose	FMC Corp., Philadelphia, PA 19103

REFERENCES

1. G. Milosovitch, *Drug Cosmet. Ind.*, 92, 557 (1963).
2. W. C. Gunsel and L. Lachman, *J. Pharm. Sci.*, 52, 178 (1963).
3. C. D. Fox et al., *Drug Cosmet. Ind.*, 92, 161 (1963).
4. P. C. Record, *Int. J. Pharm. Tech. and Prod. Mfr.*, 1)2), 32 (1980).
5. S. Pearce, *Mfr. Chemist*, 57(6), 77 (1986).
6. R. A. Castello and A. M. Mattocks, *J. Pharm. Sci.*, 51, 106 (1962).
7. J. T. Hutton and G. Palmer, U.S. Patent 3,639,170 (1972).
8. N. A. Butuyios, *J. Pharm. Sci.*, 55, 727 (1966).
9. G. K. Bolhuis et al., *Drug Dev. Ind. Pharm.*, 11(8), 1657 (1985).
10. H. Vromans et al., *Acta Pharm. Suec.*, 22, 163 (1985).
11. H. Vromans et al., *Pharm. Weekblad, Sci. Ed.*, 7, 186 (1985).
12. DeBoer et al., *Sci. Ed*, 8, 145 (1986).
13. H. V. VanKamp et al., *Int. J. Pharm.*, 28, 229 (1986).
14. H. V. VanKamp et al., *Acta Pharm. Suec.*, 23, 217 (1986).
15. C. P. Graham et al., U.S. Patent 3,642,535 (1972).
16. S. E. Tabibi and G. Hollenbeck, *Int. J. Pharm.*, 18, 169 (1984).
17. A. B. Rizzuto et al., *Pharm. Tech.*, 8(9), 132 (1984).
18. C. B. Froeg et al., U.S. Patent 3,639,169 (1972).
19. H. D. Bergman et al., *Drug Cosmet. Ind.*, 109, 55 (1971).
20. J. DuRoss, *Pharm. Tech.*, 8(9), 32 (1984).
21. A. M. Guyot-Hermann and D. Leblanc, *Drug Dev. Ind. Pharm.*, 11, 551 (1985).

22. A. Briggs, *Develop. Biol. Standards, 36,* 251 (1977).

23. A. Briggs and T. Maxwell, U.S. Patent 3,932,943 (1976).

24. B. Debord et al., *Drug Dev. Ind. Pharm., 13,* 1533 (1987).

25. R. Short and F. Verbanac, U.S. Patent 3,622,677 (1971).

26. K. S. Manudhane et al., *J. Pharm. Sci., 58,* 616 (1969).

27. G. E. Reier and R. F. Shangraw, *J. Pharm. Sci., 55,* 510 (1966).

28. J. W. Wallace et al., *Pharm. Tech.* 7(9), 94 (1983).

29. T. Personen and P. Paronen, *Drug Dev. Ind. Pharm., 12,* 2091 (1986).

30. E. Doelker et al., *Drug Dev. Ind. Pharm., 13,* 1847 (1987).

31. A. D. F. Toy, *Phosphorous Chemistry in Everyday Living,* Am. Chem. Soc. Press, Washington, D.C., 1976, p. 57.

32. X. Hou and J. T. Carstensen, *Int. J. Pharm., 25,* 207 (1985).

33. C. F. Lerk et al., *Pharm. Weekblad, 109,* 945 (1974).

34. J. Bavitz and J. B. Schwartz, *Drug Cosmet. Ind., 114,* 44 (1974).

35. A. V. Katdare and J. F. Bavitz, *Drug Dev. Ind. Pharm., 13,* 1047 (1987).

36. L. L. Augsburger and R. F. Shangraw, *J. Pharm. Sci., 55,* 418 (1966).

37. R. Ho et al., *Drug Dev. Ind. Pharm., 3,* 475 (1977).

38. J. N. Staniforth, *Int. J. Pharm. Tech. Prod. Manuf., 3*(Suppl) 1, (1982).

39. J. Verraes and R. Kinget, *Int. J. Pharm. Tech. Prod. Manuf., 1*(3), 38 (1980).

40. J. Staniforth and J. Rees, *J. Pharm. Pharmacol., 35,* 549 (1983).

41. A. C. Shah and A. R. Mlodozeniec, *J. Pharm. Sci., 66,* 1377 (1977).

42. G. K. Bolhuis et al., *Drug Dev. Ind. Pharm., 13,* 1547 (1987).

43. H. Hess, *Pharm. Tech., 2*(9), 36, (1978).

44. R. Shangraw et al., *Pharm. Tech., 5*(9), 68 (1981).

45. R. Shangraw et al., *Pharm. Tech., 5*(10), 44 (1981).

46. R. Shangraw, *Pharm. Tech., 11*(6), 144 (1987).

47. American Pharmaceutical Association and the Pharmaceutical Society of Great Britian, *Handbook of Pharmaceutical Excipients,* American Pharmaceutical Association, Washington, D.C. (1986).

48. Anil Salpekar, U.S. Patent 4,600,579 (1986).

49. Steve Vogel, U.S. Patent 4,439,453, (1984).

50. E. J. deJong, *Pharm. Weekblad, 104,* 469, (1969).

51. I. Ullah et al., *Pharm. Tech., 11*(9), 48, (1987).

52. R. Franz, U.S. Patent 4,609,675, (1986).

5
Compression-Coated and Layer Tablets

William C. Gunsel*

Ciba-Geigy Corporation
Summit, New Jersey

Robert G. Dusel

Lachman Consultant Services, Inc.
Westbury, New York

I. COMPRESSION COATING

In the early 1950s, two major developments in tableting presses occurred. Machines for compressing a coating around a tablet core and machines for making layer tablets appeared on the market. They were accepted enthusiastically through the 1960s, but the compression-coating technique is rarely employed today in the manufacture of new products because of the advent of film coating with its relative simplicity and its cost advantages.

The chief advantage was the elimination of water or other solvent in the coating procedure. Thus there is no need for a barrier coating to prevent water from penetrating the cores—possibly softening them or initiating an undesired reaction. Such barriers, if efficient, slow down disintegration and dissolution. The dry coating is applied in a single step (in contrast to the repeated applications of different syrups), reducing the time required to evaporate the water and eliminating the necessity of cleaning the coating pan each time it becomes heavily encrusted with dried syrup. With dry coating, incompatible substances can be separated by placing one of them in the core and the other in the coating. There may be some reactivity at the interface but this should be negligible in the dry state. In addition, if a drug tends to discolor readily or develop a mottled appearance because of oxidation or sunlight, these problems can be minimized by incorporating the drug in the core tablet.

Compression-coated tablets function like sugar-coated or film-coated tablets in that the coating may cover a bitter substance, conceal an unpleasant or mottled appearance, or provide a barrier for a substance irritating to the stomach or one inactivated by gastric juice. The advent of film coating

---

*Currently retired.

dissipated much of the advantage of dry coating since larger quantities of tablets can be coated in a short time with film-formers dissolved in organic or aqueous solvents. These films dry so rapidly that there is scarcely sufficient time for a reaction to occur. Most recently, the deposition of films out of aqueous solution and suspension has become feasible. Recent advances in coating equipment, such as the side vented pans, have increased the efficiency of the aqueous coating operation to a point where even asprin tablets may be aqueous coated without significant hydrolysis. This has greatly increased the popularity of film coating over compression coating. Films produce a minimal increase in the size and weight of the core tablets; monograms and other devices on the core remain legible.

While sugar coating a tablet may increase its weight by 50 to 100% of the core weight, the compression-coated tablet requires a coating that is about twice the weight of the core. If the cores are composed mainly of materials of low bulk density, such as fats and waxes, the amount of coating (by weight) must be even greater to assure a uniform volume of material surrounding the core.

Another application of the compression-coated dosage form is in sustained-release preparations. A coating containing the immediate-release portion is compressed around a slowly releasing core. This gives a far more accurate dose than is the case with sugar coating. In the latter, the immediate-release portion must be applied in increments; the cores do not pick up weight equally. As the process continues, those with increased surface area gain at the expense of those with less. Thus at the end of a coating run, tablet weights and drug content may vary as much as ±20% for individual tablets, depending on the number of coats of active ingredient required. With compression coating, monograms and other markings may be impressed in the coating—in contradistinction to the printing of sugar-coated tablets in a separate step. The latter also requires complete inspection to sort out imperfect printing.

A. History of Compression Coating

The availability of compression-coating machines in the 1950s generated great interest; nevertheless, the idea was not new. As early as 1896, P. J. Noyes of New Hampshire acquired a British patent for such a device [1]. The machine was a rotary press with two hoppers which supplied the granulation of the bottom and top coating. Between them was a third hopper from which the previously compressed core tablets passed through a tube with a reciprocating finger into the die. As each tablet was deposited on the bottom layer of coating, the die table paused in its rotation to allow good centering of the core. Then the process continued with deposition of the top layer, compression, and ejection.

The next advance occurred in 1917 when F. J. Stokes [2] patented a machine which fed the cores onto a toothed disk. The cores passed from the disk into the dies. The timing of the disk was controlled by a star-wheel, which was actuated in turn by projections on the turret. Another innovation was the embedding of the core into the bottom fill by the fall of the upper punch. The patent indicates that this was a layer press, but that a coated tablet was feasible if the cores had smaller diameters than the dies into which they were deposited.

In 1935, the DeLong Gum Company of Massachusetts obtained a British patent [3] for a machine to compress a sugar composition onto chewing gum. The purpose of the invention was to protect the gum from the atmosphere. Biconvex cores were punched out of sheets of gum and deposited by the machine between two layers of coating. The concave faces of the punches, the convexity of the cores, and the lubricity of the coating contributed to automatic centration. A device with fingers might also aid in the placement of the cores, according to the claim made; the mechanics of this unit was not described. The inventor also mentioned that the product could be distinctively embossed.

In 1937, Kilian, a German inventor, received a British patent [4] for a unit which compressed tablets on one machine and held them in the upper punches. These punches had rods passing lenthwise through them. The compression wheel was recessed so that it could compress the cores without activating the core rod. The cores were carried around the turret to the transfer mechanism. At this point the upper punches passed under a roller which pressed down the core rods, ejecting the cores onto the transfer plate. The plate carried the cores to the coating machine. It is evident that the Manesty DryCota adopted the idea of two machines running synchronously from this patent. Kilian, however, in cooperation with Evans Medical Supplies, Ltd., developed for sale the Prescoter which is a single rotary press. In the operation of this machine, the cores are fed from a vibrating hopper onto a feed plate which carries them to the dies, the process then resembling that of the Stokes machine. A reject device operating by the difference in hardness eliminates any coreless tablet.

B. Available Equipment

There are three principal designs in compression-coating machines. Two of them provide for putting the coating on cores that were compressed on another machine; one provides for the compression of the core on one side of the machine with almost instantaneous transfer to the other side of the machine for the application of the coating. An example of the first type is the Colton Model 232 (Fig. 1). Previously compressed cores are fed by a vibrating feeder unit (A) onto a circular feeding disk (B) which is rotated clockwise or counterclockwise, as desired, by a variable-speed motor. The disk is tapered slightly downward from its center to its edge. A vibrator (C) gently agitates the disk so that the core tablets separate into a single layer. Around the periphery of the disk is a plastic ring (D) which prevents the tablets from piling up or escaping from the core selector ring immediately below (not visible in the photograph). The selector ring has 33 V-shaped slots around its inner edge, which engage the cores. The cores are picked out of the slots by transfer cups (E) connected to a vacuum system through flexible tubing (F). The cups, which are spring loaded, are guided into contact with the cores by means of the cam (G) and the pins (H). The core centering ring and the transfer cups are synchronized with the speed of the die table.

In practice, a bottom layer of coating enters the die from the hopper (I) and feed frame (J). At the same time (see Fig. 2), a core is picked up by a transfer cup which is guided by another cam (A) into the die (not visible). The vacuum is interrupted, and the core rests on the bed of

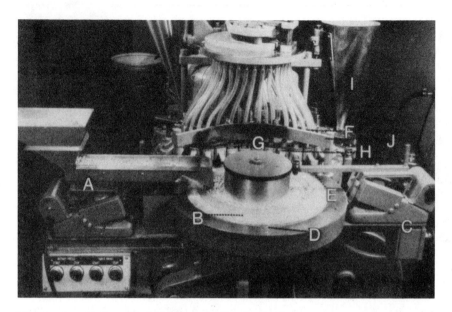

Figure 1   Colton Model 232.   Refer to text

coating. A metering feed plate (B) passes under a hopper (C) and feed
frame (D)—and over the die into which it deposits the top layer of granulation. The whole is then compressed in the usual manner by passing the
punches between the compression rolls. If a transfer cup does not contain
a core, the vacuum will suck the bottom layer of coating from the die. The
metered amount of the top layer is then insufficient to form a tablet and
will be expelled. If a core is not deposited, the pin in the transfer cup
activates a microswitch which shuts off the press. Figure 3 is a schematic
providing another view of the machine.

The machine has 33 compression stations. It can produce a maximum
of 900 tablets per minute, the largest tablet being 5/8 in. in diameter. It
can handle cores previously made with flat-faced, shallow concave, standard
concave, capsule-shaped, or oval punch tips.

There are a number of problems in the operation of this machine. When
one transfer cup fails to pick up a core, vacuum is lost—to the extent that
cores picked up by the other nozzles are held insecurely and fall out before they can be deposited in the dies. Some cores are picked up inaccu-
rately because, being constantly in motion, they do not slide all the way
into the slots of the core centering ring. They are then deposited off-
center or at a tilt and sometimes become visible in the surface of the coated
tablet. The pins in the transfer cups, which are supposed to ensure deposition of the cores in the dies, become bent or jam; then cores are
crushed, or the machine is frequently stopped by the tripping of the microswitch when the cores are retained. Parts of crushed cores can be carried
beyond the point of deposition, fall on the die table, and be swept into the
feed frame. Blockage may occur. Cores prepared with standard concave
or deep concave punches tend to *shingle* or overlap on the core centering
ring and cannot be picked up properly. Capped tablets will also disrupt
the feeder which inserts the core tablets into the transfer device, producing

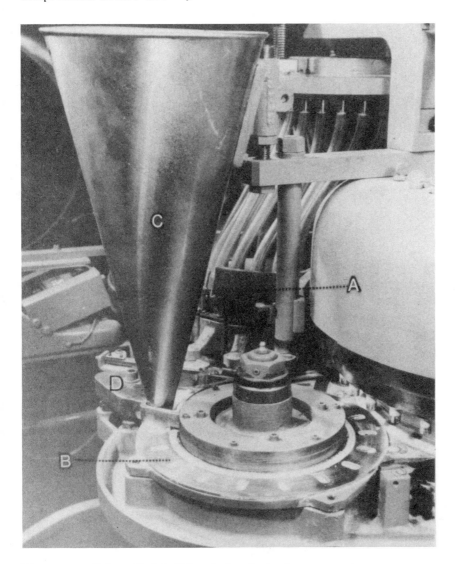

Figure 2   Colton Model 232.   Refer to text.

a high level of rejected "coreless" tablets. Tablets with flat faces or shallow convexities behave much better.

The Stokes Model 538 is a modified 27-station BB2 double rotary machine with one set of compression rolls removed. As can be seen in Figure 4, the previously manufactured cores are loaded into a vibrating hopper (A) which moves them into a flexible feeder tube (B). The cores pass down the tube against a wheel mounted vertically, behind the housing (C). The top surface of the wheel is level with the die table. It contains 9 holes bored through the center; these are connected to a vacuum system by means of which the cores are carried to a transfer mechanism (D) mounted horizontally. This device contains 14 V-shaped slots in a link-chain system. A star-wheel, which is synchronized with the die table by means of bushings

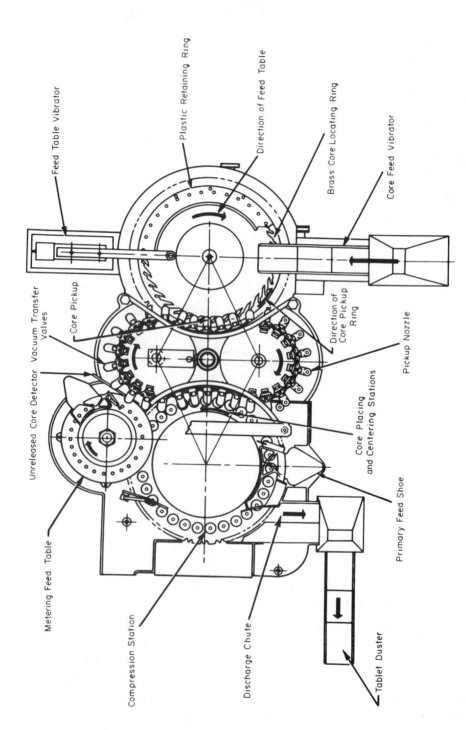

Figure 3 Colton Model 232, schematic (Vector Corp.).

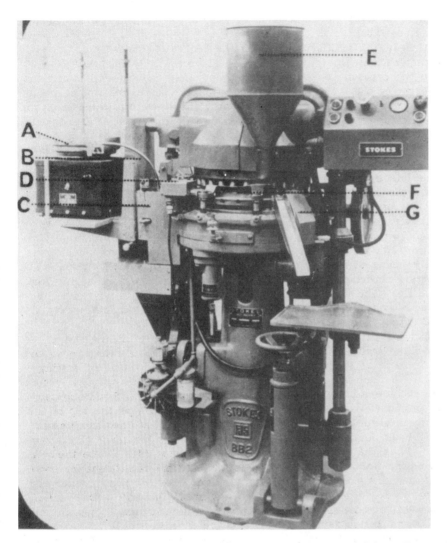

Figure 4 Stokes Model 538. Refer to text (Stokes Division, Pennwalt Corporation).

on the turret, guides the V-slots over the vacuum wheel and the dies. As the core tablet enters the V-slot, a spring-loaded pin rests with a slight pressure upon it. As the core passes over the die, which now contains the lower layer of coating from the hopper (E) and feed frame (F), the pin presses the core into the coating. At this moment the lower punch drops, leaving room for the deposition of the top layer of coating provided by a hopper and feed frame at the back of the machine. If a core is missing, an electrical sensing device on the feed mechanism detects the fact and activates a time-delay solenoid—which, in turn, releases a brief blast of compressed air, which blows the defective tablet into a reject chute (G) installed just before the normal tablet take-off. This machine can produce 700 tablets per minute, with diameters up to 5/8 in.; it can handle special shaped such as ovals and capsules; and it is much simpler to set up and operate than the Colton Model 232.

Nevertheless, difficulties occur with the Stokes machine also. Cores may clog the feeding tube; the vacuum wheel occasionally fails to hold a tablet; and the cores do not always slide accurately into the V-slots or fall into the center of the dies. In the last instance, some cores will be partially visible in the surface of the completed tablet. The reject mechanism catches more than one tablet in its jet of air and blows good as well as bad tablets into the reject chute. The good, however, can be salvaged by inspection.

The Manesty DryCota is illustrated in Figure 5. It is essentially two heavy-duty D3 presses with a transfer device between, the three parts of the machine joined and kept in synchronization by a common drive shaft. The core tablets are compressed in the normal manner on the left-hand press (A). Upon ejection, they are brought up flush with the surface of the die adjacent to the right-hand side of the feed frame. They rise up into cups (B) on transfer arms (C) and are carried across the bridge (D) to the coating side of the machine (E). The transfer arms are positioned precisely by means of rings projecting below the upper punch guides. The rings engage a semicircular recess in each arm. The arms are spring loaded for positive fit. The bridge is perforated and connected to a vacuum pump, which removes loose dust and small particles from the cores and prevents transfer of core granulation into the coating granulation.

The feed frame (F) on the coating turret is narrowed in its central portion to allow the transfer arms to pass. Granulation flows from the hopper (G) into the front of the feed frame and fills the bottom layer of coating into the die. A transfer arm is guided over this die; the core falls out of the cup as the lower punch is pulled down to make room. Simultaneously the upper punch (H) drops down on its cam track and taps the top of the transfer cup to assure positive release of the core. The die then passes beneath the back portion of the feed frame where the top layer of coating is applied. Then the whole is compressed together at (I). While the other two machines require a hopper, a feed frame, and fill adjustment for each of the bottom and top coatings, the DryCota requires only one hopper and feed frame. It does, however, have two weight adjustments. One is for the total amount of coating; the second, at (J), adjusts the bottom fill so that the top and bottom layers are of equal thickness.

In the operation of the machine, the weight and hardness of the cores are adjusted first. Once these parameters are satisfactory, the transfer arms and cups are installed. Now, as the cores are being transferred to the coating turret, the weight of the coating and the hardness of the tablets are established. Tablets are cut or broken in half to determine if the cores are centered. If not, the bottom fill is adjusted until centration is satisfactory. The weight and hardness of the cores can now be routinely checked while the machine is running. A lever behind the control box is depressed, causing a portion of the lower cam track to be raised and to eject the core and coating just before the compression wheels. A fixed blade, mounted across and close to the die table, diverts the ejected materials around the compression wheels to the discharge chute. The cores can now be separated from the coating granulation and tested for compliance with specifications, and any needed corrections can be made.

There is a positive arrangement for detecting coreless tablets. The transfer cup is actually composed of two parts; a die with a cylindrical vertical bore through it, in which the core is tapped, and a pin with a

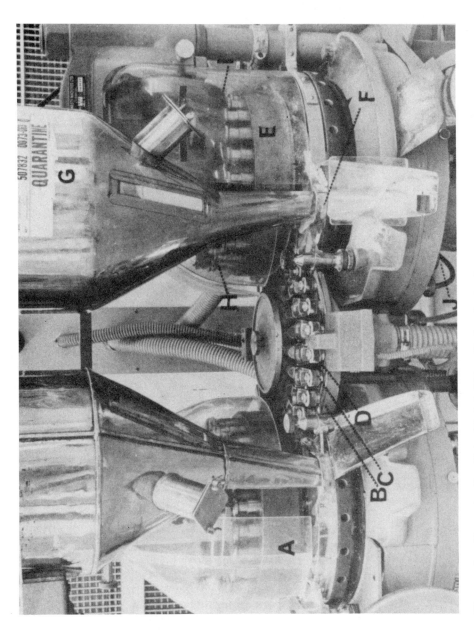

Figure 5   Manesty DryCota Model 900.   Refer to text.

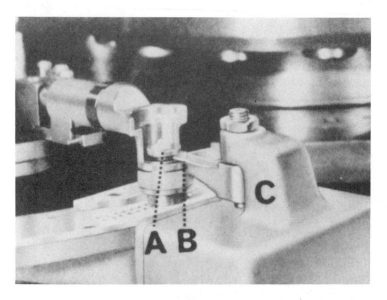

Figure 6   Manesty DryCota: front microswitch.

wide flange on top, which rests on the tablet. As Figure 6 demonstrates, when a core is in the cup, the flange (A) is raised and passes the knife blade (B) of a microswitch (C) without disturbing it. When the flange is resting on the die, signifying that a core has not been picked up, the switch is tripped and stops the machine. This switch is mounted at the front of the machine. As shown in Figure 7, at the back is another microswitch (A), which is actuated when the pin is up, indicating that the core has not been deposited. Again the machine is stopped. It is not necessary

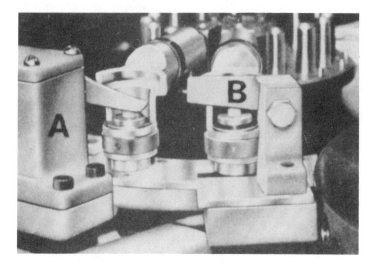

Figure 7   Manesty DryCota: rear microswitch.

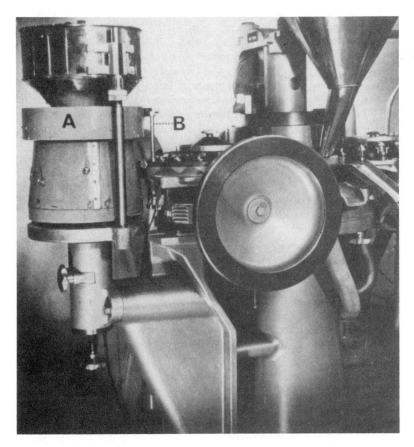

Figure 8   Manesty DryCota: CenterCota unit.   Refer to text.

that the machine be wired to stop it in case of a reject.   Alternatively, a
gate in the discharge chute can be activated to divert the reject (along with
several other tablets) into a separate receptacle while the machine continues
to run.   When the core is not deposited, it is forced out of the cup when the
pin passes under, and is depressed by, an inclined ramp (B).   The core
falls into a small depression in the bridge of the transfer unit and thus cannot return to the core turret.

The largest DryCota is a 23-station machine capable of producing 900
tablets per minute with a maximum diameter of 5/8 in.   The machine can also
be fitted with a unit called the CenterCota (Fig. 8), which enables previously
compressed cores to be dry coated.   It consists of a vibratory hopper (A)
which guides the cores to a flexible tube (B).   The cores pass down the
tube to be engaged by U-slots mounted on transfer arms like those described
above.   The slots guide the cores to the dies of what is normally the core-
forming turret.   Thus the DryCota could be used for compressing a coating
on cores that had been specially treated with a barrier coating, for example,
to obviate a reaction between the two parts of the tablet or to provide a
delayed release.

Apart from its low output, the DryCota has several drawbacks: the core tablets cannot be analyzed before they are coated, and they cannot be pretreated unless the CenterCota device is added to the machine. The first problem can be compensated for in large measure by analyzing the granulation beforehand. Although the cores are dedusted as they cross the bridge to the coating side, particles from the core granulation may be carried over to mingle with the coating and show up in the surface of the finished tablet. This event is most apt to occur if the upper core punches are worn and form a small ring (flash) around the top of the tablet. Flakes from this ring then fall off. Precompressed cores, having been vigorously vibrated beforehand on a tablet deduster, tend to be free of flash. Of course, good manufacturing practice would require the replacement of worn punches.

Another machine available is the Kilian Prescoter, which operates like the Stokes machine except that the vacuum wheel is absent. The modern Prescoter is a single rotary machine and does not resemble the machine described in the 1937 British patent mentioned above.

The newer model dry-coating machines have a number of distinctive features. Perfect feed-in of tablet cores is achieved by setting the circumferential speed of the core centering table equal to that of the turntable and employing an involute curve. A photoelectric tube is used to detect whether a tablet has its core or not; if not, the tablet is rejected. As a doublecheck, coreless tablets are detected by measuring, with a load cell, the pressure difference between tablets with cores and those without.

C. Comparison of Compression–Coating Machines

The advantage of the Colton 232 and Stokes 538 is that the cores can be compressed on machines of much greater output—as many as 10,000 tablets per minute. The cores may be assayed before coating. When the core tablet is prepared on a separate machine, the hardness must be sufficient to retain its integrity during the bulk transfer and feeding into the die. This increased hardness often requires additional lubricant which will reduce the powder coating bond strength and therefore increase the level of rejects. Such cores will be firm enough to be handled in packaging machinery without incurring damage and therefore should be able to withstand transfer on the coating machines. It is almost futile to assign a numerical standard to the hardness requirement; hardness varies with the composition, thickness, shape, and diameter of tablets. A core 3/8 in. in diameter with a hardness of 5 SC units may be very satisfactory in one instance and completely inadequate in another. Although hardness testers measure resistance to crushing, which is important in dry coating, the resistance of a tablet to transverse fracture is more important. Unfortunately, there is no satisfactory way to make this measurement; there is only the subjective test of breaking the tablet with the fingers and listening for a distinct report of breakage—the snap.

The coating granulation tends to bond poorly to hard cores because of the latter's surface density. Then the strength of the coating depends mainly on its own cohesiveness. The core may be likened to a peanut in a shell. The principal area of weakness is over the edge of the core. Increasing the coating thickness may compensate for the weakness. The advantage of the Manesty DryCota is that the core need only be firm enough to hold together while being carried a short distance across the bridge of the press to the coating turret. Thus the surface of the core is rather porous,

Table 1   Condensed Specifications for Compression-Coating Machines

Specification	Manufacturer and model designations							
	Compression coaters					Standard Machines[a]		
	Colton 232	Stokes 538	Dricota Manesty 900		Hata HT-AP44-C	Stokes 585-1	Colton 247-41	Manesty Beta Press
			Core	Coating				
Maximum tablet diameter (in.)	5/8	5/8	9/16	5/8	7/16	7/16	7/16	5/8
Maximum depth of fill (in.)	1/2	11/16		7/16	5/16	11/16	3/4	11/16
Number of compression stations	33	27	23	23	44	65	41	16
Maximum output (tablets per min)	900	500	950	900	1,540	10,000	4,300	1,500
Pressure (tons. in.$^{-2}$)	3	4	6	6	5.5	10	4.5	6.5

[a]Several standard presses for comparison.

permitting penetration by the granules of the coating. On final compression, core and coating are densified simultaneously and bound firmly together.

Since each of the machines described is a modification of equipment used in normal tablet operations, the manufacturers stress the latter use also. However, when such machines are purchased, they are usually devoted exclusively to dry coating. Only a research laboratory or a small business would employ them for multiple purposes. Their low output is extremely disadvantageous. The Manesty, being composed of two presses, is more productive than the others because it can turn out twice as many plain tablets as coated ones.

Table 1 details the manufacturers' specifications for each machine. For comparison purposes, several high-speed machines are listed.

II. FORMULATIONS (COMPRESSION COATING)

Information about formulations for compression coating is characterized by its paucity. A few workers have published some of their experiences; a few have obtained patents on compositions. Several authors have prepared review articles in which they have set down general rules for successful use of the dry-coating technique but there are few specifics.

It is no easy task to obtain optimum quality in a tablet—a task to be attacked anew for each active ingredient and sometimes for each strength of the same medicinal chemical. For compression coating, where two formulas are involved for each product, the task can be even more difficult. Also of course, no one knows what the optimum formula is; the formulator usually settles for that composition which satisfies certain standards of hardness, friability, disintegration time, dissolution time, and stability, as well as the clinical requirement of effectiveness. Almost every new therapeutic agent presents problems of formulation which cannot be solved by some pet formulation. Nevertheless, there are compositions available which can be tried and, with some changes, found satisfactory.

A. Core Tablets

Almost any formula which will produce a firm tablet is satisfactory for all the machines described. There are a number of compressible fillers and compositions on the market which may be combined with the medicament, disintegrants, glidants, dry binders, and each other in an infinite number of proportions. They are economical to use because they eliminate the need for wetting to form granules and subsequent drying. There is no need to mill them, although screening may be required to break up agglomerates. On the other hand, the presence of the drug may interfere with the cohesion of the filler. Seldom does one find a substance like sodium chloride or potassium chloride which is inherently directly compressible. When the amount of drug is small, the content uniformity may be poor; the drug may not distribute well because static charge develops during blending with the vehicle. The addition of starch, with its high moisture content, is useful for dissipating the charge. The fluidity of the vehicle may lead to segregation of the active ingredient on the tablet press. Here, the presence of microcrystalline cellulose in the formula can reduce the tendency to demix. Often also, large quantities of the compressible excipient may be needed for good cohesion. Since core tablets should be kept small, it is better to change to a wet granulation formula.

Some materials currently available are spray-dried lactose, anhydrous lactose, microcrystalline cellulose, dicalcium phosphate, granular mannitol, sucrose, hydrolyzed starch derivatives (Emdex, Starch 1500 NF), and compositions of sucrose, invert sugar, starch, and magnesium stearate (Nu-Tab). Some typical formulas using these materials are shown.

Example 1:   Typical Core Granulation

Ingredient	Quantity
Active ingredient	q.s.
Starch NF	5.0%
Magnesium stearate NF	0.5%
Lactose NF anhydrous	q.s.
	100.0%

Example 2:   Typical Core Granulation

Ingredient	Quantity
Active ingredient	q.s.
Microcrystalline cellulose NF	30.0%
Magnesium stearate NF	0.5%
Lactose NF (spray-dried)	q.s.
	100.0%

Example 3:   Typical Core Granulation

Ingredient	Quantity
Active ingredient	q.s.
Sodium starch glycolate NF	5.0%
Magnesium stearate NF	1.0%
Diabasic calcium phosphate USP	q.s.
	100.0%

Example 4:   Typical Core Granulation

Ingredient	Quantity
Active ingredient	q.s.
Sodium starch glycolate NF	4.0%
Stearic acid NF	1.0%
Emdex	q.s.
	100.0%

In these four examples the drug is comminuted
to a fine particle size, the other ingredients
are passed through a 20 mesh screen if they
are agglomerated, and the materials are blended for 15 to 20 min in a planetary, ribbon, or
double-arm blender.   The starches are included to promote disintegration.   In the second example, the microcrystalline cellulose
improves cohesion, disintegration, and compressibility.   With dicalcium phosphate, additional magnesium stearate is needed for
die release.

An example of an active ingredient which could be formulated for direct
compression is chlorisondamine chloride, a quaternary ammonium ganglionic
blocker, used for the treatment of hypertension.   It had a extremely unpleasant, bitter taste which had to be masked to make it acceptable.   It
had one physical attribute that was useful for tableting; namely, it was
readily compressible.

Example 5:   Chlorisondamine Chloride Tablets

Ingredient	Quantity per tablet
Chlorisondamine chloride[a]	55.55 mg
Lactose, NF spray-dried	43.70 mg
Magnesium stearate NF	0.75 mg
	100.00 mg

Break up any aggregates by passing all materials through a 20 mesh screen.   Blend for 20
min in a double-arm mixer.

[a] Contains 10% alcohol of crystallization.

This formulation was suitable also for 25-mg and 100-mg cores, which were other desired strengths of the drug. The 25-mg core was compressed with 3/16-in. diameter standard concave punches; the 50-mg core with 1/4-in. punches; and the 100-mg core with 5/16-in. punches. The level of magnesium stearate was established at 0.75% to overcome resistance of the tablets to extrusion. When these cores were covered with an inert composition, the 50-mg strength had a hardness value of 12 SC units and disintegrated in 10 min. The coating formula used was the same as in Example 9.

A second type of formula is a two-phased one in which the drug and the fillers are formed into granules by wetting them in the presence of an adhesive, drying the resultant moist mass, and passing it through a mill to obtain a convenient particle size. These granules are then blended with a disintegrant, if necessary, and a lubricant. It is a good idea to incorporate a disintegrant in the wet phase so that the granules will also readily disintegrate after the core tablet breaks up. Some thought must be given to the milling step since, in general, the granules should be relatively coarse so that the surfaces of the cores will be somewhat porous and permit penetration by the coating material for good bonding. Wire mesh or perforated plates for milling with openings of 10 to 16 mesh should be selected, the smaller openings for the smaller cores.

Examples of core granulations prepared by the two-phase system are shown.

Example 6:   Core Granulation (Two-Phase)

Ingredient	Quantity
Active ingredient	q.s.
Dibasic calcium phosphate NF	29.5%
Starch NF	6.0%
Lactose, NF, impalpable	q.s.
Povidone USP	2.0%
Purified water USP	q.s.
Magnesium stearate NF	0.5%
	100.0%

Note: The amount of lactose NF is reduced by the amounts of the drug.
Blend the first four ingredients and pass them through a #1 perforated plate (round-hole screen) on a Fitzmill operating at medium speed with hammers forward. Prepare a solution by suspending the povidone in water. Add this povidone solution to the blended powders and mix until the mass is

Example 6:   (Continued)

---

uniformly moist. Spread the mass on trays
and dry at 50°C to a moisture content of
2 to 3%. Pass the dried material through a
20 (wire) mesh screen on a Fitzmill running
at medium speed with knives forward.

Return the granules to a mixer and add
the magnesium stearate. Mix for 10 min. In
this formula, the lactose and calcium phosphate are the fillers; the starch is an internal disintegrant; the povidone is the
binder. The magnesium stearate is the die-
release agent.

Example 7:   Core Granulation (Two-Phase)

Ingredient	Quantity
Active ingredient	q.s.
Mannitol USP	q.s.
Hydroxypropylmethylcellulose, NF	2.0%
Purified water USP	q.s.
Sodium starch glycolate NF	4.0%
Magnesium stearate NF	1.0%
	100.0%

Blend the drug and the mannitol. Dissolve
the hydroxypropylmethylcellulose in water.
Add to the powders and mix until the batch
is uniformly moist and granular in appearance. Dry on trays at 50°C. Pass the
dried materials through a Tornado mill
equipped with a 16 (wire) mesh screen and
running at medium speed with knives forward.
Return the granules to the blender, add the
sodium starch glycolate and magnesium
stearate. Mix until uniformly dispersed (5
to 10 min). Compress into tablets.

Example 8:   Core Granulation (Two-Phase)

Ingredient	Quantity
Active ingredient	q.s.
Lactose NF implapable	q.s.
Starch 1500 NF	20.0%

Example 8:   (Continued)

Ingredient	Quantity
Purified water USP	q.s.
Sodium lauryl sulfate NF	1.0%
Magnesium stearate NF	0.5%
	100.0%

Blend the first four ingredients in a double-
arm or planetary mixer. Moisten the powders with sufficient water to form a uniformly moist, granular mass. Pass the wet
mass through a #4A screen on a Fitzmill operating at low speed with hammers forward.
Spread the batch on trays and dry at 45°C,
until the moisture content is 2 to 3%. Pass
the dried material through a #6 perforated
plate on a Tornado mill running at medium
speed with knives forward.

   Return the resultant granules to a twin-
shell blender, add the sodium lauryl sulfate,
and magnesium stearate. Mix for 10 min.
Compress at the predetermined weight and
tablet dimensions. The sodium lauryl sulfate is the disintegrant in this formula.

   An unusual type of formula is the single-step granulation patented by
Cooper et al. [5]. Also referred to as self-lubricating, the method calls
for the blending of glidant and lubricant in the wet stage.

   It may seem unusual to include the lubricants in the wet granulation
step, a procedure contrary to what is usually taught about the necessity
for fine particle size of these substances in order to obtain easy die-
release. Nevertheless, the idea is valid and is presently used in a majority
of one company's solid dosage forms. Apparently, in the comminution step,
enough of the lubricant becomes exposed to perform its intended function.
The quantities used in these one-phase formulas are the same as those in
two-phase formulas. This procedure eliminates the usual mixing step to
incorporate the lubricants. Any losses of materials in processing are in
proportion to their presence in the formula.

Example 9:   Core Granulation (One-Phase)

Ingredient	Quantity
Active ingredient	q.s.
Lactose NF impalpable	q.s.
Sucrose NF	5.0%

Example 9: (Continued)

Ingredient	Quantity
Polyethylene glycol 6000 NF	3.0%
Starch NF	6.0%
Talc USP	5.0%
Magnesium stearate NF	0.5%
Purified water USP	q.s.
Anhydrous alcohol	q.s.
	100.0%

After suitable screening to break up any
aggregates, blend drug, lactose, sucrose,
starch, talc, and magnesium stearate in a
planetary or ribbon blender. Dissolve the
polyethylene glycol in a mixture of purified
water and alcohol at 50°C. (The volume
of the mixture is 20% larger than the weight
of the polyethylene glycol.) Add this solution to the blended powders, mixing until
granules form, using additional 50% alcohol
if necessary. Dry the moist mass at 45
to 50°C until moisture content is 1.0 to
2.5%. Pass the dried material through a
#5 perforated plate on a Tornado mill
running at medium speed with knives forward. The batch is now ready for compression at the desired shape and weight.
The use of the alcohol is not essential,
but gives a better control of the wetting
of the blended powders and promotes
more rapid drying of the granulation.

B. Coating Granulations

Coating granulations also have some special requirements so that they will
make a physically stable tablet. They require excellent cohesiveness as
well as the ability to adhere tightly to the core. They should be plastic
enough to expand slightly with the slight swelling of the core after the extrusion of the completed tablet from the die. The maximum size of the
granules must be less than the space between the deposited core and the
walls of the die so that the granules will readily fill the space. Preferably
the granules should be about one-fourth the width of this space. Good
centration of the core is necessary to obtain a coating of equal strength
all around. Although it is possible to apply a coating of only 1/32 in. on
the edges of the core, 3/64 in. is better because the granulation can more

easily fill the space, and there is leeway for slight off-centering. Centration can be critical if an enteric coating is being applied. Uniformity of coverage eliminates thin areas which may break down and release the contents of the core too early. Centration is also critical if the tablet is bisected with the intent of providing a divided dose. Misalignment of cores will make for unequal doses when the tablet is halved.

Centration is affected by the mechanics of the machine, its rotational speed, and the quality of the coating granulation. The adjustment of the press must be made according to the manufacturer's specifications and will not be discussed here. The speed of the machine tends to centrifuge the core tablet toward the periphery of the table and opposite to the direction of rotation. Reducing the speed of the press will overcome this tendency. However, this is not an economical solution to the problem. The answer lies in the formulation of the coating. The granules should be relatively soft, somewhat like lactose, rather than hard like sucrose. Such granules prevent the core from sliding on the bottom layer of coating. The fall of the upper punch on top of the core while the latter is being deposited is also helpful. To provide softness in the granulation, plastic materials such as gelatin and polyethylene glycol should be included in the formula. The amount of granulating liquid should be kept to a minimum, and granulating time should be restricted, to prevent excessive activation of the binders.

Because the edges of compression-coated tablets are thicker than those of ordinary tablets, a somewhat larger amount of lubricant is needed to facilitate extrusion from the die. If 0.5% of magnesium stearate is sufficient for a plain tablet, about 50% more is necessary for dry-coated products. The amount of stearic acid or of hydrogenated vegetable oils, which are much less efficient, should be about double that of magnesium stearate. However, the amounts of these and similar lubricants may be reduced if polyethylene glycol 4000, 6000, or 20,000 is part of the formula since they also have lubricity.

Any excipient that is suitable for a standard tablet or core tablet is suitable for the dry-coating formulation. It is customery, however, to use the same materials in the coating as in the core, a practice based on the theory that like substances will bond better to like than to different ones. Nevertheless, a better criterion is the cohesiveness and plasticity of the formula: cohesiveness because the continuity of the coating depends on its strength around the edge of the core, and plasticity so that it can absorb the expansion of the core after the completed tablet is released from the die. This is especially important with the DryCota because there is only the briefest time for lateral expansion of the core, while the other machines the cores are prepared well ahead of time and can thus be *seasoned*. Wolff [6] has recommended that 2% of acacia be included in the formula to achieve bonding and has said that 1.75% of gelatin imparted satisfactory plasticity. His examples also reveal an extensive use of sugar in his coating formulas, a substance which is very cohesive. Cooper et al. [5] have relied mainly on tragacanth and sucrose for bonding and polyethylene glycol 6000 for plasticity and lubrication. Examples of typical formulas for coatings are shown in Examples 10 and 11.

A formula which is resistant to moisture penetration is Example 12.

A formula for an enteric coating given by Blubaugh et al. [7] is shown in Example 13.

Example 10:   Typical Coating Granulation

Ingredient	Quantity
Lactose NF impalpable	q.s.
Confectioners sugar NF	q.s.
Acacia NF spray dried	2.0%
Starch NF	5.0%
Gelatin NF	2.0%
Magnesium stearate NF	0.5%
Soluble dye	q.s.
Purified water USP	q.s.
	100.0%

Blend the first four materials until homo-
geneously mixed. Dissolve the dye in
sufficient water and the gelatin in 5
times its weight of water, using heat.
Combine the dye and gelatin solutions
and add to the mixed powders. Continue mixing until a moist, uniformly
colored mass is formed. Pass the mass
through a #4 perforated plate on a
Fitzmill running at low speed with hammers forward. Spread on trays and
dry at 45°C to a moisture content of
2 to 3%. Pass the dried granules
through a #27 perforated plate on a
Tornado mill operating at medium
speed, knives forward. Return the
granules to the mixer and add the
magnesium stearate. Blend for 5 min.
The granulation is ready for compression.

Example 11:   Typical Coating Granulation

Ingredient	Quantity
Lactose NF (spray-dried)	q.s.
Confectioners sugar NF	2.0%
Acacia NF (spray-dried)	2.0%
Polyethylene glycol 6000 NF	4.0%
Talc USP	3.0%
Magnesium stearate NF	0.5%

Example 11: (Continued)

Ingredient	Quantity
Soluble dye	q.s
Purified water USP	q.s.
	100.0%

Blend all ingredients except the dye and polyethylene glycol in a double-arm mixer. Dissolve the dye in a minimum amount of water and the polyethylene glycol in 1.2 times its weight of water at a temperature of 50°C. Combine the two solutions and add slowly to the mixed powders. Mix for about 30 min or until a uniformly colored and moist mass is formed. Spread on trays and dry at 45°C until the moisture content is 1 to 3%. Alternatively, the batch may be dried in a vacuum tumbler dryer with a jacket temperature ranging from 35 to 60°C. Pass the dried granules through a #5 perforated plate on a Tornado Mill operating at medium speed with knives forward. The granulation is ready for compression. (If a drug is incorporated into the coating, the amount of lactose is reduced to compensate.)

Example 12: Typical Coating Granulation (Moisture Resistant)

Ingredient	Quantity
Calcium sulfate dihydrate	q.s.
Mannitol NF	10.0%
Tragacanth NF	2.0%
Acacia NF	3.0%
Talc USP	5.0%
Magnesium stearate NF	2.0%
Colorant	q.s.
Purified water USP	q.s.
	100.0%

Example 12:   (Continued)

Blend the calcium sulfate, mannitol,
tragacanth, talc, magnesium stearate,
and colorant. Make a mucilage of the
acacia with the water and add to the
mixed powders. Pass the moist mass
through a #4A perforated plate on a
Fitzmill operating with knives forward.
Spread on trays and dry in an oven at
45°C. Pass the dried material through
a 20 mesh screen on the same mill. The
granulation is ready for compression.

Example 13:   Enteric Coating

Ingredient	Quantity
Triethanolamine cellulose acetate phthalate	20.0%
Lactose NF	78.0%
Magnesium stearate NF	1.0%
Colorant	q.s.
Purified water	q.s.
	100.0%

Mix the triethanolamine cellulose acetate
phthalate and lactose in a mixer with a
Z-type agitator. Dissolve the colorant
in the water and add to the mixed powders. Use sufficient water to make a
tacky mass. Dry to the mass at 26°C
and a relative humidity of 30%. Pass
the dried batch through a #2 perforated
plate on a Fitzmill. Blend the granules
with the magnesium stearate. Compress
around core tablets using punches and
dies 3/32 in. larger in diameter. The
coating is to be a minimum of 1/32-in.
thick. This coating withstands disintegration for 2 hr at pH 5.5. But
of pH 5.6, disintegration occurs in 100
to 110 min. At pH 7.5, it is 10 to 12
min.

In Examples 10, 11, and 12 one may substitute an active ingredient for
part of the major excipient. Typical mesh patterns for the formulations
in these examples would be:

Caught on screen	Example			
	10	11	12	13
20 mesh	0%	2.5—7.5%	0%	0%
40 mesh	15—25%	25—35%	42%	42%
60 mesh	25—35%	10—20%	20%	20%
80 mesh	10—20%	2.5—7.5%	12%	12%
100 mesh	5—15%	2.5—7.5%	3%	3%
Pan	2.5—7.5%	35—45%	23%	23%

C. Problem Solving

Since core formulations can be, and are developed on standard machines, problems relating to hardness, friability, capping, extrusion from the dies, and disintegration can be solved before resorting to compression-coating machines. But it is otherwise with the coating formulations. They must be evaluated on the specific equipment available. The coating may cap off the cores because there is an excess of fine powder in the granulation: the amount of glidants, disintegrants, and lubricants should be no more than 10% of the batch, since these are powders with little cohesiveness. An excess of fines may be due to powdering in the mill because the granulation is weak and needs more binder, or because it is too hard and brittle. When a drug is present, it may affect the adhesive quality of the binder selected and require the choice of a different one. Fines may also be caused by the selected and require the choice of a different one. Fines may also be caused by the selection of the screen for milling. It is advisable to prepare a granulation and divide it into several parts. Each part should then be passed through a different screen—and at two different speeds. Then, each part should be used to coat the same batch of cores, and the physical parameters of the tablets should be evaluated.

The granulation may be too dry; since water improves bonding, an increase would be needed. It can be obtained by adding starches or materials which tend to hold on to water, like sucrose or povidone. Perhaps the drying conditions need to be altered, with a reduction in temperature or drying time.

The cores may have been compressed too hard and their surfaces densified so that the coating cannot bond. Hard cores tend to be elastic rather than plastic. Upon release of pressure when the tablet is ejected from the die, the rebound of the core pops the top off the tablet.

Improper centration of the core either vertically or horizontally produces weak edges, and the coating will not hold together. Figure 9 illustrates faulty placement of cores within the envelope of coating. Windheuser and Cooper [8] ascribed poor centration to the poor flow characteristics of a granulation. They also believed that hard granules allowed the centrifugal force applied by the rotating turret to move the core off-center. Along the same lines, Lachman et al. [9] compared the bed of coating to a liquid.

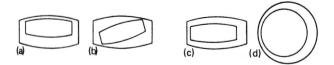

Figure 9   Examples of off-centering. Faults in compression coating: (a)
unequal coating; (b) cocking; (c) and (d) off-center.

The rotation of the press would cause the liquid to move from the level.
They found that fine granules caused the least movement of the cores.

This failure of the cores to orient themselves on the bottom bed of
coating is frequently found with those composed mainly of waxy substances.
The core fall off-center or they land in a cocked position. The fault lies
in the relative humidity in the compression booth. For good core deposition,
the relative humidity should be at least 35%, and preferably between 40 and
50%. Temperatures above 75°F can soften wax cores and cause sticking in
the transfer cups or V-slots. Either the temperature in the booth should
be kept under control or the core granulation should be refrigerated for
24 to 48 hr before being compressed. One drum of granulation should be
used up before a second drum is removed from the refrigerator and brought
into the compression room.

If there is an incompatibility between the drugs in a combination tablet,
or if the core is sensitive to moisture, the moisture content of the granulations should be kept to a minimum. Excipients such as mannitol and anhydrous lactose are preferable to sucrose in such cases. Longer drying times
or more severe drying conditions are useful. The relative humidity in the
compression area may need to be lowered also.

When steel dies have been used for some time, they develop compression
rings. The diameter of the ring is larger than that of the rest of the die.
The tablet is slightly imprisoned by the ring, and a greater force than normal is applied to the circumference of the tablet during ejection. The bond
at the top of the tablet weakens, and capping results. One must be sure
that the dies are in good condition or invest in carbide insert dies which
have an extremely long life without showing wear. The use of deep cup
punches may also result in capping because the compression force is so unequal between the edge and the center of the tablet that, again, the adhesion
of coating to core is weakened.

Capping is not always obvious at the time that the tablets are being
compressed. It may occur at some time later. To determine quickly if this
event may occur, the formulator has several means. One common way is to
attempt to force the coating off by pressing the thumbnail at the point
where the top (or bottom) of the tablet meets the side. The tablet may be
cut in half with a sharp knife or razor blade, and then an attempt may be
made to pull off the coating. Another common test is to shake 20 or 30
tablets vigorously in the cupped hands. More scientifically, a friability test
may be performed. This test can be continued beyond the normal 4 min
until the tablets do break up. This longer trial can be used to compare
formulations. An even more pertinent test is to run the tablets two or more
times through an automatic tablet counter and bottling machine and examine
the tablets for damage.

As a rule of thumb, the weight of the coating is about twice the weight of the core, provided that the granulations of both have similar bulk densities and the coating diameter is 3/32 in. larger than that of the core. This ratio provides enough material for a covering about 3/64 in. thick around the core. This margin can be made greater if the amount of drug in the coating is large. To make it less means risking cores that show through the coating or weakness at the tablet edge. If the core contains materials of low bulk density, then the amount of coating must be increased to give adequate coverage.

III. INLAY TABLETS

A variation of the compression-coated tablet is the *inlay, dot,* or *bull's-eye* tablet. Instead of the core tablet being completely surrounded by the coating, its top surface is completely exposed. With a yellow core and a white coating, the tablet resembles a fried egg. The preparation of such tablets requires that the top layer of coating be eliminated. Only the bottom layer of coating is deposited in the die and the core is placed upon it. The compression wheels then embed the core in the granulation, displacing some of the latter to form the sides, and finally press the whole into a tablet. Figure 10 shows two views of inlay tablets. With the Stokes, Colton, or Kilian machines, no alterations in equipment are needed. The feed frame and hopper which normally provide the top coating are not installed. With the Manesty DryCota, which utilizes a two-compartment feed frame for coating, it is necessary to block off the second part so that the granulation is diverted away from the dies and around the turret.

This dosage form has a number of advantages over the compression-coated tablet. It requires less coating material, only about 25 to 50% more than the weight of the core. The core is visible, so coreless tablets are readily detected. The reduction in the amount of coating makes for a thinner tablet. There is (of course) no concern with the capping of the top coating.

This form can be useful in sustained-release preparations to reduce the size and weight of the tablet. The slow-release portion, which contains 2 to 3 times the amount of active ingredient, becomes the coating, and the immediate-release portion becomes the core. A specific example is the 100-mg PBZ Lontab. As marketed, it was composed of a slow-releasing core weighing 200 mg and containing 67 mg of tripelennamine hydrochloride USP. The coating weighed 350 mg and contained 33 mg of the drug. The complete tablet weighed 550 mg and was 7/16 in. in diameter and 5.7 mm thick. When

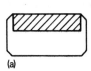
(a)

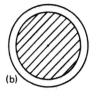
(b)

Figure 10   Inlay tablet: (a) cross-section; (b) view from above.

the core became the outer shell, the immediate-release portion could be reduced to 130 mg at 9/32-in. diameter, and the complete tablet made 3/8 in.
in diameter with a thickness of only 4.2 mm, a tablet more easily swallowed.
The 100 mg PBZ Lontab is no longer marketed. It has been replaced by a
conventional wax matrix release tablet. Another example is a European preparation containing 25 mg of hydrochlorothiazide in the bull's-eye and 600
mg of potassium chloride in the outside portion. The latter contains a
waxy substance to retard release and obviate gastrointestinal irritation.
Thus the inlay is available immediately for its diuretic activity. To surround the potassium chloride with a granulation containing the hydrochlorothiazide would result in a tablet at least 1/2 in. in diameter—and in a
great waste of materials. Only a layer tablet would be a reasonable alternative.

The inlay tablet requires the use of the same equipment as the
dry-coated tablet, the problems encountered are similar. Poor centration
is a much more obvious defect in the inlay tablet, however. Also, any
color reactions due to incompatibility between the core and coating are
obvious.

The types of formulations previously cited are suitable for this kind of
product.* There will be no difference in the output of the machines.

IV. LAYER TABLETS

Layer tablets are composed of two or three layers of granulation compressed
together. They have the appearance of a sandwich because the edges of
each layer are exposed. This dosage form has the advantage of separating
two incompatible substances with an inert barrier between them. It makes
possible sustained-release preparations with the immediate-release quantity
in one layer and the slow-release portion in the second. A third layer
with an intermediate release might be added. The weight of each layer can
be accurately controlled, in contrast to putting one drug of a combination
product in a sugar coating. Two-layer tablets require fewer materials than
compression-coated tablets, weigh less, and may be thinner. Monograms
and other distinctive markings may be impressed in the surfaces of the
multilayer tablets. Coloring the separate layers provides many possibilities
for unique tablet identity. Analytical work may be simplified by a separation of the layers prior to assay. Since there is no transfer to a second
set of punches and dies, as with the dry-coating machine, odd shapes
(such as triangles, squares, and ovals) present no operating problems except for those common to keyed tooling.

A. History of Layer-Tablet Presses

F. J. Stokes, in his 1917 patent [2], indicated that his machine was a layer
press, the first layer or tablet being compressed on another machine. The
idea was apparently not pursued by the pharmaceutical industry at that time,

---

*Dorsey Laboratories of Lincoln, Nebraska hold a patent [10] on the inlay
concept and marketed several products in this dosage form.

but the electrical industry developed the idea for the production of bimetallic contacts, which are actually two layers of metal bonded together.

The earliest machines fed controlled volumes of each separate granulation on top of each other and compressed them together at one pressing station. The later machines were engineered to compress each layer separately before the deposition of the next granulation, with a final compression for the complete tablet. Since, in these machines, the excess granulation from each feed frame could not be permitted to circulate around the turret and commingle, wipe-off blades covering the entire face of the die table had to be installed. The excess was thus directed into pots at the side of the press and manually returned to the appropriate hopper. Suction tubes were needed to remove any fine dust that escaped under the scraper blades. The latest refinement has been the force feeders which retain the individual granulations. But some powder escapes from these also, and the same arrangement as described above is installed on the presses to prevent one granulation from contaminating the other.

In the operation of the older type of machine, the granulation for the first layer is placed in the hopper, and the machine is adjusted until the desired weight is achieved with consistency; then the second hopper is filled with its granulation, and the same procedure is followed until the correct total tablet weight is obtained. In this, the single-compression method, the delineation between layers tends to be a little uneven. It is also difficult to make weight adjustments during a run.

B. Layer-Tablet Presses

Of the modern machines, there are two types which differ mainly in the way the layers are removed for weight and hardness checking. In one, the first layer of the first two layers are diverted from the machine; in the other, the first layer is made so hard that the second layer will not bond to it or will bond only weakly; upon ejection of the completed tablet, the layers may be easily separated and tested individually.

Figure 11 illustrates the operation of a three-layer press with force feeders. The line (A) represents the die table. A granulation is placed in the first hopper and flows into the feed frame (B). The machine is started, and the volume of granulation in the die is adjusted by the weight-adjustment cam (C). The upper and lower punches are brought together by the precompression rolls (D) and (E) to form a weak compact. Part of the lower cam track (F) is then raised hydraulically to eject the first layer, which is swept off the die table (A) by a wipe-off blade (G) affixed to the back edge of the second feeder (H). Samples are weighed, and hardness is determined. The operator makes any necessary corrections. When conditions are satisfactory, the ejection cam is lowered, and the entire procedure is repeated for the second layer, using feed frame (H), weight-adjusting cam (I), tamping rolls (J) and (K), ejection cam (L), and wipe-off blade (M). The weight of the second layer is determined by the difference between the two weighings. The sequence is again repeated for the third layer by means of feed frame (N), weight adjustment (O) and final compression rolls (P) and (Q), with the completed tablet being removed from the machine by the wipe-off blade (R) [to the right of the first feed frame (B)].

When a layer is ejected, the upper tamping roll is lowered slightly to exert more pressure upon the layer. This action will prevent damage to

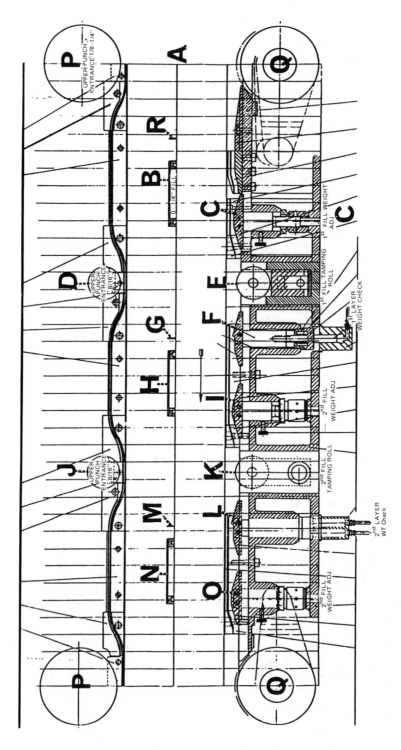

Figure 11   Schematic of a layer press.   Refer to text (Thomas Engineering).

Table 3   Specifications for Some Layer Presses

Specification	Manesty Layerpress	Manesty Rotapress mk IIa	Killian RU-3S	Stokes Versapress 560-1	Fette P-3002	Hata HT AP55L-DU	Vector Magna
				Manufacturer and model designation			
Number of dies	47	61	20	45	55	55	90
Maximum pressure (tons)	6.5	6.5	8.5	4	20(kN)	9	10
Maximum tablet diameter (in.)	7/16	7/16	3/4	7/16	1/2	1/2	7/16
Maximum depth of fill (in.)	11/16	11/16	9.16	11/16	5/16	5/16	—
Maximum layer thickness (prior to pressing) (in.)							
First layer	1/4	7/16	1/4	7/16	11/16	—	3/4
Second layer	1/4	1/4	1/4	1/4	11/16	—	3/4
Third layer	1/4	—	1/4	—	—	—	3/4
Maximum output (TPM)	1,500	5,550	417	2,100	4,125	3,850	5,000

the layer as strikes the take-off blade and is directed into the collection box. Once the lower punches have cleared the next filling station, they are quickly pulled down by a lowering cam so that they are not struck by the upper punches. The latter are already descending into the dies to make the next tamping or compression stroke.

The leading and trailing edges of each feed frame are equipped with wipe-off blades which divert any powders that escape from the feeders into collection boxes. The blade on the trailing edge of the first feed frame guides the completed tablets down the chute (G) to the collection bin. Vacuum tubes at each filling unit suck away any powder or granulation that remains in the lower punch faces during weight checks. Although the punches are raised flush with the die table at this time and do not drop as they pass under the feed frames, they do trap a small amount of material in the depressions in their tips.

If an adjustment in the weight or thickness of the first or second layer is necessary, then the weight of each succeeding layer will probably need correction, since weight is related to the fill volume.

The second type of machine is similar to the one described above, except for the manner in which weight checking is handled. Instead of a cam arrangement for ejecting the layers, the pressure on the first layer is increased, and the layer is made so hard that the next layer will not bond to it. Thus both layers are easily separated for weighing. This effect is achieved by activating a pneumatic cylinder which raises the lower tamping roll. There is an adjustment to control the distance that the compression roll may rise. Embossed or engraved upper punches provide a key between layers and tend to hold them together. Gentle shaking may be required to separate the layers in this case. Table 3 provides specifications for several typical layer presses currently available.

V. FORMULATIONS (LAYER)

As with compression-coated tablets, the granulation for layer tablets should be readily compressible for good bonding between layers. Dustlike fines should be kept to a minimum; the less dust, the cleaner the scrape-off at each feed frame. It may be necessary to separate out that fraction of a granulation which is finer than 70 or 80 mesh. Such material is not discarded but added to the next lot and regranulated. Lubricants, however, must be finely divided, their efficiency depending on the degree of fineness. Since these lubricant fines cannot be avoided, the quantities used should be kept minimal. The metallic stearates present an additional difficulty in that they interfere with the bonding of the layers. Stearic acid and the hydrogenated fats are better lubricants from this point of view. Nevertheless, granules should be small, less than half the thickness of the layers; otherwise, the lines of demarcation between layers will be uneven.

Equal weights of granulation will not necessarily lead to equal thickness of the layers. That will depend on the compression ratios of the formulations. It may be compensated for by adjusting the weights required for each layer. (It is not necessary, however, that each layer have the same thickness.) The shape of the punches also plays a role: punches with

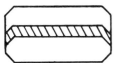 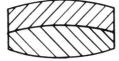

Figure 12   Cross sections of layer tablets.

beveled edges or concave faces will make the top and bottom layers of a three-layer tablet appear thinner than the middle one. Flat-faced tooling will produce equal thickness of the layers, but unfortunately the edges of the tablets will tend to chip readily. Figure 12 shows cross sections of layer tablets and illustrates how the shape of the upper punch determines the shape of the layers. If the upper punch faces have monograms or other markings, the bonding between layers will be strengthened because the devices will act as keys between the layers. Additionally, precompression lengthens dwell time and aids in bonding. The formulas previously given for compression-coated tablets will serve as a guide for the development of formulations for layer tablets, with the exception of two of those for direct compression (Examples 1 and 2), which are composed entirely of fine substances.

An illustrative formula is one for an analgesic-antipyretic decongestant containing aspirin and phenylpropanolamine. A thin layer of placebo is placed between them to negate the chemical incompatibility of the active ingredients.

Example 14: First Layer of
Analgesic-Antipyretic Decongestant

Ingredient	Quantity per tablet
Phenylpropanolamine HCl USP	12.50 mg
Lactose NF (spray-dried)	55.00 mg
Microcrystalline cellulose NF	28.00 mg
Colloidal silicon dioxide NF	1.25 mg
Stearic acid NF	1.25 mg

Screen where necessary to break down agglomerates or lumps (30 mesh screen is satisfactory) and blend the phenylpropanolamine, lactose, colloidal silicon dioxide and stearic acid.

Example 15: Second Layer of
Analgesic–Antipyretic Decongestant

Ingredient	Quantity per tablet
Lactose NF (spray-dried)	26.00 mg
Microcrystalline Cellulose NF	54.00 mg
Colloidal silicon dioxide NF	1.00 mg
Stearic acid NF	1.00 mg

Pass the lactose and microcrystalline cellulose
through a 30 mesh screen and blend them in
a suitable mixer. Add the stearic acid and
colloidal silicon dioxide. Mix for 10 min.

Example 16: Third Layer of
Analgesic–Antipyretic Decongestant

Ingredient	Quantity per tablet
Aspirin 40 mesh crystals	81.0 mg
Starch 1500 NF	19.0 mg
Colloidal silicon dioxide NF	0.5 mg
Stearic acid NF	1.0 mg

Blend in a suitable mixer until homogeneous
(10 to 15 min). Compress the three layers
together using 3/8-in. diameter, flat-faced,
beveled-edge punches. The weight of each
layer is:

    First layer, 98 mg
    Second layer, 82 mg
    Third layer, 101.5 mg

The top layer is the last layer to be pressed.
Since it is the aspirin portion, it will be most
resistant to extrusion from the dies.

Layer presses find employment in the manufacture of chewable antacid
tablets. A possible formula for such a product follows. The mannitol provides pleasant mouth-feel and sweetness, and the saccharin enhances the
latter. Peppermint flavoring has a long and honorable association with antacid preparations. The sucrose acts as the binder, although, of course, it
also contributes to the taste of the tablet.

Example 17: First Layer of Chewable
Antacid Tablet

Ingredient	Quantity
Magnesium oxide heavy USP	200.0 mg
Mannitol USP	400.0 mg
Sucrose NF	60.0 mg
Saccharin sodium USP	1.0 mg
Purified water USP	q.s.
Magnesium stearate NF	7.0 mg
Peppermint oil NF	4.0 mg

Blend the magnesium oxide, mannitol, and
saccharin in a double-arm mixer. Dissolve
the sucrose in double its weight of water
and add to the blended powders. Continue mixing until a moist, granular mass
is formed, using additional purified water
if necessary. Pass the batch through a
#5 perforated plate on a Fitzmill oper-
ating at low speed with hammers forward.
Spread the material on trays and dry at
50°C. Pass the dried granules through
a 12-mesh screen on a Fitzmill running at
medium speed with knives forward. Return the granules to the mixing machine
and add the peppermint oil. When the
oil has been thoroughly dispersed, add
the magnesium stearate. (If the oil is
not added before the lubricant, the tablet will have oil spots on its surface.)
Compress the layer at 672 mg using
5/8-in. diameter punches with flat faces
and beveled edges.

Example 18: Second Layer of Chewable
Antacid Tablet

Ingredient	Quantity
Aluminum hydroxide (dried gel) USP	200.0 mg
Mannitol USP	400.0 mg
Saccharin sodium USP	0.6 mg
Starch NF	32.0 mg
Purified water	160.0 mg

Example 18:   (Continued)

Ingredient	Quantity
Peppermint oil NF	3.4 mg
Magnesium stearate NF	7.0 mg
Color	q.s.

Blend the aluminum hydroxide, mannitol, and saccharin. Dissolve the color in the water and add the starch. Heat the mixture on a waterbath until the starch jells and forms a paste. Use the paste to granulate the blended powders. Add more water, if necessary, to form a lumpy mass. Pass this mass through a #5 perforated plate on a Fitzmill running at low speed with hammers forward. Spread the material on trays and dry at 50°C. Pass the dried granules through a 12 mesh screen on a Fitzmill running at medium speed with knives forward. Return the granules to the mixer. Add the flavor first and then the magnesium stearate. Compress at 643 mg onto the first layer.

A recent search of the literature has shown that no significant advances have been reported in the field of three-layer tablets.

From the older literature [11] there is this example of a three-layer tablet. Today, this formulation would be unacceptable from a safety standpoint because of the FD&C Yellow #5, chloroform, and phenacetin. However, it is a good example of a typical three-layer tablet.

Example 19:   Bottom Layer of Three-Layer Tablet

Ingredient	Quantity
Acetylsalicylic acid	210.0 g
FD&C Yellow No. 5	4.0 g
Cornstarch	30.0 g
Talc	10.0 g
Chloroform	q.s.

Mix thoroughly and pass the mixture through a hammer mill. Add sufficient

Example 19: (Continued)

chloroform to obtain a wet granulation. Reduce the granules to a range of 20 to 40 mesh and dry overnight at a temperature of 120 to 140°F.

Example 20: Middle Layer of Three-Layer Tablet

Ingredient	Quantity
Phenacetin	150.0 g
Caffeine	15.0 g
Phenyltoloxamine dihydrogen citrate	25.0 g
Cornstarch	4.0 g
Powdered sugar	0.4 g
Distilled water	3.3 g
Magnesium stearate	3.0 g

Blend the phenacetin, caffeine, and phenyltoloxamine dihydrogen citrate. Prepare a paste by heating the starch and sugar in the water. Add the paste to the powders and form granules. Dry the moist mass overnight at 120 to 140°F. Reduce the mass to granules of about 20 mesh. Blend the granules with the magnesium stearate.

Example 21: Top Layer of Three-Layer Tablet

Ingredient	Quantity
Potassium phenethicillin	125.00 g
FD&C Red No. 3	0.03 g
Chloroform	q.s.
Magnesium stearate	3.00 g

Blend the first two ingredients and pass them through a hammer mill. Add sufficient chloroform to make a hard rubber-like mass. Break up the mass and dry overnight at 120 to 140°F. Reduce the dried

Example 21:   (Continued)

---

material to about 20 mesh granules. Blend
the granules with the magnesium stearate.

Using a three-layer press, compress
the bottom layer at 254 mg, the middle
layer at 197.4 mg, and the top layer at
128.03 mg.

Today FD&C Yellow No. 5 would not
be used with acetylsalicylic acid because
of the possibility of allergic reactions.

Although compression-coated and layer tablets are a modest fraction of
solid oral dosage forms, they provide two additional alternatives in solving
formulation problems. They tend to be more expensive to manufacture than
other tablets (except tablet triturates) because of the multiple granulations
needed and the slowness of the special presses used.

REFERENCES

1.   Noyes, P. J., British Patent 859996 (1896).
2.   Stokes, F. J., U.S. Patent 1,248,571 (1917).
3.   DeLong Gum Company, British Patent 439,534 (1935).
4.   Kilian, F., British Patent 464,903 (1937).
5.   Cooper, J., Pasquale, D., and Windheuser, J., U.S. Patent 2,857,313
     (1958).
6.   Wolff, J., U.S. Patent 2,757,124 (1956).
7.   Blubaugh, F., Zapapas, J., and Sparks, M., J. Amer. Phram. Assoc.
     [Sci. Ed.], 47,12:857—870 (1958).
8.   Windheuser, J. and Cooper, J., J. Amer. Pharm. Assoc. [Sci. Ed.],
     45,8:543 (1956).
9.   Lachman, L., Speiser, P., and Sylwestrowicz, H., J. Pharm. Sci.,
     52,4:379—390 (1963).
10. Boswell, C., U.S. Patent 3,048,526 (1962).
11. Buchwalter, F., Granatek, A., and DeMurio, M., U.S. Patent
     3,121,044 (1964).

SUGGESTED READING

Remington's Practice of Pharmacy, 17th ed., Mack Pub., Easton, Pa., 1985.
Ritschel, W. A., Die Tablette, Editio Cantor KG, Aulendorf i. Wuertt.,
     Germany, 1966.

6

Effervescent Tablets

Raymond Mohrle

Warner-Lambert Company, Morris Plains, New Jersey

I. INTRODUCTION

Effervescence is defined as the evolution of bubbles of gas from a liquid as the result of a chemical reaction. Effervescent mixtures have been known and used medicinally for many years. Effervescent powders used as saline cathartics were available in the eighteenth century and were subsequently listed in the official compendia as compound effervescent powders. These were more commonly known commercially as "Seidlitz Powders." Effervescent mixtures have been moderately popular over the years since along with the medicinal value of the particular preparation, they offered the public a unique dosage form that was interesting to prepare. In addition, they provided a pleasant taste due to carbonation which helped to mask the taste of objectionable medicaments. When tableting equipment was developed, these granular materials began to be compressed into tablets that offer some advantages over the powdered dosage forms. Effervescent tablets are convenient, easy-to-use, premeasured dosage forms. They cannot spill as can the powdered preparations. They can be individually packaged to exclude moisture, thereby avoiding the problem of product instability of the unused contents during storage.

Only two effervescent tablets (both potassium supplements) are listed in the current USP [1]. However, a wide range of effervescent tablets have been formulated over the years. These include dental compositions containing enzymes [2], contact lens cleaners [3], washing powder compositions [4], beverage sweetening tablets [5], chewable dentifrices [6], denture cleansers [7], surgical instrument sterilizers [8], analgesics [9], effervescent candy [10], as well as many preparations of prescription pharmaceuticals such as antibiotics [11,12], ergotamines [13], digoxin [14], methadone [15] and L-dopa [16]. Preparations for veterinary use have also been developed [17].

Some types of effervescent tablets are illustrated by the formulations in Section VIII of this chapter; however, all of them can generally be categorized into two distinct classes depending on the intended use of their solutions (i.e., is the resultant solution ingestible or not suitable for ingestion?). Effervescent tablets are not meant to be ingested or used without prior dissolution, usually in water. The ultimate use of the tablet solution plays a major role in the formulation of the product, specifically in the choice of raw materials to be used. Many substances have useful properties in the formulation of tablets whose solutions are not ingestible while possessing at the same time additional properties that render them useless if the solution is to be ingested (i.e., boric acid as a tablet lubricant, sodium bisulfite as an acid source, or sodium bicarbonate as a source of carbon dioxide in a sodium-free potassium supplement).

Several investigators have studied changes in the bioavailability of a drug when delivered from an effervescent tablet. Many studies have been done with aspirin. Some indicated that significant differences in the absorption kinetics of aspirin were observed between effervescent and conventional or enteric coated tablets [18-20] and that the differences could be attributed to gastric emptying rate and rapid tablet dissolution [21]. No significant differences were observed in other studies with aspirin [22,23] or acetaminophen [24] effervescent tablets. Another investigator reported increased bioavailability of phenylbutazone from an effervescent dosage form [25].

The use of enteric coated effervescent tablets to improve the absorption of sodium aminosalicylate or L-dopa from the intestine has also been studied [26,27]. As the cellulose acetate phthalate- or hydroxypropyl methylcellulose phthalate-coated tablets reached the upper part of the intestine, rapid disintegration ensued causing an increased rate of absorption and a more prolonged blood level of the drugs as compared to conventional compressed tablets. The clinical effectiveness of a foaming antacid tablet was reported to be significantly higher than that of placebo in a study using a chewable tablet containing an effervescent matrix of alginic acid and sodium bicarbonate [28].

II. RAW MATERIALS

A. General Characteristics

In many respects, the principles that apply to the production of conventional, noneffervescent tablets apply to the production of effervescent tablets, and are covered in greater detail in other sections of this volume. Much of the processing and process equipment are the same, as are the general properties of tablet granulations needed to produce a satisfactory tablet, such as particle shape, particle size, and uniformity of distribution to produce a free-flowing granulation suitable for use with high-speed rotary tablet presses. In addition, the granulations must be compressible either through the inherent properties of the raw materials or through the use of additives or specialized processing to impart the desired compressive properties.

One property of the raw materials chosen for use in effervescent tablets, perhaps somewhat more important than for conventional tablets, is moisture content. The reaction most often employed for tablet disintegration in an effervescent tablet formulation is that between a soluble acid source and an alkali metal carbonate to produce carbon dioxide gas, the latter serving as the tablet disintegrant. This reaction proceeds spontaneously when the acid and carbonate components are mixed in water. The reaction can also occur—to a lesser degree—in the presence of small amounts of water bound to or adsorbed on the raw materials used in the formulation. If this reaction does occur after the tablet is prepared and packaged, it will cause the product to become physically unstable and decompose. Once initiated, the reaction will proceed even more rapidly since a byproduct of the reaction is additional water. For these reasons, raw materials either in the anhydrous state, with little or no adsorbed moisture, or with water molecules bound in a stable hydrate are preferred. Some water is needed, however, for binding purposes since a completely anhydrous granulation usually will not be compressible. Raw materials can be carefully chosen to provide the water needed for binding purposes as explained further in Section III of this chapter.

Solubility is another raw material property especially important in the formulation of effervescent tablets. If the tablet components are not soluble, the effervescent reaction will not occur and the tablet will not disintegrate quickly. The rate of solubility is perhaps even more important than solubility per se since a slowly dissolving soluble substance can hinder tablet disintegration and provide a slowly soluble, often objectionable residue after the tablet disintegrates. Ideally, all the tablet components should have similar rates of solubility.

B. Acid Sources

The acidity needed for the effervescent reaction can be derived from three main sources: food acids, acid anhydrides, and acid salts. The food acids are the most commonly used. They occur in nature and are used as food additives; they are all ingestible.

Food Acids

Citric Acid

Citric acid is the most commonly used food acid, being readily abundant and relatively inexpensive. It is highly soluble, of high acid strength, and available in fine granular, free-flowing, anhydrous, and monohydrate food grade forms. Powdered forms are also commercially available. It is very hygroscopic, and care must be taken to prevent exposure to and storage in high-humidity areas if it is removed from its original container and not suitably repackaged.

Tartaric Acid

Tartaric acid is also used in many effervescent preparations, being readily available commercially. It is more soluble than citric acid and is also more hygroscopic. It is as strong an acid as citric acid, but more must be used to achieve equivalent acid concentration since it is diprotic, whereas citric acid is triprotic.

Malic Acid

Malic acid is also available in sufficient quantity for possible use in effervescent preparations. It is also hygroscopic and readily soluble. Its acid strength is less than citric or tartaric acids but high enough to provide sufficient effervescence when combined with a carbonate source. It has a smooth, tart taste that does not "burst" in flavor as does the tart taste of citric acid.

Fumaric Acid

Fumaric acid, although as strong an acid as citric acid, is not generally useful in effervescent tablets due to its extremely low solubility in water. It is virtually nonhygroscopic in nature and is the most economical of the food acids. A cold water soluble form of furmaric acid is available (Monsanto Co., St. Louis, Missouri). The increase in solubility is due to the addition of 0.3% dioctyl sodium sulfosuccinate; however, even this additive has not made fumaric acid adaptable for effervescent products.

Adipic and Succinic Acids

Neither of these food acids has been used extensively in effervescent products since they are far less soluble than citric acid in the temperature range in which most effervescent products are used. They are also less available and less economical. Both have the advantage, however, of being nonhygroscopic. Both have been reported to be useful as tablet lubricants as discussed in Section II.G.

Acid Anhydrides

Anhydrides of food acids are of possible value in effervescent products. When mixed with water, they are hydrolyzed to the corresponding acid, which can react with the carbonate source present to produce effervescence. If the hydrolytic rate is controlled, acid will be continuously produced throughout the solution, resulting in a sustained, high-volume, effervescent effect. Water cannot be used in the manufacture of products containing anhydrides since they would be converted to the acid prior to product use. Succinic anhydride is commercially available and has been used in a denture soak composition. It is reported that the acid anhydride reduces caking tendencies by acting as an internal desiccant in addition to increasing carbon dioxide evolution [29]. Citric anhydride has been reported in the literature [30].

Acid Salts

Certain acid salts are useful in the formulation of effervescent products.

Sodium Dihydrogen Phosphate

This compound, also known as monosodium phosphate, is available commercially in granular and powdered anhydrous forms. It is readily soluble in water, producing an acid solution of about pH 4.5. It readily reacts with carbonate or bicarbonate to produce effervescence when dissolved.

Disodium Dihydrogen Pyrophosphate

This compound, also called sodium acid pyrophosphate, is another acid salt that has been used in effervescent tablets. It is also readily available and is soluble in water, producing an acid solution.

Acid Citrate Salts

Use of both sodium dihydrogen citrate and disodium hydrogen citrate has been reported in an effervescent composition [31]. Both are readily soluble and produce acid solutions suitable for ingestion.

Sodium Acid Sulfite

This raw material, also known as sodium bisulfite, produces an acid so-lution capable of releasing carbon dioxide gas from a carbonate source. Sodium bisulfite is not suitable for ingestion but may have application in the formulation of effervescent tablets for uses such as toilet bowl cleaners. It is a strong reducing agent and is not compatible with oxidizing agents.

C. Carbonate Sources

Dry, solid carbonate salts provide the effervescent in most effervescent tablets—carbon dioxide gas. Both the bicarbonate and carbonate forms are useful with the former being more reactive and used most often.

Sodium Bicarbonate

Sodium bicarbonate is the major source of carbon dioxide in effervescent systems. It is completely soluble in water, nonhygroscopic, inexpensive, abundant, and available commercially in five particle size grades ranging from a fine powder to a free-flowing uniform granule. It is ingestible and is, in fact, widely used as an antacid either alone or as part of antacid products. It is used extensively in food products as baking soda, and as a component of dry chemical and soda/acid fire extinguishers. It is the mildest of the sodium alkalies, having a pH of 8.3 in an aqueous solution of 0.85% concentration. It yields approximately 52% carbon dioxide.

Sodium Carbonate

Sodium carbonate, also known as soda ash, can be a useful raw material to the formulator of effervescent tablets. In addition to its effect as a source of carbon dioxide, it is useful as an alkalizing agent due to its high pH of 11.5 in an aqueous solution of 1% concentration. Sodium carbonate also exhibits a stabilizing effect when compounded into effervescent tablets due to its ability to absorb moisture preferentially, preventing the initiation of the effervescent reaction. (This phenomenon is discussed in more detail in Section VI.) For this reason, the anhydrous form is preferred over the hydrated forms that are also available.

Potassium Bicarbonate and Potassium Carbonate

Both of these salts can be used in effervescent tablets, especially when the sodium ion is undesirable or needs to be limited, as in the case of ant-acid products in which dosage is dependent on the amount of sodium recom-mended for ingestion. They are more soluble than their sodium counterparts and are significantly more expensive. The range of commercially available forms may be less satisfactory to the formulator than the wide range avail-able for the sodium salts.

Sodium Sesquicarbonate

This material, used primarily in the laundry industry, is a compound consisting of equal molar amounts of sodium carbonate and sodium bicarbo-nate and twice the molar amount of water. It is soluble in water, with a pH of 10.1 at a 2% concentration. It may be useful in effervescent tablets; however, mixtures of sodium bicarbonate and sodium carbonate will usually suffice in this application. The dihydrate form may also present a stability problem in some applications.

Sodium Glycine Carbonate

This material is a complex of aminoacetic acid and sodium carbonate. It is reported [32] to have the following advantages over other carbon dioxide sources: directly compressible granules; greater water solubility; less alkalinity; more heat stability; does not yield free water or reaction, and therefore provides the tablet with greater stability in the presence of trace amounts of water. The economics of the product may be a disadvantage in some formulations.

L-Lysine Carbonate

The preparation of this material is described in the literature [33]. It can be used in effervescent mixtures for preparing sparkling drinks and pharmaceutical compositions, especially when alkali metal ions are not desired. The material is a white crystalline powder that is very soluble in water. However, commercial availability is not apparent.

Arginine Carbonate

Use of this material has been reported [34] in an effervescent product free from alkaline earth metals. Tablets incorporating citric acid and arginine carbonate provided a source of the amino acid for various medicinal uses.

Amorphous Calcium Carbonate

Preparation and use of this material has been described in the literature [35]; however, it is not yet commercially available. This material, which does not show a crystalline state upon X-ray analysis, remains stable without reverting to a crystalline form for a significant period of time. The preparation was reported for effervescent compositions that are sodium-free and highly palatable with excellent carbonation.

D. Other Effervescent Sources

The gas produced during effervescence need not always be carbon dioxide, although this is the one most frequently used. The evolution of oxygen gas can be used as a source of effervescence in certain products, particularly denture cleansers. Tablets have been compounded [36] in which a raw material known as anhydrous sodium perborate or effervescent perborate has been used. This raw material is prepared by heating either sodium perborate monohydrate or tetrahydrate under controlled conditions to drive off the hydrated water molecules. When it is mixed with water, copious volumes of oxygen gas are liberated, producing effervescence.

Another method of generating oxygen gas to serve as an effervescent tablet disintegrant is the reaction between a peroxygen compound that yields active oxygen on mixture with water, e.g., sodium perborate monohydrate or sodium percarbonate, and a chlorine compound that liberates hypochlorite on contact with water, e.g., sodium dichloroisocyanurate or calcium hypochlorite [37]. The evolution of oxygen gas, which occurs best in alkaline media, proceeds as the peroxygen compound is decomposed by the chlorine compound.

A recent U.S. patent [38] describes the preparation and use of an effervescent material prepared by the absorption of a gas, such as carbon dioxide, into an anhydrous base medium composed of an inorganic oxide material, such as zeolite aluminosilicate. Upon contact with water, the gas is desorbed from the inorganic matrix producing effervescence. This process is most useful for semisolid applications such as toothpastes and hand cleaners.

E. Binders and Granulating Agents

Binders are materials that help to hold other materials together. Most materials require some binder to assist in the formulation of a granulation suitable for tablet compression. Compared to conventional tablets, the use of binders in effervescent tablet formulation is limited, not because binders are unnecessary but because of the two-way action of the binders themselves. The use of any binder, even one that is water-soluble, will retard the disintegration of an effervescent tablet. In granulations that require a binder for tableting, a proper balance must be chosen between granule cohesiveness and desired tablet disintegration. Binders such as the natural and cellulose gums, gelatin, and starch paste are generally not useful due to their slow solubility or high residual water content. Dry binders such as lactose, dextrose, and mannitol can be used but are often not effective in the low concentrations normally permissible in effervescent tablets due to their disintegration-hindering properties as well as weight/volume restraints.

Most effervescent tablets are composed primarily of ingredients needed to produce effervescence or to carry out the function of the tablet.

Usually there is little room for excipients, which are needed in large concentrations to be effective. Polyvinylpyrrolidone (PVP) is an effective effervescent tablet binder. This material is usually added to the powders to be granulated either dry, and subsequently wetted with the granulating fluid, or in a solution with aqueous, alcoholic, or hydroalcoholic granulating fluids. Isopropanol and ethanol exert no binding effects themselves but are used in granulating fluids as solvents for the dry binders such as PVP. Water is useful both as a solvent for dry binders and as a binder itself. A small amount of water carefully added, and controlled to prevent initiation of the effervescent reaction, is very effective as a binder because of a partial dissolution of the raw materials followed by subsequent crystallization on drying. Procedures for manufacturing effervescent tablets using this technique are discussed in Section III. The hazards and solvent recovery problems associated with the organic solvents are common to the manufacture of both effervescent and conventional tablets.

F. Diluents

Due to the nature of the ingredients in an effervescent tablet, there is normally little need for added diluents. The effervescent materials themselves are usually present in large enough quantity to preclude the use of diluents to achieve the desired tablet bulk. Sodium bicarbonate is as useful and inexpensive a filler as any, provided the extra effervescence and solution pH effects do not pose a problem. Other materials that are considered should be readily soluble, available in a particle size similar to that of the other ingredients in the product, and crystalline in nature to provide adequate compressibility. Examples are sodium chloride and sodium sulfate. Both of these substances are relatively dense and may be useful in producing a more dense tablet compaction if desired.

G. Lubricants

Of all the ingredients compounded into effervescent tablets, the lubricant
is one of the most important because without this material production of
effervescent tablets on high-speed equipment would not be possible. Effervescent granulations are inherently difficult to lubricate, partly due to
the nature of the raw materials used and partly due to the rapid tablet
disintegration usually required. Many substances are effective lubricants
in certain concentrations but inhibit tablet disintegration at these same
concentrations. When the concentration is lowered to permit the tablet to
properly disintegrate, the lubricating efficiency of the material is lost or
so greatly diminished that it is no longer useful. If a clear solution is
desired when the tablet disintegrates, the problem is even greater since
the most efficient lubricants are water-insoluble and will leave a cloudy
solution once dispersed.

Excellent articles pertaining to the fundamental aspects of tablet lubrication and the mechanism of action and evaluation of tablet lubricants have
been published [39,40]. In the latter article, 70 materials were evaluated
as tablet lubricants, some of them water-soluble and therefore of particular
interest to the effervescent tablet formulator.

Intrinsic lubrication is provided by those materials that are compounded
directly into the tablet as the granulation is being prepared. This is the
most efficient and most used method. The magnesium, calcium, and zinc
salts of stearic acid are the most efficient substances commonly used. Concentrations of 1% or less are usually effective; however, they are not water-
soluble, can hinder tablet disintegration, and produce cloudy solutions.
Talc and powdered polytetrafluoroethylene are also insoluble in water but
generally permit more rapid tablet disintegration. The water-soluble or
dispersible materials discussed in the remaining paragraphs of this section
can be used. All are less efficient than the stearates but may provide the
needed properties if the concentration is high enough. All solid materials
must be finely divided, and in some cases micronized, to act efficiently.
Liquids are more easily handled if they are dispersed on a granulation component prior to addition.

Powdered sodium benzoate and micronized polyethylene glycol 8000 are
effective water-soluble lubricants. It has been found in one case that the
addition of sodium benzoate promotes tablet disintegration rather than producing an inhibiting effect [41]. An improvement in the efficiency of
sodium benzoate was seen by the incorporation of paraffins, dimethicone,
or polyoxyethylene glycols [42].

Sodium stearate and sodium oleate are soluble in low concentrations;
therefore, a combination of small amounts of both may be effective. The
taste of these materials may be objectionable for an ingested product. Cottonseed, corn, and mineral oils all have lubricating properties and will disperse in water. Polyvinylpyrrolidone [43], powdered sodium acetate, and
impalpable boric acid have also been used as soluble lubricants as well as
powdered adipic acid [44], powdered succinic acid [45], and powdered
fumaric acid [46]. An interesting soluble lubricant, although rarely used
in effervescent tablets due to its extremely high cost, is L-lycine. This
amino acid is highly efficient, having a stereochemical structure similar to
that of graphite. It is most often used to lubricate noneffervescent hypodermic tablets that must completely dissolve prior to injection.

The surfactants that are contained in some formulations to provide cleaning or detergent solutions also act as lubricants. Sodium lauryl sulfate is an effective lubricant but can hinder tablet disintegration if present in too high a concentration. Magnesium lauryl sulfate will also provide lubricating properties with a minimal disintegration-hindering effect. A mixture of spray-dried magnesium lauryl sulfate powder and micronized polyethylene glycol polymers has been found to be an excellent water-soluble lubricant for effervescent denture cleanser tablets [47].

Acetylsalicylic acid crystals provide adequate lubricating properties so that effervescent analgesic formulations containing this substance at effective dose levels usually do not require additional lubricants.

Extrinsic lubrication is provided by a mechanism that applies a lubricating substance to the tableting tool surface during processing. In one method, a film of melted wax is sprayed onto the tool surfaces after one tablet is ejected and before the granulation for the next tablet enters the die cavity. Accurate spray synchronization with minimal volume delivery and precise spray placement were troublesome when this experimental system was adopted for high-speed tablet production. Another method makes use of an oiled felt washer attached to the lower punch below the tip, which wipes the die cavity with each tablet ejection. Neither of these methods is as good as adding lubricating substances directly to the granulation, as directed above.

Another lubricating procedure can be used with tablet presses having two compression cycles used for the production of multilayer tablets [48,49]. A tablet containing a high concentration of lubricant is compressed at the first compression station. As this tablet is ejected, a film of lubricant is deposited over the die wall and punch surfaces.

The effervescent tablet of interest is compressed at the second compression station, lubricated by the thin film previously deposited. Elegant effervescent tablets can be produced in this manner; however, the output of the double-rotary press is cut in half. The lubricating tablets can be milled and reused but this further adds to the cost of the effervescent tablets. In addition, it is necessary to use care to prevent the lubricant and effervescent granulation from becoming mixed.

The role of the lubricating substances can be eased somewhat if the following mechanical means are employed. All tablets expand slightly after compression due to the elasticity of their ingredients. The use of outward-tapered dies can promote an easier escape for an expanding compaction as it leaves the die cavity. It is also beneficial if the tableting tools are coated with materials having a low frictional resistance. Many materials, such as polytetrafluoroethylene, have been applied to tableting tools but have rapidly worn off during processing. Electroplating all compression surfaces with chromium, which resists wear, is helpful.

H. Other Ingredients

Effervescent tablets may contain ingredients other than those previously mentioned. All are related to some function of the tablet other than its effervescent system, and in some cases may consist of a large portion of the tablet. These ingredients include drugs such as analgesics, decongestants, antihistamines, potassium supplements, and antacids; oxidizing agents such as sodium perborate or potassium monopersulfate are commonly found in denture cleaning compositions; flavoring, coloring, or sweetening agents are usually contained in tablets whose solutions are ingested. Often these materials can influence the perceived attractiveness of the effervescent solution. As with any formulation, all ingredients of an effervescent tablet must be carefully balanced to achieve the desired properties.

III. PROCESSING

A. Special Conditions

The processing of effervescent tablets, although similar in many ways to the processing of conventional tablets, presents certain problems and employs methods that are not often found with the latter. Special environmental conditions are required. Low relative humidity and moderate-to-cool temperatures in the processing areas are essential to prevent the granulations or tablets from sticking to machinery and from picking up moisture from the air, which can lead to tablet instability.

The storage of unopened containers of raw materials need not be restricted to a low relative humidity area. Normal warehouse conditions are usually sufficient since the containers of most hygroscopic raw materials contain moisture barriers of some type to protect their contents. Once the container is opened, however, the unused portion should be protected from moisture by transfer to suitable containers or by storage in a low-humidity area. Once effervescent reactants are mixed, storage in a low-humidity area is essential, since adsorbed moisture can initiate the effervescent reaction.

A maximum of 25% relative humidity at a controlled room temperature of 25°C (72°F) or less is usually satisfactory to avoid problems due to atmospheric moisture. Relative humidity is more correctly expressed as grains of moisture per pound of air at a specified temperature. If the amount of moisture remains constant while the temperature increases, the volume a pound of air occupies will increase and the relative humidity will fall. As such, relative humidity expressed in terms of percent or grains of moisture per pound of air must be accompanied by a value for temperature; otherwise the term lacks definition. A study of the geographic and chronological distribution of relative humidity in an effervescent manufacturing area illustrates the need to pay particular attention to environmental moisture control [50].

B. Equipment

The processing equipment used to produce conventional tablets is adaptable to the production of effervescent tablets provided the operations conducted with the various mixers, blenders, mills, granulators, tablet presses, and ovens are done in a low-moisture atmosphere. Specialized equipment known as a Topo granulator has also been used [51]. In order to produce effervescent granules, this self-contained device controls the effervescent reaction which occurs during processing with the addition of a solvent to the dry ingredients following by quick vacuum drying. This process is repeated until a surface passivation is reached that increases product stability. This phenomenon is discussed further in Section VI of this chapter.

C. Wet Granulation

The principle in preparing a granulation for effervescent tablets is basically the same as for conventional tablets. Wet-granulating techniques involve mixing the dry ingredients with a granulating fluid to produce a workable mass. The mass, which may be plastic and cohesive in nature, is reduced to an optimum particle size distribution and dried to produce a compressible granulation. Alternate procedures in which the formed mass is dried before particle size reduction are also possible.

A more unconventional granulation for effervescent tablets is simply a mixture of loosely adhering particles to which a very small amount of granulating fluid (0.1 to 0.5%) has been added. The mixture, which appears dry, is tableted, directly followed by drying. A discussion of this process appears in Section III.C.3. Wet granulations can be prepared in three different manners: with the use of heat, with nonreactive liquids, and with reactive liquids.

With Heat

This classical method of preparing effervescent granulations involves the release of water from hydrated formulation ingredients at a low temperature to form the workable mass. The ingredient most often used for this purpose is hydrous citric acid which, when fully hydrated, contains about 8.5% water. This process is very sporatic and difficult to control to achieve reproducible results. Often done in a static bed, the reaction is not uniform throughout the bed because the release of water, being temperature-dependent, is not uniform throughout the depth of the bed. A different approach to the preparation of effervescent granules with heat, not intended for, but adaptable to, granulations for tableting, has been reported in the literature [52]. The use of a special mixer, which generates the heat required to start the effervescent reaction solely by the frictional resistance of the mixer contents to turbulent, high-speed mixing, is described.

With Nonreactive Liquids

This method is more commonly employed and is similar to that used to prepare granulations for conventional tablets. Granulating fluids such as ethanol or isopropanol, in which the effervescent ingredients and most of the remaining ingredients are not soluble, are most often used. The granulating fluid is slowly added to the premixed formulation components in a suitable mixer until the fluid is uniformly distributed. Binders, which are required in many formulations, can be added to the dry ingredients and activated as the mass is wetted. Alcohol-soluble binders, such as PVP, can be dissolved in the granulating fluid prior to addition to the bulk. Binders added in this manner are usually more effective and can be used in lower concentrations with fewer negative effects on tablet disintegration. Once the mass is uniformly wetted, it is manually transferred to trays and dried in an oven. Automated systems have been designed to remove the granulation from the mixer and pass it through an oven on a continuous basis. (The latter method is more suitable for loosely bound particulate granulations.) After the granulations are dried, they are reduced to the desired particle size by using appropriate mills or granulators, and are collected in containers for future use or transferred directly to other mixers

for further processing prior to tableting. The denture cleanser tablet
formulation (Example 7) is an example of this process.

The characteristics (e.g., uniformity, compressibility, and flowability)
of a granulation to be tableted are the same for effervescent tablets as for
conventional tablets, and are discussed elsewhere in this volume.

An advantage of granulating with nonreactive liquids is that not all the
ingredients of a formulation need to be subjected to contact with the granulating fluids or to the heat of the drying process. In some formulations,
it may be desirable to granulate the acidic and basic effervescent components separately to eliminate any reaction. Heat-labile compounds can be
added subsequently to the granulation phase, and bulk raw material-handling
requirements can be reduced if some of the formulation components have inherently suitable tableting characteristics and need not be granulated.

One disadvantage is that some processing is still required after the
granulation has been dried and ground. Most often, this entails additional
mixing to blend more of the separate granulations or add heat-labile compounds or tableting lubricants. Additional grinding of the granulations
can occur due to the attrition in the mixers, which may be detrimental to
the granulation particles. Another disadvantage is that the vapors from
the granulating fluids are often hazardous and must be exhausted or condensed and collected. In any case, suitable ventilation must be provided
to prevent dangerous levels of these solvents from accumulating.

With Reactive Fluids

One of the most effective granulating agents for effervescent mixtures is
water. Due to the fact that the effervescent reaction is initiated with
water, obvious care must be taken to adequately control such a process if
the effervescent character of the finished tablet is to be maintained. Often
this process is difficult to control since the granulated mass must be quickly
dried to stop the effervescent reaction. A process using water as a granulating agent for a mass-produced effervescent tablet has been developed
and used for many years to produce tablets with final uses ranging from
antacids to reconstitutable mouthwashes to denture cleanser tablets.

This granulation process is based on the addition of small amounts of
water (0.1 to 0.5%) to a blend of raw materials that possesses the uniformity,
compressibility, and flowability needed to produce good-quality tablets, but
which lacks the needed binding properties. The added free water acts as
a binder. In practice, the water is usually added in the form of a fine
spray to selected formulation components while mixing in a ribbon blender.
When uniform distribution of the water has been achieved, the remaining
constituents are consecutively added with adequate mixing to distribute the
water throughout the mass. The formulation and process described for bath
salt tablets (Example 8) illustrates this method.

The ingredients selected to receive the water spray should readily release the adsorbed water to the rest of the formulation components rather
than adsorb and bind it internally. After the formulation is complete, the
free-flowing granulation is transferred directly to the tablet-compressing
machines and tableted while moist. The compressed tablets are then passed
through an oven, which causes the water to be removed or bound internally
as water of crystallization and thus stabilized. Substantial increases in
tablet hardness are usually experienced during the heating process. By
using more than one blender to feed a common granulation transfer system,
a continuous flow of granulation can be directed to the tablet presses from

granulation prepared on a batch-to-batch basis. One distinct disadvantage of this process is that formulations which contain ingredients susceptible to attack from moisture and/or heat cannot be prepared without some degradation occurring.

A wet granulation method using the simultaneous addition of water and application of heat in a vacuum oven has been described [53]. It is claimed that the tablets produced from the granulation had better carbon dioxide release properties with more rapid effervescence than from tablets produced by conventional means.

D. Dry Granulation

Dry granulation can be accomplished with the use of special processing equipment known as a roller compactor or chilsonator. These machines compress premixed powders between two counterrotating rollers under extreme pressure. The resultant material is in the form of a brittle ribbon, sheet, or piece—depending on the configuration of the roller. The compressed material is reduced to the proper size for tablet granulation purposes. The toilet bowl cleanser tablets described in Example 10 are prepared by this process.

Another dry granulation procedure is slugging, in which slugs or large tablets are compressed using heavy-duty tablet-compacting equipment and are subsequently ground to the desired granulation characteristics. Both of these processes are used for materials that ordinarily will not compress using the more conventional wet granulation techniques and require precompression to increase density or exclude entrapped air due to porosity.

A simple blending of raw materials, which after mixing are suitable for direct compression into tablets, can also be considered a form of dry granulation. Measurements have been made of the mechanical properties of effervescent raw materials and mixtures to predict compressibility when directly compressed [54]. Fumaric acid had the best compression properties among the acids tested, while sodium bicarbonate was the best among the carbonates.

E. Fluidized Bed Granulation

The production of effervescent granules that can be used to prepare effervescent tablets has been accomplished using fluidized bed granulation.

A dry mixture of the powdered form of an acid and carbonate source is suspended in a stream of hot air, forming a constantly agitated, fluidized bed. An amount of granulating fluid, usually water, is introduced in a finely dispersed form causing momentary reaction before it is vaporized. This causes the ingredients to react to a limited extent forming single granules of the two reactive components. The granules are larger than the powder particles of the starting materials and suitable for compression into tablets after drying has been completed in the fluidized bed apparatus. This procedure has the advantage of ingredient mixing, granulating, and drying all in one piece of equipment with minimal loss of carbon dioxide. Preparations containing aspirin and acetaminophen have been made using a fluidized bed temperature of 60 to 64°C [55,56] with the effervescent granulation dried to a water content of 0.25%. The effect of the ratio of citric acid, sodium bicarbonate, and the PVP content of the granulating fluid as

well as the temperature and rate of the input air was studied in a factorial
design using a fluidized bed apparatus [57]. Granule size, fine-powder
content, and the dissolution rate of aspirin tablets made using the resultant granules were measured. All the parameters affected the value of the
fine-powder content; however, only the ratio of the reactants and the PVP
concentration in the granulation fluid affected the dissolution rate of the
tablets. It was concluded that a maximum content of 20% fine powder was
optimum to achieve the desired tablet dissolution time of 120 sec.

F. Pretableting Operations

In many cases, after the effervescent portion of the granulation is prepared,
certain materials are added that were purposely withheld during the granulation process. These materials are most often those that would be degraded by the heat or moisture present in granulation preparation (e.g.,
acetylsalicylic acid, enzymes, and gragrance oils) or are those added in
the final stages before tableting, such as lubricants. Lubricating powders
are added as near to the end of the granulation process as possible in order to coat the rest of the granulation and provide their maximum effect.
Ingredients present in small amounts should be added using geometric dilution techniques to ensure even distribution throughout the granulation.
If liquid ingredients such as fragrances or oil lubricants are to be incorporated into the formulation, it is desirable to separately mix them thoroughly
with a small portion of the total granulation or one of the formulation ingredients, and then add this wetted mixture to the remainder of the granulation. If the oils are added directly to the granulation, an even distribution is difficult to obtain, and small lumps are likely to occur throughout
the granulation. Oils are effectively distributed when premixed with granular sodium bicarbonate.

The ideal granulating and tableting operation from a cost and efficiency
point of view is one of direct compression without prior granulation. This
process, which may be feasible for some effervescent tablets, is difficult
to carry out in general. In order to be directly compressible, the particle
size distribution of the raw materials used in the formulation should be
roughly the same and have inherent compressible properties. Many of the
raw materials used in effervescent tablets are available in a fine granular
form. Others, which are available in larger particle sizes, can be ground
to the desired size. The problem occurs when a large portion of the formulation is composed of particles that are smaller than average. In this case
granulation is required. The addition of small amounts of finely powdered
substances can usually be accommodated if the bulk of the formulation is
granular and free flowing, in which case the fine particles fill in the voids
among the larger particles and become thoroughly mixed throughout the
granulation. If the granulations are properly prepared, tableting operations
will run smoothly.

G. Tableting

Effervescent granulations are tableted in the same manner as conventional
tablet granulations (discussed in detail in other sections of this volume).
Common process controls are tablet weight, thickness, and hardness.

Once the tablet presses are operating and have been properly adjusted, these parameters will be relatively constant if the granulation is of good quality. Significant variations indicate the development of problems, and the tablets leaving the press should be examined closely for signs of difficulty. If problems occur, they will most often be caused by insufficient binding (evidenced by laminating or capped tablets) and inadequate lubrication (evidenced by tablet surface picking and die wall sticking). Since many effervescent tablets are large in diameter, laminations or capping can be detected easily by snapping the tablet between the thumb, forefinger, and middle finger across the diameter of the circular surface of the tablet. Examination of the broken interface will reveal the presence of a lamination if definite layers or striations can be seen within the tablet. As the severity of lamination increases, capping becomes evident (i.e., the top surface of the tablet splits from the body of the tablet). A downward adjustment in tablet hardness may eliminate this problem if tablets of adequate quality can be produced at hardness levels below that at which capping occurs. A sudden drop in tablet hardness with a concomitant increase in the pressure adjustment (which normally raises the hardness) is indicative of the failure of the binding system at that pressure. A reduction in pressure should result in a return to tablets of expected quality.

Evidence of lubrication difficulties can be observed by a loss in the gloss or shine on the surface of the tablet when held so that light is seen reflecting from it. Granulation sticking to the tablet tools will produce, in the tablet surface, small indentations called picking. Careful observation of the tablet edge can detect early stages of die wall sticking, seen as lines or scratches perpendicular to the tablet face. These are caused by small amounts of granulation adhering to the die wall. If not remedied, this situation will increase in severity and the tablets will not eject freely from the die cavity.

Modifications in the binder and lubrication systems contained in the formulation can solve these problems; but as previously mentioned, the effects of both binders and lubricants are detrimental to tablet disintegration and, in the case of lubricants, the hardness of tablets. Formulations must be individually tailored to achieve adequate binding and lubrication with minimal negative effects to the finished tablets. A complete factorial design experiment has been carried out to study the influence of compression force, drug content, and particle size of ingredients on the hardness of effervescent aspirin tablets [58]. The interactions between compression force and drug content as well as compression force and ingredient particle size were found to be significant. The interactions between drug content and ingredient particle size as well as the interaction among all three parameters had no marked effect on tablet hardness. Information gathered from studies of this type can be useful in preparing high-quality effervescent tablets.

The preparation of two-layer effervescent tablets is possible but requires special tableting equipment. It is more difficult since adequate binding and lubrication are needed for both layers, which usually differ from each other in composition. This technique is used to separate active ingredients for stability purposes and to create a visual difference between layers with the use of colors [59]. Compositional differences will allow each layer to effervesce at a different rate. This is useful for a color effect in solution when different dyes are used or for functional reasons

when release of one ingredient into solution prior to a second is desired.
The pH of the solution can be controlled in this manner if, for instance,
the more rapidly soluble layer is acidic, which is subsequently neutralized
ane even alkalinized as the basic layer dissolves. In conventional tablets,
the separation of drugs for stability reasons is usually accomplished by
encapsulation. Encapsulated materials frequently are not acceptable in effervescent preparations, if clear solutions are desired, due to their slow
rates of solubility in water.

Molded rather than compressed effervescent tablets have been prepared
[60]. These tablets, which contain about 30% void space, are rapidly soluble in iced liquids. They are formed by triturating acid and carbonate
powders with a limited amount of water containing up to 10% of a volatile
organic solvent such as ethanol. The wet mass is molded into a tablet form
and dried at 50°C. Evaporation of the volatile solvent causes the void
space, which permits very rapid solution in cold liquids. Tablets containing sweetening agents, analgesics, and disinfectants have been produced
using this procedure.

IV. MANUFACTURING OPERATIONS

The large-scale manufacture of effervescent tablets is best done using a
batch-continuous type of procedure. As with most tablet-making processes
that require a granulation step, a continuous feed-in and feed-out system
is not suitable. An exception would be an extrusion process that allows
for a continuous flow of material during granulation.

Two different processes are illustrated in Figures 1 and 2. The process
in Figure 1 requires more equipment and space than that depicted in

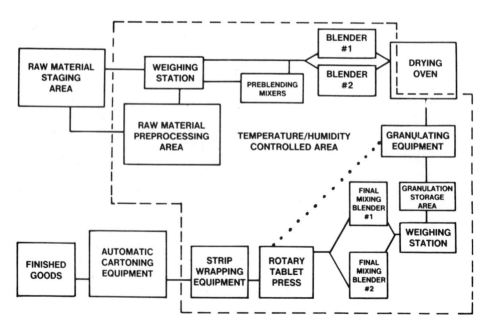

Figure 1   Manufacturing flow chart.

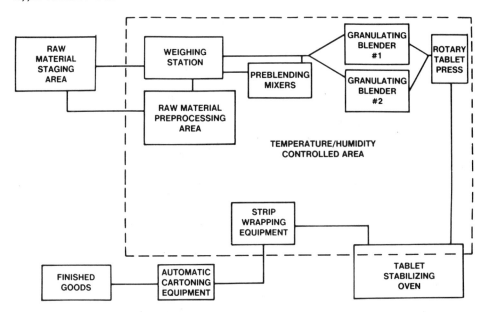

Figure 2   Manufacturing flow chart.

Figure 2 if a continuous flow of material is to be obtained. In this process, the raw materials are brought from a storage or staging area to the manu- facturing area and weighed into proper batch quantities. Any preprocessing that may be required, such as grinding, is done before weighing takes place, since the yield from exact batch quantities subjected to preprocessing will be less than 100% due to factors such as loss in the equipment, spillage, and dust generation.

Some manufacturers prefer to weigh the raw materials in an area other than the manufacturing area to reduce the chances of a compounding error in the quantity or in the specific raw material weighed. Once weighed, the raw materials are transferred to the appropriate mixers and the mass to be granulated is prepared. Smaller mixers are used for blending raw materials such as liquids or coloring substances prior to transfer to the larger blend- ers. Two blenders are used to prepare the granulation to provide a con- tinuous flow of material. As one batch, just prepared, is being transferred to the drying ovens, a second batch is in the process of preparation. The time needed to prepare one batch should not be longer than the time needed to empty the other blender if a continuous flow of granulation is to be main- tained. After passing through the drying oven, the mass is passed through appropriate equipment to produce the granules of desired size satisfactory for tableting. At this point, the granulation must be collected if heat- labile ingredients have been withheld for addition after the heating process has been completed. Appropriate quantities of the granulation are then re- weighed and mixed with the withheld ingredients in the final blenders. Two blenders are also used at this point to provide a continuous flow of material as described above. Once mixed, the just completed granulation is transferred to the tablet press; the compressed tablets to the strip- wrapping equipment (see Section VII.C for details of this operation); and the wrapped tablets to automatic cartoning and finally to storage as finished goods ready for shipment, after the needed quality assurance approval.

If no additional materials are to be added after granulating, the granulation can be transferred directly to the tablet press for compaction, as indicated by the dotted line in Figure 1, bypassing the second weighing and mixing operations. All process areas contained in the dashed line area should be maintained at the proper temperature and low humidity as described in Section III.A. The strip-wrapping equipment should be separated from the granulating and tableting equipment to minimize the possiblity of poor sealing characteristics due to airborne dust.

The process illustrated in Figure 2 is that used when the granulation is prepared with a reactive fluid and no additional components are added after the granulation is completed as described in Section III.C.3. This process is similar to that described above, up to the point when the granulation leaves the blenders in which it is mixed. From the blender, the loosely bound granulation is transferred directly to the tablet press and the compacted tablets are passed through the stabilizing oven, the last portion of which is actually a cooling area to reduce temperature of the tablets before packaging. Note that in both processes, only the oven inlet and outlet are in the dehumidified area. Due to the high cost of temperature and humidity control equipment and the energy required for its operation, economic advantages can be realized if the environmental controlled area is kept to a minimum. The strip-wrapping and cartoning procedures are as previously described, with a separate area provided for the strip-wrapping equipment.

V. TABLET EVALUATION

The important parameters in the evaluation of effervescent tablets can be divided into physical and chemical properties. The evaluation of their effectiveness in their intended use (e.g., whether a denture cleanser tablet solution actually cleans dentures) is not discussed.

A. Physical Parameters

Tablet disintegration time is one of the most important characteristics since the visual effect of the dissolving tablet and its subsequent carbonation are the main reasons for the use of effervescent systems, other than providing a mechanism for tablet disintegration. Obviously, there is little advantage over compressed, noneffervescent tablets if rapid disintegration is not obtained. Previously discussed factors that can hinder tablet disintegration are excessive concentrations of water-insoluble materials or too efficient binder systems. Excessive tablet hardness can also reduce the expected rapidity of tablet disintegration. As with conventional tablets, disintegration is distinct from dissolution, since an effervescent tablet can disintegrate into slowly soluble fragments or particles. Usually this is a distinct negative since a slowly soluble residue is unsightly and the full effect of the functional ingredients is not obtained unless they are in solution. A properly formulated effervescent tablet will disintegrate and dissolve quickly, usually in 1 or 2 min.

Table 1 Volume and Temperature of Water Used in Effervescent Tablet
Disintegration Testing

Tablet	Water volume (ml)	Water temperature (°C)
Antacid/analgesic	120–180	15–20
Denture cleanser	120–150	40–45
Flavored beverage	180–240	10–15
Mouthwash	20–30	25–25
Toilet bowl cleaner	4000–6000	20–25

Disintegration time tests involve placing the tablet in a standard volume
of water at a specified initial water temperature and recording the time in
which the tablet disintegrates. The volume and temperature of the water
depend on the type of product being tested. It is most realistic if both
are those to be used by the consumer. Examples are given in Table 1.
Often, effervescent tablets will float to the top of the solution prior to
complete disintegration, making accurate disintegration time determination
difficult. This occurs when the density of the tablet mass and bubbles adhering to it become less than the density of the solution in which it is disintegrating. Careful observation of the floating tablet as it crumbles is
needed at this point to determine the actual disintegration time.

Two other important effervescent tablet physical parameters are hardness and friability. As with conventional tablets, these criteria are inter-
related, depending on the formulation components. Generally with effervescent tablets, the harder the tablet, the lower the friability. Both of
these parameters are indicative of how well the tablet will withstand the
rigors of handling after compression. Automated packaging systems provide the most abuse to the tablet surfaces after compression. Many marketed effervescent tablets are large in diameter and chip easily at the edges
during handling.

The choice of proper tableting tools, especially beveled edge configurations, can minimize edge chipping. The relative hardness of effervescent
tablets can be modified by adjusting the ratio of tablet thickness to tablet
diameter. The closer this ratio is to 1, the harder the tablet will be.
Often this approach is not useful, however, because thick tablets are difficult to properly package in individual, hermetically sealed pouches. As
the tablet becomes thicker, a greater strain is placed on the pouch seal
area, increasing the probability of leaking pouches. This will be discussed
in greater detail in the Section VII.C.5 of this chapter. Tablet hardness
is measured using standard hardness testers available to the pharmaceutical
industry. A Roche friabilator is useful in measuring tablet friability.

Another important physical parameter is tablet weight. This is a function of the formulation and compressing equipment adjustments, as is the
case with conventional tablets. Good manufacturing practice will result in
tablets that conform to compendial weight variation tests discussed elsewhere in this volume.

B. Chemical Parameters

An interesting chemical property, perhaps unique to effervescent tablets, is the solution pH generated when the tablet dissolves. Due to the nature of the effervescent system components, buffer systems are formed, and thus discrete pH readings can be obtained. The consistent measurement of solution pH is a sign of good distribution of raw materials within the tablet. A wide variation in solution pH from tablet to tablet is indicative of a nonhomogeneous granulation directly prior to tableting. A consistent pH difference from that normally observed for a product in a particular batch of tablets is indicative of a compounding or raw material weighing error. The pH of the solution is important for taste reasons in a product meant for ingestion. Often antacid products are formulated to yield a slightly acidic pH to augment the taste of the solution, particularly if citrus or berry flavors are used. Products that are mint flavored are best formulated so that the solution is neutral or slightly alkaline. Solution pH can be functionally important for some effervescent products. A toilet bowl cleaner should be acidic rather than alkaline to dissolve calcium and iron deposits from the porcelain fixture.

A denture cleanser can be acidic for maximum calculus solubility, or neutral to slightly alkaline for potentiation of the typical oxidizing agents used in these formulations.

Solution pH is measured with suitable instrumentation in standardized water volumes and temperatures. It is conveniently done following disintegration time measurements. The pH should be measured at a specific time after the tablet has been placed in the water since it is not unusual for effervescent solutions to change in pH on standing. This is due to the constant breakdown of carbonic acid to carbon dioxide gas and water within the solution. If slowly soluble materials are present, adequate time should be given for the ingredients to dissolve (after tablet disintegration occurs) before pH measurements are made.

Another important chemical parameter for tablets containing assayable active ingredients is content uniformity assay. This is the same for any tableted dosage form and is discussed elsewhere in this volume. A 10% variation from the theoretical amount of the active ingredient compounded into the product is usually acceptable.

VI. EFFERVESCENT STABILITY

The stability of effervescent tablets can be discussed in two distinct parts. One deals with the degradation of drugs or other functionally active ingredients, the other with the stability of the effervescent system itself. They are not mutually exclusive, however, since if the portion of the tablet is unstable and has decomposed, the stability of the active assayable components is of little concern to the formulator. This section deals with the stability of the effervescent system common to all effervescent tablets and not the stability of particular components compounded into effervescent systems that are peculiar to each formulation.

Effervescent systems are not stable in the presence of moisture. Trace amounts of moisture can activate the effervescent system during prolonged storage and decompose the tablet prior to use. To make matters worse, effervescent tablets are hygroscopic and will absorb enough water to initiate degradation if not properly packaged.

A. Methods of Achieving Stability

The elimination or inactivation of free water within the effervescent system is the key to stability, aside from manufacturing effervescent tablets in controlled low-humidity atmospheres. A choice of the proper types of raw materials is essential. Unless a hydrated form of a raw material is chosen purposely, all raw materials used should be in their anhydrous form. Many anhydrous raw materials that are prepared from hydrated forms become hygroscopic and readily adsorb water vapor from the air. In such cases, drying of these raw materials prior to use can be critical. The knowledge of possible hydrates formed during processing (which are not present at the outset) is useful, especially if free water is used as a granulating agent.

Materials such as citric acid and sodium carbonate will form hydrates readily. It is possible that the tablets containing hydrates formed during processing will appear to be stable when first examined but will slowly decompose as these hydrates are released with time. Some materials, such as anhydrous citrate salts, will form stable hydrates and act as effective internal desiccants to actually increase the stability of the tablet with time under certain conditions. Finely divided silica gel has also been used as an internal desiccant in effervescent tablets [61].

Finely divided anhydrous sodium carbonate has been found to be an effective stabilizing agent for effervescent tablets when incorporated into formulations at about 10% w/w of the sodium bicarbonate concentration. It is theorized that the anhydrous salt preferentially absorbs any minute trace of free water present, producing stable hydrated forms. Another method of sodium carbonate stabilization is found in the patent literature [62]. In this method, the sodium bicarbonate used in the formulation is heated so that 2 to 10% w/w is converted to sodium carbonate. Stabilization of the effervescent system results from the chemical change that occurs on the outer particle surface forming a barrier to hinder reaction with the acid source contained in the formulation.

Surface passivation of a solid acid has been found to improve effervescent product stability [63,64]. The acid and a carbonate source are heated from 40 to 80°C in a closed vessel. A polar solvent such as water is introduced and rapidly vacuum-dried. The degree of passivation is measured by monitoring the pressure increase in the vessel during processing. The procedure is repeated until no further pressure increase is observed, indicating that surface passivation has been achieved. It is claimed that the dry mixtures are highly stable even on storage under tropical conditions. In another case [65], crystals of solid acid are coated with calcium carbonate which adheres to the acid crystal surface by a bonding layer formed during processing.

The addition of substances that decrease the hygroscopicity of the effervescent mixtures can also provide a stabilizing effect. Encapsulation of the acid and/or carbonate phases has been accomplished using PVP and hydroxypropylcellulose [66], methacrylic acid polymers [67], and maltodextrin [68]. In general, however, tablet solubility is reduced due to the slowly soluble nature of the encapsulating materials. Stabilization of the effervescent system is also possible if the sodium bicarbonate is mixed with a dilute solution of gum followed by drying and particle size reduction [69], or if as little as 0.5% of lactic albumin, casein, or soya bean albumin is mixed with the total effervescent preparation [70].

Another method of achieving effervescent stability was accomplished by
producing a cored tablet in which the inner core of effervescent materials
was protected from moisutre absorption by coating with a sugar alcohol
such as sorbitol [71]. This tablet was meant for oral use rather than for
dissolution in water.

B. Stability Testing and Shelf-Life

The stability testing and shelf-life prediction of effervescent tablets are not
complicated, and the usual Arrhenius equation kinetic principles can be applied to the data obtained from the following tests. Each tablet is hermetically
sealed in a standard size aluminum foil laminate pouch. The pouches are
placed at 25, 37, 45, and 60°C after the thickness of the tablet and the
foil pouch is measured and recorded. If decomposition occurs, small amounts
of carbon dioxide gas will be released into the pouch, causing it to swell.
The degree of swelling, as measured by increase in pouch thickness, is related to the amount of gas evolved. An apparatus can be constructed so
that the initial thickness of the packaged tablet is assigned a zero reading
on an adjustable measurement scale while a constant weight is applied. An
increase less than 1/16 in. is considered negligible. Even though the decomposition of the product may be small, pouch swelling is considered an
important criterion of stability. Most effervescent products are sold packaged in this manner, and swollen packages are not readily accepted by the
consumer.

Another method of measuring the stability of the effervescent system
with time is to assay the tablet themselves for total carbon dioxide content.
This is easily done following established procedures for baking powder assays as developed by the Association of Agricultural Chemists [72]. This
method uses liquid volume displacement equipment known as the Chittick
apparatus. A tablet sample is crushed, and a portion of powder is accurately weighed and placed in a flask, into which is introduced an acid-water
solution. The amount of carbon dioxide liberated from the sample is measured volumetrically by the displacement of a non-carbon-dioxide-adsorbing
solution contained in a graduated cylinder. It is essential that the solution
be nonabsorbent of carbon dioxide. The weight percent of carbon dioxide
is then calculated using temperature and pressure corrections.

Tablet disintegration time is another measure of effervescent stability.
If carbon dioxide is lost due to chemical decomposition within the dosage
form, the tablet will not disintegrate as rapidly as when it was initially
prepared. Using the techniques to measure disintegration time previously
described in this chapter, a record is kept of the tablets' disintegration
characteristics when stored at elevated temperatures for varying lengths
of time. If the disintegration time exceeds the previously established acceptable limit when stored for less than 3 months at 45°C, 6 months at 37°C,
or 24 months at 25°C, evidence of decomposition exists and should be investigated.

Quantification of an effervescent reaction to monitor the stability of
selected effervescent tablet systems has been studied [73]. Two devices
were developed to monitor the reactivity of pharmaceutical effervescent systems. The first device monitored carbon dioxide pressure generation during
the effervescent reaction in a specially constructed cylindrical plastic pressure vessel that allowed mixing of the sample tablet and water after the

unit had been sealed. At standard time intervals the pressure was read
from the pressure gage fitted to the vessel and recorded. The dissolution
time of the tablet was observed through a transparent position of the pressure vessel and was also recorded. The second device utilized a double-
cantilever beam and an electomagnetic proximity transducer to measure the
weight loss attributed to carbon dioxide loss to the atmosphere. Tablet
dissolution time was also observed and recorded. A correlation coefficient
of 0.937 was calculated from a plot of the relationship of pressure generated
versus weight loss for a series of experimental effervescent tablets. Using
these data an index of reactivity was calculated that can be used to quanti-
tate the effervescent activity from a particular system. Loss of reactivity
with time as a quantitative measure of stability of the system can therefore
be monitored using this technique.

Further work was done combining these techniques with mercury intru-
sion porosity measurements to determine the effects of compression pressure,
water vapor, and high temperature on effervescent tablet stability [74]. It
was found that compression pressure was not a factor in tablet stability.
The stability was dependent, however, on the tablet formulation, storage
conditions, and the length of time the tablet was stored.

C. In-Process Stability Measurements

Obviously, it is not an acceptable technique to place samples of each batch
of tablets at elevated temperatures and wait for swelling to occur to determine if the tablets are unstable. Quick, accurate, in-process quality assurance methods are needed to determine if each batch of tablets will be
stable for the expected shelf life of the product. Since any decomposition
is triggered by trace amounts of water, several methods have been devised
to measure the residual water content either directly or indirectly.

Conventional loss-on-drying methods are not useful for effervescent
systems containing carbonates since the heat generated in the test apparatus
will drive off carbon dioxide gas, producing false weight-loss readings.
Water assay using the Karl Fischer titration procedure usually is not useful
since the water content being measured is too low to be determined accurately. A better method, but still not ideal, is vacuum drying to a constant
tablet weight over concentrated sulfuric acid. This procedure, aside from
being time consuming and potentially hazardous due to the acid used, lacks
the accuracy needed. It also probably would not detect initially stable
hydrates formed during processing, which could subsequently decompose
and release free water, initiating the effervescent reaction.

An acceptable technique using a modified Parr calorimeter (illustrated
in Fig. 3) has been used for many years. The tablets are sealed inside a
closed chamber fitted with a pressure gage with a scale ranging from 0 to
60 lb in.$^{-2}$. Enough tablets should be placed in the chamber so as to leave
a minimum air space in order to avoid erroneous readings due to air expansion. As heat is applied externally from a constant temperature source,
any trace amount of water will be liberated, causing the effervescent reaction to begin and release carbon dioxide. The pressure from the gas
evolved is measured on the gage, being directly related to the amount of
potentially troublesome water contained in the tablet. Through experimentation, it is possible to produce a stable effervescent tablet that, when tested
using this procedure, gives a mid-range reading on the pressure gage. To

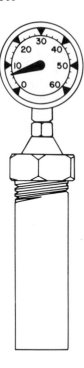

Figure 3   Modified calorimeter used for stability measurement.

do this, a correlation among the moisture content of the tablets, elevated-
temperature stability testing, the test bath temperature, and the time of
exposure in the bath must be made.

In practice, several batches of the product are prepared with moisture
content varying from batch to batch. These are packaged and placed in
environments with a range of controlled temperatures such as 25, 37, 45,
and 60°C. With time, differences in the stability of the test products will
become evident, and a dividing line between a stable and an unstable product can be determined. Concurrently, calorimeter tests are conducted at
varying temperatures and lengths of exposure to the temperatures until a
reasonable range of values relating to the moisture content of each batch
of product is determined. These data are then correlated with those of
the elevated temperature tests, resulting in a specification for a stable
product as measured by the calorimeter test. The established specification
and test method can easily be incorporated into quality assurance procedures
since the calorimeter method is rapid and reliable. In a comparison of two
products, data accumulated for one product—even though both are similar
in effervescent composition—should not be related to the other, especially
if additives in the first differ from those in the second. Each product
should be thoroughly tested according to the above procedure and assigned
its own stability specification. An example of determining a specification
for an effervescent tablet with a diameter of 0.75 in. and thickness of 0.20
in. follows.

Enough tablets are placed in a stainless tube with an internal diameter
of 0.90 in. so that the top tablet is 0.25 in. below the top of the tube, in

this case 10 tablets. The pressure gage is attached, the device is sealed and placed in a constant temperature bath so that the liquid in the bath covers the stainless steel tube. Trials are conducted at 75, 80, and 85°C and pressure readings are recorded at 30, 45, 60, 90, and 120 min. Similar data are obtained for two additional batches of the same formulation with different moisture contents resulting from varying oven-drying procedures. The data obtained are shown in Table 2. Additional stability testing with these same products using the packet puffing and carbon dioxide measurement testing described above indicate that only the low moisture level tablets were acceptably stable after 3 months storage at 45°C. Therefore the data in Table 2 for the low moisture level tablets can be used to determine the specification. A good choice for this example would be to accept any batch whose readings are not greater than 15 psig when tested for 60 min.

Any of the values could be used. However, it is best to avoid the low or very high pressure readings on the pressure gage scale for accuracy and to allow enough time in the bath to adequately heat the tube contents causing decomposition, if it is to occur.

Table 2   Pressure Readings (psig) Obtained During Stability Specification Determination Testing for a Particular Effervescent Tablet Formulation

Bath temperature (°C)	Time (min)				
	30	45	60	90	120
High Moisture Level Tablets					
75	8	14	18	27	37
80	12	20	27	40	54
85	15	26	38	51	60+
Medium Moisture Level Tablets					
75	6	12	16	22	28
80	9	17	23	31	41
85	13	24	33	46	52
Low Moisture Level Tablets					
75	4	6	10	13	16
80	5	8	15	18	23
85	7	9	20	26	34

VII. PACKAGING

A. Moisture Control

Since effervescent tablets are hygroscopic, they must be protected from atmospheric moisture if a reasonable shelf life is to be expected. Any absorption of moisture will initiate the effervescent reaction; therefore packages for effervescent tablets must have hermetic seals regardless of the type of container. Multiuse containers, such as tubes or bottles, must have closures that can be resealed after each tablet is removed. Packaging operations must be conducted in low-humidity environments (maximum 25% relative humidity at 25°C) similar to those required for granulating and tableting if the long-term stability of the tablets is to be maintained.

B. Packaging Configurations and Materials

Effervescent tablets are usually packaged in glass, plastic, or metal tubes or individual foil pouches joined to form a conveniently sized strip of tablets.
     Glass offers the highest degree of moisture protection of the nonflexible packaging materials; however, inherent limitations exist, such as breakage and cost of shipping a heavy package. Since individual packaging in glass is economically infeasible, moisture-proof closures for these multiple-use containers must be used. Metal caps with a waxed, aluminum foil, pulp-backed cap liner usually prove satisfactory when repeatedly opened and closed. If properly closed after each use, moisture is excluded from the interior of the package. Many effervescent tablets are rather large, approaching 1 in. in diameter, and do not lend themselves to random filling in a glass bottle as would smaller tablets. These tablets are packaged by stacking them one on another in a glass or plastic tube slightly larger in diameter than the tablets and about 5 in. high.
     In this manner, a minimum of air space surrounds the tablet prior to use. Since moisture can enter a glass container only through the closure, the top tablet serves as a desiccant and protects the rest of the tablets in the package. Once opened, however, protection from moisture is diminished because the air space becomes greater and greater as the tablets are used. This can be especially troublesome if humid air is permitted to enter the tube. In any event, the tablets should be used promptly or the last few will be nonreactive when placed in water, due to complete reaction which has slowly occurred in the container prior to use. Plastic tubes are not as protective as glass due to the moisture vapor permeability of plastic packaging materials. Tablets with a low order of hygroscopicity can be satisfactorily packaged in plastic tubes with moisture-proof closures. Special caps can be constructed with a chamber containing silica gel or some other desiccant that will preferentially absorb moisture vapor entering through the closure. Extruded, seamless metal tubes, often made from aluminum, have been used commonly in Europe to package effervescent tablets. These are impervious to moisture as are glass tubes. Tightly fitting plastic snap caps that may contain a desiccant chamber are used as closures.
     Effervescent tablets are most frequently strip-wrapped in individual pouches arranged in conveniently sized strips and stacked in a paperboard box. Each tablet is hermetically sealed in its own container and is not exposed to the atmosphere until the time of use. Many different flexible packaging materials are available for packaging, but few are suitable for

protecting effervescent tablets from moisture vapor or physical damage.
Some effervescent tablets produced in Europe are available packaged in
thermoformed plastic blisters with foil backing. This type of packaging requires that the tablets be pushed through the foil backing by pressing on
the blister. The tablets packaged in this manner must be hard enough so
as not to break when they are removed from their package. Most large-
diameter, relatively thin effervescent tablets cannot be made hard enough
to withstand the force required to remove them from this type of packaging.
A transparent film known as Aclar has a very low moisture-vapor transmission rate and will suitably protect effervescent tablets, but it is too
expensive to be competitive with the standard material used industrywide
(i.e., heat-sealable, aluminum foil laminates).

Aluminum foil is a flexible, absolute barrier to gases, water vapor, and
light. It is nontoxic and immune to microbiological attack. It has excellent
heat conductivity, thereby making it an excellent choice for heat-sealing
strip-packaging operations.

Aluminum foil laminates are composed of several layers of different materials bonded together. A primer or wash is applied to the surface of
one layer to promote bonding of the adjacent layer. Shellac or ethyl acrylic
acid copolymers are commonly used as primers. The outside layer of the
laminate is typically some form of paper, perhaps glassine, bond, or calen-
dered (compressed) pouch paper. This layer provides a surface for printing, protects the foil against abrasion, and provides mechanical support for
the entire laminate. A printed laminate allows identification of each tablet
unit after removal from the strip. The next layer is polyethylene—about
0.005 in. thick—which bonds the paper to the aluminum foil layer. The
aluminum foil can range in thickness from 0.00035 in. to 0.002 in. Foil of
0.001 in. thickness will impart the needed barrier properties to the packaging laminate. Thinner materials can be used, but a loss in moisture protection can occur due to the possibility of pinholes in the foil through
which moisture vapor will pass. The thinner the foil is rolled, the more
pinholes will be present. The inside layer consists of a heat-sealable material such as polyethylene, also about 0.001 in. thick. Laminates are also
available with heat seals consisting of acrylic copolymers such as Surlyn.
A typical laminate structure is illustrated in Figure 4.

New laminates containing a stretchable aluminum foil alloy sandwiched
between two plastic stretchable films have been developed in Europe
(Alusuisse Metals Company, Singen, West Germany) for use on equipment
which produces a foil blister by mechanically drawing the laminate into a
machined cavity without the use of heat. The outer film, which is usually
biaxially oriented nylon or polypropylene, provides strength to the laminate
to prevent foil rupture during the cold forming process. The inside layer,
which comes in contact with the product, is usually made from polyvinyl-
chloride or polyethylene depending on the compatability requirements of
the product.

C. Strip Wrapping

In a typical packaging operation, a diagram of which is shown in Figure 5,
two sheets (or webs) of the laminate converge and pass between a pair of
matching heated cylinders, each containing exactly corresponding cavities
appropriate in depth and dimension to the tablet to be packaged. The

Effervescent Tablets

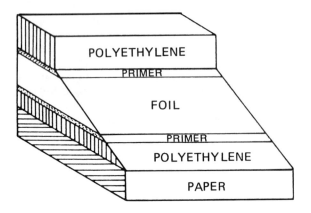

Figure 4   Typical packaging laminate structure.

tablets are fed between the converging sheets synchronously with the cylinder cavities so that they are not crushed.   The two sheets of foil laminate
around each cavity are heated by contact with the cylinder surface and
subjected to pressure between the cylinders, forming the heat seal.   The
cylinders are engraved with a knurled or cross-hatched pattern to ensure
an effective seal.   As the formed pouch leaves the heated cylinders, the
temperature of the laminate falls, causing the two heat seal layers to bond.
The sheet is then automatically cut into the proper configuration and perforated to allow the removal of one pouch without disturbing the sealed area

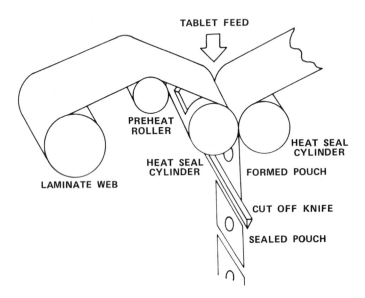

Figure 5   Strip wrap packaging.

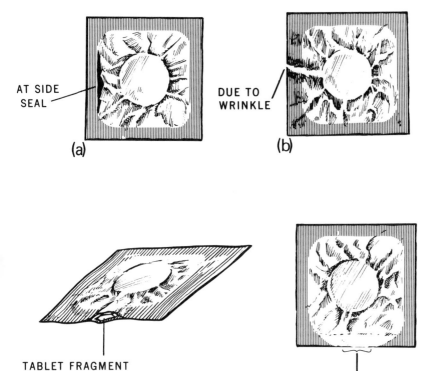

Figure 6 Poor foil laminate seals: (a) foil fracture, (b) wrinkling in the laminate, (c) foreign matter in seal, and (d) stress on the foil.

of the adjacent pouch. The seal integrity of the completed pouches is of prime importance because without a good seal, moisture will enter the pouch and decompose the tablet prior to use by the customer.

Poor seals in high-speed strip-wrapping operations can result from a number of sources, illustrated in Figure 6 and discussed in the following paragraphs.

Temperature of Sealing Roller Too Low

High-speed equipment is capable of wrapping in excess of 800 tablets per minute. At these speeds, the contact time between the foil laminate and the heat sealing roller is short. Even though aluminum is a good conductor of heat, it may not transfer the heat from the sealing roller to the thermoplastic heat-seal material fast enough to effect a good seal. If, at a maximum sealing roller temperature, adequate sealing does not take place and production speeds cannot be decreased to extend the contact time between the laminate and the roller, preheating of the laminate is advisable. This can be accomplished by the use of preheat rollers over which the laminate passes immediately prior to contact with the sealing roller. The preheat rollers will heat the laminate to a point just below the melting point of the thermoplastic heat seal and facilitate complete sealing in a relatively short period of time.

Foreign Matter in Seal Area

A common problem leading to poor seals is the presence of dust or tablet chips or pieces in the seal area. This is especially true if the tablets are not hard enough to possess a low order of friability and easily chip or break when subjected to the rigors of the packaging equipment. If tablets are vertically fed and dropped between the sealing rollers, it is possible for troublesome quantities of dust to fall onto the heat seal surface of the laminate prior to sealing. Adequate vacuum systems along the tablet feed track will minimize, if not eliminate, this problem.

Wrinkling in the Laminate

Uneven tension for the foil rolls or misregistration of the two laminates as they feed between the sealing rollers can cause a puckering, folding, or wrinkling of the foil laminate. Leaks are possible in this area due to the formation of a channel from the atmosphere to the interior of the pouch through which moisture can pass. A defect-free laminate and careful packaging equipment adjustment can remedy this problem.

Foil Fracture

Often foil fractures are found parallel to the inside seals, but not parallel to the cross-seals, as the packaged tablets leave the sealing rollers. This is caused by too much sealing pressure between the heat seal rollers. The pressure between the rollers is constant; therefore, much greater pressure is applied to the laminate at the side seals when the rollers are sealing an area across the nonsealed centers of the pouches. While the cross-seals are being formed, the rollers are completely touching and the pressure is less and evenly distributed across the roller. This phenomenon can be eliminated by careful packaging equipment adjustment.

Stress on the Foil

Pouch size in relation to the tablet diameter and thickness is an important factor in producing adequately packaged tablets. The tablet thickness must not be so great as to put an undue stress on the foil laminate during the sealing operation and immediately afterward. At this point, the thermoplastic heat-seal materials are still hot and in the process of binding. A thick tablet can physically pull them apart and seriously lessen the seal integrity. Coordination of tablet size and pouch configuration will obviate this problem. Satisfactory relationships between tablet and pouch size are shown in Table 3.

A change in tablet shape from flat-faced to one with a deeply beveled edge may help also. Design patents [75-77] have been issued for tablets of this shape. Due to an extreme bevel on the tablet, the angle at the point of laminate contact is much less than that present with a flat-faced tablet. Less stress is transferred to the side seal area, thereby reducing the possibility of laminate separation before heat-seal binding occurs.

A recent innovation from European packaging machine manufacturers has been the modification of thermoform plastic, blister pack equipment to produce a packet containing a formed aluminum blister (Uhlmann Packaging Systems, Fairfield, NJ). An example of this equipment is shown in Figure 7. The vacuum-draw, heated dies used to form plastic blisters have been replaced with a unit that mechanically draws the laminate into a machined

Table 3   Satisfactory Dimensional Relationships Between Tablets
and Foil Laminate Pouch to Avoid Excessive Laminate Stress

Pouch size (in. × in.)	Tablet diameter (in.)	Tablet thickness (in.)
2.25 × 2.25	1.00	0.22
2.00 × 2.00	1.00	0.16
2.00 × 2.00	0.75	0.19
1.50 × 1.50	0.63	0.16

cavity to form the aluminum laminate packets. Tablets are fed into the
packets while the laminate containing the formed packets moves through the
machine in a horizontal plane rather than vertically as with the strip-
wrapping equipment described above. After the tablets have been placed
in the packets, a printed, thin, lidding foil laminate is positioned on top of
the tablet packets, heat is applied, and a sealed packet is produced. Tablets can be removed by tearing the laminate from the edge or pushing the
tablet through the lidding laminate.

In addition to its modern appearance, this package is more economical
to produce since less laminate is required to package a given number of
tablets due to the orientation of the tablets in the package. It is also
possible to package tablets that are thicker than vertical strip-wrapping
equipment can accommodate. The cavity depth is limited only by the degree
to which the foil laminate can be stretched during packet formation. Examples of formed aluminum packages for tablets are shown in Figure 8.

D. Package Integrity Testing

To be certain an effervescent tablet reaches the ultimate user with the
same quality as originally produced and packaged, tests are performed on
the seal integrity of various packaging configurations. Clearly, the integrity of any package is only as good as its closure. For effervescent
tablets, an impervious package with a loose-fitting cap or imperfect heat
seal is as good as if the cap were left off or the heat seal area left un-
bounded. Hermetic packaging is required if effervescent tablets are to
attain a reasonable shelf life of 2 to 3 years. The ultimate testing procedure is to store packages for their expected shelf life under the most
severe humidity and temperature conditions that they will encounter, once
sold. Since this is not practical, accelerated testing procedures have been
developed that simulate long-term storage in adverse environments. Packages containing effervescent tablets are stored in chambers regulated at
constant high humidity and temperatures, such as 80% relative humidity at
37°C and 80% relative humidity at 25°C. If the relative moisture content of
the product is determined before the study is started, changes in moisture
content with time can be monitored. These changes may be due to moisture
seeping into the product through the closure or through the package itself

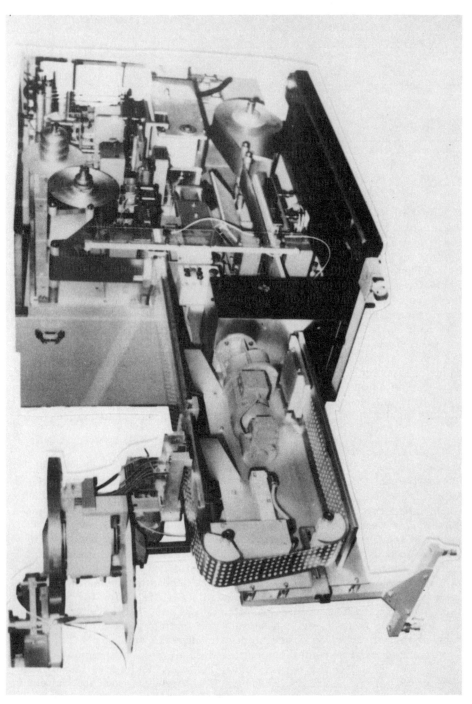

Figure 7   Aluminum blister-forming machine.   (Courtesy Uhlmann Packaging Systems, Inc., Fairfield, NJ.)

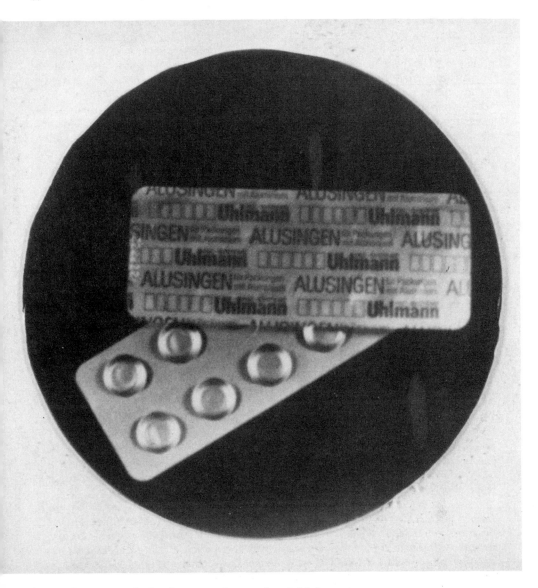

Figure 8 Formed aluminum packages for tablets.

if it is made of a material not completely impervious to moisture-vapor transmission, such as polyethylene bottles or thin aluminum foil with pinholes.

The point at which the package is no longer protective will be determined by the rise in moisture content of each particular tablet formulation and is governed by the relative hygroscopicity of the tablet. Since this is so, tablets that have low hygroscopicity may be suitably packaged in less expensive, less protective containers. If a product shows little or no moisture pickup after being stored in a chamber at 80% relative humidity at 37°C for 3 months, the package is considered satisfactory. Test conditions in the high-humidity and high-temperature chambers should be dynamic and not static. Air should be freely circulating about the packages to maximize the similarities between the test conditions and those that would actually occur in the field. Products and packaging that can pass the most severe laboratory testing are sure to be stable in the field.

An extrapolation of accelerated test data to actual field conditions can be made after some testing under field conditions to ensure the predictive accuracy of laboratory testing. It is important that packages prepared on production equipment be used for any testing that will be the basis of projections to field conditions. Data gathered for packages wrapped on laboratory or experimental equipment should only be used as a guide, due to differences among machinery and the speeds at which they operate.

Obviously, one cannot afford the expense or the time to wait 3 months to test representative samples of the packages produced on a day-to-day basis; therefore, several methods to test seal integrity rapidly (especially seals of aluminum foil laminates) have been devised.

Vacuum Underwater Method

The most commonly used method involves the application of vacuum to the pouches while they are submerged in water. A representative sample of pouches is placed in a water-filled chamber under a weighted plate to keep the pouches from floating during the test. The chamber is sealed and a 500- to 635-mmHg vacuum drawn and maintained for 3 min. The vacuum is then slowly released over an additional 2- to 3-min period.

Seal and foil defects can be located by a small stream of bubbles rising from a particular point on the pouch. After testing, the pouches should be removed from the water, allowed to dry, and carefully opened for examination. Water that has been drawn into the pouch during the decreasing vacuum phase will initiate the effervescent reaction. Tablets enclosed in leaking pouches can be identified easily in this manner. This method, although indicative of truly leaking pouches, has a distinct disadvantage: the difficult balance that must be made between (a) the vacuum needed to put enough stress on the seal to promote failure of poorly sealed pouches and (b) the maximum vacuum allowable without creating additional leaking pouches due to distortion of the foil laminate. Whether this balance is possible to achieve is open to question. This problem does not exist with the alternative methods that follow.

Detection of Tracer Material Sealed Within the Pouch

In this method a tracer material such as dry carbon dioxide or helium gas is sealed into the pouch with the tablets. The pouches to be tested are placed in a small, sealed chamber to which a vacuum is applied. The effluent from the chamber is passed through an infrared spectrophotometer sensing device calibrated for the specific tracer being used (Modern Controls, Minneapolis, MN). If the pouches are adequately sealed, none of the tracer escapes from the pouches and no response is given by the instrument.

If a leak exists, the tracer is detected and an alarm is sounded. Systems can be devised for various tracer substances, some of which, perhaps, may be part of the formulation, thereby obviating the need for extraneous addition of the tracer. This method will not detect grossly unsealed areas from which the tracer has escaped prior to testing. However, customary visual examination will detect these gross defects.

Purging with Detectable Gas

This method is similar to the one just described, except that the pouches are placed in a vessel that is *subsequently* pressurized with the tracer gas as noted above. If the pouches have seal or foil defects, the gas will enter the pouch and mix with the contents. The pressure is released, and the pouches are tested as described above. The sensitivity of the instrument must be such that the concentration of the tracer gas, now diluted with the gaseous contents of the pouch, can still be detected.

Infrared Seal Inspection

A nondestructive infrared test method has been developed to detect sealing flaws (Barnes Engineering Co., Stamford, CT). A transport mechanism holds the sealed package and passes the seal across a focused radiation heat source that produces a thermal gradient in the seal. An infrared microscope located opposite the heat source can directly measure the temperature differences along the heated strip of the flexible seal. When the seal is uniform, heat dissipates at a uniform rate and the infrared microscope output is uniform. If there are voids, occluded matter, or wrinkles in the seal, the heat transfer rate is reduced and a sharp negative change is recorded by the microscope. Each unit produced can be screened in this manner with an automatic system designed to reject only those strips that contain defects. This system is not designed to detect defects other than those in the seal area. Tests with knurled or cross-hatch seals have presented problems in the past due to uneven heat distribution caused by the seal configuration. This method is most applicable to flat-seal areas without distortion—seldom used to package effervescent tablets.

Electronic Airtightness Tester

This relatively new, patented test method [78] was developed at the Warner–Lambert Company to quickly and nondestructively test the hermetic seal integrity of packages and containers. Using vacuum and position sensors and analog and digital processing techniques, the unit will quickly and accurately determine the seal integrity of a wide variety of packages including those used for effervescent products. The instrument features include nondestructive testing with no package preconditioning necessary. It is simple to operate and produces objective results. This instrument utilizes a microprocessor controller and associated software to determine the degree of package airtightness based on the package's response to an external vacuum. The unit includes a vacuum chamber, pump, microprocessor, and both vacuum and displacement transducers. The package that has at least one flexible

surface is positioned inside the vacuum chamber and the door is latched.
A linear displacement transducer is lowered into contact with the expandable
surface of the package. The unit is activated and a dedicated microprocessor begins the test sequence. The chamber air is gradually evacuated and
the package thickness is monitored in response to the changing vacuum.
Over the course of 5 to 30 sec, the microprocessor analyzes the data and,
based on the expansion and contraction of the package in response to the
vacuum, determines whether or not the package is airtight. As the test
proceeds, the data points collected are graphically displayed on a monitor
screen and a go/no-go determination appears. The microprocessor also
computes a linear regression of the package expansion as a function of
vacuum. The principle of the test is that if the package is airtight, the
expansion of the package will track the applied vacuum, expanding and
contracting as the vacuum increases or decreases. Consequently, the linear
regression will have a high degree of correlation. If the package is not
airtight, it either will not expand or will expand initially and begin to col-
lapse as the head space is vented under the external vacuum. In either
case, the expansion of the package will not behave as a linear function of
vacuum and the correlation will be low. The decision regarding the acceptability of the package seal integrity is made based on the variables measured during the test.

   This test instrumentation is being used in a manufacturing environment
to provide a quick determination of the suitability of the package coming
off the packaging line. It can provide the line operator important information regarding the performance of the packaging machine so that corrective
actions can be accomplished before a large quantity of defective goods are
produced.

   This instrument has been tested against the gas detection methods described above and was found to be as accurate without the need to purge
or fill the packages with a tracer or detection gas. A limited number of
units are under fabrication and are available to the pharmaceutical, food,
and confectionery industries from the Consumer Products Package Development Department, Warner-Lambert Company, Morris Plains, NJ 07950.

VIII. EFFERVESCENT FORMULATIONS

The following formulations and suggested manufacturing procedures illustrate
the principles discussed in the text of this chapter.

Example 1: Antacid Effervescent Tablets

Ingredient	Quantity
1. Citric acid, anhydrous (granular)	1180 g
2. Sodium bicarbonate (granular)	1700 g
3. Sodium bicarbonate (powder)	175 g
4. Citrus flavor (spray-dried)	50 g
5. Water	30 g

Example 1: (Continued)

Thoroughly blend 1, 2, and 4 in a planetary mixer.
Quickly add all of 5 and mix until a workable mass
is formed. Granulate through a 10-mesh screen using
an oscillating granulator. Spread evenly on a paper-
lined drying tray and dry in a forced-draft oven at
70°C for 2 hr. Remove from oven, cool, and re-
granulate through a 16-mesh screen. Place granulation in a tumble blender and add 3. Mix well.
Compress 1-in. flat-faced, beveled edge tablets
each weighing 3.10 g. Package in glass tubes or
aluminum foil.

Example 2: Antacid-Analgesic Effervescent Tablets

Ingredient	Quantity
1. Acetylsalicylic acid (80-mesh crystals)	325 g
2. Monobasic calcium phosphate (powder)	165 g
3. Sodium bicarbonate (granular)	1700 g
4. Citric acid, anhydrous (granular)	1060 g

Convert 3 to 7—9% sodium carbonate by placing in a
forced-draft oven set at 100°C for 45 min, with two
mixings at 15-min intervals. Cool the converted bicarbonate and mix with 2 and 4 in a tumble blender. Add
1 and mix for 10 min. Compress 1-in.-diameter flat-
faced, beveled edge tablets each weighing 3.25 g.
Stabilize tablets in a forced-draft oven at 60°C for 1 hr.
Cool and package in glass tubes or aluminum foil.

Example 3: Potassium Chloride Effervescent Tablets [79]

Ingredient	Quantity
1. Glycine hydrochloride	1338 g
2. Potassium chloride	597 g
3. Potassium bicarbonate	1001 g
4. Potassium citrate	216 g
5. Polyvinylpyrrolidone	77 g
6. Polyethylene glycol 8000 (powder)	115 g
7. Saccharin	20 g
8. Silica gel (fumed)	5 g

Example 3:   (Continued)

Ingredient	Quantity
9. L-Leucine (pulverized)	34 g
10. Citrus color	3 g
11. Citrus flavor (spray-dried)	5 g
12. Isopropyl alcohol	6 g

Grind together 1, 2, 3, and 4. Mix the ground materials
in a tumble blender for 15 to 20 min. Granulate the
mixed powders with a solution of 5, 6, and 7 dissolved in
12. Spread the granulation on trays and dry in a forced-
air oven at 50 to 55°C until the alcohol odor is gone.
Pass through a 12-mesh screen. Place granulation in a
tumble blender and blend in 8, 11, and 9. Compress
1-in.-diameter, flat-faced, beveled edge tablets each
weighing 3.41 g. Package in aluminum foil.

Example 4:   Flavored Beverage Effervescent Tablets

Ingredient	Quantity
1. Sodium bicarbonate (granular)	735 g
2. Sodium carbonate, anhydrous	80 g
3. Citric acid, anhydrous (granular)	1300 g
4. Aminoacetic acid	50 g
5. Flavor (spray-dried)	50 g
6. Color	5 g
7. Light mineral oil	15 g
8. Water	4 g

Premix 7 with 200 g of 1. Disperse 6 on 35 g of 1.
Place 3 in the bowl of a planetary mixer. Start mixer
and slowly add 8; mix thoroughly. Add to mixer in sequence, while mixing, the remainder of 1, 2, 4, 5, the
color dispersion, and the mineral oil dispersion; mix until
uniform. Compress 3/4-in., flat-faced, beveled edge tablets weighing 2.23 g each. Pass through curing oven;
cool; and package in aluminum foil.

Example 5:   Stannous Fluoride Mouthwash Effervescent
Tablets [80]

Ingredient	Quantity
1. Malic acid	420 g
2. Sodium bicarbonate	290 g
3. Sodium carbonate	70 g
4. Stannous fluoride	21 g
5. Color	3 g
6. Flavor	20 g
7. Sweetener	4 g
8. Sorbitol	110 g
9. Polyethylene glycol 8000 (powder)	30 g
10. Sodium benzoate (fine powder)	30 g
11. Simethicone	2 g

Coat 10 with 11 using a twin-shell blender with intensifier bar activated. Blend 1, 2, 3, 4, 9, the blend
of 10 and 11, 8, 5, 7, and 6 in a ribbon blender.
Compress 11.1-mm-diameter, shallow concave tablets
each weighing 480 to 500 mg. Package in aluminum
foil.

Example 6:   Children's Decongestant Effervescent
Cold Tablets

Ingredient	Quantity
1. Acetylsalicylic acid, USP (crystals)	81 g
2. Pseudoephedrine hydrochloride	30 g
3. Fruit flavor (spray-dried)	20 g
4. Fruit color	2 g
5. Sodium bicarbonate (granular)	550 g
6. Citric acid, anhydrous (granular)	325 g
7. Citric acid, anhydrous (powder)	325 g
8. Water	

Convert 5 to 7—9% sodium carbonate by placing in a
forced-draft oven at 100°C for 45 min, with two mixings at 15-min intervals. Cool the converted bicarbonate and mix with 6 and 7 in a planetary mixer for 10
min. Quickly add 8 and mix until the water is evenly

Example 6:   (Continued)

distributed and a mild reaction occurs. Immediately
transfer to paper-lined drying trays and spread evenly.
Place trays in a forced-draft oven at 70°C for 2 hr.
Remove from oven, cool, and granulate through a
12-mesh screen. Mix together 2, 3, and 4. Mix the
dried granulation, the 2-3-4 premix and 1 in a tumble
blender until uniform. Compress 5/8-in.-diameter,
flat-faced, beveled edge tablets weighing 1.33 g each.
Stabilize the tablets by heating in a forced-draft oven
at 60°C for 1 hr. Cool and package in aluminum foil.

Example 7:   Denture Cleanser Effervescent Tablets

Ingredient	Quantity
1. Potassium monopersulfate	800 g
2. Citric acid, anhydrous (granular)	575 g
3. Sodium bicarbonate (granular)	800 g
4. Sodium chloride	320 g
5. Sodium perborate monohydrate	320 g
6. Sodium sulfate	225 g
7. Polyvinylpyrrolidone	100 g
8. Isopropyl alcohol	170 g
9. Sodium lauryl sulfate	10 g
10. Color	2 g
11. Oil of peppermint	16 g
12. Magnesium stearate	20 g

Blend 3, 4, 5, 6, and 7 in a planetary mixer. Add
8 and mix until the mass is uniformly wet. Spread
wetted mixture on trays about 1-in. deep. Dry in
forced-draft oven at 70°C for 16 hr. Pass dried
granulation through an 18-mesh screen using an
oscillating granulator. Mix 1 and 2 in a tumble blender. Add 1500 g of the dried, screened granulation
and tumble until well mixed. Distribute 9, 10, and
11 in 265 g of the dried, screened granulation and
add to the tumble blender. Mix thoroughly. Add
12 to the tumble blender and mix well. Compress
1-in.-diameter flat-faced, beveled edge tablets
weighing 3.19 g each. Package in aluminum foil.

Example 8:   Bath Salt Effervescent Tablets

Ingredients	Quantity
1. Monosodium phosphate anhydrous	3200 g
2. Citric acid, anhydrous	630 g
3. Sodium bicarbonate (fine granular)	2500 g
4. Surfactant	17 g
5. Blue color	1 g
6. Simethicone	1 g
7. Encapsulated fragrance	50 g
8. Water	16 g

Thoroughly mix 6 with 100 g of 3 on which 5 has been previously distributed. Add 7 and mix thoroughly; set aside. Place 1 in a ribbon blender. Slowly add 8 while mixing and mix thoroughly. While mixing, slowly add 2, 2400 g of 3, the 3-5-6-7 premix, and 5. Mix well. Compress 1-in.-diameter flat-faced, beveled edge tablets each weighing 6.4 g. Pass through a forced-draft oven to stabilize, cool, and package six tablets to a container. (Six tablets are dissolved in a 25-gallon tub to yield a water softening, lightly colored, and lightly fragranced bath.)

Example 9:   Feminine Hygiene Solution Effervescent Tablets

Ingredient	Quantity
1. Sodium lauryl sulfate	70 g
2. Simethicone	15 g
3. Sodium bicarbonate	345 g
4. Monosodium phosphate, anhydrous (granular)	440 g
5. Citric acid, anhydrous (granular)	655 g
6. Sodium chloride	865 g
7. Water	2 g

Thoroughly blend 2 with 145 g of 3 in a planetary mixer. Place 5 and 6 in a pony mixer; energize the mixer and blend for 1 min. Continue mixing and slowly add 7. Mix for 1 min or until uniform. Continue mixing and add consecutively 4, simethicone premix, 300 g of 3 and 1. Mix for 3 min until

Example 9:   (Continued)

---

thoroughly blended.   Compress 3/4-in.-diameter flat-
faced, beveled edge tablets each weighing 2.39 g.
Place tablets on a paper-lined drying tray and stabilize
in a forced-draft oven at 90°C for 30 min.   Remove
from oven, cool, and package in aluminum foil.   (Each
tablet is dissolved in 1000 ml of 40°C water prior to
use.)

Example 10:   Toilet Bowl Cleaner Effervescent Tablets

Ingredient	Quantity
1. Sodium bisulfate	1200 g
2. Sodium bicarbonate	250 g
3. Detergent	30 g
4. Color	2 g
5. Fragrance oil	10 g

Disperse 4 and 5 on 3, using geometric dilution techniques.   Place 600 g of 1 in a tumble blender.   Add
the color/fragrance premix and blend for 1 min.   Add
20 g of 3 and blend for 1 min.   Add 600 g of 1 and
blend for 2 min.   Roller-compact or slug the granulation to densify.   Granulate the compacted sheets or
slugs by passing through a 12-mesh screen.   Place
granulation in the tumble blender and add 10 g of 3.
Blend thoroughly.   Compress on heavy-duty tablet
equipment or form compacts using briquetting equipment,
each compact weighing 149.2 g.   A suitable tablet size
would be 2-3/4 in. in diameter and about 7/8 in. thick.
Individually wrap each tablet in an aluminum foil pouch.

REFERENCES

1.   *United States Pharmacopeia XXI*, 854, United States Pharmacopeial Con-
     vention, Inc., Rockville, MD (1985).
2.   U.S. Patent 3,590,121 (1971).
3.   Eur. Patent 93784A (1983).
4.   Fr. Patent 2,477,174 (1980).
5.   U.S. Patent 4,552,771 (1985).
6.   U.S. Patent 3,962,417 (1976).
7.   U.S. Patent 4,417,993 (1983).
8.   Br. Patent application 2,095,556 (1982).
9.   Br. Patent 1,328,591 (1970).
10.   U.S. Patent 4,127,645 (1976).
11.   R. Gaedeke, C. Sander, P. Schmidt, and H. Steinitz, *Med. Klin.*
     (Munich), 67:1173–1175 (1972).

12. U.S. Patent 4,289,751 (1981).
13. A. J. Blowers, E. G. Cameron, and E. R. Lawrence, *Br. J. Clin. Pract.*, *35*:188–190 (1981).
14. U.S. Patent 4,147,768 (1976).
15. U.S. Patent 3,980,766 (1976).
16. U.S. Patent 3,961,041 (1976).
17. U.S. Patent 4,153,678 (1979).
18. W. D. Mason and N. Winer, *J. Pharm. Sci.*, *72*:819–821 (1983).
19. G. Ekenved, R. Elofsson, and L. Solvell, *Acta Pharm. Suec.*, *12*:323–332 (1975).
20. L. M. Ross-Lee, M. J. Elms, B. E. Cham, F. Bochner, I. H. Bunce, and M. J. Eadie, *Eur. J. Clin. Pharmacol.*, *23*:545–551 (1982).
21. W. D. Mason and N. Winer, *J. Pharm. Sci.*, *70*:262–265 (1981).
22. D. Orton, R. Treharne Jones, T. Kaspi, and R. Richardson, *Br. J. Clin. Pharmacol.*, *7*:410–412 (1979).
23. M. Zdrakovic, G. T. Pedersen, N. A. Klitgaard, and E. Rasmussen, *Arch. Pharm. Chemi, Sci. Ed.*, *9*:25–33 (1981).
24. V. Sanno, J. Tuomisto, and M. Airaksinen, *Acta. Pharm. Fenn.*, *92*:77–83 (1983).
25. Z. El-Din, A. T. Nouth, A. H. El-Gawad, and M. El-Shaboury, *Biopharm. Pharmacokinet. Eur. Congr.*, *2nd, 1*:395–399 (1984).
26. U.S. Patent 3,131,123 (1964).
27. K. Nishimura, K. Sasahara, M. Arai, T. Nitanai, I. Yoshihiko, T. Morioka, and E. Nakajima, *J. Pharm. Sci.*, *73*:942–946 (1984).
28. F. L. Lanza, V. Smith, J. A. Page-Castell, and D. O. Castell, *So. Med. J.*, *79*:327–330 (1986).
29. U.S. Patent 4,180,467 (1979).
30. A. J. Repta and T. Higuchi, *J. Pharm. Sci.*, *58*:1110–1113 (1969).
31. Eur. Patent 11,489 (1978).
32. Technical Bulletin, Edward Mendell Co., Carmel, N.Y.
33. Belg. Patent 880,749 (1978).
34. Fr. Patent 2,547,501 (1983).
35. U.S. Patent 4,237,147 (1980).
36. U.S. Patent 2,931,776 (1960).
37. U.S. Patent 3,936,385 (1976).
38. U.S. Patent 4,592,855 (1986).
39. W. A. Strickland, Jr., E. Nelson, L. Busse, and T. Higuchi, *J. Am. Pharm. Assoc. Sci. Ed.*, *45*:51–55 (1956).
40. W. A. Strickland Jr., T. Higuchi, and L. Busse, *J. Am. Pharm. Assoc. Sci. Ed.*, *49*:35–40 (1960).
41. U.S. Patent 3,821,117 (1974).
42. Br. Patent 1,255,437 (1969).
43. U.S. Patent 3,136,692 (1961).
44. Br. Patent 1,221,038 (1971).
45. U.S. Patent 4,536,389 (1985).
46. Br. Patent 1,178,294 (1967).
47. U.S. Patent 3,976,601 (1976).
48. F. E. J. Sendall, J. N. Staniforth, J. E. Rees, and M. J. Leatham, *Pharm. J.*, *230*:289–294 (1983).
49. U.S. Patent 4,007,052 (1976).
50. J. P. Armandou and A. G. Mattha, *Pharm. Acta. Helv.*, *57*:287–289 (1982).
51. Braz. Patent 8,150 (1982).

52. R. W. Murray, *J. Pharm. Sci.*, 57:1776–1779 (1968).

53. J. Joachim, J. Corboda, G. Joachim, and H. Delonca, *J. Pharm. Belg.*, *38*:251–257 (1983).

54. S. I. Saleh, A. Aboutaleb, C. Boymond, and A. Stamm, *Expo.-Congr. Int. Technol. Pharm.*, *3rd*, 2:38–48 (1983).

55. U.S. Patent 4,614,648 (1986).

56. Belg. Patent 781,358 (1971).

57. A. Devay, J. Uderazky, and I. Racz, *Acta. Pharm. Technol.*, 30: 239–242 (1981).

58. H. M. El-Banna and S. N. Savtin, *Sci. Pharm.*, 48:369–377 (1980).

59. U.S. Patent 4,256,599 (1981).

60. U.S. Patent 4,004,036 (1977).

61. Br. Patent, 1,374,105 (1970).

62. U.S. Patent 3,105,792 (1963).

63. Eur. Patent 76,340A (1983).

64. Eur. Patent 76,340B (1984).

65. Br. Patent, 2,148,117 (1985).

66. Br. Patent, 1,270,781 (1969).

67. U.S. Patent 4,579,742 (1986).

68. Technical Bulletin, Durkee Industrial Foods, Cleveland, OH.

69. U.S. Patent 2,984,543 (1961).

70. U.S. Patent 3,875,073 (1975).

71. U.S. Patent 4,127,645 (1978).

72. W. Horowitz, (ed.), *Official Methods of Analysis of the Association of Official Agricultural Chemists*, *9th ed.*, 1960, pp. 97–98, Association of Official Agricultural Chemists, Washington, D.C.

73. N. R. Anderson, G. S. Banker, and G. E. Peck, *J. Pharm. Sci.*, *71*:3–6 (1982).

74. N. R. Anderson, G. S. Banker, and G. E. Peck, *J. Pharm. Sci.*, *71*:7–13 (1982).

75. U.S. Design Patent 274,846 (1984).

76. U.S. Design Patent 275,614 (1984).

77. U.S. Design Patent 275,615 (1984).

78. U.S. Patent 4,663,964 (1987).

79. U.S. Patent 3,903,255 (1975).

80. U.S. Patent 4,267,164 (1981).

7
Special Tablets

James W. Conine* and Michael J. Pikal

Eli Lilly and Company, Indianapolis, Indiana

Most tablets are intended to be swallowed, the active ingredients being absorbed from the gastrointestinal tract. There are some special types of tablets, however, which are intended for administration in other ways. Most of
the tablets discussed in this chapter are intended for adsorption through the
mucosal lining of the mouth, either sublingually (i.e., from the area beneath
the tongue) or buccally (i.e., from the area between the cheek and gum) [1].
In addition, molded tablets for other applications and other modes of administration will be briefly discussed.

I. DRUG ABSORPTION THROUGH THE ORAL MUCOSA

A. Effect of the Site on Absorption

Drugs can be absorbed into the bloodstream from many of the surfaces of
the body (e.g., gastrointestinal, nasal, rectal, dermal) to which the drug
can be applied and held in position for a sufficient time for absorption to
take place. A compound should be formulated so that it can be properly
administered for the particular surface through which it will be absorbed.
The use of swallowed medication is by far the most common means of intro-
ducing drugs into the general circulatory system. When absorbed from
the stomach or intestinal tract, the drug passes through the membrane
lining into the capillaries to the superior mesenteric vein, then through
the portal vein and liver into the inferior vena cava, before reaching the
heart and arterial circulation which distributes the drug throughout the
body. This route selectively channels compounds through the liver, which
is the body's major organ of detoxication. Metabolism by the liver can
greatly reduce the amount of active compound ultimately reaching the target organs.

---

*Currently retired.

Absorption of drugs through the highly vascular mucosal lining of the
mouth moves the drug through the sublingual or buccal capillaries and
veins to the jugular vein and superior vena cava—directly into the heart
and arteria circulation without first passing through the liver. This
route can be effective when drugs absorbed through the gastrointestinal
tract are destroyed by extensive hepatic detoxication. For example, 'n
rats naltrexone and naloxone were found to have less than 1% bioavailability from oral dosage as a result of extensive first-pass metabolism,
while buccal availability was 63 and 71%, respectively [2]. The sublingual
and buccal areas offer convenient sites to deposit and hold a tablet on an
absorbing surface over a time sufficient for absorption to take place.

Some recent work has been directed toward the determination of the
degree of enzymatic hydrolysis of peptides that occurs at different mucosal
sites. In a study in rabbits using enkephalins as models, peptide hydrolysis was found to be twice as great in nasal compared to buccal mucosa,
and in both of these areas it was much less than that found in ileal mucosa
[3]. Inhibition of aminopeptidase activity has been shown to occur in the
presence of the penetration enhancers sodium desoxycholate, sodium glycolate, and polyoxyethylene-9-lauryl ether [4].

B. Effect of the Drug on Absorption

The practice of chewing leaves or other parts of plants so that alkaloids
or other compounds are absorbed through the lining of the mouth to produce central or systemic effects is common in several cultures. In Malays-
ia and the South Pacific the areca or betel nut is chewed in combination
with shell lime and the leaves of Piper betel. The natives of Peru have
a history of chewing coca leaves with or without lime, which predates the
Spanish conquest. In our own society there is an appreciable market for
smokeless tobacco products. Also the use of nicotine chewing gum and
other buccally absorbed nicotine products have been used to help break
the tobacco-smoking habit.

Absorption of drugs through the mucous membrane lining of the mouth
has been described as the passive diffusion of the un-ionized form of the
drug from the aqueous phase (in the saliva) to the lipid phase (in the
membrane) [5]. The work of Walton and Lacy [6] and of Walton [7,9]
established that there is a direct relationship between the oil/water partition coefficient and drug absorption. Absorption of the drug is more
or less independent of the absolute solubility of the drug in either the
aqueous or lipid phase.

Table 1 shows the inverse relationship between the oil/water partition
coefficient and the ratio of sublingual to subcutaneous dose for some of
the drugs studied by Walton. A comparison of the sublingual and subcutaneous dose is used since this is a measure of the ability of the drug
to penetrate the membrane lining of the mouth. Satisfactory absorption
of compounds over a wide oil/water partition coefficient range of 40 to
2000 has been observed. Compounds with coefficients in the 20 to 30
range are borderline for effective administration by the sublingual route.
For compounds with oil/water partition coefficients of less than 20, the
effective sublingual doses are several times the subcutaneous doses.

Buccal administration of morphine sulfate has been reported to provide
a similar degree of postoperative analgesia to an equal dose administered
intramuscularly [10]. Peak plasma levels were somewhat lower following

Table 1 Comparison of Oil/Water Partition Coefficient
Compared to Sublingual/Subcutaneous Dosage Ratio [9]

Drug	Oil/water partition coefficient	Sublingual/subcutaneous ratio
Cocaine	28	2
Apomorphine	20	2
Heroin	17	3
Strychnine	21	4
Thebaine	12	>4
Emetine	9	>6
Atropine	7	8
Morphine	0.15	10
Hydromorphine hydrochloride	0.2	15
Codeine	2.0	15

buccal dosage, but total bioavailability was 40 to 50% greater. Nitroglycerin has a very high partition coefficient of 1820 [9] and is extremely effective when administered sublingually. However, as the oil/water partition coefficient increases beyond 2000, the solubility in the saliva is usually not enough to supply an adequate concentration for transfer through the mucous membrane. Since nitroglycerin is a liquid, absorption of the undissolved compound directly into the membrane possibly explains its very rapid absorption and pharmacological response.

A number of studies by Beckett and coworkers [5,11,12] demonstrated that the relationship of pK_a to absorption from the lining of the mouth is similar to the results observed in the gastrointestinal tract [13]. It has been found that, by buffering a solution of the drug which is held in the mouth, absorption depends on partitioning the un-ionized form into the lipid phase. Basic drugs which are administered as salts become better absorbed as the pH is raised, thereby converting more of the salt into the base. For example, buccal absorption of amphetamine does not occur below pH 6.6, but over 60% absorption occurs at pH 9.0 [11]. The saliva ordinarily maintains the pH of the mouth between 5.6 and 7.6. The use of buffered solutions or tablets makes it possible to control the pH somewhat outside this range in order to enhance the absorption of some drugs. When two compounds have the same pK_a, the compound with the greater oil/water solubility ratio will be better absorbed (Fig. 1). In this series of n-alkanoic acids (from 4 to 12 carbons), all with pK_a from 4.82 to 4.85 at 25°C, the absorption increases as the chain length and oil/water solubility ratio increase. Compounds which contain no ionizable groups are less affected by pH changes, although buccal absorption of nitroglycerin is greater below pH 5.0 [14].

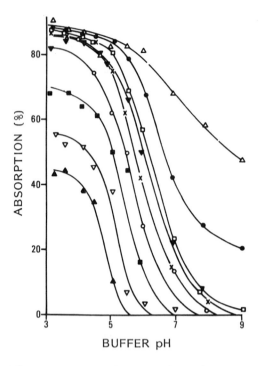

Figure 1 Buccal absorption of n-alkanoic acid in humans. Key: ▲ butyric; ▽ Valeric; ■ hexanoic; ○ heptanoic; × octanoic; ▼ nonanoic; □ decanoic; ● undecanoic; △ dodecanoic. [From Ho, N. F. H., and Higuchi, W. I., *J. Pharm. Sci.*, 60:537 (1971). Reproduced with permission of the copyright owner.]

There is good evidence that peptides are absorbed buccally. The thyrotropin-releasing hormone protirelin when administed through buccal absorption from a paper disk produced increases in the thyrotropin and prolactin levels of human subjects [15]. However, buccal doses were 100 times the intravenous doses used in the study [15].

Theoretical physical models have been proposed to accurately describe the mechanism of absorption from the lining of the mouth [16,17]. The model for the n-alkanoic acids whose absorption is described in Figure 1 consists of a three-compartment system where the first and third are aqueous compartments separated by the second, which is a lipid layer. The first compartment or mucosal side is the bulk aqueous drug solution, and the third or sclerosal side is an aqueous layer at pH 7.4, which is the pH of the blood. There is assumed to be a perfect sink after the third compartment. The pH of the first compartment is either the natural pH or one adjusted by buffers.

C. Currently Marketed Buccal and Sublingual Drugs

In addition to good absorption, the ideal drug for sublingual or buccal use should be small in dose, usually not more than 10 to 15 mg. The drug

Table 2 Drugs Marketed as Sublingual or Buccal Tablets

Tablet	Dose	Equivalent oral dose
Sublingual		
Ergoloid mesylates	0.5–1 mg	—
Ergotamine tartrate	2 mg	0.6–1 mg
Erythrityl tetranitrate	5–10 mg	30 mg
Isoproterenol hydrochloride	10–15 mg	—
Isosorbide dinitrate	2.5–5 mg	10–20 mg
Nitroglycerin	0.15–0.6 mg	2.5–6 mg (propylactic)
Buccal		
Methyltestosterone	5–20 mg	10–40 mg
Nitroglycerin	1–3 mg	2.5–6 mg (propylactic)

should not be highly ionic or at least should be capable of being buffered in tablet form if it is to result in satisfactory absorption. The ideal compound should not have an undesirable taste, since bitter or bad-tasting compounds will stimulate saliva flow. The major drugs which are currently marketed as sublingual or buccal tablets are listed in Table 2. These consist of nitrate esters, isoproterenol hydrochloride, and hormones. They represent a select group of compounds for which this is currently the most effective means of administration. Nitroglycerin, which is the most widely used sublingual drug, has placed in the top 100 of most prescribed drugs for the past several years [18]. The sublingual response to nitroglycerine is more rapid than that from the gastrointestinal tract and more effective, since it avoids the destructive first passage through the liver [19].

A number of other products besides those listed in Table 2 have at one time or another been commercially available either as sublingual or buccal tablets. Estradiol and progesterone, which were once administered buccally have been replaced by orally active agents having the same activity. Because there is some inconvenience in the administration of sublingual and buccal tablets, particularly in the latter, products designed for absorption through the mucosal lining of the mouth are usually those for which this is the only satisfactory nonparenteral method of administration. After the sublingual or buccal tablet has been placed in position, the patient should avoid eating, drinking, chewing, smoking, and possibly talking, in order to keep the tablet in place. Swallowing of saliva should also be avoided, since the saliva may contain dissolved drug, and ingestion through the gastrointestinal tract is usually much less efficient than absorption through the oral mucosa.

II. MOLDED SUBLINGUAL TABLETS

The molded tablet was originally introduced by Fuller in 1878 [20]. Only a year earlier Brunton [21] described the first use of sublingual drug therapy when he utilized nitroglycerin in the treatment of angina pectoris. Sublingual tablets are intended to be placed beneath the tongue and held there until absorption has taken place. They must dissolve or disintegrate quickly, allowing the medicament to be rapidly absorbed. Therefore, sublingual tablets are frequently formulated as molded tablets.

Molded tablets may also be used for buccal absorption, may be swallowed, may be used to prepare solutions for topical application, or (as in the past) may be used for injection. Molded tablets are also referred to as tablet triturates; the designation comes from the early practice of preparing tablets from triturations. Official triturations were 10% dilutions of finely divided potent drugs in lactose. A dilution of this type made it easier to handle the drug and divide it more accurately into single doses. The trituration could be further diluted with lactose to make the correct tablet weight.

Molded tablets designed to be dissolved in a small amount of water to make an aqueous solution which can be administered parenterally are known as hypodermic tablets. Current standards of sterility cannot be met by by the usual method of handling hypodermic tablets in multiple-dose containers. The removal of one tablet would—under most conditions—expose the remaining tablets to possible contamination. Technical advances which have increased the availability of sterile parenteral products have eliminated the need which once existed for the hypodermic tablet [22]. The formulations for hypodermic tablets are similar to those which will be described for tablets triturates.

A. Formulations for Molded Tablets

Molded tablets are usually prepared from soluble ingredients so that the tablets are completely and rapidly soluble. They contain, in addition to the drug, an excipient or base of lactose, dextrose, sucrose, mannitol, or other rapidly soluble materials or mixtures of these ingredients. Commercial lactose is the monohydrate or α form and is the most common excipient. β-Lactose, which is an anhydrous form produced by crystallization above 93.5°C, has been also used as an excipient and is reported to be more readily soluble than α-lactose. Tablets containing insoluble excipients may be prepared from finely divided kaolin, calcium carbonate, calcium phosphate, or other insoluble powders; but such tablets are not often encountered today. To insure rapid solubility of the soluble tablets, the excipients are usually put through a fine screen or 120-mesh bolting cloth.

After the excipient is blended with the drug, the powder mix is moistened with the solvent, which is most commonly aqueous alcohol. Other volatile solvents such as acetone or hydrocarbons might also be used. Antioxidants, such as sodium bisulfite, and buffers or other ingredients may be added to improve the physical and chemical stability of the product.

A variety of materials have been tested in nitroglycerine tablets to stabilize them against decreases in the content uniformity of the tablets which occur during aging. Problems unique to nitroglycerin tablets will be discussed in Section III of this chapter. To increase the hardness and reduce the erosion on the edges of the tablets during handling, agents such as glucose, sucrose, acacia, or povidone have been added to the solvent mixture. This should be done with care, since, if used in excessive amounts, such agents can decrease the rate of solubility of the tablets.

Formulations for molded tablets are usually very simple and contain no insoluble ingredients. Placebo tablets can be prepared which contain only lactose. Typical formulas for several molded tablets are listed here.

Example 1: Codeine Phosphate Tablets (30 mg)

Ingredient	Quantity per tablet
Codeine phosphate powder	30.0 mg
Lactose (bolted)	17.5 mg
Sucrose (powder)	1.5 mg
Alcohol-water (60:40)	q.s.

Screen and blend the powders; add alcohol-water (60:40) to moisten and mold tablets.

Example 2: Scopolamine Hydrobromide Tablets (0.4 mg)

Ingredient	Quantity per tablet
Scopolamine hydrobromide	0.4 mg
Lactose (bolted)	35.0 mg
Sucrose (as 85% syrup)	0.3 mg
Alcohol-water (60:40)	q.s.

Screen and blend the powders: moisten the blend with alcohol-water (60:40) to which the surcrose syrup has been added, and mold the tablets.

Example 3: Nitroglycerine Tablets (0.4 mg)

Ingredient	Quantity per tablet
Trituration of nitroglycerin (10% on lactose)	4.4 mg
Lacotose (bolted)	32.25 mg
Polyethylene glycol 4000	0.35 mg
Alcohol-water (60:40)	q.s.

Screen and blend the powders; moisten the blend with alcohol-water (60:40) to which the polyethylene glycol 4000 has been added, and mold the tablets.

B. Hand Molding of Tablets

The method and equipment used for hand molding tablets have changed little since they were originally described by Fuller [20]. The powder mixture must be blended carefully to insure that a homogeneous mixture is obtained. On a very small scale, this is usually done in a mortar. The solvent mixture is added to make a workable mass without overwetting the powder. The mold plate is placed on a smooth tile or glass plate, and the mass is forced into the tablet mold with sufficient pressure, uniformly applied, to insure that all tablets have the same weight (Fig. 2). This can be done with either an ordinary spatula or a special spatula resembling a short-bladed putty knife. The mold plates contain anywhere from 50 to several hundred die holes and are made of metal, hard rubber, or plastic. To remove the tablets for drying, the mold plate is placed on top of a plate which has projecting pegs that coincide with the die holes (Fig. 3). By pressing the mold plate down onto the pegs, the tablets are forced out of the dies onto the tops of the pegs. The tablets are then removed from the pegs to drying. There are usually two longer guide pins (one at each

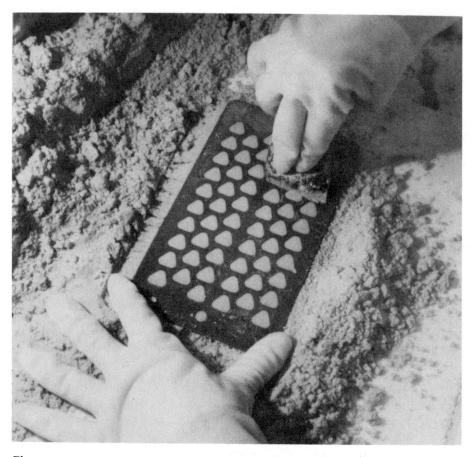

Figure 2   Hand molding of dispensing tablets.

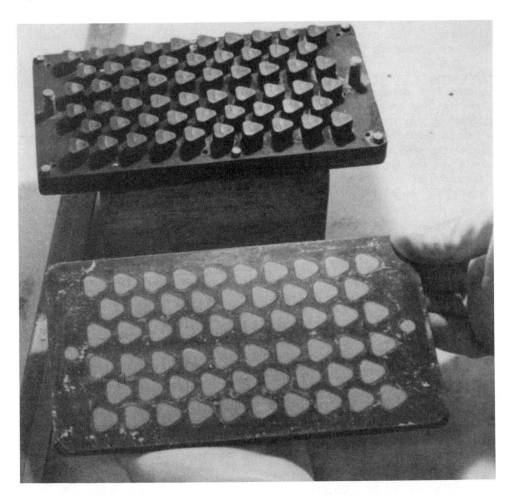

Figure 3   Molded dispensing tablets ready for removal from mold plate.

end of the peg plate) which coincide with the holes in the mold plate so
that the pegs can be precisely guided, and no damage to the soft tablets
results. The ends of the plates differ in shape so that they can be put
together correctly in only one way. This feature gives the process better
reproducibility and the tablets greater uniformity. Since the weight uniformity normally increases with tablet density, the molds should be packed
fairly tightly to minimize the weight variation. However, the uniformity of
weight normally attained with compressed tablets cannot be achieved with
molded tablets.

Some molding problems can be related directly to the solvent. Application of too little solvent may result in a soft tablet. On the other hand, too
much solvent will result in tablet shrinkage upon drying. In addition to
the irregular shape due to shrinkage, the tablets may become case-hardened
and less readily soluble. Similiar problems result if aqueous alcohol of incorrect solvent proportions is used. The most satisfactory range for lactose-
based tablets is 50 to 60% alcohol. When the water content is low, the

resulting tablets are poorly bonded and will tend to powder and wear on
the edges. With high water content, the tablets will become harder and
less readily soluble.

The tablets are removed from the pegs and allowed to dry in ambient
air currents, or the drying may be accelerated by placing the tablets in
a forced-air oven. As the tablets dry, the solvent migrates to the surface
and may carry the active ingredient or other soluble components to the
tablet surface [23,24]. This can produce a nonhomogeneous distribution
of drug throughout the tablet. Solvent-mediated migration of the drug may
affect the stability, particularly if the active component is photosensitive
or is subject to oxidation [23]. Although drug migration has been reported
in studies of granulation drying [25,26] and can be readily demonstrated
in the migration of soluble dyes during drying, drug migration in molded
tablets has received little attention. A change to a different solvent or
mixture can minimize migration and thereby result in an improved tablet.
Also, a change to an excipient which has greater attraction for the drug
in the solvent system will also reduce the amount of migration which occurs
during tablet drying. Care should be exercised to avoid choosing an excipient which will bind the drug so tightly that it is not easily removed
from the excipient in vivo.

When formulating tablets, a placebo can be made in order to determine
the expected tablet weight. If the dose is quite small (for example, less
than 1 mg) a direct substitution of drug for excipient can be made. If a
larger portion of the tablet consists of the drug itself, the density of the
drug as well as that of the excipient needs to be considered in determining
the finished tablet weight.

C. Machine Molding of Tablets

Equipment is available for the large-scale production of molded tablets.
The blending of the dry mix may be carried out in any of the pharmaceutical mixers capable of producing a homogeneous mixture of dry powders.
Depending on the lot size, the entire lot or only a portion of the dry mix
may be moistened for molding at one time. A Colton production-size molding
machine is shown in Figure 4. The dampened mass is placed in a hopper
(A) which is equipped with a revolving blade, and the mass is allowed to
drop into one of four circular sections in the rotating circular feed plate
(B). The feed plate is set above the mold or die plate (C), but they are
on different centers so that only about 30% of the mold plate is covered by
the feed plate. The mold plate contains four sets of die holes. In the
first step of the molding operation, the mass which was dropped into the
feed plate is moved over one set of dies into which the foot of the packing
spinner (D) uniformly forces the tablet mass. The packing spinner has a
spring which can be adjusted to regulate the force (and correspondingly
the amount of tablet mass filled into the die) and thus to control the tablet
weight. The mold plate moves to the second position, in which the top
surfaces of the tablets are smoothed off by the foot of the smoothing spinner (E). Any excess powder is removed from the die plate by a rake-off
(F) in the third position. At the fourth and final position, the tablets
are ejected onto a conveyer belt (G) by a nest of carefully fitted punches
(H) which match the dies. The tablets are air dried at room temperature
as they move along the belt to drop onto a drying tray. Depending on

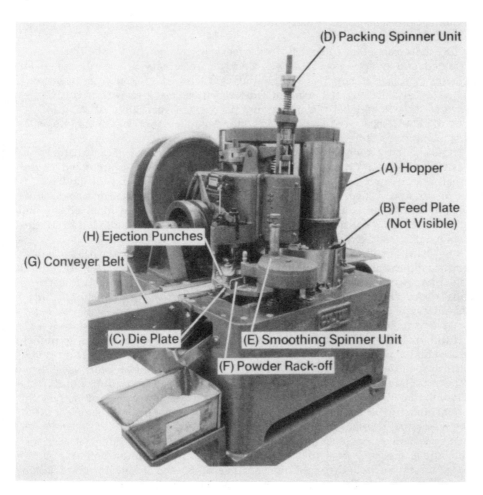

Figure 4   Colton machine for preparing molded tablets.

the tablet size and the number of dies in a set, the production rate varies from 100,000 to 150,000 tablets per hour. The belt drying can be accelerated by electrical heating units, warm air currents, or infrared heat lamps which are directed onto the conveyer belt.

At the end of the conveyer belt, the tablets are dropped onto a drying tray where they will undergo completion of the drying process. They are sampled at this time to check the tablet weight. Weighing of the damp tablets at this point gives an estimate of what the dry weight will be and can be used to determine what packing spinner adjustments need to be made to achieve the correct tablet weight.

The remaining solvent in the tablets can be removed by air drying on trays in a rack or in a circulating-air oven at 100 to 120°F for up to 1 hr. Microwave drying of 1 to 3 min may be used to reduce the exposure time during the drying process. The tablets should be dedusted on a vibrating screen or by passing the screen holding the tablets over an exhaust unit prior to final evaluation and packaging.

D. Evaluation of Molded Tablets

The USP now recognizes separate uniformity of dosage unit specifications
for molded and compressed tablets. Content uniformity standards for molded tablets are met if not less than 9 out of 10 tablets taken from a sample
of 30 as determined by the content uniformity method lies within the range
of 85.0 to 115.0% of label claim, no unit is outside the range of 75.0 to
125.0% of label claim, and the relative standard deviation of 10 tablets is
less than or equal to 6.0%.

If two or three dosage units are outside the range of 85.0 to 115.0%
but not outside the 75.0 to 125.0% range, or if the relative standard deviation is greater than 6.0%, or if both conditions prevail, an additional 20
units are tested. The uniformity requirement is met if not more than three
tablets of the 30 are outside the range of 85.0 to 115.0% of label claim, and
none lies outside 75.0 to 125.0%, and the relative standard deviation of the
30 tablets does not exceed 7.8%.

The disintegration test for sublingual tablets is run in the USP disintegration apparatus without disks, using water at 37 ± 2°C. All six tablets
should disintegrate completely within the time limit specified in the monograph (2 min for nitroglycerin tablets). If one or two of the tablets fail
to disintegrate completely, a repeat test is made on 12 more, and not less
than 16 of the total 18 tablets should disintegrate in the specified time [27].

If the molded tablets are intended to be completely soluble, a solubility
test should be required which includes both rate and completeness of solution in a specified amount of water. Dissolution tests have been established
for many tablets, but they usually are done in large volumes of water.
For sublingual nitroglycerin tablets, where only small volumes of saliva
would ordinarily be encountered in actual use, methods have been established using very small amounts of media [28,29].

One method places the individual tablet on a Millipore filter (0.45 mm)
in the upper chamber of a plastic Millipore Swinnex 25 filter holder. One
ml of water is flushed through the chamber at 30-sec intervals up to 2 min,
and samples at each time interval are collected and assayed [28].

In a second method designed specifically for nitroglycerin, a tablet is
dropped into 5 ml of water purged with nitrogen to remove any oxygen, in
a cell containing a rotating platinum electrode. The system is operated until no further increase in reduction potential is observed. From the data,
the amount of nitroglycerin in solution at any time interval is obtained [29].

Stability studies on each formulation are needed to establish the shelf
life of the product for both physical and chemical evaluation. Specific procedures and methods are in the literature for many drugs. Potency changes
on aging should be monitored, and special attention should be paid to physical changes such as color development, decreased solubility of the tablet,
and changes in disintegration time and dissolution rate. Special tests developed for the evaluation of sublingual nitroglycerin tablets will be discussed in the next section.

III. SPECIAL PROBLEMS WITH MOLDED NITROGLYCERIN TABLETS

A. Mechanisms of Potency Loss

Since nitroglycerin is a liquid with a significant vapor pressure at ambient
temperatures, and since each tablet contains only a small amount of

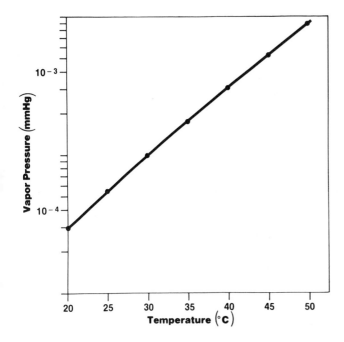

Figure 5 Vapor pressure of pure nitroglycerin as a function of temperature.

nitroglycerin (0.15 to 0.6 mg), the formulation, manufacture, and packaging of nitroglycerin tablets present some special problems. Nitroglycerin tablets potentially can lose potency in four ways: loss to the atmosphere by evaporation, intertablet migration, sorption by packaging materials, and chemical decomposition. The first three mechanisms of potency loss, although perhaps not unique to nitroglycerin, are certainly not common modes of potency loss in pharmaceuticals.

Evaporation

The vapor pressure of pure nitroglycerin (Fig. 5), although it increases sharply with an increase in temperature, is equal to only about $10^{-4} \times$ the vapor pressure of water [30]. Due to the minute levels of nitroglycerin in tablets, even this slight volatility is sufficient to result in significant losses in potency when nitroglycerin tablets are exposed to ambient air currents for a few days. Loss of nitroglycerin from conventional tablets spread in a monolayer and exposed to ambient ($\sim 25°C$) air currents is illustrated in Figure 6. The term *conventional tablets* refers to molded tablets formulated only with nitroglycerin and lactose, and perhaps a small amount of sucrose to serve as a binder.

The "drafty" environment (Fig. 6) is a location near an air vent while the "draft-free" location represents more normal room air circulation. The vertical lines represent the 90% confidence error limits for the mean value of 30 single-tablet assays. The increases in error limits as the tablets age reflect the decrease in content uniformity observed as the tablets lose potency. The data shown in Figure 6 are qualitatively similar to corresponding data reported by other workers [29,31], although exact agreement

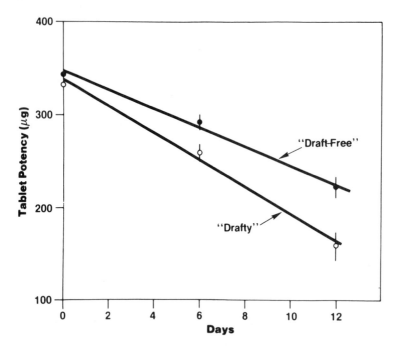

Figure 6   Potency loss of nitroglycerin from conventional tablets exposed
to ambient air currents ($\sim 25°C$).

between different laboratories cannot be expected due to variations in air
currents.   Clearly, the unnecessary exposure of tablets to air currents
during manufacture or storage should be avoided.   However, with reasonable care in the manufacturing process, the drying step is the only phase
of manufacturing where potency losses via evaporation could be significant.
    During drying, the storage air currents and elevated temperatures
needed to remove water and alcohol from the freshly molded tablets will
also remove a measurable amount of nitroglycerin—the amount volatilized
depending on the drying methodology and the tablet formulation.   Data
typical of potency loss in a forced-air drying oven operated at 40°C are
shown in Figure 7 [32].   The tablets are 0.4-mg stabilized tablets which
contain povidone at a level of 1% of the tablet weight.   The povidone is included to stabilize the content uniformity.   The tablets not only show a
significant loss in potency beyond about 1 hr but, as might be expected,
the potency loss depends on the tablet location within the dryer.   Since
essentially all the alcohol and excess water is removed after about 1 hr of
drying, drying in excess of 1 hr serves only to decrease the mean potency
and to magnify the effect of tablet location on tablet potency.
    Since the rate of nitroglycerin loss for a given tablet will depend on
the temperature, air velocity, and partial pressure of nitroglycerin in the
immediate vicinity of that tablet, these variables should be uniform throughout the drying oven.   The difference between the two curves in Figure 7
is probably due to a lower temperature and a higher pressure of nitroglycerin for the air near the air exhaust port.   Prolonged drying and lack
of uniform drying will result in tablets suffering variable potency loss, resulting in poor content uniformity.

Although, in principle, nitroglycerin will leak from loosely sealed containers, the leak rate would be negligible for any closure likely to be used. For example, Fusari [31] found that 100 tablets stored in a glass bottle *without* a closure lost only about 2% in potency during 1 month of storage at ambient conditions. Thus, heroic efforts to seal the containers are unnecessary. (Nitroglycerin sorption by packaging components is a more serious problem and will be discussed later.)

Intertablet Migration

On aging for several months, conventional nitroglycerin tablets normally develop very poor content uniformity with only minor losses in potency [30, 33]. This phenomenon is illustrated in Figure 8 for a lot consisting of 0.3-mg conventional tablets. For fresh tablets (8 days old), the assays (wt% nitroglycerin in each of 30 tablets) are clustered tightly around the mean value and the content uniformity parameter σ, defined as the relative standard deviation for assay (wt% nitroglycerin) of 30 tablets, in only 3.9%. As the tablets age (at 25°C in closed glass containers), a greater range of assay values is observed until, at 50 days, a significant number of both subpotent and superpotent tablets are found. The content uniformity parameter σ is 13.3%, significantly higher than found for the fresh tablets.

Most of the loss in content uniformity occurs during the first 2 months after manufacture (Fig. 9). The data shown represent mean values for 2 lots (153 days), 3 lots (88 days), and between 7 and 11 lots for all other points. Although all single lots show qualitatively the same behavior as

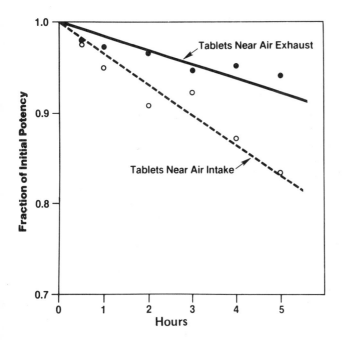

Figure 7   Potency loss of tablets (0.4-mg nitroglycerin) in a forced-air drying oven at 40°C. Tablets contain 0.36 mg povidone added to stabilize content uniformity.

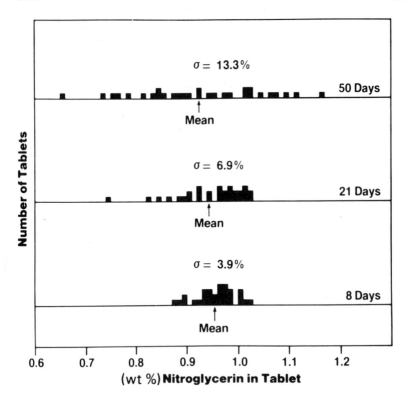

Figure 8   Loss of content uniformity on aging: 0.3-mg conventional tablets.

shown in Figure 9, significant quantitative differences do exist (i.e., some
lots develop poorer content uniformity than others).   While the data shown
in Figure 9 refer only to conventional tablets manufactured by Eli Lilly
(prior to December 1972), conventional tablets manufactured by Parke-Davis
exhibit qualitatively the same behavior [33].

The observation that some tablets increase in potency while others decrease is a most unusual observation that is attributed to the phenomenon
of capillary condensation [30].   Any liquid that is condensed in a capillary
tube will have a lower vapor pressure and, therefore, lower free energy G
than the same liquid in the bulk state.   This reduction in vapor pressure
becomes more pronounced the smaller the diameter of the capillary, and it
is significant only for very small capillaries.   Nitroglycerin tablets contain
a significant number of cracks and pores which behave as small capillary
tubes; due to nonuniformity in the molding process, the volume of such
small pores exhibits significant variation within a group of nominally equivalent tablets.   Thus, freshly prepared tablets exhibit significant and variable
deviations from equilibrium due to a number of empty or partially filled
small pores.   As the tablet system (e.g., 100 tablets in a bottle) ages and
approaches equilibrium, nitroglycerin is transferred from regions of high
free energy (i.e., nitroglycerin coated on the lactose surface) to the empty
or partially filled small pores, which are states of lower free energy.   This

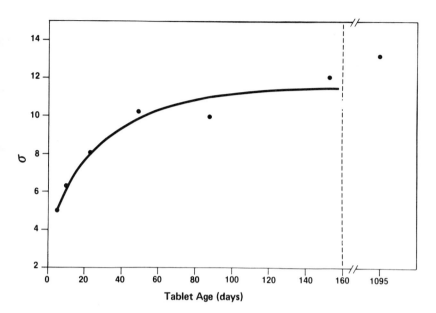

Figure 9   The content uniformity parameter σ as a function of tablet age: Conventional tablets (0.3-mg nitroglycerin).

transfer is shown schematically in Figure 10.   Here, the relative vapor pressure P/P', where P is the vapor pressure of nitroglycerin in a given state and P' is the vapor pressure of bulk nitroglycerin (where surface effects are negligible), is lowered from about 1.0 to 0.9 by the transfer process.   Thus ΔG, the free energy change for this process is negative and the change is spontaneous in the thermodynamic sense.

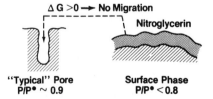

Figure 10   Mechanism for the migration effect (illustrated for transfer to empty pores).   Top, conventional tablet.   Bottom, stabilized tablet.

Table 3   Nitroglycerin Absorption by Polymer Films

Polymer type[a]	Crystallinity (X-ray)	Absorption of nitroglycerin (wt%)	
		25°C	37°C
Vinyl (I)	Amorphous	28.9	24.8
Vinyl (II)	Amorphous	25.6	20.8
Vinyl (III)	Amorphous	25.6	20.8
High-density polyethylene (IV)	Highly crystalline	0.030	0.028
Low-density polyethylene (V)	Very weak crystalline	3.0	2.3
Ionomer (IX)	Essentially amorphous	0.81	0.89

[a]The film numbers in parentheses correspond to those in reference [37]. The ionomer is Surlyn 1604 (DuPont).

Since a given tablet is not an isolated system, intertablet as well as intratablet transfer takes place, resulting in intertablet potency variations of the same order of magnitude as the intertablet variations in the volume of small pores. In summary, the migration effect is a direct result of the volatility of nitroglycerin, the presence of small pores, and an intertablet variation in the volume of small pores. The mechanism of stabilization shown in Figure 10 will be discussed in Section III.B.

Sorption by Packaging

Because nitroglycerin is volatile and has a great affinity for many common packaging materials, nitroglycerin tablets may suffer significant potency losses via sorption by the packaging [31,33,34–37]. For example, conventional tablets strip packaged in an aluminum foil and low-density polyethylene laminate lost about 90% of their nitroglycerin to the package [35].

As the data in Table 3 illustrate, plastics vary greatly in their affinity for nitroglycerin. These data were generated [37] by allowing the polymer films (or plastics) to absorb nitroglycerin from a 10% trituration of nitroglycerin and lactose until equilibrium was attained, and thus indicate the solubility of nitroglycerin in the plastic. Vinyls absorb the most nitroglycerin, and high-density polyethylene, due to its high crystallinity, absorbs the least. The ionomer (IX), although less crystalline than the low-density polyethylene film (V), absorbs significantly less nitroglycerin. This effect is believed due to the chemical composition of the ionomer. An ionomer has a chemical composition similar to that of polyethylene except that the ionomer contains structurally bound anions (i.e., carboxyl ions) and their corresponding counterions (i.e., Na^+ ions). One might speculate [37] that the electrostatic field of the ions is sufficient to "salt out" nitroglycerin in much the same way that electrolytes decrease the aqueous solubility of many nonpolar solutes.

While stabilized tablets show less nitroglycerin loss to packaging [29, 37] even stabilized molded tablets show excessive loss of potency in most types of strip packaging [29,37]. An aluminum foil and thermoplastic polymer laminate appears to be necessary for achievement of stability in a unit-dose strip package comparable to the stability in conventional packaging (100 tablets in a screw-capped glass bottle) [37]. The aluminum foil is necessary to eliminate potency loss by diffusion through the package and evaporation to the atmosphere. The thermoplastic polymer is needed to allow the package to be sealed by a heat-sealing process. Obviously, the thermoplastic polymer must not absorb excessive amounts of nitroglycerin. Stabilized nitroglycerin tablets do maintain acceptable potency and content uniformity when strip packaged in an aluminum foil and Surlyn 1604 laminate [37].

Not even the standard commercial package (100 tablets in an amber glass bottle with a screw cap) is free of package absorption problems. The stuffing used to retard tablet breakage absorbs nitroglycerin, and the cap liners cause some loss of nitroglycerin by absorption—and perhaps by diffusion through the liner facing into the bulk of the liner. Cotton stuffing appears to absorb about 5 times as much nitroglycerin as rayon stuffing [33], at least with 0.4-mg conventional tablets. Rayon stuffing absorbs about the equivalent of two 0.4-mg tablets when packaged with 0.4-mg conventional tablets [33]. Tablets packaged with vinyl cap liners offer the least protection against potency loss while Excelloseal is only slightly better. Tin foil, Mylar (polyethylene terephthalate), and Aclar (a fluorohalocarbon) offer the best protection against potency loss [33].

Chemical Decomposition

Although chemical stability is normally not a problem with conventional nitroglycerin tablets, both polyethylene glycol 400 and povidone (molecular weight $\sim 35,000$), which are used to stabilize content uniformity, may accelerate the hydrolysis of nitroglycerin.

Chemical decomposition via hydrolysis is illustrated by the data in Table 4 [37] for nitroglycerin—povidone—lactose systems. Both 1,2-dinitroglycerin and 1,3-dinitroglycerin were present in the aged samples in roughly equal amounts. Dinitroglycerin content is expressed as weight percent of the total nitroglycerin compounds. Within the uncertainty of the data, both the nitroglycerin loss and the dinitroglycerin content were independent of the povidone concentration above a weight ratio of 0.6. Although the thin-layer chromatographic assay [37] is only semiquantitative, the data demonstrate that a significant fraction of the nitroglycerin loss was due to hydrolysis of the trinitroester to dinitroglycerin species.

The high-temperature stability of tablets containing povidone is compared with that of other formulations in Table 5 [37]. Potency loss at high temperature was significantly greater with the povidone-containing formulation. Analysis by thin-layer chromatography showed significant amounts of the 1,2- and 1,3-dinitroglycerin species in the aged povidone formulation but only trace amounts in the other formulations. Although povidone-containing tablets show poor high-temperature stability, the stability at 25°C is satisfactory (approximately 3 to 4% potency loss per year) [37,38].

Polyethylene glycol 400 has also been shown to accelerate potency loss of nitroglycerin from tablets [39] and from solution [40]. However, tablets with satisfactory stability have been formulated with PEG 400 at a

Table 4   Hydrolysis of Nitroglycerin in Nitroglycerin-Polyvinylpyrrolidone Systems

PVP/Nitro weight ratio	Nitro loss (%)[a]		Dinitroglycerin content (%)[b]	
	1.5 yr/25°C	1.5 yr/25°C + 1 mo/50°C	1.5 yr/25°C	1.5 yr/25°C + 1 mo/50°C
0.22	2	11	1	2
0.65	7	22	4	7
1.04	12	22	3	9
1.56	—	—	4	8
2.13	—	—	5	8

Note: Samples were prepared by dry-blending polyvinylpyrrolidone (PVP) and 10% nitroglycerin trituration on β-lactose.

[a]Determined from nitroglycerin assay on initial and aged samples.

[b]Expressed as weight percent of total nitroglycerin compounds (i.e., dinitroglycerin and trinitroglycerin), determined by semiquantitative thin-layer chromatography.

Source: From Pikal, M. J. Bibler, D. A., and Rutherford, B., *J. Pharm. Sci.*, 66:1293 (1977).   Reproduced with permission of the copyright owner.

Table 5   Potency Loss of 0.3-mg Tablets at High Temperature: A Comparison of Formulations

Formulation	Potency loss (%)	
	6 mo/37°C	6 mo/45°C
Conventional tablet (no stabilizer)	9	7
Stabilized tablet (1% polyvinylpyrrolidone)	17	36
Stabilized tablet (polyethylene glycol)[a]	—	8

Note: Tablets stored in screw-cap glass bottles with rayon stuffing, 100 tablets per bottle.

[a]Nitrostat (Parke Davis).

Source: From Pikal, M. J., Bibler, D. A., and Rutherford, B., *J. Pharm. Sci.*, 66:1293 (1977).   Reproduced with permission of the copyright owner.

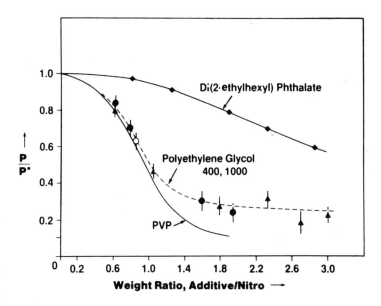

Figure 11   Nitroglycerin vapor pressure reduction at 25°C by selected additives (▲, PEG 1000 powder; ○, PEG 400 tablet; ●, PEG 400 powder). [From Pikal, M. J., Lukes, A. L., and Ellis, L. F., *J. Pharm. Sci.*, *65*: 1278 (1976).]

weight ratio of glycol to nitroglycerin of 0.85 [31]. This apparent anomaly is resolved when stability is examined as a function of the weight ratio of PEG 400 to nitroglycerin. It appears that below a weight ratio of approximately 1, PEG does not significantly affect the stability of nitroglycerin, but at high weight ratios (∿2), PEG 400 causes extensive hydrolysis of nitroglycerin even at 25°C [41].

B.   Stabilization of Content Uniformity

Empirical observations have indicated that the addition of PEG 400 or 4000 at a weight ratio of glycol to nitroglycerin of 0.85 would stabilize the content uniformity. Similar observations have been made for the addition of povidone [38]. These additives are soluble in nitroglycerin [30] at the levels used and decrease the vapor pressure of nitroglycerin (Fig. 11). Polyethylene glycol 4000 data, not shown in Figure 11, are nearly identical to the data shown for the other glycols up to the maximum solubility of PEG 4000 in nitroglycerin (weight ratio of 0.9) [41]. The data for di-(2-ethylhexyl) phthalate are included only for comparison. This material is not used as a tablet additive.

The vapor pressures of nitroglycerin in aged tablets and the corresponding content uniformity parameters are summarized in Table 6 [30]. The first three rows refer to conventional tablets, and the last four rows refer to commercial stabilized tablets (povidone or PEG additive). The relative vapor pressure $P/P^{\cdot}$ is the vapor pressure of nitroglycerin in the tablet P divided by $P^{\cdot}$, the vapor pressure of pure bulk liquid nitroglycerin.

Table 6 Vapor Pressure and Content Uniformity of Aged Nitroglycerin Tablet Formulations

Additive	Potency (mg)	Weight ratio (additive/NG)	Relative vapor pressure $P/P^{\cdot}$ at 25°C	Content uniformity σ (%)	Content uniformity Number of lots
None[a]	0.6	0	0.97	12	(2)
None[a]	0.4	0	1.01	12	(3)
None[a]	0.3	0	0.90	13	(6)
Povidone[a]	0.6	0.59	0.76	5.4	(8)
Povidone[a]	0.4	0.89	0.52	5.7	(13)
Povidone[a]	0.3	1.19	0.31	5.8	(5)
Polyethylene[b] glycol (400 or 4000)	0.6	0.85	0.64	4.3[c]	(12)

Note: Tablet age 6 months to 5 years.

[a]Eli Lilly.

[b]Parke Davis.

[c]Estimated from the published [31] relative standard deviation data calculated from nitroglycerin content per tablet and the weight variation given for one lot.

The number in parentheses after the content uniformity parameter σ is the number of lots used to generate the average content uniformity listed.

The value of σ is approximately 3% at the date of manufacture for both conventional tablets (Fig. 9) and povidone-stabilized tablets [38]. Thus, while conventional tablets show an increase in the content uniformity parameter of about 11% on aging, povidone-stabilized tablets (Table 6) and PEG-stabilized tablets [31] show an increase of only 2 to 3%. Note that, although the stabilized formulations yield reduced nitroglycerin vapor pressures from 24 to 69%, all stabilized formulations are equally effective in preventing the large increase in content uniformity parameter characteristic of conventional tablets.

The role of the additive in content uniformity stabilization is believed to be a reduction of vapor pressure sufficient to make it *thermodynamically* impossible for a significant quantity of nitroglycerin to be transferred from the lactose surface to a small pore. This mechanism is illustrated (bottom of Fig. 10) for transfer to an empty pore. Here the nitroglycerin on the lactose surface is in solution with the additive, giving a relative vapor pressure less than 0.76 (Table 6). Most of the small pores in a tablet are only small enough to lower the vapor pressure of nitroglycerin by about 15% [30]. For purposes of illustration, a typical pore in Figure 10 is assumed to be small enough to lower the vapor pressure by 10% (i.e.,

P/P˙ = 0.9). Thus the transfer of nitroglycerin from a system of lower vapor pressure (P/P˙ ⩽ 0.76) to a region of higher vapor pressure (P/P˙ = 0.9) would result in a positive free-energy change ($\Delta G > 0$), and the process is therefore thermodynamically impossible. Note that the role of the stabilizing additive is *not* to minimize the migration rate by slowing the rate of volatilization. Reduction of the rate of volatilization is not particularly important within the context of the migration effect.

Although absorption by the packaging materials is not normally the major cause of poor content uniformity, it should be noted that reduction of the vapor pressure of nitroglycerin in the tablet will reduce the extent of package absorption and, therefore, will also reduce content uniformity problems arising from package absorption.

C. Testing Procedures

Vapor Pressure

Since all mechanisms of potency loss except chemical decomposition depend directly on the vapor pressure of nitroglycerin in the tablet, any evaluation of a proposed formulation should include vapor pressure measurement or determination of some property strongly correlated with vapor pressure.

The vapor pressure of nitroglycerin in molded tablets may be measured directly by a modification of the gravimetric Knudsen effusion technique [30,42]. Here the sample is placed in a chamber having a small orifice in the top, and the chamber is suspended from one arm of a high-vacuum microbalance. The rate of mass loss through the orifice is determined in a high vacuum (10^{-6} torr). For pure materials the vapor pressure is calculated directly from the proportionality between the rate of mass loss and the vapor pressure. However, for nitroglycerin tablets, vaporization of water present as an impurity may result in an appreciable "background" mass loss, and nonequilibrium effects may be present (i.e., the nitroglycerin vapor may be unable to escape from the sample rapidly enough to maintain the equilibrium vapor pressure in the Knudsen cell). Thus, the rate of nitroglycerin loss is not directly proportional to the vapor pressure. Special procedures and data analysis are needed to extract vapor pressure data from the rates of mass loss [42].

In view of the special equipment and complex data analysis needed for the direct measurement of vapor pressure, convenience may dictate that an alternate property be measured that is strongly correlated with vapor pressure. The *open dish evaporation* test used for this purpose has been described in promotional literature as well as scientific literature [29,31]. Here tablets are placed in a single layer in an open glass dish and are exposed to normal laboratory air currents. Circulating air evaporates some of the nitroglycerin, causing loss of potency, which is monitored by assay for nitroglycerin as a function of time. Results of such a test may be seen in Figure 6. Although the test is simple and, if carefully done, capable of providing evaporation rates which are, as a first approximation, proportional to the initial vapor pressure of nitroglycerin in the tablets [41], great care must be exercised to insure that the air currents are uniform and reproducible or the data obtained are too imprecise to be useful. For example, the data in Figure 6 illustrate qualitatively the difference observed when the air currents differ.

A modified open dish evaporation test [43] is illustrated by the schematic shown in Figure 12. The flow of air over a set of tablets is measured

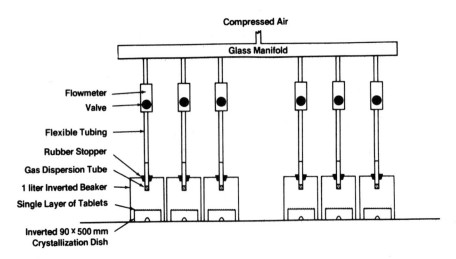

Figure 12   Controlled flow rate evaporation test: schematic diagram.

and controlled by the flow meter valve. Moreover, placing the tablets inside the inverted beaker ensures that only air initially devoid of nitroglycerin is being passed over the tablets. Thus, the modified evaporation test standardizes the evaporation conditions and allows more reproducible data to be obtained. An example of data obtained [43] with this procedure is shown in Figure 13. The tablets were 0.4-mg, stabilized with 0.36 mg of povidone. An increase in flow rate from 2 to 4 ft^3 hr^{-1} clearly increases the evaporation rate. Data obtained at 6 ft^3 hr^{-1} (not shown) were essentially the same as the data for 4 ft^3 hr^{-1}. Evidently, at flow rates greater than approximately 4 ft^3 hr^{-1}, gas phase diffusion of nitroglycerin through the tablet matrix is rate controlling for loss of nitroglycerin.

Isothermal thermogravimetric analysis has also been used as a measure of nitroglycerin volatility [44]. The weight loss of two tablets is followed for 1.5 to 4 hr at 80°C with a nitrogen flow rate of 20 ml min^{-1}. To avoid loss of water of hydration, anhydrous lactose should be used to formulate the tablets. If loss of nitroglycerin via decomposition is ignored, the thermogravimetric experiment at 80°C is probably equivalent to a controlled open dish evaporation test where the rate is accelerated by increased temperature. Thus, it is reasonable to assume that the rate is proportional to the vapor pressure of nitroglycerin (at 80°C), with the proportionality constant being some unknown function of the nitroglycerin diffusion coefficient and the tablet porosity. To the extent that the rate is sensitive to porosity, intertablet variation in porosity could result in variable results since only two tablets are used in a given experiment.

The authors of the foregoing study [44] did not address either decomposition or variations of rate with tablet porosity. If one assumes that these potential problems are minor, thermogravimetric analysis offers a rapid method for a relative measurement of nitroglycerin vapor pressure at elevated temperatures.

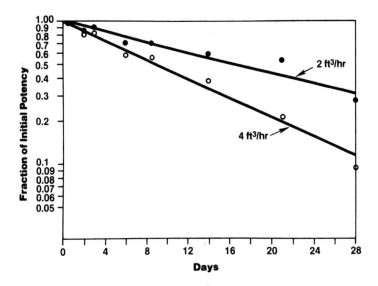

Figure 13   Potency loss of 0.4-mg tablets at selected air flow rates at
25°C. Nitroglycerin tablets containing 0.36 mg povidone added to stabilize
content uniformity.

Package Adsorption

So-called package adsorption may be detected by a solvent extraction of
all packaging material which is in vapor phase contact with the tablets,
followed by an assay for nitroglycerin. Ethanol was found to be a suitable
solvent for most types of strip packaging [37]. Simple rinsing of the packaging is normally not sufficient to remove absorbed nitroglycerin. Extraction times of 1 to 2 days may be necessary [37].

Content Uniformity Stability

The content uniformity should be determined shortly after manufacture by
single-tablet assay [30,33] of large tablet samples (about 30 or more).
The content uniformity parameter σ should be about 5% or less for freshly
manufactured tablets. After the tablets are packaged in the containers
of interest, σ should be determined at monthly intervals for several months.
Normally, if poor content uniformity is going to develop, a significant increase is σ will be obvious after 2 to 3 months of storage of 25°C (Figs. 8
and 9).

Chemical Stability

The chemical stability is best studied by storage of a large number of tablets (more than 100), in glass bottles with no stuffing and with foil cap
liners, so that package absorption is negligible. Thus, any potency loss
can be attributed to chemical decomposition. Thin-layer chromatography
is also useful in that trace levels (about 2%) of dinitroglycerin and

mononitroglycern may be detected—to confirm decomposition via hydrolysis
[36,41]. Since the decomposition rate increases sharply with increasing
temperature (Table 4) [37,41], accelerated stability studies may be used
for a preliminary evaluation of any proposed formulations. Storage at
50°C for 1 to 2 months normally results in decomposition at least as extensive as that of storage at 25°C for 2 years.

The effect of humidity (moisture content) on stability may be studied
by first placing bottles of tablets without caps in a closed chamber of
fixed relative humidity to equilibrate for about 24 hr. Constant humidity
is conveniently maintained by a mixture of a salt and its saturated aqueous
solution. The bottles are then closed, and the stability test is started.

Simulated Patient Use Tests

Tests designed to simulate the conditions generated when a patient repeatedly opens the bottle and removes a tablet have also been used. For
example, a bottle is opened, the rayon stuffing is descarded, and an initial assay is obtained for a small tablet sample (perhaps 3 tablets). The
bottle is then opened daily for a fixed time to simulate a patient's removal
of a tablet. Each week a small tablet sample is taken for assay until approximately 15 tablets remain, at which time the remaining tablets are
assayed to obtain a measure of average potency and content uniformity.
However, since no measurable nitroglycerin will evaporate during this procedure (the entire bottle volume contains less than 0.2 µg nitroglycerin
in the vapor state), this type of test offers no real scientific advantage
over the testing procedures described previously.

IV. COMPRESSED SUBLINGUAL TABLETS

The requirements for sublingual tablets are speed of absorption and a correspondingly rapid physiological response, which are normally best achieved
with a rapidly soluble molded tablet. However, compressed sublingual tablets have also been prepared which disintegrate quickly and allow the active ingredient to dissolve rapidly in the saliva—and to be available for
absorption without requiring the complete solution of all the ingredients of
the formulation. Erythrityl tetranitrate, isosorbide dinitrate, and isoproterenol hydrochloride are marketed as compressed tablets for sublingual
use. Compressed nitroglycerin tablets have been described in the literature [22,24]; formulations for these tablets contain large amounts of cellu-
losic material and may also contain lubricants, glidants, flavors, coloring
agents, and stabilizers.

Compared to molded tablets, compressed tablets of this type normally
have less weight variation and better content uniformity. The USP [27]
requirement for the uniformity of dosage units is met if each of the 10
tablets tested lies within the range of 85.0 to 115.0% of label claim and the
relative standard deviation is less than or equal to 6.0%. If one unit is
outside the 85.0 to 115.0% range and no unit is outside 75.0 to 125.0% of
label claim, an additional 20 tablets are tested, and the requirements are
met if not more than one out of 30 tablets is outside the 85.0 to 115.0%
range but none lies outside of 75.0 to 125.0% of label claim and the relative standard deviation of the 30 dosage units does not exceed 7.8%. The
tablets are also harder and less fragile, thereby avoiding weight and potency loss that occur by the erosion of the molded target edges.

George Green Library - Issue Receipt

Customer name: Siddiqui, Nabil Ahmad

Title: Pharmaceutical dosage forms and drug
delivery systems / Howard C. Ansel, Loyd V.
Allen, Jr., Nichola
ID: 1002224303
Due: 12/05/2011 23:59

Title: Pharmaceutical dosage forms : tablets.
ID: 100041650X
Due: 12/05/2011 23:59

Title: Pharmaceutical dosage forms : tablets.
ID: 6100973666
Due: 12/05/2011 23:59

Total items: 3
17/03/2011 16:43

All items must be returned before the due date
and time.
The Loan period may be shortened if the item is
requested.

WWW.nottingham.ac.uk/is

Example 4: Nitroglycerin Tablets (0.3 mg,
Direct-Compression)

Ingredient	Quantity per tablet
Nitroglycerin (10% of microcrystalline cellulose)	3.0 mg
Mannitol	2.0 mg
Microcrystalline cellulose	29.0 mg
Flavor	q.s.
Sweetener	q.s.
Coloring agent	q.s.

Screen and blend the powders and compress
into tablets.

Compressed nitroglycerin tablets were reported to have a rapid disintegration time of from 3 to 7 sec by the USP method for sublingual tablets
[27], as well as rapid response time as measured by an increase in pulse
rate of 10 to 13 beats/min within 3 min in human volunteers [24]. However, in some clinical patients, these compressed tablets did not appear
to disintegrate or release the medication for absorption. In these subjects,
the compressed tablets either gave no response or gave a delayed response
when compared with molded tablets [45,46].

Example 5: Nitroglycerin Tablets (0.3 mg,
Granulation)

Ingredient	Quantity per tablet
Microcrystalline cellulose	21.00 mg
Anhydrous lactose	5.25 mg
Starch, USP	3.00 mg
Coloring agent	q.s.
Povidone	0.30 mg
Nitroglycerin (as the spirit)	0.30 mg
Calcium stearate	0.15 mg

Blend the excipients and the coloring agent,
and granulate with an ethanol solution of
povidone and nitroglycerin. After the
granulation is dried and milled, it is
blended with the calcium stearate and
compressed.

Perhaps insufficient saliva is present to allow complete removal of nitro-glycerin from the absorbent cellulose. A strong negative psychological effect resulting from the presence of undissolved cellulose in the patient's mouth has also been suggested as the reason for product failure [29,47]. The methods for evaluation of compressed sublingual tablets are the same as those given for molded sublingual tablets.

V. BUCCAL TABLETS

The purpose of buccal tablets is the same as that of sublingual tablets (i.e., absorption of the drug through the lining of the mouth). While the advantage of sublingual medication is rapid response, buccal tablets are most often used when replacement hormonal therapy is the goal. Although *completeness* of absorption is desired, a high *rate* of absorption is not de-sirable. Flat, ellipitcal or capsule-shaped tablets are usually selected for buccal tablets, since they can be most easily held between the gum and cheek. The parotid duct empties into the mouth at a point opposite the crown of the second upper molar, near the spot where buccal tablets are usually placed. This location provides the medium to dissolve the tablet and to provide for release of the medication.

Methyl testosterone and testosterone propionate are the most commonly used buccal tablets. The following formulation is an example of a typical buccal tablet.

Example 6: Methyltestosterone Buccal
Tablets (10 mg)

Ingredient	Quantity per tablet
Methyltestosterone	10 mg
Lactose, USP	86 mg
Sucrose, USP	87 mg
Acacia, USP	10 mg
Talc, USP	6 mg
Magnesium stearate, USP	1 mg
Water	q.s.

Put the drug and excipients through a
60-mesh screen and blend. Moisten with
water to make a stiff mass; pass through
an 8-mesh screen and dry at 40°C. Reduce the particle size by passing the dried
granulation throguh a 10-mesh screen;
blend in lubricants and compress.

Compressed buccal tablets are prepared either by the procedures used for granulation (as described) or by direct compression. In Example 6 the formulation contains no disintegrants, so the tablet will dissolve slowly. Flavoring agents and sweeteners are sometimes added to make the tablets more palatable, but this practice has been criticized since increased flow of saliva may result. It is important to minimize the swallowing of saliva during the time that the buccal tablet is held in place, since compounds administered by the buccal route are either not absorbed from the gastrointestinal tract or are rapidly metabolized on the first pass through the liver. Since buccal tablets are to be held in the mouth for relatively long periods of time (from 30 to 60 min), particular care should be taken to see that all the ingredients are finely divided so that the tablets are not gritty or irritating.

Water-soluble cyclodextrans have been used as adjuvants to enhance the absorption of steroidal hormones from the lining of the mouth. To prepare these materials a 40% aqueous solution of 2-hydroxypropyl or poly-β-cyclodextran was saturated with the steroid, freeze-dried, and compressed into tablets. Testosterone derivatives administered sublingually as either tablets or solutions produced serum levels two to three times greater than that of the drug alone or when it was solubilized with polyethylene glycol 20 sorbitan monooleate [48]. This elevated serum level was seen only when the adsorption took place from the oral cavety but not from the GI tract where the absorbed steroid would be removed on first pass through the liver and by direct metabolism in the intestinal tissues.

A number of formulations designed as long-acting buccal tablets have been published in the patent literature. The basis for these formulations is the use of viscous natural or synthetic gums or mixtures of gums which when present in the formulations, can be compressed to form tablets which absorb moisture slowly to form a hydrated surface layer from which the medicament slowly diffuses and is available for absorption through the buccal mucosa. If the tablet can be maintained in place, absorption can take place for periods up to 8 hr.

Several patents cover the use of hydroxypropylmethylcellulose (HPMC) alone or blended with hydroxypropylcellulose (HPC), ethylcellulose (EC), or sodium carboxymethylcellulose (SCMC) as Synchron carriers [49–52]. Some restrictions are made on the USP type, viscosity, or moisture level of the HPMC. The HPMC may be treated with oxygen or moisture to oxidize or hydrolyze it prior to incorporating it into the formulation or it may be used in the untreated form. Release profiles of the drug from tablets of this type follow a zero-order rate [53].

Tablets have also been prepared using polyacrylic copolymer (Carbapol 934, B. F. Goodrich Chemical Co.) blended with HPC [54] or sodium caseinate [55] for long-acting buccal absorption. Other tablet bases include sodium polyacrylate (PANA) combined with carriers such as lactose, microcrystalline cellulose, and mannitol [56]. Natural gums such as locust bean gum, xanthan, and guar gum have also been utilized [57,58].

Some polymers have mucosal adhesive properties that aid in holding the tablet in position at the adsorption site between the gum and the cheek or lip. PANA and Carbapol 934 have been reported to possess these properties [54,56]. Two-layer tablets have been prepared with an adhesive and a nonadhesive layer [54]. An in vitro method to measure the adhesiveness of various materials to mucus has been developed based

on the force required to detach a glass plate coated with the test substance from isolated mucous gel [59]. Time must be allowed to hydrate
the materials in order to obtain a satisfactory evaluation. Carbapol 934,
SCMC, tragacanth and sodium alginate had good mucosal adhesive properties, whereas povidone and acacia were poor when measured by this method.
Following are examples of long-acting buccal tablets:

Example 7: Nitroglycerin Buccal Tablets
(2 mg) [50]

Ingredient	Quantity per tablets
Nitroglycerin on lactose (1:9)	20 mg
HPMC E50	16 mg
HPMC E4M	10 mg
HPC	2 mg
Stearic acid	0.4 mg
Lactose anhydrous spray-dried	q.s. 70 mg

The cellulose ethers are blended with the lactose and then the nitroglycerin dilution and
lubricant are added and mixed. The tablets
are then compressed from the powder blend.

Example 8: Prochlorperazine Maleate Buccal
Tablets (5 mg) [57]

Ingredient	Quantity per tablet
Prochlorperazine maleate	5.mg
Locust bean gum	1.5 mg
Xanthan gum	1.5 mg
Povidone	3 mg
Sucrose powder	47.5 mg
Magnesium stearate	0.5 mg
Talc	1.0 mg

A blend of prochloperazine maleate, the gums,
and sucrose is granulated with a solution of
povidone in aqueous alcohol. After the granulation is sized and blended with the lubricants,
it is compressed into tablets.

Weight variation, content uniformity, hardness, and friability are determined by the same procedures used for compressed tablets. The disintegration evaluation differs in that the test for buccal tablets is run in
water at 37°C, according to the USP emthod [27] for uncoated tablets
using disks. The requirement is that 16 out of 18 tablets should disintegrate within 4 hr. A long dissolution time is allowed since buccal tablets are normally designed to release the medication slowly. The usual
disintegration time for a compressed tablet would be between 30 and 60
min.

VI. VAGINAL TABLETS

Tablets have been designed for vaginal administration in the treatment of
local infections as well as for systemic absorption and absorption into the
vaginal tissue. The vaginal wall consists of highly vascular tissue providing the potential for excellent absorption across the membrane lining.
The venous circulation from this area drains through the hypogastric vein
directly into the inferior vena cava thus bypassing the portal vein and
avoiding the rapid destruction of those drugs which are susceptible to
first-pass metabolism in the liver.

Only those compounds that have specific use in treating the femal re-
productive system are usually administered by the vaginal route, although
many drugs are well absorbed this way and would give effective blood
levels. The absorption of compounds used to treat local vaginal infections
is not necessarily desirable, since this could lower the effective concentration of the drug directly in contact with the infecting organism. Many
types of products have been designed for vaginal administration including
creams, gels, suppositories, powders, solutions, suspensions, and sponges
as well as tablets, which are the subject of this discussion. Estrogens
have been administered to increase the level in the vaginal tissue in the
treatment of atropic vaginitis and further absorption into the system is
not seen as beneficial. Progesterones such as flugestone acetate have
been administered intravaginally on sponges to syncronize estrus in sheep
and other domestic animals [60]. Tablets could also be used but are not
considered the dosage form of choice for this purpose.

Vaginal absorption follows first-order kinetics and has been described
as two parallel pathways, a lipoidal and an aqueous pore pathway. This
is based on a study of absorption of aliphatic acids and alcohols in the
rabbit [61]. The plasma level of propranolol in women after vaginal administration has been shown to be much higher than when the product is
given orally [62]. Cyclodextran formulations of hydrophilic drugs such as
aminoglycosides, β-lactam antibiotics, and peptides are reported to be
more readily absorbed from the nasal cavity, vagina, and rectum than
when the drug is administered alone [63].

Despite the demonstrated effectiveness of systemic absorption through
the vaginal wall, the most frequent use of vaginally administered medication and especially tablets is in the treatment of localized vaginal infections
such as *Candida albicans*, yeast, and *Haemophilus vaginalis*. The most
commonly used drugs in the treatment of these infections are nystatin,
clotrimazole, and sulfonamides. The formula and design of vaginal tablets
should aim for the slow dissolution or erosion of the tablet in the vaginal

Example 9: Triple-Sulfa Vaginal Tablets

Ingredient	Quantity per tablet
Sulfathiazole	166.7 mg
Sulfacetamide	166.7 mg
Sulfabenzamide	166.7 mg
Urea	400 mg
Lactose	400 mg
Guar gum	60 mg
Starch	30 mg
Magnesium stearate	10 mg

The sulfonamides, urea, lactose, and guar gum
are blended together and granulated with water.
After drying, the granulation is sized and
blended with the starch and lubricant and then
compressed.

secretions, as a rate sufficient to provide an effective level of medication
for as long a time as possible. The same approach is also used in the formulation of buccal tablets and troches. The tablet should remain in one
piece during dissolution and not break into fragments. Vaginal tablets
weigh from 1 to 1-1/2 g, are flat with an oval-, pear-, or bullet-shaped
silhouette, and are usually not coated. They can be inserted with the aid
of an applicator that is provided by the manufacturer. The treatment for
these infections usually is one to two tablets once or twice daily for 2
weeks.

Since these tablets are not subject to peristaltic action, a method of
testing tablet disintegration under static conditions has been devised that
should give a more realistic measure of what could be expected in actual
use and also serve as a quality control test [64]. The apparatus is simple
and consists of two pieces of no. 9 mesh screen wire. The tablet is
placed on a screen and covered with the second screen and placed in distilled water at 37°C in the horizontal position. The disintegration time is
defined as the time when the two screens touch. This method has been
used for both effervescent and noneffervescent tablets.

Sustained release-type formulations that were previously described
under buccal tablets also include references to and examples of vaginal
tablets using HPMC or vegetable gums [49,65].

VII. RECTAL TABLETS

Rectal administration of drugs is an old and accepted means of treatment
for both conditions requiring systemic absorption and the alleviation of
local symptoms. The small veins of the lower colon drain through the

inferior mesentaric vein into the portal vein thus exposing any absorbed compound to potential first-pass metabolism. Other veins from this part of the colon flow into the vena cava so that first-pass metabolism is avoided. The proportion of absorbed compound channeled through each of these two pathways has not been determined [66]. The availability of the medication for absorption depends on the release of the drug from the dosage form and its dissolution. The volume and nature of the rectal fluid, its buffer capacity, pH, and surface tension play a large part in this but are subject to wide variation, even within single subjects, resulting in variability of absorption by this route of administration [66]. There is also the possibility of premature expulsion of the dosage form before sufficient absorption takes place.

The suppository has been the customary means of rectal administration of medication. Suppository vehicles are most often cocoa butter or some other fatty material with similar properties that depend on melting at body temperature to release the drug. Water-soluble solid PEG vehicles have been used, but the rate of solution controls the release. PEG bases have been criticized as being irritating [67]. The limitations of theobroma oil and the PEG vehicles, which include the promotion of decomposition of some drugs, and the handling requirements, such as the necessity of refrigeration, have restricted the usage of the suppository dosage form.

The physician, when treating illnesses in which the patient may be temporarily unable to swallow tablets or capsules due to nausea, asthmatic attacks, or other conditions that make swallowing difficult, may instruct the patient as an alternative to administer the tablet or capsule rectally. Although this is usually an emergency measure, some consideration should be given to the design of tablets for rectal administration. In the review article of de Bleay and Polderman [66], the rational for the design of rectal delivery forms including capsules is discussed but fails to consider tablets.

Tablets, which disintegrate rapidly in very small volumes of water to form pastes, can be formulated. Such tablets, which disintegrate under static conditions in an amount of water equal to only a few times the tablet weight, present the drug in a form for absorption equivalent to that from the suppository, unless the presence of a lipid base promotes absorption. Unfortunately, little is known about rectal delivery from tablets and additional studies would be required to demonstrate the extent of bioavailability. Tablets offer some distinct advantages over suppositories [66] in not requiring refrigeration as well as demonstrating better product stability, even at room temperature. Suppositories containing such compounds as aspirin and penicillin G sodium have limited product stability, even under refrigeration. Tablets of these products are quite stable and can be readily formulated.

The oil or PEG suppository bases act as their own lubricants for insertion, but the HPMC film coat on the tablet could also provide some lubricant action, especially in the presence of water, even in small amounts. If this should prove to be inadequate, further lubrication could be supplied by a jelly. The ultimate usefulness and acceptability of rectal tablets awaits further studies.

The following formulation for tablets will disintegrate to form a paste within a few minutes in the presence of four to five times its weight in water under static conditions in a water bath. The addition of high-efficiency disintegrants, such as croscarmellose sodium and crosslinked povidone, will also produce a rapid tablet disintegration.

Example 10:   Rectal tablet Prochlorperazine
(25 mg)

Ingredient	Quantity per tablet
Core Tablet	
Prochlorperazine	25 mg
Lactose	600 mg
Starch	210 mg
Povidone	30 mg
Starch	52 mg
Talc	14 mg
Magnesium stearate	8 mg
Coating (aqueous solution)	
Hydroxypropylmethylcellulose	7%
PEG 6000	1.5%
Propylene glycol	2.5%

The prochlorperazine is blended with the lactose
and starch and the mixture granulated is with
an aqueous solution of povidone. After drying
and sizing, the granulation is blended with the
lubricants and additional starch and then compressed. The tablets can then be film-coated
with the HPMC solution.

VIII.   DISPENSING TABLETS

Tablets which are to be added to water or other solvents to make a solution containing a fixed concentration of the active ingredient are known
as *dispensing tablets*. Most commonly they are used to prepare antiseptic
solutions such as mercuric chloride or cyanide at dilutions of 1/1000. The
tablets are usually large and contain no insoluble materials since they will
be made into a clear solution. Because of their toxic nature, they are
made in disinctive, unusual shapes such as diamond, triangle, or coffin-
shaped. In order to call further attention to their toxicity, they are
marked either with the word *poison* or with skull and crossbones. They
are also packaged in bottles of distinctive shape with knurled or rough
edges, so that anyone picking up the container would be aware that it is
a toxic item.

The following is a formula for a dispensing tablet suitable for preparing 1 pint of 1/1000 mercuric chloride solution.

Example 11: Mercuric Chloride Dispensing
Tablets

Ingredient	Quantity per tablet
Mercury bichloride	475 mg
Potassium alum (powdered)	510 mg
Tartaric acid	65 mg
Soluble dyes	q.s.
Ethanol-water (75:25)	q.s.

The preparation of dispensing tablets is similar
to that described for small hand-molded tablets. The powders are screened, blended,
then moistened with ethanol-water (75:25),
and molded—as described earlier and shown in
Figures 2 and 3.

A tablet can also be made for the preparation of eye drops.

Example 12: Tablet for Ophthalmic Drops of
Neomycin Sulfate [68]

Ingredient	Quantity per tablet
Boric acid	100 mg
Neomycin sulfate	125 mg
Sodium sulfate	275 mg
Phenyl mercuric nitrate	2.5 mg

The powders are finely milled and blended, and
the blend is then compressed into tablets. The
tablet is dissolved into sufficient sterile water to
make 50 ml of solution.

Other types of dispensing tablets which have also been used include
topical local anesthetics, such as cocaine, and antibiotics, such as bacitra-
cin, which are used for topical application or irrigation.

IX. TABLETS FOR MISCELLANEOUS USES

The technology of tablet production offers an economical and efficient
means of manufacturing solid units of accurate weight and composition.
The use of the tablet form has spread far beyond pharmaceutical usage
into almost every aspect of daily life. These tablets cover a wide range

of shapes and sizes from molded tablets through a variety of compressed tablets designed to fill specific needs.

Reagent tablets have been prepared that are relatively stable and provide the ingredients as a single unit to conveniently perform qualitative and quantitative tests away from the laboratory. Tablets have been formulated to be used to enable diabetics to estimate urinary sugar levels and the presence of acetone and other aldehydes or ketones in the urine. The addition of the tablet to a premeasured amount of water yields a standard reagent solution for a single test. Other tablets are available to determine the presence of albumin in the urine and for the detection of occult blood. The tablets contain all the ingredients required for the test and, if necessary, any lubricants or binders that will not interfere with the sensitivity of the test. Although tests utilizing reagent tablets have provided useful information over the years, their use is now being challenged by the convenient and sophisticated paper strip tests and rapid tests utilizing biotechnology.

Tablets fulfill countless other needs (e.g., Halizone for water purification, artificial sweeteners, nutritional ingredients for diet control, cleaners for dentures, general cleaners and disinfectants, fertilizers for house plants, and even Easter egg colors. These represent but a few examples of the extension of tablet utilization into nonpharmaceutical areas.

REFERENCES

1. M. Gibaldi and J. L. Kanig, *J. Oral Ther. Pharmacol.*, 1:440 (1965).
2. M. A. Hussain, B. J. Aungst, A. Kearney, and E. Shefter, *Pharm. Res.*, 3(Suppl), 97S (1986).
3. H. Choi and V. H. L. Lee, *Pharm. Res.*, 3(Suppl), 70S (1986).
4. D. Gallardo and V. H. L. Lee, *Pharm. Res.*, 3(Suppl), 73S (1986).
5. A. H. Beckett, R. N. Boyes, and E. J. Triggs, *J. Pharm. Pharmacol.*, 20:92 (1968).
6. R. P. Walton and C. F. Lacey, *J. Pharmacol. Exp. Ther.*, 54:61 (1935).
7. R. P. Walton, *Proc. Soc. Exp. Biol. Med.*, 32:1486 (1935).
8. R. P. Walton, *Proc. Soc. Exp. Biol. Med.*, 32:1488 (1935).
9. R. P. Walton, *J. Am. Med. Assn.*, 124:138 (1944).
10. M. D. D. Bell et al., *Lancet*, Vol. I, 71 (1985).
11. A. H. Beckett and E. J. Triggs, *J. Pharm. Pharmacol.*, 19(Suppl), 31S (1967).
12. A. H. Beckett and A. C. Moffat, *J. Pharm. Pharmacol.*, 20(Suppl), 239S (1968).
13. L. S. Shanker, *J. Med. Pharm. Chem.*, 2:343 (1960).
14. W. A. Ritschel, *J. Pharm. Sci.*, 60:1683 (1971).
15. R. Anders, H. P. Merkle, W. Schurr, and R. Ziegler, *J. Pharm. Sci.*, 72:1481 (1983).
16. N. F. H. Ho and W. I. Higuchi, *J. Pharm. Sci.*, 60:537 (1971).
17. K. R. M. Vora, W. I. Higuchi, and N. F. H. Ho, *J. Pharm. Sci.*, 61:1785 (1972).
18. *Am. Druggist*, Feb. 1987, p. 19.
19. M. H. Litchfield, *J. Pharm. Sci.*, 60:1599 (1971).
20. R. M. Fuller, *New Remedies*, 7:69 (1878). Republished from *Medical Record*, 13:185 (1878).

21. R. L. Brunton, The Gaulsonian Lectures Delivered before the Royal College of Surgeons, Macmillan, London, 1877.
22. M. D. Richmond, C. D. Fox, and R. F. Shangraw, *J. Pharm. Sci.*, *54*:447 (1965).
23. I. A. Chaudry and R. E. King, *J. Pharm. Sci.*, *61*:1121 (1972).
24. F. W. Goodhart, H. Gucluyildiz, R. E. Daly, L. Chefetz, and F. C. Ninger, *J. Pharm. Sci.*, *65*:1466 (1976).
25. J. W. Warren and J. C. Price, *J. Pharm. Sci.*, *66*:1406 (1977).
26. J. W. Warren and J. C. Price, *J. Pharm. Sci.*, *66*:1409 (1977).
27. *United States Pharmacopeia XXI*, Mack Publishing, Easton, PA 1984.
28. C. A. Gaglia, Jr., J. J. Lomner, B. L. Leonard, and L. Chefetz, *J. Pharm. Sci.*, *65*:1691 (1976).
29. B. Dorsch and R. Shangraw, *Am. J. Hosp. Pharm.*, *32*:795 (1975).
30. M. J. Pikal, A. L. Lukes, and L. F. Ellis, *J. Pharm. Sci.*, *65*:1278 (1976).
31. S. A. Fusari, *J. Pharm. Sci.*, *62*:2012 (1973).
32. M. L. Broderick, Eli Lilly & Co., unpublished data.
33. S. A. Fusari, *J. Pharm. Sci.*, *62*:122 (1973).
34. D. Banes, *J. Pharm. Sci.*, *57*:893 (1968).
35. B. A. Edelman, A. M. Contractor, and R. F. Shangraw, *J. Am. Pharm. Assn.*, *NS11*, 30 (1971).
36. D. P. Page, N. A. Carson, C. A. Buhr, P. E. Flinn, C. E. Wells, and M. T. Randall, *J. Pharm. Sci.*, *64*:140 (1975).
37. M. J. Pikal, D. A. Bibler, and B. Rutherford, *J. Pharm. Sci.*, *66*: 1293 (1977).
38. M. J. Pikal, Eli Lilly & Co., unpublished data.
39. D. Stephenson and J. F. Humphreys-Jones, *J. Pharm. Pharmacol.*, *3*:767 (1951).
40. P. Suphajettra, J. Strohl, and J. Lim, *J. Pharm. Sci.*, *67*:1394 (1978).
41. M. J. Pikal, A. L. Lukes, and J. W. Conine, *J. Pharm. Sci.* *73*: 1608 (1984).
42. M. J. Pikal and A. L. Lukes, *J. Pharm. Sci.*, *65*:1269 (1976).
43. S. Shah, Eli Lilly & Co., unpublished results.
44. H. Gucluyildiz, F. W. Goodhart, and F. C. Ninger, *J. Pharm. Sci.*, *66*:265 (1977).
45. B. Greer, *Am. J. Hosp. Pharm.*, *32*:979 (1975).
46. J. Zeitz and N. Schwartz, *Am. J. Hosp. Pharm.*, *33*:209 (1976).
47. R. M. Gabrielson, *Am. J. Hosp. Pharm.*, *33*:209 (1976).
48. J. Pitha, S. M. Harmon, and M. E. Michel, *J. Pharm. Sci.*, *75*:165 (1986).
49. H. Lowery, U.S. Patent 3,870,790 (1975).
50. H. Lowery, U.S. Patent 4,259,314 (1981).
51. J. M. Schor, U.S. Patent 4,357,469 (1982).
52. J. M. Schor, A. Nigalaye, and N. G. Gaylord, U.S. Patent 4,389,393 (1983).
53. S. S. Davis, J. W. Kennerley, M. J. Taylor, J. G. Hardy, and C. G. Wilson, *Int. Congr. Symp. Ser.-R. Soc. Med. 1983*, 54(Mod. Concepts Nitrate Delivery Syst.) 29—37. Through *C.A. 99*:110574s (1983).
54. Y. Suzuki, H. Ikura, and G. Yamashita, U.S. Patent 4,292,299 (1981).
55. G. L. Christenson and H. E. Huber, U.S. Patent 3,594,467 (1971).

56. W. Tanaka, A. K. Yoshida, T. Terada, and H. Ninomiya, U.S. Patent 4,059,686 (1977). Through *Transdermal and Related Delivery Systems*, (D. A. Jones, ed.), Noyes Data Corp., Park Ridge, NJ, 1984.

57. K. Sugden, Br. Patent Appl. GB 2,165,451. Through *C.A.* *105*: 30103q (1986).

58. G. L. Christenson and H. E. Huber, U.S. Patent 3,590,117 (1971).

59. J. D. Smart, J. W. Kellaway, and H. E. C. Worthington, *J. Pharm. Pharmacol.*, *36*:295 (1984).

60. M. B. Kabadi and Y. W. Chien, *J. Pharm. Sci.*, *73*:1464 (1984).

61. S. Hwang, E. Owada, L. Suhardja, N. F. H. Ho, and G. L. Flynn, *J. Pharm. Sci.*, *66*:781 (1977).

62. L. G. Patel, S. J. Warrington, and R. N. Pearson, *Br. Med. J.*, *287*:1247 (1983).

63. Y. Uda, S. Hirai, and T. Yashiki, U.S. Patent 4,670,419 (1987).

64. M. Yamaguchi and K. Tanno, *Yakauzaigaku*, *45*:41 (1985). Through *C.A.*, *103*:59192n (1985).

65. J. M. Schor, U.S. Patent 4,226,849 (1980).

66. C. J. deBlaey and J. Polderman, in *Drug Design*, Vol. 9 (E. J. Ariens, ed.), Academic Press, New York, 1980.

67. J. G. Wagner, *Biopharmaceutics and Relevant Pharmacokinetics*, Drug Intelligence Publications, Hamilton, ILL, 1971.

68. I. Smazynski and L. Krowizynski, *Acta Pol. Pharm.*, *25*:291 (1968). Through *C.A.*, *70*:31654r (1969).

8
Chewable Tablets

Robert W. Mendes   *Massachusetts College of Pharmacy and Allied Health Sciences, Boston, Massachusetts*

Aloysius O. Anaebonam   *Fisons Corporation, Rochester, New York*

Jahan B. Daruwala   *E. I. du Pont de Nemours & Company, Inc., Wilmington, Delaware*

I. INTRODUCTION

Chewable dosage forms, such as soft pills, tablets, gums, and, most recently, "chewy squares," have long been part of the pharmacist's armamentarium. Their possible advantages, compared to solid dosage forms intended to be swallowed, include better bioavailability through bypassing disintegration (and perhaps enhancing dissolution), patient convenience through the elimination of the need for water for swallowing, possible use as a substitute for liquid dosage forms where rapid onset of action is needed, improved patient acceptance (especially in pediatrics) through pleasant taste, and product distinctiveness from a marketing perspective.

There are, of course, limitations to the use of chewable tablets. Bad-tasting drugs and those having extremely high dosage levels present the formulator with significant obstacles to be overcome. These will be discussed in considerable detail throughout this chapter.

Chewable tablets represent the largest market segment of the chewable dosage forms, with chewing gums and the new chewy squares accounting for a much smaller percentage. Of the chewable market, from a therapeutic perspective, antacids account for the largest segment, with pediatric vitamins next. For both physiological and psychological reasons, children up to the young teens usually have trouble swallowing tablets and capsules; often, this problem continues into adulthood. As a result, most products for children are formulated as liquids. A notable exception to this is represented by the over-the-counter (OTC) and prescription (Rx) vitamin products. For these, chewable tablets are preferable because of their patient acceptability and better stability. Additionally, several OTC cough/cold products and some analgesics are alternatively available as chewables.

Formulation considerations of importance primarily revolve around taste; children tend to be particularly sensitive in their preferences for various flavors, sweetness levels, etc.

The swallowing problems associated with the very young may also be assumed to exist among the elderly. Despite this, the authors have been unable to identify a single drug product formulated as a chewable and specifically targeted to this population.

Formulation considerations here would be similar, except that the preference would be different: less sweet, less flavor emphasis, etc.

II. FORMULATION FACTORS

Various factors involved in the formulation of a chewable tablet can be schematically represented as shown in Figure 1. The first four formulation factors shown in the schematic diagram are common to regular (swallowed) and chewable tablets; however, the organoleptic properties of the active drug substance (or substances) are of primary concern here. A formulator may use one or more approaches to arrive at a combination of formula and process that results in a product with good organoleptic properties. Such a product must have acceptable flow, compressibility, and stability characteristics. Generally as the required amount of active substance per tablet gets smaller and less bad tasting, the task of arriving at an acceptable formulation becomes easier due to the fact that a greater number of formulation options are available. Conversely, extremely bad-tasting and/or high-dose drugs are difficult to formulate into chewable tablets.

The factors of flow, lubrication, disintegration, compressibility, and compatibility-stability have been described in depth in Chapters 1 through 4. The organoleptic considerations will be elaborated here.

A. Taste and Flavor

Physiologically, *taste* is a sensory response resulting from a chemical stimulation of the taste buds on the tongue. There are four basic types of tastes: salty, sour, sweet, and bitter. Salty or sour tastes are derived from substances capable of ionizing in solution [1]. Many organic medicinal compounds stimulate a bitter response even though they may not be capable of ionizing in an aqueous medium. Most saccharides, disaccharides, some aldehydes, and a few alcohols give a sweet taste. Substances incapable of producing a sensory stimulation of the buds are referred to as bland or tasteless.

The term *flavor* generally refers to a specific combined sensation of taste *and* smell (olfaction). For example, sugar has a sweet taste but no flavor whereas honey has a sweet taste and a characteristic smell—the combination of the two being known as honey flavor.

B. Aroma

Pleasant smells are generally referred to as aromas. For example, a well-formulated, orange-flavored, chewable tablet should have a characteristic sweet and sour taste *and* an aroma of fresh orange.

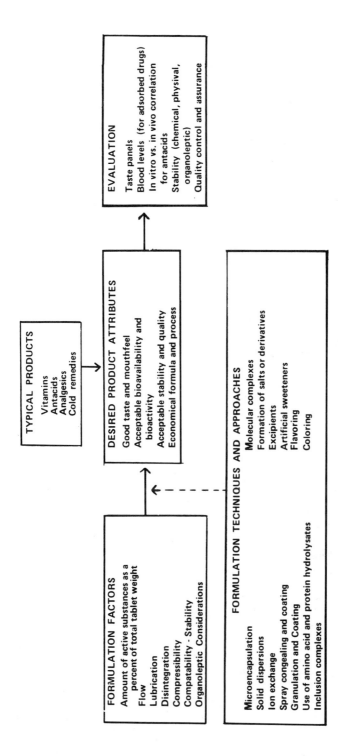

Figure 1 Flow chart of various aspects to be considered in connection with chewable tablets.

C. Mouth-feel

The term *mouth-feel* is related to the type of sensation or touch that a tablet produces in the mouth upon chewing. As such, it has nothing to do with chemical stimulation of olfactory nerves or taste buds. However, for a formulation to be successful, the overall effect in the mouth is important. In general, gritty (e.g., calcium carbonate) or gummy textures are undesirable, whereas a soothing and cooling sensation (e.g., mannitol) with smooth texture is preferred.

D. After Effects

The most common after effect of many compounds is aftertaste. For example, some iron salts leave a "rusty" aftertaste; saccharin in high amounts tends to leave a bitter aftertaste.

Another common after effect is a numbing sensation of a portion of the whole surface of the tongue and mouth. Bitter antihistamines such as pyribenzamine hydrochloride and promethazine hydrochloride are typical of this class of drugs.

E. Assessment of the Formulation Problems

Wherever feasible and practical, the first step in the formulation of a chewable tablet is to obtain a complete profile of the active drug. This usually leads to the most efficient formulation of a stable and quality product as the drug usually dictates the choice of fillers, carriers, sweeteners, flavor compounds, and other product modifiers.

The drug profile ideally should contain information on the following:

Physical properties
    Color
    Odor
    Taste, aftertaste, and mouth-feel
    Physical form: crystal, powder, amorphous solid, oily liquid, etc.
    Melting or congealing temperature
    Existence of polymorphs
    Moisture content
    Aqueous solubility
    Active drug's stability on its own
    Compressibility if applicable
Chemical properties
    Chemical structure and chemical class
    Major reactions of this chemical class
    Major incompatible compounds or class of compounds
Drug dose and any limit on final dosage size
Any other relevant information

This active drug profile would eliminate potentially incompatible excipients, flavors, and the like at the outset, leading to the use of excipients that would best compliment the drug chemically, physically, and organoleptically. The choice of excipients and other product modifiers would involve judgment, balancing their cost with their functionality. The use of low-calorie and non-sugar-based excipients may represent a marketing advantage, especially with consumers concerned about calorie intake and dental caries.

III. FORMULATION TECHNIQUES

Almost invariably, the formulation problem involves at least one of the following: undesirable taste, bad mouth-feel, or aftertaste. The desired product should prevent or minimize stimulation of the taste buds, contain a suitable flavor and sweetener, and achieve good mouth-feel and compressibility. The following techniques are used to solve one or more of the above.

A. Coating by Wet Granulation

Wet granulation, which is discussed in detail in Chapter 3, historically has been the method of choice for preparing drugs for compression.

This process may be described as one which agglomerates drug particles through a combination of adhesion and cohesion using a wetting agent and binder. Generally, binders are classified as hydrophilic gums (e.g., acacia), sugars (e.g., sucrose), starches (e.g., natural or modified corn), and polymers (e.g., povidone, cellulose derivatives, gelatin), which have the property of becoming sticky when wetted with water or another suitable solvent. This method consists of the mixing of the ingredients in a solids-liquids processor to form a dampened, agglomerated mass that may then be subdivided, dried, and sized to form a suitable free-flowing and compressible granulation.

Although this process is primarily intended to impart flowability and compressibility to impalpable substances, under certain conditions it may be useful in the application of coatings to drug particles in order to mask or reduce their taste. Example 10 illustrates the use of ethylcellulose (a water-insoluble polymer) to coat ascorbic acid through wet granulation to improve its stability and assist in taste masking. In this case, the drug is wet-granulated with an anhydrous solution of polymer in a planetary processor, dried, sized, and blended with a directly compressible sweetener and other ingredients to produce a material suitable for compressing.

In general, this is the simplest approach to taste masking. Wet granulation may be accomplished as described above with or without the inclusion of additional excipients such as lactose, sucrose, mannitol, sorbitol, other sugars, or starches. Although this approach is similar to that for the wet granulation of nonchewable tablets, some fundamental concepts should be kept in mind. Whenever possible, the granulating/coating agent should form a flexible rather than brittle film, have no unpleasant taste or odor of its own, be insoluble in saliva but not interfere with drug dissolution after swallowing. Ideally, sweet fillers, such as sugars, should be included in the granulation. Disintegrant should preferably be included in the wet granulation to ensure proper dissolution of the granules after chewing.

While the procedure described above involves the use of classical wet granulation processing, the desirability of utilizing more modern techniques should not be overlooked. The use of *fluidized bed* or *air suspension coating* may represent a more efficient approach.

In this technique, drug particles to be coated are fluidized by means of suspension in a controlled, high-velocity, warm air stream directed through a perforated plate into a coating chamber. The drug particles undergo cyclic flow past an atomizing nozzle delivering coating agent in solution or suspension. The sprayer may be mounted either to spray upward from the bottom (Wurster style) or downward from the top, as depicted in Figure 2. As the particles become coated, they are removed from the spray field, dried by the warm air stream, and returned for recoating. This cycling continues until the desired coating thickness has been achieved. Fluidization of the drug particles provides increased surface exposure for more efficient and uniform coating and drying. Since evaporation occurs over the entire surface in a very short time, particle temperature does not increase. This permits the coating of heat-labile drugs without concern for degradation. Figure 3 is a comparative electron micrograph showing acetaminophen particles before and after air suspension coating.

Although it is not within the scope of this discussion to detail the optimization of the process, the formulator should recognize the importance of factors such as particulate properties of the drug, viscosity of the coating liquid, design and placement of the spray nozzle, and velocity and temperature of the fluidizing air.

Although taste improvement by coating is attractive in its simplicity, it should be understood that this method may only suffice for mildly to moderately unpleasant tasting drugs. For those that are extremely bitter, sour, or otherwise difficult, more heroic methods will most certainly be required.

B. Microencapsulation

Microencapsulation is a method of coating drug particles or liquid droplets with edible polymeric materials, thereby masking the taste and forming relatively free-flowing microcapsules of 5- to 5000-μm size [2−4]. A number of methods have been described in the literature [5,6], but phase separation or coacervation technique appears to be more relevant and suitable for taste-masking applications. The process essentially consists of three steps [5]:

1. Formation of three immiscible phases: a liquid-manufacturing vehicle phase, a core material drug phase, and a coating material phase
2. Depositing the liquid polymer coating by sorption around the core material under controlled physical mixing of the three phases
3. Rigidizing the coating, usually by thermal crosslinking or desolvation techniques, to form a rigid microcapsule

The resultant coated granules not only mask the taste of a drug but also minimize any physical and chemical incompatibility between ingredients [2]. The size distribution of the drug can be narrow or relatively broad, and the process is applicable to a variety of compounds regardless of pharmacological classification. Typical coating materials include carboxymethylcellulose, cellulose acetate phthalate, ethylcellulose, gelatin, polyvinyl alcohol, gelatin-acacia, shellac, and some waxes—with the choice depending on the specific application. The encapsulated drug is isolated from the liquid-manufacturing vehicle as a free-flowing powder. In general, the encapsulated drug is then blended with direct-compression vehicles

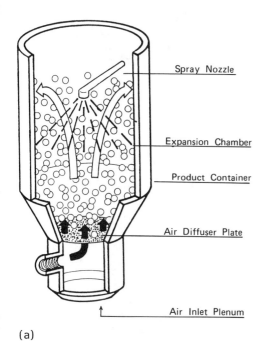

(a)

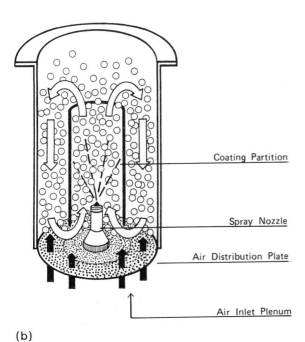

(b)

Figure 2 (a) Top spray fluidized bed system. (b) Bottom spray fluidized system. (Courtesy Nortec Development Associates, Inc.)

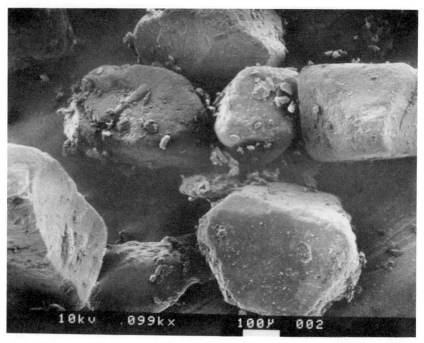

(a)

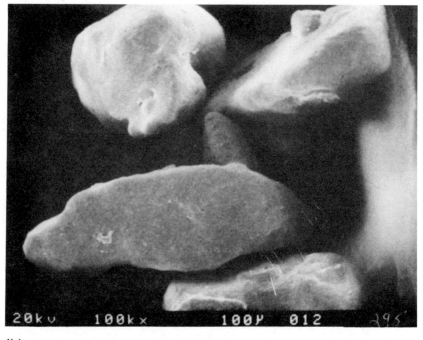

(b)

Figure 3   (a) Uncoated acetaminophen.   (b) Coated (taste-masked)
acetaminophen.   (Courtesy Nortec Development Associates, Inc.)

(described later in this chapter), other diluents, artificial sweeteners, flavors, and lubricants for tableting.

A typical taste-masking application of microencapsulation has been described by Bakan and Sloan [2] for acetaminophen tablets (Example 1).

It must be borne in mind that, upon compression, the structure of the coating is disrupted and should be expected to lose some of its protective barrier. Furthermore, the extent of mastication and the length of time that a drug remains in the mouth also play an important role in determining the extent of taste masking, especially for very bitter drugs. Appropriate compensatory measures, such as choosing the right coating material and the extent of the applied coat, along with the solubility and particle size considerations, must be taken into account before arriving at an acceptable microencapsulated form suitable for further blending with excipients and subsequent tableting. As discussed earlier, the mouth-feel characteristics of a chewable tablet formulation are important; it is noteworthy that microcapsules larger than 60 mesh are unsatisfactory [2], and that smaller particle sizes (about 100 to 120 mesh) should give a good mouthfeel, and at the same time have adequate flow for uniform blending and compression. Eliminating or minimizing a potential incompatibility is also an inherent advantage with this technique.

Farhadieh [4] has used coagulable water-soluble egg albumin as the coating medium for masking the taste of erythromycin derivatives. The process involves suspending the drug particles in an aqueous solution of egg albumin at pH 7 to 10, and stirring the suspension with a liquid alkane containing a surfactant to form an emulsion. The emulsion is then heated to 50 to 80°C with stirring, so as to coagulate the albumin in the form of

Example 1: Acetaminophen Tablets (Microencapsulated, Chewable)

Ingredient	Quantity per tablet
Microcapsules (∿100 mesh)	
Acetaminophen	327 mg
Coating (cellulose–wax)	35 mg
Excipients	
Mannitol (major diluent)	
Microcrystalline cellulose (Avicel)	
Talc	
Saccharin	393 mg
Guar gum	
Mint, spice, and peppermint flavors	
Magnesium stearate	
	755 mg

microcapsules around the drug. The solid microcapsules are separated from the suspension and dried. This can be made into chewable tablets by dilution with direct-compression grade mannitol, flavor, artificial sweeteners, and lubricant and subsequent compression. Heat stability (physical and chemical) of the tablets made with denatured protein should be carefully evaluated along with flavor retention characteristics of the formulation over a prolonged period of time before considering the formulation as acceptable.

The above discussion points out certain obvious advantages of the process, such as considerable flexibility in the choice of coating materials, particle size, and minimization of incompatibilities. However, it should be pointed out that compared to the conventional wet granulation process, microencapsulation is more expensive and does require specialized equipment and knowledgeable personnel. The economics of the process and its practicality for a given drug should be expected to improve as the required dose per tablet decreases. Limitations imposed due to extensive patent coverage should also be taken into account.

C. Solid Dispersions

Bad-tasting drugs can be prevented from stimulating the taste buds by adsorption onto substrates capable of keeping the drugs adsorbed while in the mouth but releasing them eventually in the stomach or gastrointestinal tract. A good example of such an application is the adsorption of dextromethorphan hydrobromide onto magnesium trisilicate substrate (Example 2) [7]. The adsorbate is commercially available in the form of micronized powder with a drug content of 10% w/w. It must be noted that besides the dextromethorphan portion of the compound, the bromide ion contributes significantly to the undesirable taste of the drug. This is indeed true of many other bromide salts of medicinal compounds. A formulator attempting to formulate an adsorbate may consider many substrates such as bentonite, Veegum, and silica gel.

D. Adsorbate Formation Techniques

Solvent Method

Generally the formation of an adsorbate involves dissolving the drug in a solvent, mixing the solution with the substrate, and evaporating the solvent—leaving the drug molecules adsorbed upon the substrate. The variables of the process, such as choice of solvent, substrate, proportions, mixing conditions, rate of evaporation, and temperature, must be optimized to give the desired product.

Melting Method

Here the drug or drugs and a carrier are melted together by heating. The melted mixture is then cooled and rapidly solidified in an ice bath with vigorous stirring. The product is then pulverized and sized. Heat-labile drugs, volatile drugs, and drugs that decompose on melting are obviously unsuitable for this method. The method is simple with low cost and no problem of residual solvents as are encountered in the solvent evaporation method.

Example 2:   Cough Preparation (Chewable)

Ingredient	Quantity per tablet
10% Dextromethorphan HBr adsorbate (micronized)	76.5 mg*
Benzocaine	2.5 mg
Mouthwash flavor (Givaudan F5098)	10.0 mg
Magnesium stearate	10.0 mg
Sorbitol (crystalline)	1301.0 mg
	1400.0 mg

*Contains 7.5 mg active drug plus 2% excess.

Pass the sorbitol through a 10-mesh screen to deagglomerate the particles.   Premix the adsorbate, benzocaine, and flavor with one-fourth of
the required amount of sorbitol for 10 min.   Add the rest of the sorbitol
and mix for another 10 min.   Finally, add the magnesium stearate and
mix for a further 3 min.   Compress to a hardness of about 6 kp using
5/8-in. diameter tooling.

Comments: A noteworthy feature of the above example is that the total
drug content (dextromethorphan HBr and benzocaine) of the tablet is
about 10 mg, which requires a tablet of 1,400 mg weight to give satisfactory taste-masking and mouth-feel characteristics.   It must also be
pointed out that the compression hardness of 6 kp gives the tablet
chewable characteristics.   Furthermore, the required 5/8-in. tooling
would put some restriction on the tablet press that could be used for
the product.

Chiou and Riegelman [8] reported a third method of preparing solid
dispersions with limited application.   This method is a combination of certain aspects of the solvent and melting methods.

E.   Ion Exchange

Ion exchange has been defined by Wheaton and Seamster [9] as the reversible interchange of ions between a solid and a liquid phase in which there
is no permanent change in the structure of the solid.   The solid is the
ion exchange material while the ion could be a drug.   When used as a drug
carrier, ion exchange materials provide a means for binding drugs onto an
insoluble polymeric matrix and can effectively mask the problems of taste
and odor, in drugs to be formulated into chewable tablets.

Ion exchange resins can be classified in four major groups: strong
acid cation, weak acid cation, strong base anion, and weak base anion
exchange resins.

(1) Strong acid cation exchange resins are best exemplified by the
principal sulfonated styrene-divinylbenzene copolymer products such as
Amberlite IRP-69 (Rhom and Haas) and DOWEX MSC-1 (Dow Chemical).

These resins can be used for masking the taste and odor of cationic (amine-containing) drugs prior to their formulation into chewable tablets. These resins are spherical products prepared by the sulfonation of styrene-divinylbenzene copolymer beads with the sulfonating agent of choice: sulfuric acid, chlorosulfonic acid, or sulfur trioxide. The use of a nonreactive swelling agent is generally required for rapid and uniform swelling with minimum breakage.

Strong acid cation exchange resins function throughout the entire pH range. A schematic of a strong acid cation exchange resin in use follows:

$$\text{Resin } (SO_3)^- A^+ + D^+ \longrightarrow \text{resin } (SO_3)^- D^+ + A^+$$

Cation exchange resin + drug ⟶ resin–drug complex + displaced ion

(2) The most common weak acid cation exchange resins are those prepared by crosslinking an unsaturated carboxylic acid such as methacrylic acid with a crosslinking agent such as divinylbenzene.

Examples include DOWEX CCR-2 (Dow Chemical) and Amberlite IRP-65 (Rhom and Haas). Weak acid cation exchange resins function at pH values above 6.

(3) Strong base anion exchange resins are quaternized amine resins resulting from the reaction of triethylamine with chloromethylated copolymer of styrene and divinylbenzene. Examples include Amberlite IRP-276 (Rhom and Haas) and DOWEX MSA-A (Dow Chemical). These strong base anion exchange resins function throughout the entire pH range.

(4) Weak base anion exchange resins are formed by reacting primary and secondary amines or ammonia with chloromethylated copolymer of styrene and divinylbenzene. Dimethylamine is usually used. These weak base anion exchange resins function well below pH 7.

Important properties to be considered when using an ion exchange resin include particle size, shape, density, porosity, chemical and physical stability, and ionic capacity.

The rate and extent of drug desorption from these resins in vivo will be controlled by the diffusion rate of the drug through the polymer phase of the resin, as well as the selectivity coefficient between the drug and the resin.

Ion exchange resins, especially weakly acidic cation exchange resins, have certain adsorptive mechanisms that have been utilized in the stabilization of the nonionic vitamin B_{12} (cyanocobalamin) for many years [10].

A formulator must thoroughly investigate the various available types of pharmaceutical grade resins available for specific applications and check their approval status for oral use in the amounts anticipated. The quantity of resin required per unit quantity of drug to achieve effective taste masking and/or stability improvement is a limiting factor as the dose of drug per tablet increases.

F. Spray Congealing and Spray Coating

In a broad sense, the process of spray congealing involves cooling (or congealing) of melted substances in the form of fine particles during their travel from a spray nozzle to the distant vicinity of a spraying chamber held at a temperature below their melting point. If a slurry of drug material insoluble in a melted mass is spray-congealed, one obtains discrete particles of the insoluble material coated with the congealed substance.

The application is best exemplified by the taste masking of thiamine mononitrate, riboflavin, pyridoxine hydrochloride, and niacinamide by fatty acids or monoglycerides and diglycerides of edible fatty acids. These are commonly available (as Rocoat vitamins) in the form of relatively free-flowing powders having the composition shown in Table 1.

It must be noted that the weight of the active substance is approximately one-third that of the spray-congealed preparation. For small-dose entities, such as the vitamins, spray congealing is ideally suited. The influence of the coating on the bioavailability of the drug must be considered before considering this method as the means of improving the taste of the drug. Polyethylene glycols (Carbowaxes) of molecular weights between 4000 and 20,000 are suitable for spray congealing especially where their solubility would represent an added advantage.

As opposed to spray congealing, the *spray-coating* process involves the spraying of a suspension of the drug particles in a solution of the coating material through an atomizer into a high-velocity stream of warm air. The coarse droplets delivered by the atomizer consist of drug

Table 1   Examples of Coated Vitamins

Vitamin	Coating agent	Vitamin content (% w/w)
Thiamine mononitrate (B_1)	Mono- and diglycerides of edible fatty acids	33.3
Riboflavin (B_2)	Mono- and diglycerides of edible fatty acids	33.3
Pyridoxine HCl (B_6)	Mono- and diglycerides of edible fatty acids	33.3
Niacinamide	Stearic acid	33.3

particles enveloped by coating solution.   As the solvent evaporates, the coating material encapsulates the drug particle.

The atomizers typically used in such a system may be of the pneumatic type in which atomization is accomplished through pressurization through an orifice, or the rotating disk which functions through centrifugal force. Since drying is nearly instantaneous, the drug particle is subjected to little temperature increase, making this process suitable for heat-labile drugs.   As with all spray-drying techniques, concentration, viscosity, spray rate, temperature, and velocity are factors that require optimization. Examples of applications of the method include the spray coating of flavor oils and the coating of sodium dicloxacillin [11] and vitamins A and D.

The coating of the antibiotic sodium dicloxacillin, or some other tetra-cyclines, involves a mixture of ethylcellulose and spermaceti wax (as coating materials) dissolved in methylene chloride.   A suspension of micronized antibiotic in this solution, upon spray drying, results in a free-flowing product suitable for further compounding into a chewable formulation.   [It should be noted that in July 1987 the United States Consumer Product Safety Commission (CPSC) rejected a proposed rule that would have declared methylene chloride a hazardous substance in consumer products. Instead, the commission voted to require chronic hazard warning labels on consumer products containing more than 1% methylene chloride.   This points up the significant interest among various regulatory agencies with regard to the use of organic solvents.   It is encumbant on the formulator to ascertain the regulatory status of solvents with respect to their use in pharmaceutical products and processes, as well as possible restrictions due to environmental concerns.]

Vitamins A and D are fat-soluble and, as such, are unsuitable (too oily) for incorporation into chewable formulations, primarily because of their physical form and poor stability due to oxidation.   Two commercially available, protectively coated forms of vitamin A or vitamins A and D together exemplify the application of the technology under discussion.

Crystalets: Contain vitamin A acetate, available with or without vitamin D_2 as fine, free-flowing particles in a matrix of gelatin, sugar, and cottonseed oil, stabilized with BHT, BHA, and sodium bisulfite.

Beadlets: Contain vitamin A acetate and vitamin D_2 beadlets as fine, free-flowing particles in a gelatin matrix with sugar and modified food starch, stabilized with BHT, BHA, methylparaben, propyl-paraben, and potassium sorbate.

It should be noted that the coating method for antibiotics described above was primarily for masking the taste, whereas vitamins A and D are essential-ly tasteless and are spray-dried for reasons of stability and ease of processing.

G.   Formation of Different Salts or Derivatives

This approach differs from the others previously discussed in that an attempt is made to modify the chemical composition of the drug substance itself, so as to render it less soluble in saliva and thereby less stimulating for the taste buds, or to obtain a tasteless or less bitter form.   Even if one is successful in preparing a new salt or a derivative of a bitter drug, the legalities of its new drug status from a regulatory point of view must be considered.   Moreover, the solubility, stability, compatibility, and bio-availability aspects of the "new" compound must also be kept in mind.   If a less bitter tasting salt form or a tasteless derivative can be obtained, this would represent the best approach to taste masking.   Since there is no coating that can be broken during chewing, no problem will be encoun-tered with respect to unpleasant aftertaste.

H.   Use of Amino Acids and Protein Hydrolysates

By combining amino acids, their salts, or a mixture of the two [12], it is possible to substantially reduce the bitter taste of penicillin.   Some of the preferred amino acids are sarcosine, alanine, taurine, glutamic acid, and especially glycine.   The taste of ampicillin is markedly improved by granu-lating with glycine in the usual manner and subsequently blending this mixture with additional glycine, starch, lubricants, glidants, sweeteners, and flavors before compression.

I.   Inclusion Complexes

In inclusion complex formation, the drug molecule (guest molecule) fits into the cavity of a complexing agent (host molecule) forming a stable complex. The complex is capable of masking the bitter taste of the drug by both decreasing the amount of drug particles exposed to the taste buds and/or by decreasing the drug solubility on ingestion, both activities leading to a decrease in the obtained bitterness associated with the drug.   The forces involved in inclusion complexes are usually of the Van der Waals type, and one of the most widely used complexing agents in inclusion type complexes is β-cyclodextrin, a sweet, nontoxic, cyclic oligosaccharide obtained from starch.

Three primary methods have been reported for the preparation of cyclodextrin inclusion compounds [13].   Two of these are laboratory scale, while the other is industrial scale.

Laboratory Methods

(1) Equimolar quantities, or a 10-fold excess of water-soluble sub-stances, are dissolved directly in concentrated hot or cold aqueous solu-tions of the cyclodextrins. The inclusion compounds crystallize out immedi-ately or upon slow cooling and evaporation.

(2) Water-insoluble drugs are dissolved in a non-water-miscible organic solvent and shaken with a concentrated aqueous solution of cyclodextrins. The inclusion compounds crystallize at the interface between the layers, or as a precipitate. The crystals must then be washed with solvent to remove uncomplexed drug and dried under appropriate conditions to remove residual solvents.

Industrial Method

The drug substance is added to the cyclodextrin and water to form a slurry which undergoes an increase in viscosity with continued mixing. This may concentrate to a paste that can be dried, powdered, and washed. If the inclusion compounds are readily soluble in water, or decompose on drying, it may be advisable to use lyophilization to accomplish drying. This may provide the additional advantages of easy redispersibility and improved dissolution rate.

Inclusion-type complexes can also increase the stability of the guest molecule by shielding it from moisture, oxygen, and light, which can de-grade the drug molecule via hydrolysis, oxidation, and photodegradation, respectively.

J. Molecular Complexes

Molecular complex formation involves a drug and a complexing organic mole-cule and, like inclusion complexes, can be used in the masking of the bitter taste or odor of drugs by forming complexes that would lower the aqueous solubility of the drug and thus the amount of drug in contact with the taste buds.

Higuchi and Pitman [14] reported the formation of a molecular complex between caffeine and gentisic acid leading to a decrease in caffeine solu-bility. One would consequently expect a decrease in the bitter taste of caffeine if the above complex were used in a chewable caffeine tablet formulation.

IV. EXCIPIENTS

The subject of tablet excipients in general has been extensively covered in Chapters 3 and 4. Special consideration, however, needs to be given to those materials that form the basis for chewable tablet formulation. The acceptability in the marketplace of chewable tablets will be primarily deter-mined by taste and, to a lesser degree, appearance. Therefore, appro-priate selection and use of components that impact on these properties are of extreme importance. Of course, the formulator must not become so con-cerned with these properties as to lose sight of other pharmaceutical and biomedical considerations; the resultant product must be as pure, safe, efficacious, and stable as any other.

The processes described in Chapters 3 and 4 (wet granulation, dry granulation, direct compaction) are as applicable to chewables as to any other type of tablet. The concerns such as moisture content and uptake, particle size distribution, blending and loading potentials, flow and compressibility are no less important, and must be addressed by the formulation/process development pharmacist as for any product. However, in the case of chewables, the new concerns of sweetness, chewability, mouthfeel, and taste must also be considered. Major excipients, such as fillers or direct-compaction vehicles, have the major role in the outcome of these concerns; process, a lesser (but certainly not minor) role.

Many of the excipients commonly used in tablet formulation are especially applicable for use in chewable tablets due to their ability to provide the necessary properties of sweetness and chewability. In general, these fall into the sugar category, although a combination of bland excipient with artificial sweeteners may provide a satisfactory alternative.

The following descriptions of chewable excipients have been compiled from general references [15—19] and from other specific references as noted.

Uko-Nne and Mendes [20] reported on the development of dried honey and molasses products marketed for use in chewable tablets. *Hony-Tab* [21] and *Mola-Tab* [22] are marketed by Ingredient Technology Corporation, and consist of 60 to 70% honey or molasses solids codried with wheat flour and wheat bran. Both are free-flowing compressible materials with characteristic colors, odors, and tastes that limit their primary applicability to the vitamin/food supplement field. These were evaluated with vitamin C, vitamin E, and vitamin B complex, as well as with wheat germ and bran.

Two other molasses derivatives are also available that may have applicability to specialized chewable tablets. Granular molasses is a cocrystallized aggregate of molasses, syrup, and caramel marketed as *CrystaFlo* by Amstar Corporation. It contains up to 94% sucrose and 2% invert, with no carriers or flow agents [23]. It is a coarse, free-flowing, granular material with the color and taste of molasses. Moisture content is not more than 1%. *Brownulated*, also marketed by Amstar Corporation, has similar properties [24]. Neither has been reported on, relative to evaluation as tableting agents.

Compressible sugar, which may or may not be designated "N.F.," consists chiefly of sucrose that has been processed and combined with other constituents in such a way as to render the product directly compressible. The N.F. permits the addition of starch, dextrin, invert sugar, and lubricants. Compressible sugar is white, odorless, has a sweet taste (equal to that of sucrose) and acceptable mouth-feel, a high degree of water solubility, and demonstrates good compressibility under normal conditions. It has a moisture content of less than 1% and is nonhygroscopic, thus contributing to good overall product compatibility and chemical stability, despite a tendency toward discoloration when stored at high temperature. Its compressibility is markedly effected by moisture content and lubricant concentration.

Generally, equilibrium moisture content is approximately 0.4%; higher levels usually produce harder tablets with reduced chewability, while lower levels may produce unacceptably soft tablets. Tablet strength also may be adversely affected by increased lubricant levels; normally, a magnesium stearate concentration between 0.5 and 0.75% is adequate.

Table 2 Common Chewable Tablet Excipients

Common name	Trade name	Source	Particle size	LOD	Comments
Brown sugar	Brownulated	Amstar	92% on 50 mesh	0.7%	Dark brown 92% sucrose bulk density 0.67 g/ml
Molasses granules	CrystaFlo	Amstar	100% on 12 mesh	1%	Dark brown 92% sucrose bulk density 0.67 g/ml
Compressible molasses	Mola-Tab	Ingredient Technology	50% on 60 mesh 10% thru 120 mesh	4%	Dark brown 70% solids
Compressible honey	Hony-Tab	Ingredient Technology	50% on 60 mesh 10% thru 120 mesh	4%	Golden yellow 60% solids
Compressible sugar	Di-Pac	Amstar	75% on 100 mesh	0.5%	Bulk density 0.64 g/ml
	NuTab	Ingredient Technology	50% on 60 mesh 10% thru 120 mesh	0.5%	Bulk density 0.72 g/ml

Dextrose/fructose/maltose	Sweetrex	Mendell	3% on 20 mesh 25% thru 100 mesh	7%	Bulk density 0.6–0.9 g/ml heat of solution −18 cal/g
Dextrates	Emdex	Mendell	3% on 20 mesh 25% thru 100 mesh	9%	Bulk density 0.68 g/ml
Lactose	DT	Sheffield	20% on 60 mesh 50% thru 100 mesh	1%	
	Fast-Flo	Foremost	25–65% on 140 mesh	5.5%	
Mannitol	—	ICI-Americas	75% on 80 mesh	0.3%	Bulk density 0.6 g/ml heat of solution −28.9 cal/g
Sorbitol	Sorb-Tab	ICI-Americas	—	—	
	Tablet type	Pfizer	33% on 60 mesh 22% thru 120 mesh	1%	Heat of solution −26.5 cal/g bulk density 0.7 g/ml

Each of the major suppliers produces a different product based on composition and process. *Di-Pac* (Amstar Corporation) consists of a co-crystallized 3% highly modified dextrins and 97% sucrose [25]. The former acts to interrupt the crystal structure of the latter, thereby improving its compressibility. *NuTab* (Ingredient Technology Corporation) is a chilsonated mixture of 4% invert sugar (dextrose and levulose) and 96% sucrose, with approximately 0.1% each cornstarch and magnesium stearate as processing aids [26]. The agglomerates thus formed are very dense and compressible. Several other products are also available from other suppliers; they tend to be very similar in their properties.

Dextrose is the sugar obtained through the complete hydrolysis of starch. Its sweetness level is approximately 70% that of sucrose, and it is available in both anhydrous (but more hygroscopic) and a monohydrated form. Equilibrium moisture content of the former is approximately 1% at up to 75% relative humidity; the latter, approximately 10% at up to 80% RH. It occurs as a colorless to white crystal or as a white granular powder. Dextrose is suitable for use in wet granulation with added binder; its compressibility is not sufficient for direct compression. For the latter use, Dextrates, a spray-crystallized combination of 95% dextrose with various maltoses and higher glucose saccharides, is marketed as *Emdex* (Edward Mendell Co.) [27]. It is free-flowing, compressible, moderately hygroscopic (except at high relative humidity where liquification may occur), and stable. Deformation during compression occurs over many planes, resulting in extremely hard tablets at relatively low compressional force levels. Tablets harden markedly during the first few hours after compression. Because of the high equilibrium moisture content of dextrose and its potential for reaction with amines, dextrose and Dextrates may present problems in some applications. A related commercially available product is *Sweetrex* (Edward Mendell Co.), a combination of approximately 70% dextrose and 30% fructose with minor amounts of related saccharides [28]. It is slightly sweeter than sucrose, and its other properties are similar to other dextrose-related excipients.

Lactose is a monosaccharide produced from whey, a byproduct of the processing of cheese. Although generally acknowledged as the most widely used pharmaceutical excipient in the world, its applicability to chewable tablets is minor at best, due to its extremely low sweetness level (15% of sucrose). This deficiency requires the addition of an artificial sweetener of sufficient potency to overcome lactose's blandness. Assuming that such an addition is acceptable, lactose may be considered a very useful filler. For wet granulation applications, regular pharmaceutical grades (hydrous fine powders) are available.

For direct compression, an anhydrous grade having good flow and compressional characteristics is available as *Lactose DT* (Sheffield Products Co.). This product has the appearance of granulated fine crystals that easily deform under pressure, providing excellent compressibility [29]. Another directly compressible form is *Fast-Flo* Lactose (Foremost Foods Co.), an aggregated microcrystalline α-lactose [30]. Although more flowable, it is less compressible than anhydrous lactose. It is also more prone to discoloration upon exposure to high temperature and humidity. Both often require higher than normal lubricant levels in their formulations.

Mannitol is a white, crystalline polyol approximately 50% as sweet as sucrose. It is freely soluble in water and, when chewed or dissolved in

the mouth, imparts a mild cooling sensation due to its negative heat of
solution. This combined with an exceptionally smooth consistency has
made mannitol the excipient of choice for chewable tablet formulations.
In powder form, it is suitable only for wet granulation in combination
with an auxiliary binder. For direct-compression applications, a granular
form ("tablet grade") is available (ICI Americas). Mannitol has a low
moisture content, is nonhygroscopic, and the equilibrium moisture content
remains at approximately 0.5% up to a relative humidity of approximately
85% [17]; these properties, combined with those related to sweetness and
mouth-feel, represent significant advantages for the formulation of chewable tablets.

Sorbitol is a slightly sweeter and considerably more hygroscopic isomer
of mannitol. For direct compression, it is available commercially as *Sorb-
Tab* (ICI Americas) and *Crystalline Tablet Type* (Pfizer Chemical). Although similar in that both are aggregated microcrystals covered with den-
drites, the structures of these materials are sufficiently different to provide somewhat different compressional characteristics. Relative humidities
greater than 50% at 25°C should be avoided. Equilibrium moisture content
rises 10-fold (from 2.7 to 28.4%) between 64 and 75% RH [17].

Artificial sweeteners are a class of excipients that are of significant
importance to chewable tablet formulations. As noted above, none of the
other sugars are as sweet as sucrose, which itself is often not sweet
enough to mask the bitterness or sourness of many drugs. Presently,
there is considerable regulatory disagreement worldwide concerning the
use of these materials; some are approved for use in some countries but
not others. Although this formulation problem is not related solely to
artificial sweeteners, but in fact to virtually all classes of excipients (and
drugs), it is probably a greater problem only with colorants. Three
materials appear to be usable from other than a regulatory perspective:
aspartame, cyclamate, and saccharin. All have potency (sweetness) levels
many times that of sucrose, permitting the use of very low concentrations
(less than 1%) to cover most bitter drugs. Other semisynthetic sweeteners,
derived from glycyrrhiza, have enjoyed some degree of popularity over the
years. These are much sweeter than sucrose but less sweet than saccharin.
It is recommended that the formulator validate the current regulatory acceptance of the intended sweetener prior to its use for a particular product
and market country.

V. FLAVORING

From the perspective of consumer acceptance, taste is almost certainly the
most important parameter of the evaluation of chewable tablets. Taste is a
combination of the perceptions of mouth-feel, sweetness, and flavor.

Mouth-feel is affected by the heat of solution of the soluble components
(negative being preferable), smoothness of the combination during chewing,
and hardness of the tablet. These factors are directly and almost entirely
related to the active ingredient and major excipients.

Sweetness, at an appropriate level, is a necessary background to any
flavor. The primary contributors to sweetness in a chewable tablet are
the drug, natural sweeteners, and artificial sweetness enhancers that may
be incorporated in the formulation.

A. Sweeteners

Most of the excipients described in the previous section as appropriate
bases for chewable tablets have, as their major property, a level of sweetness that contributes positively to the overall taste of the product. Often,
the sweetness imparted by these excipients is insufficient to overcome the
bad taste of the drug. In these cases, the formulator must often use
artificial enhancers to increase the overall sweetness impact.

Table 3 presents a compilation of the most common artificial and synthetic sweeteners used in pharmaceutical products, their relative sweetness
levels, and pertinent comments. It is important to note that, with all excipient materials, it is the responsibility of the formulator to ascertain the current regulatory status of the material in the country for which the product
is intended. At the present time, the acceptability of saccharins and cyclamates varies from country to country, while aspartame and glycyrrhizin
are generally (though perhaps not universally) recognized as safe. In
addition to use restrictions, label requirements may apply.

The obvious major advantage to the use of artificial sweeteners is their
relative potencies, which may range from 50 to 700 (compared to sucrose)
depending on choice and conditions of use. For example, the relative
sweetness of saccharin decreases as the sweetener level is increased. Furthermore, as the saccharin concentration is increased, the level of unpleasant aftertaste increases.

Glycyrrhizin (Magnasweet) is a licorice derivative with an intense, late,
long-lasting sweetness [31]. These properties permit its use as an auxiliary
sweetener to boost sweetness level while overcoming aftertaste. Typical use
levels are 0.005 to 0.1%, with higher concentrations tending to lend a
slight licorice flavor.

Aspartame (NutraSweet) is the most recently introduced artificial
sweetener, having been approved for use in the United States in 1981.
Its relative sweetness level is approximately 200, and its duration is
greater than that of natural sweeteners [32]. It enhances and extends
citrus flavors. Aspartame's dry stability is said to be excellent at room
temperature and a relative humidity of 50%, while in solution it is most
stable at pH 4. Its typical usage level in chewable tablets is 3 to 8 mg
per tablet.

B. Flavors

Flavoring agents, both natural and artificial, are available in a variety of
physical forms from a large number of suppliers specializing in these
materials. Virtually all offer technical support services, which will be
addressed in the section on flavor formulation. Forms available include
water-miscible solutions, oil bases, emulsions, dry powders, spray-dried
beadlets, and dry adsorbates. A typical flavor house might catalog 50 or
more basic flavors, while having the capability of producing several
hundred combinations for a given application.

C. Flavor Selection and Formulation

Initially, the inherent taste of the active drug must be evaluated to determine its probable contribution to the formulation. Next, a decision must

Table 3 Approximate Relative Sweetness of
Different Vehicles and Auxiliary Sweeteners

Material	Relative sweetness[b]
Aspartame[a]	200
Cyclamates[a]	30–50
Glycyrrhizin[a]	50
Saccharins[a]	450
Dextrose (glucose)	0.7
Fructose (levulose)	1.7
Lactose	0.2
Maltose	0.3
Mannitol	0.5–0.7
Sorbitol	0.5–0.6
Sucrose	1

[a]Regulatory status must be checked before use.

[b]Sucrose is taken as a standard of 1 for comparison.

be made relative to formulation components that would impact on both the pharmaceutical properties and organoleptic characteristics of the tablet. Throughout the steps in formulation development, these considerations must be maintained and eventually optimized. The goal must be a baseline formulation having acceptable properties such as hardness, friability, and dissolution, while providing a suitable mouth-feel and sweetness background for flavoring. Appropriate selection of processes and excipients discussed earlier in this chapter, and others, will lead to the development of such a base.

Having succeeded in the preparation of one or more unflavored bases, the development pharmacist should next prepare several basic flavored preference samples. These should be designed to narrow the flavor focus to one or more groups or categories of flavor preferred by decision makers within the company. Tables 4 and 5 provide general guidelines for such preliminary choices based on baseline taste and drug product type.

In creating the preliminary flavor samples, the pharmacist should recognize age-dependent preferences. Children have a high tolerance for sweet and low tolerance for bitter; as age progresses, tolerance for bitter taste increases as the taste buds and olfactory centers lose sensitivity. Generally, mild tastes are less fatiguing and therefore better choices. Menthol, spices, and mint flavors tend to anesthetize the taste buds and reduce flavor reaction. Vanilla, on the other hand, tends to enhance other flavors [33].

As stated previously, flavor houses generally provide flavor development services to their customers. Once preliminary samples have been

Table 4   Suggested Flavor Groups for General Baseline Taste Types

Sweet	Vanilla, stone fruits, grape, berries, maple, honey
Sour (acidic)	Citrus, cherry, raspberry, strawberry, root beer, anise, licorice
Salty	Nutty, buttery, butterscotch, spice, maple, melon, raspberry, mixed citrus, mixed fruit
Bitter	Licorice, anise, coffee, chocolate, wine, mint, grapefruit, cherry, peach, raspberry, nut, fennel, spice
Alkaline	Mint, chocolate, cream, vanilla
Metallic	Grape, burgundy, lemon-lime

Source: Adapted from Refs. 34 and 35.

used to determine flavor category, the pharmacist should turn the remaining flavor development activities over to the flavor chemists. This will require that the company provide samples of the baseline granulation (and tablets) for the chemist to use. The more information that can be provided (under confidentiality agreements or other arrangements), the greater the probability that the supplier can produce the desired result.

Usually a broad range of samples will be created for evaluation by small, informal groups within the company. As development progresses, tablet samples should be evaluated by formal taste panels with appropriate statistical planning to assure final selection of a product with a high probability of success in the marketplace.

D. Flavor Quality Assurance

The qualification of multiple vendors for a specific flavor is a virtual impossibility. Each supplier will produce and provide a proprietary combination

Table 5   Several Commonly Recommended Flavor Applications

Antacids	Cough/cold	Vitamins
Chocolate	Anise birch	Fresh pineapple
Mint (peppermint, spearmint)	Black currant	Grape
Mint anise	Rum peach	Passion fruit
Orange	Spice vanilla	Raspberry
Vanilla	Wild cherry	Strawberry
Bavarian cream	Clove	Almond
Butterscotch	Honey-lemon	Blueberry
Cherry cream punch	Menthol-eucalyptus	Toasted nut

Source: Adapted from Refs. 34 and 35.

with similar, but not absolutely identical, flavors. While the application of
these flavors should be interchangeable, they should be processed through
the raw materials quality control system as unique components. Purchasing contracts and acceptance specifications should be tightly drawn to
assure that batch-to-batch variation is minimized, since these complex
materials are critical to the market acceptance of the product.

This complexity also leads to a potential for instability. Flavors are
highly susceptible to decomposition and/or loss of potency through exposure
to elevated temperature and humidity. The supplier should provide
storage and shelf life information, and such instructions should be followed.

The stability of a flavor compound, in its raw form or in a finished
product, is difficult to follow. Although gas chromatography may be
capable of determining the myriad of components in the flavor, very minor
chemical changes which are analytically undetectable could alter the taste.

In reality, unlike most pharmaceutical ingredients for which the user
shares responsibility with the supplier, the flavor user must rely almost
entirely on the reputation and integrity of the supplier.

E. Flavor/Color Integration

The final aspect of taste psychology requires that the flavor and color
match or correspond. A mismatch may detract from consumer acceptance.
Table 6 provides a general guideline for such matching.

Table 6 Flavors and Corresponding Color Guidelines

Flavor	Color
Cherry, wild cherry, tutti-frutti, raspberry, strawberry, apple	Pink to red
Chocolate, maple, honey, molasses, butterscotch, walnut, burgundy, nut, caramel	Brown
Lemon, lime, orange, mixed citrus, custard, banana, cherry, butterscotch	Yellow to orange
Lime, mint, menthol, peppermint, spearmint, pistachio	Green
Vanilla, custard, mint, spearmint, peppermint, nut, banana, caramel	Off white to white
Grape, plum, licorice	Violet to purple
Mint, blueberry, plum, licorice, mixed fruit	Blue

For speckled tablets, color of speckling or background should correspond to
flavors chosen.

VI. COLORANTS

Colorants are used in the manufacture of chewable tablets for the following reasons:

1. To increase aesthetic appeal to the consumer
2. To aid in product identification and differentiation
3. To mask unappealing or nonuniform color of raw materials
4. To complement and match the flavor used in the formulation

Colorants are available either as natural pigments or synthetic dyes. However, due to their complexity and variability, the natural pigments cannot be certified by the Food and Drug Administration (FDA) as are the synthetic dyes. Certification is the process by which the FDA analyzes batches of certifiable dyes to ascertain their purity levels and compliance with specifications and issues a certified lot number.

The Food Drug and Cosmetic Act of 1938 created three categories of coal tar dyes, of which only the first two are applicable to the manufacture of chewable tablets.

1. FD&C colors: These are colorants that are certifiable for use in foods, drugs, and cosmetics.
2. D&C colors: These are dyes and pigments considered safe for use in drugs and cosmetics when in contact with mucous membranes or when ingested.
3. External D&C: These colorants, due to their oral toxicity, are not certifiable for use in products intended for ingestion but are considered safe for use in products applied externally.

Two main forms of colorants are used in the manufacture of chewable tablets depending on whether the process of manufacture is by wet granulation or direct compression.

A. Dyes

Dyes are chemical compounds that exhibit their coloring power or tinctorial strength when dissolved in a solvent [36]. They are usually 80 to 93% (rarely 94 to 99%) pure colorant material. Dyes are also soluble in propylene glycol and glycerine.

Certifiable colorants, both "primary" and "blends" of two or more primary colorants, are available for use in a number of forms including powder, liquid, granules, plating blends, nonflashing blends, pastes, and dispersions [37]. For the formulation of chewable tablets the powders, liquids or dispersions are used in the wet granulation stage of tablet manufacture. The powders are first dissolved in water or appropriate solvent and used in the granulation process.

Dyes are synthetic, usually cheaper, and are available in a wider range of shades or hues with higher coloring power than the natural pigments.

The physical properties of dyes (particle size, variation in the grinding and drying process, different suppliers) are usually not critical in terms of their ability to produce identically colored systems. The tinctorial strength of a dye is directly proportional to its pure dye content. This means that 1 unit of a 92% pure dye is equivalent to 2 units of a 46% pure dye. Dyes are generally used in the range of 0.01 to 0.03% in chewable tablet formulations, and the particle size range of dyes is usually between 12 and 200 mesh. Dyes used in the wet granulation step are usually dissolved in the granulation fluid; the granulation and drying operations must be optimized to prevent or minimize dye migration. This problem is exceptionally important when dye blends are used, since a "chromatographic" effect may be obtained as the different primary dyes migrate through the granules at different rates leading to nonuniform colored granules.

Solutions of dyes should be made in stainless steel or glass-lined tanks (for minimization of dye—container incompatibility) with moderate mixing and should routinely be filtered to remove any undissolved dye particles. Dye solutions in water that are intended to be stored for 24 hr or more should be adequately preserved to prevent microbial contamination. Suitable preservatives include propylene glycol, sodium benzoate with phosphoric acid or with citric acid.

During storage, use, and processing, dyes should be protected against

1. Oxidizing agents, especially chlorine and hypochlorites.
2. Reducing agents, especially invert sugars, some flavors, metallic ions (especially aluminum, zinc, tin, and iron), and ascorbic acid.
3. Microorganisms, especially mold and reducing bacteria.
4. Extreme pH levels; especially FD&C Red #3 which is insoluble in acid media and should not be used below pH 5.0. Also, effects of fading agents such as metals are greatly enhanced by either very high or low pH values.
5. Prolonged high heat—only FD&C Red #3 is stable on exposure to prolonged high heat. Thus, dyes should be processed at low to moderate temperatures and should have only very brief exposure to moderate or high heat levels. The negative activity of reducing and oxidizing agents is greatly enhanced by elevated temperatures.
6. Exposure to direct sunlight—FD&C Red #40 and FD&C Yellow #5 have moderate stability to light, while FD&C Blue #2 and FD&C Red #3 have poor light stability. It is important to minimize the exposure of products to direct sunlight, especially products containing dye blends.

To compensate for losses due to fading and other dye loss during processing and storage, some formulators add a slight excess of dye at the beginning. This approach should be cautiously employed since one can obtain unattractive shades when too much color is added at the beginning in an attempt to provide for time-dependent or processing color loss.

Regulations covering all aspects of colorants, including their procedures for use, provisionally and permanently certified and uncertified color additives, and use levels and restrictions for each coloring additive, are covered in the Code of Federal Regulations 21 CFR parts 70 through 82.

Regulatory updates on color additives should be monitored by formulators using colorants. These updates and revisions are published in the Federal Register.

Concerns still persist about the safety of absorbable dyes despite completed studies done so far. This has led dye manufacturers and suppliers to develop and test nonabsorbable dyes, which are considered safer by virtue of their nonabsorption from the gastrointestinal tract. Long-term feeding studies using animals are continuing since 1977 and, if the profiles are good, approvals may be expected in the not too distant future.

B. Lakes

Lakes have been defined by the FDA as the "aluminum salts of FD&C water-soluble dyes extended on a substratum of alumina." Lakes prepared by extending the calcium salts of the FD&C dyes are also permitted but to date none has been made. Lakes also must be certified by the FDA.

Lakes, unlike dyes, are insoluble and color by dispersion. Consequently, the particle size of lakes is very critical to their coloring capacity or tinctorial strength. Generally, the smaller the particle size, the higher the tinctorial strength of lakes due to increased surface area for reflected light.

Lakes are formed by the precipitation and absorption of a dye on an insoluble base or substrate. The base for the FD&C lakes is alumina hydrate. The method of preparation of the alumina hydrate and the conditions under which the dye is added or absorbed determines the shade, particle size, dispersability, as well as tinctorial strength. Other important variables are the temperature, concentration of reactants, final pH, and the speed and type of agitation [36].

Lakes contain 1 to 45% pure dye but, unlike dyes, the tinctorial strength is not proportional to the pure dye content. Also, the shade or hue of a lake varies with the pure dye content.

Particle size of lakes is in the range of 0.5 to 5 μm, but the micrometer and submicrometer size leads to significant electrostatic cohesive forces causing particles to agglomerate to 40 to 100 μm. For effective use in direct-compression formulation of chewable tablets, lakes should preferably be deagglomerated to their original particle size ranges by premixing them with some of the inert ingredients in a formulation using high-shear mixers and finally incorporating the rest of the ingredients.

FD&C lakes are available in six basic colors: one yellow, one orange, two reds (a pink-red and an orange-red), and two blues (a green-blue and a royal blue). Blends are available to provide more lake colors as needed including brown, green, orange, red, yellow, and purple.

Lakes are used in chewable tablets made by direct compression in a concentration range of 0.1 to 0.3%. They possess a higher light and heat stability than dyes, are quite inert, and are compatible with most ingredients used in chewable tablets.

Lakes are usually used in the direct-compression method of chewable tablet manufacturing. However, some unique cases of wet granulation may also call for the use of lakes. These unique cases involve "chromatographic effects" previously described when blends of soluble dyes are used in the granulation step. This problem can be resolved by using lake blends instead of dye blends since lakes, being insoluble, do not migrate during massing and drying of granules.

Table 7 gives some physical and chemical properties of certified colors.

Table 7   Physical and Chemical Properties of Certified Colors

FD&C Name (common name)	Chemical class	Stability to			Tinctorial strength	Hue	Solubility (g/100 ml) at 25°C	
		Light	Oxidation	pH Change			Water	25% EtOH
Red No. 3 (Erythrosine)	Xanthine	Poor	Fair	Poor	V. good	Bluish pink	9	8
Red No. 40	Monoazo	V. good	Fair	Good	V. good	Yellowish red	22	9.5
Yellow No. 6 (Sunset Yellow FCF)	Monoazo	Moderate	Fair	Good	Good	Reddish	19	10
Yellow No. 5 (Tartrazine)	Pyrazolone	Good	Fair	Good	Good	Lemon yellow	20	12
Green No. 3 (Fast Green FCF)	TPM[a]	Fair	Poor	Good	Excellent	Bluish green	20	20
Blue No. 1 (Brilliant Blue FCF)	TPM[a]	Fair	Poor	Good	Excellent	Greenish blue	20	20
Blue No. 2 (Indigotine)	Indigoid	V. Poor	Poor	Poor	Poor	Deep blue	1.6	0.5

[a]Triphenyl methane.
Source: Adapted from Ref. 37.

VII. MANUFACTURING

A. General Considerations

Four important aspects of chewable tablet manufacture are the proper incorporation of the coloring agent, assurance of necessary particle size distribution, maintenance of correct moisture content, and achievement of proper
tablet hardness. All of these are the routine responsibility of the manufacturing department once the parameters have been established during
development. It is therefore critical that process development and scale-up
considerations be thoroughly explored in order to ensure the establishment
of proper specifications.

As with all types of tablets, if the granulating process involves wet
granulation, the extent of wetting and the rate and extent of drying must
be defined. Overwetting can be expected to produce harder granules that
may have poor compressional characteristics, resulting in softer and more
friable tablets. Due to the lesser degree of particle deformation, these
tablets often have a gritty mouth-feel when chewed. Overwetting during
granulation also leads to longer drying times in order to achieve the
desired moisture level or, worse, a higher moisture level due to failure to
compensate through adjustment of the drying cycle. Improper wetting
and drying may also adversely affect the particle size distribution, leading
to ineffective postgranulation blending, poorer flow, and increased weight
variation.

Also, the method and appropriate order for the addition of the flavor
and color must be determined if wet granulation is being used. Since most
flavor substances are volatile, they cannot be subjected to elevated temperature. For this reason, they cannot be incorporated prior to granulation;
rather, flavors are added (often as premixes) in the final blending operation of the process. The color, if in the form of a lake, would be incorporated in the same step. The concentrations of these ingredients normally
do not exceed 0.1% and generally would be even lower. An important consideration is the assurance of uniform blending; rarely would analytical
methods be used to establish flavor or color uniformity. Since the final
blending step may require the combining of a 99:1 materials ratio, the
establishment and validation of this operation is extremely important.

The uniformity of color incorporation needs to be viewed from the perspective of performance. If color is used in the form of a dye added to a
wet granulation, the final blending operation usually consists of the addition of uncolored (white?) powders (lubricants, etc.) to colored granules.
It is assumed that the white powder will uniformly coat the colored granules,
thus resulting in an even distribution of color. However, when these
granules fracture during compression, the uniformity will often be disturbed,
resulting in tablets having lighter or deeper color on the opposite background; this is referred to as "mottling."

On the other hand, if color is added as a lake following granulation
(or to a direct-compression blend), then the blending operation consists
of the addition of colored powder to uncolored (white?) granules. Again,
it is assumed that the colored powder will uniformly coat the white
granules. However, during compression, the granules fracture and release
fresh white material to the surface, resulting in white spots on a colored
background, or vice versa ("speckling"). In either case, the result is a
less than elegant finished product. Since the visible problem in both cases

may be reduced through lessening the color contrast between the materials, two common approaches are the use of low concentrations of light colors and the use of high-intensity mixing of reduced particle size materials in order to assure thorough blending.

B. Antacids

Antacid products compose a rather large percentage of the over-the-counter (OTC) drug market. Efficacy studies [38,39] have questioned the comparative efficacy of chewable antacid tablets to their suspension antacid counterparts due to the state of hydration of the latter. However, the inconvenience of carrying a bottle of liquid and a measuring device is obvious. Consequently, the user is faced with a choice between convenience and possibly greater efficacy. Most choose the convenience of the solid form at least when away from home, and probably all of the time.

Few antacid tablets specifically formulated for swallowing are presently marketed. All other solid antacid products currently available are in the form of chewable tablets, chewing gum, or chewy squares.

From a formulation perspective, antacids present extreme difficulty due to the nature and quantity of the active ingredients. They are generally metallic, astringent, chalky, and/or gritty, thus providing a combination of bad taste and bad mouth-feel to be overcome. In addition, the usually high dosage levels required result in very large tablets (typically 5/8-in. diameter, 700 to 1000 mg weight), with two tablets the normal dose. This quantity of material, coupled with the frequency of dosing, may lead to taste fatigue even with a good-tasting product; one that is poor or mediocre will quickly lose acceptability in the marketplace.

Table 8 provides a list of the commonly used antacids; generally, these are used in combinations of two or more to provide better therapeutic action.

Table 8 Common Antacid Drugs and Some Typical
Dose Ranges

Aluminum hydroxide	80–600 mg
Calcium carbonate	194–850 mg
Magnesium hydroxide/oxide	65–400 mg
Magnesium trisilicate	20–500 mg
Others	
Aluminum carbonate	—
Dihydroxyaluminum aminoacetate	—
Dihydroxyaluminum sodium carbonate	—
Magnesium carbonate	—
Magnesium gluconate	—
Potassium bicarbonate	—
Sodium bicarbonate	—

Source: Compiled from Ref. 40.

In addition to the antacid components, other ingredients are often found in these products as adjunct actives. These include simethicone (dimethicone, dimethyl polysiloxane) at a level of 20 to 40 mg per tablet as an antiflatulent. Peppermint oil, approximately 3 mg per tablet, is sometimes used as a carminative. Alginic acid, 200 to 400 mg, is also used by at least one company.

Following are two examples of antacid tablet formulations. Example 3 is a dextrose (Dextrates)-based direct-compaction system, while Example 4 is a sucrose (compressible sugar)-based product.

Example 3:   Chewable Antacid Tablets

Ingredient	mg/tablet
FMA-11* (Reheis Chemical)	400.00
Syloid 244	50.00
Emdex	1100.00
Pharmasweet Powder (Crompton and Knowles)	20.00
Magnesium stearate	16.00
Total Weight	1586.00

1. Mix FMA-11 and Syloid together for 5 min. Screen through 30-mesh screen (if ingredients not already pre-screened) and mix for 10 to 15 min.
2. Add Emdex and Pharmasweet to step 1 and blend thoroughly for 10 to 15 min.
3. Add magnesium stearate to step 2, blend 5 min, and compress.

*Aluminum hydroxide/magnesium carbonate codried gel.
Note: An appropriate flavor may be added in step 2.
Source: Ref. 27.
Comments: FMA-11 is a very fine powder that tends to "slip" rather than flow, thereby leading to blending problems and overfilling of the tablet machine feed frame. Syloid, a synthetic silica, acts as a glidant to improve flow characteristics. Pharmasweet, in conjunction with Emdex, provides sufficient sweetness to compensate for the bland chalkiness of the antacid.

Example 4:   Antacid Tablet Direct Compression

Ingredient	mg/tablet
Aluminum hydroxide and magnesium carbonate codried gel (Reheis FMA-11)	325.0
Di-Pac DTE	675.0
Microcrystalline cellulose (Avicel)	75.0
Starch	30.0
Calcium stearate	22.0
Flavor	q.s.

Mix all ingredients and compress on standard 5/8-in. flat-face bevel edge punch to a hardness of 8–11 SCA units.
Source: Ref. 25.
Comments: This formulation is similar to Example 3. Two differences are the slightly higher drug load (29% versus 25%) and the replacement of Dextrates with Compressible Sugar. If desired, the formula could alternatively be wet-granulated using water to wet the sugar and cellulose.

C.   Cough/Cold Analgesics

The primary appeal of products in this category is the pediatric market into the teens. Generally, levels of the drugs are one-quarter or less of the adult dose, which would require the use of a large number of tablets by an adult. Despite the extremely large market, the industry has failed to exploit the potential of adult strength chewable tablets and the patient convenience such products might provide.

Drugs commonly encountered include aspirin, acetaminophen, chlorpheniramine, phenylpropanolamine, pseudoephedrine, and dextromethorphan. These may be used alone or in various combinations with appropriate attention to possible incompatibilities. The one common property all of these drugs share is unpleasant taste. Aspirin is acidic and astringent; the others are all very bitter.

None, except acetaminophen, present compressibility problems; aspirin is relatively compressible, and the others are used in low doses and therefore low percentage compositions. Acetaminophen has inherently poor compressibility, although newer, directly compressible forms are marketed by some suppliers. These have previously been granulated by the producer to prepare them for tableting; the alternative for chewable tablets is a wet granulation process, as illustrated in Example 5.

The other drug products mentioned can be produced by direct compression, as shown in Examples 6 and 7.

Incompatible drugs that may be desirable in combination, such as aspirin and phenylpropanolamine, require special treatment as they would in a nonchewable tablet. The drugs must be kept separated; this can be accomplished through the multilayer technology or through coating one or both drugs prior to blending.

Example 5:   Chewable Acetaminophen Tablet (Wet Granulation)

Ingredient	Quantity per tablet
Mannitol, USP	720.0 mg
Sodium saccharin	6.0 mg
Acetaminophen, N.F. (S. B. Penick, coarse granular)	120.0 mg
Binder solution	21.6 mg*
Peppermint oil	0.5 mg
Syloid 244	0.5 mg
Banana, Permaseal F-4932	2.0 mg
Anise, Permaseal F-2837	2.0 mg
Sodium chloride (powdered)	6.0 mg
Magnesium stearate	27.5 mg
	906.0 mg

*Includes 5.4 mg acacia and 16.2 mg gelatin.
First, prepare a binder solution consisting of:

Acacia (powdered)	15 g
Gelatin (granular)	45 g
Water	q.s. ad 400 ml

Screen the mannitol and sodium saccharin through a 40-mesh screen.
Blend thoroughly with the acetaminophen. Using 180 ml of binder solution
per 1000 tablets, granulate and dry overnight at 140 to 150°F.   Screen
through a 12-mesh screen.   Adsorb the peppermint oil onto the Syloid 244
and mix with the flavors and sodium chloride. Blend this flavor mixture,
the dried granulation, and the magnesium stearate. Compress on 1/2-in.
flat-face bevel edge punches to a hardness of 12 to 15 kg.
Comments: Acetaminophen is generally regarded as very difficult to compress, and usually is processed by wet granulation in order to permit
higher drug loading. The acacia-gelatin binder provides high tablet
strength; the solution should be freshly prepared to prevent microbial
growth.

Example 6: Chewable Children's Antihistamine Tablets

Ingredients	mg/tablet
Phenylpropanolamine HCl	9.375
Chlorpheniramine maleate	1.000
Emdex	363.365
Magna Sweet 165 (MacAndrews & Forbes)	0.960
Flavor, Artificial Red Punch. S.D. (Crompton & Knowles)	1.900
Color, cherry (Crompton & Knowles)	0.560
Magnesium stearate	2.840
Total weight	380.000

1. Mix phenylpropanolamine and Emdex together for 10 min.
2. To a small portion of 1 add chlorpheniramine and Magna Sweet and mix for 15 to 20 min.
3. Mix 1 and 2 together. Add flavor and blend for 10 to 15 min.
4. To 3 add color and mix for 20 to 25 min.
5. Add magnesium stearate, blend 5 min and compress.

Source: Ref. 27.

Comments: The combination antihistamine-decongestant is commonly used for both allergy and upper respiratory tract infections. The apparent potential incompatibility between the amine drugs and dextrate excipient does not cause discoloration except in the presence of moisture and heat. Often, it is desirable to add aspirin or another analgesic for pain and fever; the combination should be expected to exhibit poor stability unless separated by techniques such as the use of multilayer tablets.

D. Vitamins/Minerals/Food Supplements

It has long been common medical practice to supplement the diet with vitamin-mineral products from infancy into elderliness. Although such products may be presumed unnecessary for those who consume an appropriate diet, it is generally recognized that the likelihood of widespread proper dietary habit is low.

In infancy, vitamin supplements are provided as liquids for "dropper" dosage. Usually, at around the age of 2 or 3, children are switched to a chewable multivitamin, with or without fluoride depending on local water supplies. Because of the age group for which these products are intended, the combinations tend to be limited and of relatively low dosage. At least one manufacturer, however, produces a higher strength product for older children. There appears to be no product in the marketplace intended for adults.

Children's vitamins in recent years have become extremely complex from a manufacturing and tooling perspective. Marketing pressures have dictated the adoption of extraordinarily detailed shapes such as cartoon characters, animals, etc., designed to stimulate sales through appeal to children. Such tablets require punches and dies with numerous compound

Example 7:   Children's Buffered Aspirin
Chewable Tablet

Ingredients	mg/tablet
Aluminum hydroxide dried gel	13 mg
Aspirin, 40-mesh crystals	81 mg
Talc	2 mg
Primogel	8 mg
NuTab	93.4 mg
Mafco Magnasweet-150	0.6 mg
Orange flavor (F&F no. 11598)	2 mg

1.   Blend the NuTab and aluminum hydroxide
     dried gel for 10 min.
2.   Add the aspirin and blend for an addi-
     tional 5 min.
3.   Premix the Primogel, talc, flavor, and
     Magnasweet and pass through a 60-mesh
     screen.
4.   Add the premix and blend for an addi-
     tional 5 min.
Comments: The combination of NuTab and
Magnasweet adds sufficient sweetness to offset the tartness of the aspirin and the orange
flavor.   In the dry state, there is no incompatible reactivity between the acidic aspirin
and alkaline aluminum hydroxide.

curves and punch faces with many detail markings.   These require optimized formulations and manufacturing processes in order to ensure acceptable appearance quality levels.

The total active ingredient content is high and consists of a combination of difficult tastes.   Barry and Weiss [41] described the basic taste
characteristics of various vitamins as follows:

Vitamin A acetate, vitamin D_2 (ergocalciferol), and vitamin E (DL-
   tocopheryl acetate):   "substantially tasteless"
Vitamin B_1 (thiamine hydrochloride or nitrate):   "yeasty," bitter
Vitamin B_6 (pyridoxine hydrochloride):   slightly bitter, slightly salty
Vitamin B_{12} (cyanocobalamin):   tasteless
Niacinamide: very bitter
Vitamin C (ascorbic acid):   sour
Vitamin C (sodium ascorbate):   less sour, salty, somewhat "soapy"
Calcium pantothenate: bitter
Biotin: tasteless
Folic acid: nearly tasteless
Minerals (e.g., iron salts):   metallic

A multivitamin and mineral mixture will have a combination of bitter plus sour plus salty plus metallic tastes. The sourness can be depressed by adding sweetness via the vehicle (e.g., mannitol) and additional sweetener (e.g., saccharin sodium). The sourness is further depressed by a careful choice of the ratio of ascorbic acid to sodium ascorbate so as to retard the acidity, and by adding a citrus flavor that corresponds to the degree of tartness chosen [41]. Ferrous fumarate and ferric pyrophosphate are relatively tasteless compared to other iron salts. A further reduction in the metallic taste of ferrous fumarate has been accomplished by a patented coating process in which the iron salt is coated with at least one of the following: a monoglyceride or a diglyceride of a saturated fatty acid, using spray-congealing technique [42]. Other mineral salts that are "practically nonmetallic" in taste include manganese glycerophosphate, zinc oxide, magnesium oxide, and dibasic calcium phosphate, all of which can be used to provide the corresponding trace metals desired in the vitamin-mineral combination formula. Finally, the bitterness must be masked. For best results, the B-complex group of vitamins are chosen in individually coated forms known as Rocoat vitamins, which are prepared by spray congealing of the vitamins with monoglycerides and diglycerides of edible fatty acids. The end product has a vitamin/fat ratio of 1:3. Niacinamide is also available in this form. Vitamin B_{12} is available in gelatin (0.1%) or as Stablets (1%). Vitamins A and D are also available as free-flowing powders protected in a matrix of gelatin, sugars or starches, and preservatives—and are known as Crystalets or Beadlets. Vitamin E is available as an adsorbed dry powder or as microbeadlets [41]. After a choice has been made of the minerals, the physical form of the B-complex vitamins, niacinamide, vitamins A, E, and D, and the ratio of ascorbic acid to sodium ascorbate, the final flavoring must be chosen. The approach [41,43] is to blend out the overall taste of the formula so that the vitamin taste becomes part of the flavor impression by adding appropriate flavors and flavor enhancers that complement the tartness, saltiness, sourness, and sweetness already present in the baseline formulation. The complementary flavors recommended [41,43] are citrus, mint, apricot, cherry, orange, peach, strawberry, raspberry, wintergreen, pineapple, and cherry (among many other potential candidates).

A typical directly compressible multivitamin with iron is illustrated in Example 8.

The most common single-vitamin product is vitamin C, which often is desirable in chewable tablet form. Since ascorbic acid is extremely sour tasting, additional steps are usually taken to improve the flavor. A combination of ascorbic acid and sodium ascorbate, both of which are available in direct-compression form, is less sour and therefore easier to flavor (see Example 9). Another approach (Example 10) requires coating the ascorbic acid with ethylcellulose to reduce its solubility and therefore its sourness. Generally, citrus flavors are preferred to compliment the taste.

An excellent account of the stability and incompatibility of various vitamins has been given by Macek [45]. The following is a brief summary of the most pertinent aspects as they relate to chewable tablets.

General: Minimum exposure to heat and moisture during processing and in final product (around 1%) is highly desirable. Vitamins A, B_1, B_2, B_{12}, C, and pantothenic acid are relatively more unstable.

Example 8:   Chewable Multivitamin Tablets

Ingredients	mg/tablet	Equivalent to
Vitamin A acetate (Roche)	12.50	5000 IU
Vitamin D_1 (Roche)	4.50	
Vitamin D_2 (Roche)	0.58	400 IU
Vitamin E, 50% SD (Roche)	33.00	15 IU
Ascorbic acid 90% (Roche)	67.00	60 mg vit. C
Folic acid	0.40	0.4 mg
Vitamin B_2 (Rocoat 33-1/3%)	5.20	1.7 mg
Vitamin B_6 (Rocoat 33-1/3%)	6.00	2.0 mg
Vitamin B_{12} (0.1% SD—Roche)	6.00	6.0 μg
Niacinamide (Rocoat 33-1/3%)	60.00	20.0 mg
Ferrous fumarate, coated	18.00	
Pharmasweet Powder (Crompton & Knowles)	8.70	
Natural orange flavor S.D. (Crompton & Knowles)	10.90	
Emdex	938.52	
Color Orange No. S3182 (Crompton & Knowles)	q.s.	
Magnesium stearate	8.70	
Total weight	1180.00	

1. Mix Vitamins D_1, D_2, folic acid, and B_{12} with niacinamide for 15 min.
2. To 1 add vitamins A, E, ascorbic acid, B_2, B_6, ferrous fumarate, small portion of Emdex, and mix thoroughly for 15 min.
3. To 2 add remaining Emdex, flavor, and Pharmasweet and mix for 10 to 15 min.
4. Add color to 3 and blend thoroughly until it is evenly distributed.
5. Add magnesium stearate to 3, blend 5 min, and compress.
Source: Ref. 27.
Comments: Common practice for multivitamin preparation is to use wet granulation in order to process the large amount and number of multiple active ingredients. This example demonstrates the feasibility of using direct compaction—in this case based on Emdex—despite the presence of 11 actives.

Example 9: Vitamin C Chewable Tablets (250 mg)

Ingredients	A	B	C
Sodium ascorbate (SA-99)[1]	170.5	170.5	170.5
Ascorbic acid (C-97)[1]	103.5	103.5	103.5
Compressible sucrose[2]	336.0	—	—
Compressible natural sugar[3]	—	389.8	—
Crystalline sorbitol	—	—	335.3
Sodium saccharin	—	—	0.7
FD&C Yellow #6 Lake (jet-milled)	2.0	2.2	2.0
Flavoring	5.0	5.5	5.0
Magnesium stearate	3.0	4.0	3.0
Total	620.0	675.5	620.0

[1]Takeda Chemical Industries.

[2]Di-Pac, Amstar Corp.

[3]Sweetrex, Edward Mendell Co.
Actives, lake, flavor, and sweeteners are mixed for 25 min in a P-K blender. Magnesium stearate is screened, added, and blended for an additional 10 min.
Source: Ref. 44.

Example 10: Ascorbic Acid Chewable Tablets (250 mg)

Ingredients	mg/tablet
Ascorbic acid (10% excess)	275.0
Ethocel 7 cps, 10% in isopropanol	q.s.
NuTab	275.0
Sta-Rx 1500	50.0
Sodium saccharin	1.0
FD&C lake	q.s.
Flavor	q.s.
Magnesium stearate	5.0

1. Granulate the ascorbic acid with the ethyl-cellulose in isopropanol in a planetary mixer.
2. Dry overnight at 50°C; screen through a 16-mesh.
3. Add the NuTab and Sta-Rx 1500 and mix for 15 min in a P-K blender without intensifier.
4. Add the sodium saccharin, lake, flavor, and magnesium stearate, previously premixed and screened.
5. Blend for 5 additional min.

Coating vitamins individually or together in compatible groups is desirable to minimize incompatibilities.

Vitamin A: Sensitive to oxidation. Palmitate and, more commonly, acetate esters coated with gelatin or gelatin-starch are used (Crystalets and Beadlets). The all-trans isomer is most active biologically but chemical assay will not differentiate it from the other isomers.

Vitamin B_1: Sensitive to oxidation and reduction. A pH environment above 3 to 4 is undesirable. Thiamine mononitrate is preferred since incompatibility with pantothenic acid is diminished by the nitrate salt. Pentothenyl alcohol or calcium pantothenate and thiamine mononitrate are preferred. Coated vitamin is preferable.

Vitamin B_2: Sensitive to light. The riboflavin base of 5'-phosphate sodium salt is used. Coated vitamin is preferable. A pH in the alkaline range is undesirable. Protection from reducing agents is desirable.

Vitamin C: Very sensitive to oxidation, and is a strong reducing agent. Presence of copper or iron increases oxidation rate. Sodium ascorbate or a mixture of the salt and free acid may be preferable.

Vitamin B_{12}: Susceptible to loss of activity by reducing agent (e.g., ascorbic acid). A pH environment of 4 to 7 is optimal. Other detrimental factors could be ferrous salts, decomposition products of thiamine, and some flavors. Vitamin B_{12} resin complex, 1% (Stablets) or 0.1% in gelatin concentrate is preferred.

Pantothenic acid: The acid itself is not used. Calcium salt is preferred since it is a soluble crystalline powder as opposed to the acid or the alcohol, both of which are viscous oils. The salt and the acid are sensitive to acid, base, and heat. The optimal pH is 6. The incompatibility with thiamine is discussed above.

Davis [46] prepared vitamin C and multivitamin formulations to evaluate coarse powder sorbitol as a chewable tablet base. Of concern was the potential of hardness gain and attempts to ameliorate the problem through the incorporation of various starch excipients. He found that the inclusion of 5 to 8% pregelatinized modified cornstarch (Dura Gel DGD) helped maintain proper hardness during storage without affecting hygroscopicity/weight gain.

VIII.   EVALUATION OF CHEWABLE TABLETS

A.   In-Process Organoleptic Evaluation

Organoleptic evaluation takes place at various stages in the development of a chewable tablet. These follow in sequence at various stages as shown in Table 9.

The evaluation of the drug substance itself (stage 1) has already been briefly discussed in this chapter. Stages 1, 2, and 3 are generally carried out by the formulating pharmacist either alone or in collaboration with a small taste panel within a development laboratory. Since organoleptic evaluation is subjective in nature, it is necessary to have the terminology, comparative standards, and test conditions well defined and controlled for

Table 9 Various Stages of Organoleptic Evaluation

Designation	Stage of organoleptic evaluation	It involves:
1	Evaluation of the drug substance itself	Characterization and comparison of the drug substance in an absolute sense or against a known reference standard
2	Evaluation of coated (e.g., granulated) or treated (e.g., adsorbed) drug	Comparison against the pure drug as well as different coatings or treatment approaches
3	Evaluation of unflavored baseline formulation	Comparisons among different vehicles, proportions of vehicles, or other formulation variables (except flavors) in presence of coated or treated drug
4	Evaluation of flavored baseline formulation	Comparison among different flavored formulations
5	Final selection and product acceptance test	Comparison between two "top-candidate" formulations and/or a competitive product

meaningful results. For example, Borodkin and Sundberg [47] evaluated methapyrilene, dextromethorphan, ephedrine, and pseudoephedrine for their basic bitterness (stage 1), followed by the taste comparison of these drugs after adsorption onto a polycarboxylic acid ion exchange resin (stage 2). The resin adsorbates were further coated with a 4:1 ethyl cellulose—hydroxypropylmethylcellulose polymer at various concentrations of coatings. Comparisons were made against pure drug, adsorbed drug, and adsorbed drug with variable coating percentages (stage 2). The coated adsorbates were blended with other tableting excipients, such as a sweetener, magnesium stearate, and mannitol vehicle in standard proportions (i.e., baseline unflavored formulations). These formulations, in tableted forms, were compared with the respective coated and uncoated adsorbates and the pure drugs (stage 3). For comparative quantitation, caffeine solutions were chosen as the standards for bitterness intensity on a scale of 0 to 3, 3 being strong bitterness (0.2% caffeine), 2 being moderate (0.1% caffeine), 1 being slight (0.05% caffeine), x being threshold (0.001% caffeine), and 0 being no taste (water) [47].

The panel in the caffeine-dextromethorphan study consisted of at least seven members of each sample, using a so-called time intensity method in which the sample equivalent to one dose is held in the mouth (or chewed, in the case of tablets) for 10 sec. The readings are taken immediately and at several intervals over a period of 15 min. The type of quantitative information generated in the study is shown, using the bitterness scale of 0 to 3, in Table 10.

Table 10 Bitterness Evaluation of Dextromethorphan HBr at Various Stages of Product Development

Form of dextromethorphan hydrobromide	Degree of bitterness after time					
	10 sec	1 min	2 min	5 min	10 min	15 min
Uncoated drug *powder*	>3	>3	2.5	1.5	1	0.5
Uncoated adsorbate *powder*	2	2	1.5	0.5	x	0
Uncoated adsorbate in *tablet*	1.5	1.5	1.5 to 2	1.5	1	x
Powder adsorbate coated with 25.4% polymer	0.5	x to 0.5	x	x	0	0
Adsorbate powder coated with 25.4% polymer in *tablet*	x to 0.5	0.5	x	x	x	0

Source: From Ref. 47.

Table 10 serves to illustrate that, although adsorption does reduce bitterness, it is necessary to reduce it further by polymeric coating. The uncoated adsorbate in the mannitol-based tablet formulation is much more bitter than the tablet made with the coated adsorbate. Another interesting observation is that there is apparently little or no difference in the bitterness of the coated adsorbate in powder form or when compounded with the mannitol-based tablet formulation under the conditions of this evaluation. A possible explanation is the fact that the coating is disrupted to some extent during compression as well as during mastication of the tablet, thus exposing the bitter substance. At this point in development the formulator should overcome the residual bitterness by a proper choice of flavors. Stages 1, 2, and 3 (Table 9) involve the evaluation of the *extent* of taste masking in *unflavored* preparations while stages 4 and 5 involve the evaluation of the *preferences* among *flavored* baseline formulations. Although the extent of testing is a matter of relative quantitation, and hence relatively easy to control, the preference testing is a matter of determining individual choices of the panelists, which are subject to significant variability. Thus, the selection of the panelists and their number are important factors in establishing a preference-testing panel. For example, during the final selection and product acceptance test (stage 5, Table 9) of a chewable multivitamin product for children, as many as 100 or more panelists representing the ultimate consumer age group are necessary [41]. Certain additional guidelines are noteworthy insofar as taste panels are concerned.

1. Conditions of testing must be optimized. These conditions include the temperature of the sample (e.g., a freshly removed sample from a refrigerator or a 40°C stability oven will taste *significantly*

different than the same sample at 25°C), a well-ventilated room, the absence of distracting noise, and the presence of muted light.

2. Rapid succession (frequency) of samples quickly fatigues the tongue, thus leading to erroneous conclusions. Sampling time should be standardized.

3. A certain "washout" treatment between samples is often recommended (e.g., fixed quantity of water with a saltine cracker).

4. Any unsolicited comments (e.g., chalky, cooling, delicious, tangy, gritty) must be recorded.

5. The panelists should not be grouped but rather should be individualized (e.g., in a compartmented room), and the panel should reflect the age and sex of the eventual consumer [41].

6. Whenever possible, the dosage should be close to the actual intended dose.

7. It is imperative that a statistician be involved in the design of the test protocol.

8. For chewable vitamin formulations, no more than two samples should be given for comparison, and the order of submission should be randomized.

9. It is best to have panelists who have had no prior experience with the test products.

10. Questions concerning acceptance, rejection, preference, and similar items should be reserved until after the panelist has made the selection.

B. Chemical Evaluation

This aspect involves total drug assay and content uniformity testing if applicable.

Assay for Drug Content

A suitable analytical method (chromatographic, titrimetric, spectrophotometric, etc.) is used to determine the active drug content on a representative sample (usually an aliquot of 20 randomly selected tablets after pulverization). The recovered amount of active drug is then expressed as percent of labeled drug content. The obtained value of drug content should be within established limits.

Dosage Uniformity

This test is done to ensure that the batch of tablets is uniform as to the content of active ingredient per dosage unit within specified limits. If the drug level in the dosage unit is high, then a weight variation test is sufficient to indicate uniformity of drug content in the dosage units. However, if the drug dose is low compared to the weight of the dosage unit, as is usually the case with chewable tablets where provision is made for a large use of sweet excipients, coating agents, and/or for taste masking and mouth-feel, then individual assay of the given number of randomly selected dosage units is done to obtain drug content in the various samples tested. The coefficient of variation gives an indication of the uniformity or non-uniformity of the tested units in the batch. The U.S. Pharmacopeia (USP) gives in detail the protocol and acceptance criteria for the determination of dosage form uniformity for conventional tablets, which is also applicable to chewable tablets.

In Vitro and In Vivo Evaluation (Antacid Tablets)

Since antacids represent a sizable proportion of chewable tablets, a description of their in vitro and in vivo evaluation is considered important.

Antacid tablets are meant to exert their effect *in* the stomach, and hence the *gastric bioactivity* is of prime concern. Analogous to the rate and extent of bioavailability, an antacid preparation should be evaluated for its rate and extent of action and total acid-consuming capacity during in vitro and in vivo testing.

In the United States a product may be labeled as an antacid only if it meets a prescribed test [48], which in principle is as follows: the tablets are comminuted to a particle size between 20 and 100 mesh (U.S. standard sieve), and an accurately weighed amount equivalent to the minimum labeled dosage is mixed with 40 ml of water under standard conditions for 1 min. Then 10 ml of 0.5 N HCl is added to the slurry and stirred under fixed conditions for 10 min. The pH of the mixture is then read. If the pH is below 3.5, the product is not permitted to be labeled as an antacid.

The U.S. Food and Drug Administration (FDA) has also defined the minimum requirement for an antacid product in terms of its acid-neutralizing capacity [48].

The sample is prepared in essentially the same manner as described above—up to the addition of water. A standard volume of 1.0 N HCl is then added and mixed for a fixed period of time, immediately followed by the back-titration of the excess acid with 0.5 N NaOH to a stable pH of 3.5. The total number of milliequivalents (mEq) of the acid neutralized by the product under test are then calculated. The requirement is that no product shall be marketed with an acid-neutralizing capacity below 5 mEq. The capacity is expressed in terms of the dosage recommended per minimum time interval or, if the labeling recommends more than one dosage, in terms of the minimum dosage recommended per minimum time interval. For compliance purposes, the value determined by this test at any time (during the expiration period of the product) must be at least 90% of the labeled value.

While the determination of the acid-neutralizing capacity is an important in vitro parameter, the onset (rate) and duration of the neutralizing action are equally important. Smyth et al. [49], for example, studied these aspects and their correlation with in vivo results in human subjects using two in vitro methods known as Bachrach titration [50] and modified Beekman procedure [51]. In principle, both methods are based on the neutralization of an acid by the antacid preparation under study.

Using Bachrach titration [50], Smyth et al. [49] showed that a fixed quantity of a tablet powder in a fixed volume of water had an initial pH of 8.66, which was initially lowered to 3.5 (onset) within 60 sec by the addition of 1.1 ml of 0.8 N HCl. To maintain the pH at 3.5 (for at least 30 sec), 4.9 ml of the acid (capacity) was required, and the endpoint was reached at 13.8 min (duration). Further addition of the acid resulted in the lowering of the pH below 3.5 (i.e., capacity exhausted). These data, when compared to those for suspension containing an equivalent stoichiometric quantity of the active ingredient, indicated that the suspension required a larger volume of the acid (1.8 ml) for initial onset, and that it took a longer time (75 sec) for the acid to initially bring the pH to 3.5.

Further, more acid (5.4 ml) was needed to reach the endpoint. Thus all observations seemed to lead to the conclusion that apparently the suspension was somewhat superior to the chewable tablets containing the same active ingredient. A similar statement is found in the literature elsewhere [52] (i.e., that antacids in tablet form are less effective than liquid or powdered preparations). In another in vitro experiment, however, Smyth et al. [49] found the two dosage forms to be comparable.

In the same study [49], the second in vitro method, known as the modified Beekman procedure [51], consisted of adding the antacid preparation (tablet, powder, or suspension) to a 50-ml volume of 0.1 N HCl at 37°C. With continuous agitation, more acid was added (by a pump) continuously at a fixed rate, and the antacid-acid mixture was continuously removed at an equal rate to keep the overall volume constant. The pH was continuously monitored with an electrode dipped in the antacid-acid mixture. The results are shown in Table 11.

The Bachrach method estimated the suspension to be slightly better in onset and capacity whereas the Beekman procedure indicated the two to be equal. Smyth et al. [49] showed by in vivo tests in human subjects that no significant difference existed between the two. The study in human subjects involved a controlled set of conditions of fasting, standard meals at specific times, a fixed volume of water, and time dosing. The criterion used for evaluation was the monitoring of the actual intragastric pH by means of a device known as a Heidelberg capsule [53,54]. The precalibrated capsule is capable of sending a radiotelemetric pH recording signal from within the stomach. The capsule is attached to a nonwettable surgical string and swallowed. The position of the capsule is controlled by the length of the string. The details of the test conditions are not within the scope of this chapter but it is sufficient to say that a fairly accurate means of intragastric pH monitoring has been clearly demonstrated and correlated with the in vitro data. The study discussed above describes the methods of comparison between antacids in two different dosage forms; however, the principles are equally applicable to the comparison of two or more chewable antacid tablet formulations.

C. Physical Evaluation

The physical evaluation involves the following:

(1) Tablet physical appearance. As one of the quality control procedures, tablets should be inspected for smoothness, absence of cracks,

Table 11   In Vitro Evaluation of Antacids by Modified Beekman Method

Preparation	Onset (time to reach pH 3 initially)	Speed (time in min to reach maximum pH)	Duration (time in min above pH 3)	Capacity for buffering (maximum pH reached)
Suspension	Immediate	5.0—7.5	26.5—27.5	5.62—5.7
Tablet	Immediate	2.5—5.0	25.5—28.0	5.72—6.1

Source: Ref. 49.

chips, and other undesirable characteristics. If the tablets are colored, this would include examination for mottling and other evidence of nonuniform color distribution except where they are used intentionally. A suitable magnifying glass may be used to appropriately view the samples.

(2) Hardness. The hardness test is performed to provide a measure of tablet strength. Tablets should be hard enough to withstand packaging and shipping but not so hard as to create undue difficulty upon chewing.

Tablet hardness is determined using equipment from various suppliers that measure the force needed to break up the tablets. Usually a random sample of tablets (10 to 20) that have been allowed to age for at least 24 hr after production (to ensure equilibration of stresses and forces within the tablet) are individually tested and the mean hardness value determined. The coefficient of variation is also determined. High variations in tablet hardness values are not unusual although abnormally high coefficients of variation may indicate excessive weight variation, blend nonuniformity, poor tooling control, etc.

(3) Friability. The friability test gives an indication of the tablets' ability to resist chipping and abrasion on handling during packaging and shipping. Usually for conventional tablets a friability value of 1% or less is desirable, while for chewable tablets (due to the lower hardness of the tablets) friability values of up to 4% are acceptable. The friability test is done using a Roche friabilator or its modification.

In this test at least 20 tablets weighing at least 6 g are accurately preweighed. The tablets are rotated in a Roche friabilator through 100 revolutions, dedusted, and reweighed. The percent friability is determined from the weight loss.

(4) Disintegration. This test initially may not appear appropriate for chewable tablets as these tablets are to be chewed before being swallowed. However, patients, especially pediatric and geriatric, have been known to swallow these chewable dosage forms. This test would thus indicate the ability of the tablet to disintegrate and still provide the benefit of the drug if it is accidentally swallowed. Tablets should preferably pass the USP disintegration test for uncoated tablets.

(5) Dissolution. The dissolution test measures the rate of dissolution of the drug from the dosage form in vitro. It is usually expressed as the extent of dissolution (percent of drug content) of the drug occurring after a given time under specified conditions. This test is necessary to help in the prediction of the behavior of the drug in the dosage form after ingestion and as a quality control tool for checking batch-to-batch uniformity. Chewable tablets should preferably be tested in two forms: intact (in case the dosage form is accidentally swallowed) and partially crushed (to simulate chewing). The USP describes the procedures for routine dissolution testing. Apparatus 1 (rotating basket) of the USP protocol may be appropriate for testing of partially crushed dosage forms while apparatus 2 (rotating paddle) may be suitable for testing whole tablets. This dissolution test on the two forms mentioned above is particularly necessary in chewable tablets formulated from active drug present in a matrix or where the active drug has been coated using different methods and means for bitter taste masking. Such treatment may alter the dissolution rate of the untreated drug.

As discussed earlier, many taste-masking applications involve some sort of coating, barrier, or adsorption to mask the taste of the drug.

As compared to regular (swallowed) tablets, such applications in chewable tablets may result in a somewhat delayed release of the drug in the stomach. The formulator should be careful to ensure that a proper balance is achieved between the desired levels of taste masking and the rate and extent of release in the stomach. Proper judgment is necessary to determine how much and what sort of testing is necessary to ensure that this balance is achieved.

D. Stability Testing

Stability testing of dosage forms or drug products is carried out to evaluate time-dependent changes, if any, occurring with the dosage form. Stability testing may be either accelerated or real time under ambient conditions. Accelerated stability testing is used to predict quickly potential changes that may occur in a product. However, it must be pointed out that results obtained under stress conditions may not be obtained under ambient conditions. Accelerated storage conditions include high temperatures, high relative humidities, and high light intensities. There are three areas of major concern in the stability testing of chewable tablets: organoleptic, chemical, and physical stability.

Data obtained from chemical evaluation of the tablets at elevated temperature and humidity stress conditions are considered most useful. The Arrhenius equation relates kinetic rates at different temperatures and, when appropriate, can be used to extrapolate and thus obtain the expected reaction rate at room temperature, which would be used to tentatively determine the stability of the product under test or for overage determination as with vitamin tablets. The FDA's Stability Guidelines [54] describe in considerable detail the appropriate conditions for conducting stability studies in order to achieve the necessary goals and objectives. The stability testing of chewable tablets would include all tests for conventional tablets plus tests unique to chewable tablets.

Fundamental to all types of stability evaluations in flavored chewable tablets is the fact that the flavor is a complex mixture, often consisting of as many as 50 or more ingredients. The picture is further complicated by the fact that the flavors are then incorporated in tablets where they come in contact with the active and inert ingredients. A flavored chewable tablet is therefore prone to many problems—with greater potential for stability problems than its nonflavored, regular (swallowed) counterpart.

Some generalization of the flavor composition is necessary to an understanding of its implication on the stability of a flavored tablet. A flavor may consist of, for example, a combination of the following:

> Alcohols (e.g., ethyl alcohol, butyl alcohol, glycerol)
> Aldehydes (e.g., benzaldehyde, butyraldehyde, citral, and vanillin)
> Ketones (e.g., methyl amyl ketone)
> Esters (e.g., ethyl acetate, butyl butyrate, methyl salicylate)
> Essential oils (e.g., anise oil, lemon oil, orange oil)
> Plant extractives (e.g., lovage, fenugreek)
> Acids (e.g., citric acid, tartaric acid)
> Carbohydrates (e.g., sugar, dextrose, molasses—used mainly as carriers)
> Others (e.g., silica gel—used as a carrier for adsorbed flavors)

These flavor compounds are either very reactive (e.g., aldehydes), volatile (e.g., the essential oils and alcohols), or prone to hydrolysis (e.g., the esters), and, as such, formulations containing them must be carefully evaluated during the stability study.

The formulator is generally responsible for the organoleptic evaluation during a given stability study. Logically and most desirably, a preliminary stability study should have been conducted after the evaluation of a flavored baseline formulation, and before the final selection, acceptance, and final stability testing. This ensures that the candidate products are marketable, pending the final selection. Conducting the final stability evaluation after the final selection and acceptance testing may be risky since a well-designed selection and testing trial is generally expensive and time consuming, requiring considerable paper work to organize.

Any stability study involves the comparison of an initial value (or an initial observation) with subsequent readings (or observations) taken at various time intervals under various conditions of storage. This definition poses a problem unique to the stability study of chewable tablets especially with regard to the organoleptic properties, since it requires the formulator to have an accurate initial reading of the organoleptic characteristics so that the future stability samples can be compared against it. This is best accomplished by comparing the stability samples with a freshly prepared lot of the same formula. The judgment of the person making such a comparison is of paramount importance in the stability study, since it is impractical to have a taste panel evaluate the flavor at each stability checkpoint. The organoleptic evaluation should be an integral part of a stability protocol, and should be conducted and recorded at reasonable intervals in the same manner as other physical and chemical results are recorded.

Other tests in the stability program would include

1. Active drug content determination using a validated stability indicating assay method.
2. Change, if any, in physical characteristics of the tablets—mottling of colored tablets, color migration, appearance of spots on tablet surfaces, crystallization of active drug on tablet surfaces, odor development, etc.
3. Changes in tablet hardness, friability, dissolution rate and/or extent of dissolution, increase in disintegration time.
4. Moisture content of tablets—moisture pickup by tablets may lead to soft tablets that crumble and are gummy upon chewing. If tablets lose moisture, they may become brittle, leading to increase in their friability. Also, the hardness of the tablet may increase.
5. Stability of the coating systems—the polymers used in taste-masking processes should not degrade, leading to exposure of the active drug particles. The coat and matrix should also be stable, thus ensuring taste protection.
6. Stability of the colorants—the color of colored tablets should not fade or shift with time. Color stability testing would include methods such as tristimulus matching with standards and with initial values.

IX. SUMMARY

Chewable tablets represent an example of a specialized tablet type specifically designed to be chewed prior to swallowing. They are primarily used for children's vitamin supplements and cough/cold/analgesic products, and for adult antacids. Despite their potential appeal to the adult population for general medicinal use, the chewable tablet form has not been exploited in the marketplace for such applications.

Chewable products must be formulated in such a way as to provide acceptable taste and mouth-feel despite the usually bad taste of most drugs. Consequently, an even greater than usual challenge is presented to the formulating pharmacist. This challenge should be looked on as an opportunity to demonstrate a full range of knowledge and skills necessary to bring a less-than-commonplace product to market acceptance.

REFERENCES

1. C. H. Best and N. B. Taylor, *Physiological Basis of Medical Practice* (J. R. Brobeck, ed.), 9th ed., Williams and Wilkins, Baltimore, 1973, Chap. 5, Sec. 8.
2. J. A. Bakan and F. D. Sloan, *Drug Cosm. Ind.*, *110*(3):34 (March 1972).
3. L. J. Luzzi, *J. Pharm. Sci.*, 59:1367 (1970).
4. B. Farhadieh, U.S. Patent 3,922,379 (1975).
5. J. A. Bakan, in *Theory and Practice of Industrial Pharmacy* (L. Lachman, H. Lieberman, and J. Kanig, eds.), 3rd ed., Lea and Febiger, Philadelphia, 1986.
6. N. N. Salib, *Pharm. Ind.*, 34:671 (1972).
7. Roche Chemical Div., Trade Literature no. STP641, Hoffmann-LaRoche, Nutley, NJ.
8. W. L. Chiou and S. Riegelman, *J. Pharm. Sci.*, 60:1281 (1971).
9. R. M. Wheaton and A. H. Seamster, A basic reference on ion exchange, form no. 177-194-86, Dow Chemical Company, Midland, MI.
10. Amberlite IRP-64 Technical Bulletin no. 5086J/232, Rhom and Haas Company, Philadelphia, PA, 1983.
11. A. P. Granatek and M. P. DeMurio, U.S. Patent 3,459,858 (1969).
12. D. Hoff and K. Bauer, U.S. Patent 3,872,227 (1975).
13. W. Saenger, *Angew. Chem. Int. Ed. Engl.*, 19:344 (1980).
14. T. Higuchi and I. H. Pitman, *J. Pharm. Sci.*, 62:55 (1973).
15. *United States Pharmacopeia XXI/National Formulary XVI*, United States Pharmacopeial Convention, Rockville, MD, 1985.
16. *The Merck Index X*, Merck and Co., Rahway, NJ, 1983.
17. *Handbook of Pharmaceutical Excipients*, American Pharmaceutical Association, Washington, DC, 1986.
18. R. W. Mendes and S. B. Roy, *Pharm. Tech.*, 2(9):61 (1978).
19. R. F. Shangraw, J. W. Wallace, and F. M. Bowers, *Pharm. Tech.*, 5(9):69 (1981).
20. S. D. UkoNne and R. W. Mendes, *Pharm. Tech.*, 6(11):104 (1982).

21. Hony-Tab Technical Literature, Ingredient Technology Corporation, Pennsauken, NJ, 1982.
22. Mola-Tab Technical Literature, Ingredient Technology Corporation, Pennsauken, NJ, 1982.
23. CrystaFlo Technical Literature, Amstar Corporation, New York, 1985.
24. Brownulated Technical Literature, Amstar Corporation, New York, 1984.
25. Di-Pac Technical Literature, Amstar Corporation, New York, 1985.
26. NuTab Technical Literature, Ingredient Technology Corporation, Pennsauken, NJ, 1982.
27. Emdex Technical Literature, Edward Mendell Co., Carmel, NY, 1986.
28. Sweetrex Technical Literature, Edward Mendell Co., Carmel, NY, 1986.
29. Lactose Technical Literature, Sheffield Products, Kraft, Inc., Norwich, NY, 1985.
30. Lactose Technical Literature, Foremost Foods Co., San Francisco, CA, 1980.
31. Magnasweet Technical Information, MacAndrews and Forbes Co., Camden, NJ, 1987.
32. Nutrasweet Technical Overview, NutraSweet Co., Skokie, IL, 1986.
33. The PFC Index, Pharmaceutical Flavor Clinic, Division of Foote and Jenks, Camden, NJ, 1986.
34. Flavor Guidelines for the Pharmaceutical Industry, Food Materials Corp., Chicago, IL, 1979.
35. F. Wesley, *Pharmaceutical Flavor Guide*, Fritzsche Brothers, Inc., New York, NY, 1957.
36. All about lake pigments, Technical Bulletin, Warner-Jenkinson Company, St. Louis, MO, 1986.
37. Certified food colors, Technical Bulletin, Warner-Jenkinson Company, St. Louis, MO, 1982.
38. J. R. B. J. Brouwers and G. N. J. Tytgat, *J. Pharm. Sci.*, *30*:148 (1978).
39. C. K. Svensson and T. H. Wiser, *Drug Intell. Clin. Pharm.*, *15*:120 (1981).
40. *Handbook of Non-Prescription Drugs*, 8th ed., American Pharmaceutical Association, Washington, DC, 1986.
41. R. H. Barry and M. S. Weiss, *J. Am. Pharm. Assn.*, *10*:601 (1970).
42. J. Raymond, U.S. Patent 3,458,623 (1969).
43. T. L. Fisher and J. F. Cassens, Presentation on Pharmaceutical Flavors, Philadelphia Discussion Group, Academy of Pharmaceutical Sciences, 1976.
44. N. Kitamori, K. Hemmi, M. Maeno, and H. Mima, *Pharm. Tech.*, *6*(10):56 (1982).
45. T. J. Macek, *Am. J. Pharm.*, *132*:433 (1960).
46. J. D. Davis, *Drug Cosm. Ind.*, *128*(1):38 (1981).
47. S. Borodkin and D. P. Sundberg, *J. Pharm. Sci.*, *60*:1523 (1971).
48. *Code of Federal Regulations*, Title 21, Food and Drugs, Sec. 331.1, pp. 132–136.
49. R. D. Smyth, T. Herczeg, T. A. Whatley, W. Hause, and N. H. Reavy-Cantwell, *J. Pharm. Sci.*, *65*:1045 (1976).
50. W. H. Steinbert, H. H. Hutchins, P. G. Pick, and J. S. Lazar, *J. Pharm. Sci.*, *54*:625 (1965).
51. S. M. Beekman, *J. Am. Pharm. Assn.*, *49*:191 (1960).

52. R. A. Locock, *Can. Pharm. J.*, *104*:86 (1971).
53. E. Johannesson, P.-O. Magnusson, N.-O. Sjoberg, and A. Skov-Jensen, *Scand. J. Gastroenterol.*, *8*:65 (1973).
54. J. C. McAlhany, Jr., D. R. Yarbrough III, M. G. Weidner, Jr., and R. Ravenel, *Am. Surg.*, *35*:836 (1969).
55. Draft guideline for stability studies for human drugs and biologics, Food and Drug Administration, Rockville, MD, 1985.

9

Medicated Lozenges

David Peters*

Warner–Lambert Company, Morris Plains, New Jersey

Lozenges are flavored medicated dosage forms intended to be sucked and held in the mouth or pharynx [1,85]. They may contain vitamins, antibiotics, antiseptics, local anesthetics, antihistamines, decongestants, corticosteroids, astringents, analgesics, aromatics, demulcents, or combinations of these ingredients [2]. The oropharyngeal symptoms which lozenges are intended to relieve are commonly caused by local infections and occasionally by allergy or drying of the mucosa from mouth breathing.

Lozenges may take various shapes, the most common being the flat, circular, octagonal, and biconvex forms. Another type, called *bacilli*, are in the form of short rods or cylinders. A soft variety of lozenge, called a *pastille*, consists of medicament in a gelatin or glycerogelatin base or in a base of acacia, sucrose, and water. Confections (now obsolete) are heavily sugared soft masses containing medicinal agents [3].

Two types of lozenge bases have gained wide usage because of their ready adaptation to modern high-speed methods of product manufacture. These two lozenge forms, which will be discussed in detail, include hard (or boiled) candy lozenges and compressed tablet lozenges.

I. HARD CANDY LOZENGES

Hard candy is a mixture of sugar and other carbohydrates that are kept in an amorphous or glassy condition [4]. This form can be considered a solid syrup of sugars generally having from 0.5 to 1.5% moisture content.

Essentially, the preparation of hard candy lozenges can be considered an art. Many of the formulations used in confectionary manufacturing, and the rationale used for solving problem areas, are based on experience and intuition rather than scientific deduction. The confectionary equipment utilized by the manufacturer of lozenges is suitable for the preparation of

---

Current affiliation: Treworgy Pharmacy, Calais, Maine

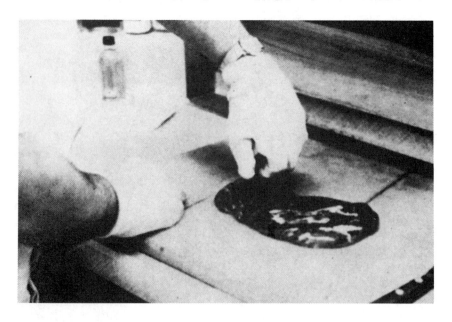

Figure 1 Mixing of flavors and medicinals by hand. Preparation of 1- or 2-kg laboratory batches enables the formulator to evaluate potential problem areas that may develop when flavor or medicament is incorporated into hard candy base. (From Ref. 24.)

candies but is not designed to produce a controlled and reproducible medicated candy with close tolerances as to size, weight, and quantity of drug concentration per unit dose. The formulator must gain a comprehensive knowledge of the physical and chemical qualities of raw materials in the product and become familiar with all aspects of candy base production in order to prepare a medicated product that conforms to the specifications for good manufacturing procedures (Figures 1 and 2). A review of possible shelf life problems must be determined through stability testing after the product is manufactured. The formulator, in essence, is required to bring a scientific approach to an empirical art.

A. Raw Materials

Sugar (Sucrose)

Various grades and types of sugars are available in commerce that may be suitable for incorporation into hard candy, but the two with the greatest utility are cane and beet sugars [4,80].

Sucrose is prepared commercially from sugar cane, beet root, or sorghum. The sugar cane is crushed and the juice (amounting to about 80%)

is expressed with roller mills, treated with lime to clear the syrup and then with carbonic acid gas to remove excess lime. The juice is then concentrated in vacuum pans until crystallization of sucrose is complete. The crystals and the syrup are separated by centrifugation—with the resulting syrup (a byproduct) known as molasses. Beet sugar is made by a similar process but is more difficult to purify.

Refined sugar from either raw cane or beet sugars is prepared by dissolving the sugar in water, clarifying, filtering, and finally decolorizing the solution by treatment with charcoal. The water-clear solution is evaporated under reduced pressure to the crystallizing point [5].

Cane and beet sugars are now chemically and physically identical and therefore cannot be distinguished from each other in the refined state. At one time, though, there were significant differences in the purity and shelf life among products prepared with each type of sugar. Beet sugar contained many impurities, producing a final product containing batch-to-batch differences in color. The candies had a tendency to grain (exhibit sugar crystallization) and pick up excessive moisture. Advances in sugar refining have led most manufacturers to indicate that these differences no longer exist, with only geographic considerations and availability determining which is used.

Today liquid sugar with a solids content of 67% w/w (Table 1) is used almost exclusively in the manufacture of confections, as all continuous candy base manufacturing equipment requires a constant supply of sugar syrup and corn syrup during cooking. Manufacturers can prepare the syrup as

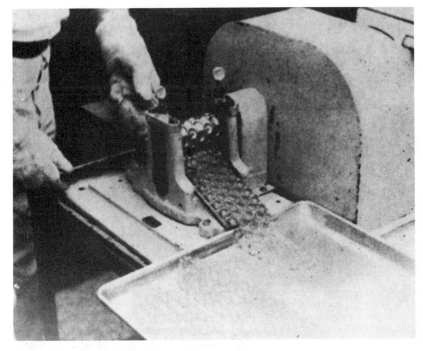

Figure 2 Motorized drop-former. Lozenges manufactured in the laboratory are suitable for stability evaluation of medicament, flavor, and color prior to manufacture of production batches. (From Ref. 24.)

Table 1   Physical Constants of Sucrose Solutions

Degrees Brix (% of sugar)	Degrees Baumé (modulus 145)	Index of refraction at 68°F	Specific gravity at 68°F	Weight (lb) of 1 US gal. at 68°F
67.0	36.05	1.4579	1.3309	11.08
68.0	36.55	1.4603	1.3371	11.13
69.0	37.06	1.4627	1.3433	11.18
70.0	37.56	1.4651	1.3496	11.23
71.0	38.06	1.4651	1.3559	11.29
72.0	38.55	1.4700	1.3622	11.34
73.0	39.05	1.4725	1.3686	11.39
74.0	39.54	1.4749	1.3750	11.45
75.0	40.03	1.4774	1.3814	11.50
76.0	40.53	1.4799	1.3879	11.55
77.0	41.01	1.4825	1.3944	11.61
78.0	41.50	1.4850	1.4010	11.66
79.0	41.99	1.4876	1.4076	11.72
80.0	42.47	1.4901	1.4142	11.77

Source: The Manufacturing Confectioner, Vol. 70, No. 7, July 1970.

needed from granular sugar or purchase liquid sugar directly from their sugar refiners.

Corn Syrup

Corn syrups are produced by either acid, enzyme, or acid–enzyme combination hydrolysis of cornstarch and are generally available in several grades, varying in degree of conversion [dextrose equivalent (DE)] and solids content (degrees Baumé) [4].

Manufacture

The manufacture of all corn sweeteners begins with the hydrolysis of cornstarch, a process involving the splitting of the starch molecules by chemical reaction with water. During the process, a thoroughly agitated slurry of purified starch granules containing the required amount of dilute acid is brought to the desired temperature by the injection of steam. A variety of acids will affect the conversion, but in the United States hydrochloric acid is used almost exclusively. Time and temperature are varied depending on the type of corn sweetener to be manufactured [6].

As the reaction progresses, the gelatinized starch is converted first to other polysaccharides and subsequently to sugars, mostly maltose and dextrose. The sugar content increases and viscosity decreases as the conversion proceeds. Complete hydrolysis produces dextrose.

The hydrolysis of the starch is halted when partially complete—to produce corn syrup, the exact degree depending on the type of syrup being made. Partial hydrolysis of starch converts part of the starch completely to dextrose; the remainder, which is not completely hydrolyzed to dextrose, consists of maltose and higher saccharides. The proportions of saccharides vary, depending on the extent and method of hydrolysis.

Two methods of hydrolysis are in commercial use for the production of corn syrup—the acid process and the acid-enzyme process. In the latter, acid hydrolysis is followed by conversion with an amylolytic enzyme, resulting in a syrup with a higher proportion of maltose than can be obtained by acid hydrolysis alone. The dextrose/maltose ratio can be varied, within certain limits, depending on the type of enzyme used and on the extent of the preliminary acid conversion.

In the acid hydrolysis process, the hydrolysis is stopped when the reaction has reached the desired DE range, by transferring the contents of the converter into a neutralizing tank where the pH is raised to the level necessary to stop the reaction. The acid acts as a catalyst and does not combine chemically with the starch. The acidified product is partially neutralized by adding a calculated quantity of sodium carbonate to the solution.

Fatty substances which rise to the surface are skimmed and then removed in centrifuges or by precoated filters. Suspended solid matter is removed by filtering the hydrolyzate in vacuum filters. The filtrate is then evaporated to a density of about 60% dry substance.

After this initial evaporation, the hydrolyzate is passed through either bone char or other carbon filters, which causes further clarification and decolorization so that the resulting syrup is clear and practically colorless. This process partially removes soluble mineral substances, which also can be removed by an ion exchange process.

After final filtration, evaporation is carried out in vacuum pans at relatively low temperature to avoid damage to the syrup. The syrup is cooled and can be stored or loaded directly in tank cars, tank trucks, steel drums, or cans.

In the production of high-conversion acid-enzyme or dual-conversion syrups, acid hydrolysis is carried to a level of 48–55 DE. The syrup then is neutralized, clarified, and partially concentrated, and the enzyme added. In other products the acid hydrolysis may be stopped at a level as low as 15 DE. When the enzyme hydrolysis has progressed to the desired degree, the enzyme is inactivated. Adjustment of the pH, further refining, and final evaporation follow as in the production of acid conversion syrup. A summary of the corn-refining process is described in Figure 3.

Dextrose Equivalent

Dextrose equivalent is a measure of the reducing-sugar content of a product calculated as dextrose and expressed as a percentage of the total dry substance [7,8]. Essentially, the dextrose equivalent is the percentage of pure dextrose that gives the same analytical effect as is given by the corn syrup. Certain sugars, such as dextrose, maltose, lactose, and levulose, are called reducing sugars because when a copper hydroxide solution (Fehling's solution) is warmed with these sugars, they react with cupric hydroxide to form cuprous oxide. Sucrose is not a reducing sugar; thus it does not react with Fehling's solution. Generally, dextrose equivalent indicates the degree of conversion in corn syrup. The higher the

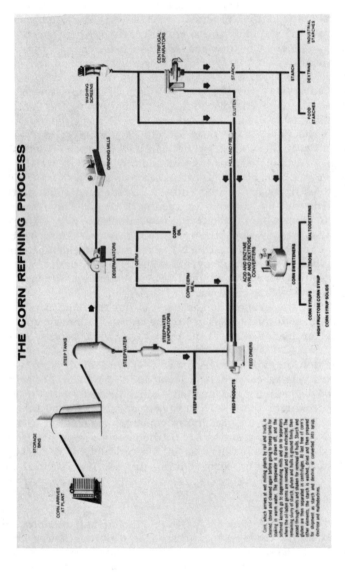

Figure 3 The corn refining process. (Corn Refiners Association, Inc., Washington, D.C.)

dextrose equivalent, the further the conversion has been carried out, resulting in less of the higher sugars (maltotriose and maltotetrose).

The classes of corn syrups categorized as to degree of conversion [8] include:

Low-conversion corn syrup	20– 38 DE
Regular conversion corn syrup	38– 48 DE
Intermediate-conversion corn syrup	48–58 DE
High-conversion corn syrup	58– 68 DE
Extra high-conversion corn syrup	68– 99 DE
Dextrose	100 DE

A typical analysis of corn syrup with representative carbohydrate composition and physical and chemical characteristics is included in Table 2.

Physical Characteristics

Corn syrups with 42– 43 DE are called normal corn syrups; those with 37– 38 DE, low-dextrose-equivalent corn syrups; and those with 58– 62 DE, high-dextrose-equivalent corn syrups. Regular- or low-conversion dextrose equivalent corn syrups are widely used in hard candy. For caramels, low-dextrose-equivalent syrup is preferred because it prevents the product from "flowing" in the cold state because of the high viscosity that low-dextrose-equivalent corn syrups impart to products to which they are added. The high viscosity prevents the caramel from losing its shape when the product is stored at elevated temperature or high-humidity conditions. High-dextrose-equivalent corn syrups are generally used for filling where a low-viscosity and higher sweetness medium is required. Since the introduction of enzyme conversion, corn syrups can be varied to best suit their application. The properties and functional applications of corn syrups based on degree of conversion may be described as follows [6].

Browning reaction. The typical brown color that candy base may develop during cooking results from a reaction between reducing sugars and proteins (Maillard reaction). As the corn syrup conversion continues, more reducing sugars are produced. The higher dextrose equivalent syrups are more prone to darkening. Some reducing sugars are more active than others. For example, dextrose is more reactive than maltose. Therefore, the more highly converted products containing maltose are selected in preference to the dextrose-containing syrups. Fructose reacts more readily than dextrose and will give a greater amount of browning than dextrose at the same solids level.

Fermentability. Yeast-raised goods, particularly bread, require fermentable sugars to serve as food for the yeast, and also some residual sugars to give good crust color and add a mild sweetness to the finished product. Because fermentable sugars increase with dextrose equivalent level, the high-DE, dextrose-rich corn syrups are always utilized in making yeast-raised products with crystalline dextrose as the ultimate ingredient.

Foam stabilizer. Because the lower dextrose equivalent syrups have a greater ability to retain incorporated air, they are always chosen as the best foam stabilizer.

Table 2   Typical Analysis of Various Corn Syrup Grades

Representative carbohydrate composition

Degree of conversion	Very low	Regular	Regular
Type of conversion	Acid-enzyme	Acid	Acid-
Dextrose equivalent (%)	26	35	43
Fermentable extract (%)	23	32	42
Dextrose (monosaccharides) (%)	5	14	20
Maltose (disaccharides) (%)	14	12	14
Maltotriose (trisaccharides) (%)	14	11	12
Higher saccharides (%)	67	63	54

Representative chemical and physical data

Baumé at 100°F (degrees	42	43	43
Total solids (%)	77.5	79.9	80.3
Moisture (%)	22.5	20.1	19.7
pH	5	5	5
Acidity as HCl (%)	0.015	0.015	0.015
Viscosity (poises at 100°F)	220	220	125
Boiling point (°F)	222	226	227
Weight (lb gal at 100°F)	11.70	11.81	11.81

Percentage ash (sulfated) of resin-refined corn syrup, less than 0.02%.

Percentage ash of vegetable-carbon refined corn syrup, 0.3%

Source: A. E. Staley Manufacturing Co., Decatur, Illinois (Tech. Data Sheet No. 110).

Freezing point depressioi. and osmotic pressure. Because freezing point depression and osmotic pressure are directly related to the number of molecules present, the highest dextrose equivalent products give the greatest freezing point depression and the highest osmotic pressure.

Hygroscopicity. The more highly converted syrups have the greatest ability to take up water and the low-conversion products the least. If a base product for preparing a dry powder with low hygroscopicity is desired, then the lowest dextrose equivalent products are used, sometimes extending below the 20-DE range into the maltodextrins.

Regular Acid-enzyme	Intermediate Acid	High Acid-enzyme	High Acid-enzyme	Very High Acid-enzyme
42	54	64	64	68
58	54	76	76	79
7	30	39	39	40
34	18	33	33	39
27	13	12	12	4
32	39	16	16	17
43	43	43	44	43
80.5	81.0	81.8	83.8	82.0
19.5	19.0	18.2	16.2	18.0
5	5	5	5	5
0.015	0.015	0.015	0.015	0.015
125	75	55	155	55
227	229	233	234	233
11.81	11.81	11.81	11.93	11.81

Nutritive solids. Since the caloric value of starch hydrolyzates is based primarily on carbon content, there is no significant difference among the various corn syrups when nutritive value is based on solids content. If a controlled rate of assimilation is required for specialty applications, such as infant foods, the lower converted products with lower rates of assimilation are used. In a special application, there could be preference for a corn syrup containing dextrose, maltose, or fructose.

Control of sugar crystallization. In the preparation of hard candies, control of the number and size of sugar crystals is required. The higher polysaccharides of the low converted corn syrups are effective agents for this purpose. By selecting syrups with the correct higher polysaccharide content and distribution, control of crystallization can be obtained.

Sweetness. Fructose is sweeter than dextrose, which is sweeter than maltose, which is sweeter than higher polysaccharides. Since the sugars, fructose, dextrose, and maltose are all reducing sugars, the higher dextrose equivalent corn syrups are generally sweeter than the lower dextrose equivalent products. However, at any dextrose equivalent level, the corn syrup containing a given amount of fructose will be sweeter than a syrup containing an equal quantity of dextrose or maltose. Where sweetness is the major functional property desired, the high-dextrose-equivalent corn syrups, especially those containing fructose, should be selected.

Viscosity. This property is basically dependent on the average molecular size. The most viscous syrups are the lowest dextrose equivalent products.

Miscellaneous. Corn syrup is transported from the manufacturer to customers or to distribution points in rail tankers as a thick, viscous, water-white syrup. The tankers are usually insulated to maintain the temperature of the syrup at 90–140°F, depending on the type of syrup being shipped. A summary of the physical characteristics available with various corn syrups appears in Figure 4 [6].

Degrees Baumé

Corn syrups are sold on a Baumé basis, which is a measure of specific gravity or dry substance content [8]. Since corn syrups are viscous at room temperature, Baumé determination is made at 140°F (60°C) with an arbitrary correction of 1.00° Baumé added to the observed reading to correct the value, which would be reported at 100°F (37.7°C). This is called *commercial Baumé* [9]. Specific gravity is an important consideration when choosing a grade of corn syrup (43° Baumé corn syrup having about 20% water, 45° Baumé about 15% water, and 37° Baumé about 30% water). For transport by tank cars, a corn syrup of 43° Baumé is preferred over one of 45° Baumé because of its superior flow characteristics. Forty-three degree Baumé corn syrup, even with improved flow vs. 45° Baumé syrup, still must be heated to 100°F to effect acceptable flow. Use of 41° Baumé corn syrup (77% solids) eliminates the heating of corn syrup during storage. This requires longer heating during candy base preparation, thus resulting in longer cooking time and possibly more browning [10]. The overall advantages of 43° Baumé corn syrup make this the syrup of choice in the preparation of hard candy lozenges.

Applications

The primary functions of corn syrup in hard candy base are (a) to control crystallization; (b) to add body; (c) to supply solids at a reduced cost; (d) to adjust sweetness level. Control of sugar crystallization is a primary application of corn syrup in hard candy. Since sugar is readily crystallized when the water of sugar solutions is boiled off, the presence of the noncrystallizable corn syrup is necessary to inhibit the *graining* or recrystallization of the sucrose. This inhibition of sugar recrystallization is accomplished by surrounding each molecule of sucrose with a film of

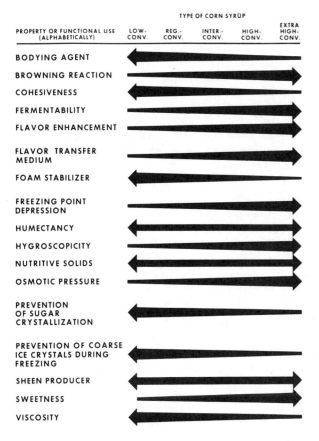

Figure 4   Properties and functional uses of corn syrup.   (Corn Refiners Association, Inc., Washington, D.C.)

uncrystallizable corn syrup. Hard candy, in essence, may be characterized as a supersaturated sugar solution in corn syrup [4]. The sugar molecules are dissolved and separated in the corn syrup, and because of the high viscosity of the corn syrup solution, movement of sugar molecules in the corn syrup is slowed. Eventually, though, molecules of sugar meet and combine, causing the formation of larger sugar crystals or the phenomenon described as graining [4].

The viscosity of the internal solution (determined by the grade of corn syrup and the moisture content of the finished candy base after cooking) and the storage conditions under which the finished lozenges are subjected (e.g., protection from moisture) determine the product's shelf life and rate of crystallization that can be expected [11]. All hard candies do eventually grain, but the speed at which this phenomenon occurs depends on the aforementioned grade of corn syrup (viscosity), moisture content of the cooked base, and storage conditions. Modification of the ratio of sugar solids to corn syrup solids in candy base will also affect the rate of graining in the finished product.

Incorporation of corn syrup solids at greater than 50% decreases graining tendencies because of the lower percentage of sugar solids dissolved in the syrup, but this increases moisture absorption, thus resulting in an increase in product stickiness and in the interactions of medicaments. Higher percentages of corn syrup reduce lozenge sweetness but allow longer processing time because of the slowed rate of candy base hardening. Addition of greater than 70% sucrose solids to candy base increases graining tendencies due to the high solids content in the corn syrup. Candy base crystallizes rapidly, thus decreasing mixing time, and increasing opacity and the brittleness of the final lozenge. Candy base formulations containing 55–65% sugar and 45–35% corn syrup solids offer the best compromise among these factors: resistance to graining, reduction of moisture absorption, and a realistic processing time period during manufacture.

Invert Sugar

Invert sugar is a mixture of two sugars (levulose and dextrose) in equal parts, produced by hydrolizing (inverting) sucrose. Molecules of sucrose combine with water to form smaller molecules during the cooking of the candy base [12].

Invert sugar has the power to absorb moisture from the air and at the same time retard crystallization. Controlling candy base cooking time will reduce the quantity of invert sugar. A standardized cooking time will result in the formation of uniform quantities of invert.

Reducing Sugars

The quantity of reducing sugar present in the corn syrup plus the quantity of reducing sugar formed during the cooking cycle determines the quantity of total reducing sugars in the final candy base. Controlling the total reducing sugars will determine how resistant the candy will be to graining and moisture absorption.

Production of hard candy base containing greater than 20% reducing sugars slows the rate of product graining by lengthening crystallization time. This attribute is advantageous during manufacturing since the candy base will harden at a slower rate. The result is a base that can be mixed longer to assure a complete distribution of medicament while entrapping less air. This allows formation of a piece of hard candy with a greater degree of clarity. Increased crystallization time also produces a candy base that is more pliable during the lozenge-forming operation. This reduces the number of rejects formed because of lozenges breaking due to candy base brittleness. The incidence of sugar dusting is also lowered, resulting in a cleaner product and a more sanitary operation.

Preparation of candy base with reducing sugar content below 14% leads to the formation of brittle candy that is susceptible to breakage, dusting, and formation of high quantities (greater than 20%) of lozenge rejects. This is the direct result of manufacturing difficulties caused from candy base hardening through rapid crystallization. The resultant lozenges, while possessing less hygroscopicity than product prepared with higher reducing sugars, are more susceptible to graining when exposed to moist conditions.

A final reducing sugar content in the 16–18% range brings to the formulator many of the advantages cited for low and high reducing sugar content while minimizing the disadvantages. Crystallization time is slow enough to assure proper incorporation of medicaments, but sufficient candy base plasticity is available for the forming and molding operation. The resultant lozenges are not brittle, resist dusting during the packaging operation, and resist both graining and excessive moisture absorption.

When selecting a grade of corn syrup suitable for lozenge manufacture, the formulator should consider a corn syrup prepared at a *regular conversion* level (41—44 DE), dual-converted (acid-enzyme) to a high maltose content (above 42%). The regular conversion imparts the proper internal viscosity to control graining, while the high-maltose-containing syrup is designed for use in products where a sweetener with minimum dextrose (less than 10%) and a resultant decrease in lozenge hygroscopicity is desired. The reduced dextrose content imparts better color stability, expecially during heating and storage, when higher dextrose contents would cause darkening.

Lozenges containing high-maltose corn syrup have increased internal viscosity. This retards sugar movement and aids in controlling crystallization of sucrose, while the lower water-pickup tendency improves and extends the lozenge shelf life—both from the chemical aspect of reducing drug decomposition and from the physical aspects of reducing graining and sticking.

High-maltose syrups were originally developed for use in hard candy, the theory being that a manufacturer using 40—50% regular conversion corn syrup (dry basis) could go to 50—60% with high-maltose syrup [13,14]. While noticeable improvements resulted in the winter months, stickiness is still a problem in the summer. Many processors who ventured to the 60% level gradually cut back to the 40—50% level. The use of high percentages (above 50%) of high-maltose corn syrup produced lozenges that exhibited increased breaking or stress cracking becuase of the high viscosity imparted by the corn syrup.

Most lozenges manufactured today possess a sugar-to-corn syrup ratio in the range of 50:50 to 70:30, with the greatest number of medicated lozenges produced with a ratio of 55—65 parts sugar to 45—35 parts corn syrup. This ratio produces lozenges with adequate sweetness, resistance to moisture pickup (with resultant stickiness), graining, and reactivity with medicinal components [15].

Acidulents

Acidulents are generally added to candy base as fortifiers to strengthen the flavor characteristics of the finished product. Acids commonly used include citric, tartaric, fumaric, and malic; of these, citric is by far the most common.

A second use for acidulents in candy base is to control pH in order to preserve the stability of selected medicaments. Since hard candy base is considered a supersaturated solution of sugar in a corn syrup medium, and because of the presence of water in the medicated lozenge base, pH is an important factor in maintaining the stability of medicaments affected by an acid or alkaline medium. The reactivity of the corn syrup and reducing sugars, the presence of moisture in the candy base, and the presence of flavors and acidulents increase the reactivity of medicament in the vehicle— to the extent that the kinetics of drug decomposition is related to liquid (as opposed to solid) dosage forms.

Regualr hard candy base has a pH of 5.0—6.0. Addition of acidulents for flavor enhancement will lower the pH to 2.5—3.0. At this pH many medicaments exhibit acceptable chemical stability, while others are subjected to rapid decomposition. A determination of the stability profiles of the medicaments intended for incorporation into the lozenge base should be carried out at various pH levels to determine that which is optimum. This determination may preclude the use of acidulents and the flavors with which they are most compatible.

In some special applications, addition of selected ingredients (calcium carbonate, sodium bicarbonate, magnesium trisilicate) to raise the lozenge pH to 7.5–8.5 will be necessary to effect the desired stability profiles.

Method of Addition

Addition of acidulents to candy base is not a random procedure. Acidulent addition should be performed under controlled conditions since, even under the best circumstances, the acidulent will react with the candy base. Addition of acid to sugar (sucrose) causes inversion, which yields by hydrolysis glucose and fructose (dextrose and levulose). As the percentage of invert sugar in the candy base increases, the internal viscosity of the lozenge decreases, and the moisture absorption characteristics increase. Both phenomena increase tendencies for lozenges to grain, absorb moisture, and become sticky [16].

A certain quantity of invert sugar is produced during the cooking cycle. The faster the cooking cycle, the lower the quantity of *cook invert* formed. Addition of acidulents to candy base during the cooking cycle— or the failure to neutralize excess acid in any salvage that may be incorporated—acts as a *sugar doctor* or inverting agent. This so-called doctor will markedly increase the quantities of invert sugar formed, negating the advantages of a low moisture content in the base preparation or the use of high-maltose corn syrup. The acidulents should be added at the completion of the cooking cycle at temperatures not exceeding 120°C. Final invert sugar levels in candy base should not exceed 2.0–2.5%.

The presence of acidulents in the completed lozenge will shorten the shelf life of the final product, since even at room temperature the acidulent will continue to invert the sugar. Thus, the rate of graining and degree of stickiness will be higher than in lozenges prepared at pH 5–6. Another drawback of acidulents in lozenges occurs with elevated temperature and humidity. Under these conditions, a localized discoloration or burning of the candy will occur. Use of finely powdered acids helps to reduce this problem but will not eliminate it.

Incorporation of the acidulents to the vehicle as a controlled procedure helps minimize the disadvantages acidulents can represent in reducing the extended shelf life of the products to which they are added. The acidulent should be added to candy base at the lowest possible workable temperature of the candy mass (100–110°C). At the same time, the acidulent should be added at the lowest effective concentration (0.1–0.5%) in a manner that will prevent direct contact of the acid with the mass. Incorporation of the acidulent as a mixture with dry, ground salvage and the flavorant will lessen contact of the acidulent with the base, and at the same time help distribute it uniformly throughout the mass. This uniform incorporation prevents reaction during the addition procedure and reduces the degree of localized discoloration or burning during storage. The use of granular acidulent instead of finely powdered material will result in localized discoloration if the lozenges are exposed to prolonged heating or high humidity during storage. The reactivity of acidulent with candy base during product manufacture is reduced because of lower overall particle surface area.

The advantages that acidulents bring to lozenge formulations through pH control and flavor enhancement usually exceed the disadvantages of discoloration and sugar inversion during storage, if the degree of inversion can be controlled during lozenge manufacture by proper addition techniques.

Colors

Incorporation of powdered or micronized dyes is not practical because of the low moisture content (less than 1.5%) and the high viscosity of the cooked candy base. Not all the dye will dissolve in the base, resulting in a nonuniform and nonreproducible colored product containing particles of undissolved dye. A method used to circumvent this difficulty involves the incorporation of colors into hard candy base as pastes, in mixtures of sugar, dextrose, corn syrup, dextrin, and glycerin; as aqueous solutions; or as commercially prepared color cubes (Figure 5) [17]. When adding colors as aqueous solutions, no more than 30.0 g of water should be added per 100 lb of candy base. More than this quantity will result in localized sticking and lumping during the mixing cycle. If more liquid is required, combinations with glycerin or propylene glycol should be used.

The formulator, during product development, should investigate the compatibility of the colorants—both at ambient temperature and at 110–115°C, the temperature at which the colors will be added to the products— since many dye systems are altered when added at the elevated temperature. A second factor that should be considered is the product pH. Addition of acidulents to candy base at elevated temperature along with, or shortly after, color addition can result in a noticeable change in the final product color as well as color differences between batches. Stability of colors in

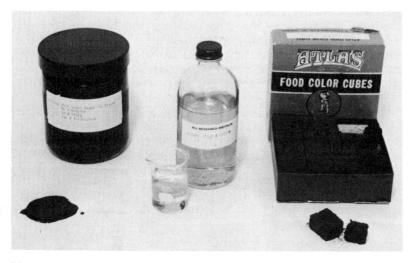

Figure 5 Colors may be added to candy base as pastes, as aqueous solutions, or as commercially prepared color cubes.

the final product (effects of moisture, sunlight, pH, and medicaments) is also a matter of concern since changes in product appearance with time are not uncommon.

Many in-process color changes result when colored liquid salvage is incorporated in the candy base. This color modification may occur because of the pH of the salvage solution before cooking or may be because of a color change effected during the candy base cooking cycle. Color changes that result from pH may be remedied by a change in salvage pH. The salvage solution pH may be adjusted anywhere in the range of 4.5–7.5. If a pH in this range can produce a stable color solution, then color change problems can be avoided. Color change problems caused by the cooking temperature of the candy base cannot be alleviated. If this problem occurs, the salvage solution may have to be decolorized before use [69]. Modification of the candy base color back to the original shade can be effected by the addition of more color to the cooked candy base. This is practical only if a uniformly color-modified product is produced each time the colored salvage solution is manufactured. Candy base colors that prove to be stable when added to candy base during the cooking cycle may be added to salvage solutions before the cooking cycle instead of to the cooked candy base during the mixing cycle.

Flavors

The addition of flavors to cooked candy base can pose a variety of problems to the formulator. These include flavor losses during processing, flavor incorporation difficulties, flavor and candy base interactions, and flavor–medicament interactions. The specific flavor-related difficulty must be determined, and remedial actions taken, if a stable and reproducible product is to result.

Addition of flavors to candy base usually takes place at temperatures from 120 to 135°C. At these temperatures, flash-off is the primary problem. Addition of flavors to the base also results in distribution difficulties because of the high viscosity of the candy base and the fact that the cooked candy base does not readily absorb liquids without rapid and continuous agitation. Separation of flavors from the cooked base will markedly increase the incidence of flavor loss, since the flavors present at the surface of the hot mass are most likely to volatilize. The ideal situation is to incorporate or surround the flavors with candy as rapidly as possible. Separation of flavors from candy base may result in the formation of bubbles of concentrated flavor in the completed lozenge. These lozenges may contain a "liquid pocket" of flavor which, when broken in the mouth, may produce excessive burning or discomfort to the user. The separation of flavor from the candy base may also cause processing difficulties because of an increase in the candy mass tackiness and a reduction in candy base elasticity. A final disadvantage of flavor separation may be a nonuniform flavor concentration among production batches. This is a negative factor, especially when flavors are medicinal in nature or are covering bitter principals. As a rule, no more than 450 g of flavor should be added to 100 lb of candy base.

A method designed to reduce the quantity of flavor flash-off and flavor separation at the surface of the candy base involves the addition of flavor components as a mixture with ground salvage. This ground salvage flavor mixture is added to the cooked candy base (125–135°C) on the mixing table and immediately folded into the hot mass.

As the ground candy melts, the flavor is drawn into the base and is rapidly mixed into the molten mass. Since the flavor is not exposed to the surface of the candy base for as long a time, flavor losses are reduced, and losses (5—15% of flavor added is lost, depending on each individual flavor) are reproducible. The resultant candy has a uniform distribution of flavors without formation of flavor pockets.

The particle size of the salvage used as a flavor carrier and extender should range from 20 to 50 mesh. If salvage particles are too large, the flavor will not be adsorbed on the surface of the candy. This will result in a separation of flavor from the salvage. If salvage is too fine, the resultant salvage-flavor mixture will set or harden, causing distribution problems.

Sufficient salvage must be utilized to adsorb the flavor in order to prevent separation from the salvage mixture—either during preparation or storage of the flavor-salvage mixture, or as the mixture is melting into the molten candy mass. The resultant mixture should consist of free-flowing, discrete granules that do not agglomerate or exhibit flavor separation during a 48-hr storage period. Depending on the type of flavor used, if the salvage is of proper particle size, 1 lb of ground salvage should adsorb 50—100 g of flavor.

A divergence from the usage of ground salvage occurs in the candy industry where the incorporation of ground salvage into a candy base is contraindicated. The explanation for this is that the addition of sugar granules or crystals to the cooling candy mass results in a medium that is suitable for crystallization of sugar (graining)]62]. The ground salvage addition may act as seed crystals which, under proper conditions (high moisture), will result in premature crystallization of sugar from the base.

The candy industry is concerned with manufacturing a product that is elegant in appearance. Refraining from addition of ground salvage produces a clear product free from excessive air entrapment and more resistant to graining than a lozenge prepared with ground candy.

Preparation of confections does not require masking of the bitter principals present in medicated products; therefore, the quantities of flavorants used are only 10—20% of those utilized in medicated lozenges. The small quantities of flavors are readily incorporated into candy base, thus minimizing losses. In instances where larger quantities of flavors are added, the candy manufacturer is not too concerned with flavor losses or nonuniform flavors between batches.

In the preparation of medicated products, the reduction in flavor losses through flash-off resulting from the use of the ground salvage is considered more important than a loss in clarity or a tendency toward premature graining. Flavors mask bitter principals and in many instances are medicinal themselves; therefore the manufacture of a product with uniform flavor content supersedes the appearance of the final product.

Another method to reduce flavor loss is the addition of selected solvents, where compatible, with the flavorants. Solvents most commonly used are propylene glycol, benzyl alcohol, polyethylene glycol [18], and glycerin. This method is most suitable when small portions (less than 100 g/100 lb candy base) of flavor are added to the product.

Use of natural or artificial flavorants [19] is left to the discretion of the formulator, but the compatibility of the flavor in the presence of heat and pressure should be evaluated. Incorporation of natural flavors containing terpenes or other materials with a low boiling point in contraindicated

in candy making because the temperature at which the flavorants are added
to candy base, along with the added heat and pressure that occur when
the mass is formed into lozenges, cause a charring or burning of these
low-boiling-point materials. The result is a formation of black specks or
black pockets of burned flavor. This phenomenon, called *dieseling* (Figure
6), does not occur in all batches, but when it does the organoleptic appeal
of the product is reduced. Elimination of low-boiling-point flavoring components (especially terpenes) will alleviate this condition.

   A third consideration in determining which flavor or flavor profiles
should be used is the compatibility of flavors with the medicaments in the
product. Different flavoring components (e.g., aldehydes, esters, ketones,
alcohols) may react with the medicaments to produce a chemical decomposition or drug instability. Adjustment of lozenge base pH to accentuate certain flavors (e.g., citrus) may also result in a situation that would be in-

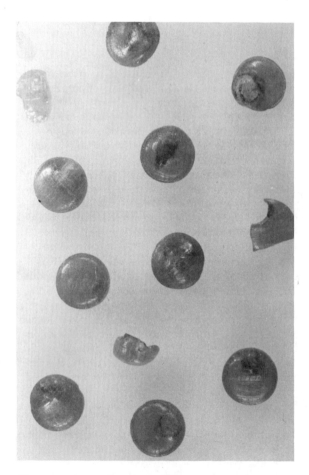

Figure 6   Lozenge diesels. Charring of low boiling point flavor components results in formation of black specks, burned areas, air pockets,
and surface irregularities. Flavor adulteration also results when dieseling
occurs.

compatible with various medicaments. The chemistry of both the flavor
and active components must be studied before choosing flavors for any
product. A classic example of flavor–drug interaction occurring in candy
base is the interaction of benzocaine with cherry, lemon, or other aldehyde-
containing flavor components. In a relatively short period (4 weeks at
45°C, or 12 weeks at 25°C), the benzocaine-aldehyde reaction causes a
Schiff's base formation:

$$RCHO + RNH_2 - RCH = NR + H_2O,$$

resulting in drug decomposition and elimination of the local anesthetic efficacy. To further aggravate the condition, the citrus flavors are usually
added with acidulants (citric or malic acid) to accentuate the citrus notes.
The resultant lozenge pH of 2.5–3.5 forces this Schiff's base reaction,
thus speeding up decomposition of the benzocaine. Elimination of the acidu-
lant slows the reaction but reduces the organoleptic appeal of the citrus
flavors.

Solid and Liquid Salvage

Preparation of a medicated product utilizing equipment that was fashioned
for production of confections requires constant control of both machinery
and production workers. Manufacture of products that require the close
tolerances and tight specifications of a medicated lozenge on machinery that
does not lend itself to these specifications leads to a high percentage of
dosage rejects.

A large number of oversized and undersized pieces are formed during
the lozenge-forming operation. Some lozenges break during the cooling
operation while others are rejected because of excessive air bubbles,
cracks, or excessive sugar dusting. Still other lozenges may be rejected
because of a high or low initial drug assay. Excess material may be produced during the cooking cycle of candy base manufacture (cooker salvage)
that cannot be immediately used. The quantity of candy base and lozenge
material rejected during normal production may range from 5% to as high
as 25%, with 15% representing a realistic figure. The necessity of discarding up to 25% of the material produced would pose a severe financial hard-
ship on a manufacturer and the consumer because of a significant increase
in cost of raw materials. In order to alleviate this situation, a system of
salvage reclamation has been developed [69].

The salvage, if properly treated, can be reused in finished product
without altering color, texture, candy base composition, or drug concentration [20]. Before any salvage can be incorporated as part of medicated
lozenge base; (a) lozenge salvage must be adjusted to a pH of 4.5–7.5 to
prevent excessive and uncontrolled inversion of sugar during the cooking
cycle; (b) stability of the active ingredients in the candy base during the
cooking cycle must be determined (some medicaments are lost through
steam distillation, some by reaction with flavors or candy base, while
others are decomposed during the candy base heating cycle); (c) heat-
sensitive colors or reactive medicaments must be removed before salvage
usage. Activated charcoal or diatomaceous earth added to the salvage
mixture, followed by filtration, will remove most color or active ingredients.
If the medicament and colorants are stable during the salvage preparation
and cooking cycle, the need for filtering the salvage is eliminated.

Salvage must be segregated as to product and incorporated only into the *same* product. If color and active ingredients can be added without treatment, a determination of how much salvage is incorporated into the candy base will also determine how much additional drug and color need be added to the completed candy base. (Flavor quantities in salvage need not be calculated as they are lost during the cooking cycle.)

Lozenge rejects can be ground and used as a carrier for flavors. Ground lozenges need not be incorporated in the final lozenge calculations for medicament, flavor, or color since the ground rejects are complete dosage entities; the addition of 5 lb of ground reject lozenges into the candy base is the same as adding 5 lb of finished lozenges. When salvage is added as ground candy, flavor loss is not a factor since the material is not involved in the cooking process.

Medicaments

The type of medicament that can be added to candy base and administered to the patient via a lozenge is restricted only by flavor, dose limitations, or chemical incompatibility. Some materials are so unpalatable or irritating to the mucous membrane that they are unsuitable for this type of administration; some active ingredients must be given at a dosage level sufficiently high to preclude their use in a hard candy lozenge; other medicaments are so reactive with candy base components that the development of a product with a reasonable shelf life is impractical.

Hard candy lozenges usually range in weight from 1.5 to 4.5 g and, depending on the solubility or the melting point of the raw materials, only 3–5% w/w can be readily incorporated. Specialized methods such as dispersing or dissolving drugs in polyethylene glycol [21] increase the quantity of medicament that can be included in candy base. These specialized procedures circumvent the normal procedures for manufacturing hard candy and tend to shorten the product shelf life. This limitation means that a maximum of only 225 mg can be incorporated into candy base using normal manufacturing procedures. The higher the concentration of active drug, the greater the problems of flavoring, mouth-feel, and processing of the candy mass. High levels of powders reduce candy base elasticity, making the lozenge-forming operation more difficult to control while at the same time increasing the percentage of lozenge rejects.

Certain medicaments may require special treatments for their addition or the use or deletion of certain raw materials to assure acceptable physicochemical stability profiles. Examples of certain classifications of medicaicaments that can be incorporated into candy base (along with the particular problems of each type) include local anesthetics, antihistamines, antitussives, analgesics, and decongestants.

B. Local Anesthetics

Ethyl Aminobenzoate (Benzocaine)

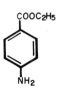

Usual dosage range: 5.0–10.0 mg per lozenge; melting point: 88–90°C; 1 g soluble in 2500 ml water; 1 g soluble in 5.0 ml alcohol. Benzocaine is extremely reactive with aldehydic components of candy base and flavor components. Addition of this material with liquid salvage is not feasible, since at 150°C (the cooking temperature of hard candy) the Schiff's base reaction is pronounced because of aldehydic components in candy and the formation of more reducing sugars during the cooking cycle [22]. As much as 90–95% of the available benzocaine will be lost if added to candy base.

Addition of acidulants to the lozenge formulation promotes degradation via the Schiff's base reaction while drug addition at lower temperatures (110–120°C), along with maximum separation from flavor oils, provides an improved stability profile. Lozenges must be protected from moisture attack as formation of higher levels of invert sugar promotes drug decomposition. Benzocaine products are not difficult to flavor because of low dose and lack of bitter taste. (Insolubility in water and poor solubility in alcohol make the addition of benzocaine as a solution in flavors and organic solvents impractical.)

Hexylresorcinol

Usual dose: 2.4 mg per lozenge; melting point 67.5–69°C; 1 g soluble in 2000 ml water; soluble in alcohol. Hexylresorcinol is less reactive than benzocaine but is still susceptible to reaction with aldehydic components. There is a 10–20% loss of drug if hexylresorcinol is added with liquid salvage, but losses are mostly due to steam distillation occurring during the candy base cooking cycle and not a chemical decomposition problem. No flavoring or mouth-feel problems are associated with this medicament because of the low dose and lack of any appreciable flavor. Hexylresorcinol is relatively easy to incorporate with flavors since the normal dose is only 25% that of benzocaine. Hexylresorcinol can be classified as either an antiseptic or a local anesthetic.

Diperidon HCl

Usual dose: 10.0 mg per lozenge; 1 g soluble in 100 ml water: soluble in alcohol.   Diperidon HCl is not used to any extent in current practice. The local anesthetic activity of diperidon HCl is about equal to that of cocaine.   Although incorporation of this medicament in candy base poses little difficulty, flavoring problems are great due to a bitter, metallic aftertaste.   Lozenges containing diperidon HCl tend to discolor with age.

Benzyl Alcohol

Usual dose: 10% w/w; boiling point: 205°C; 1 g soluble in 25 ml water. A liquid with a faint aromatic odor and sharp, burning taste, benzyl alcohol has an effective anesthetic dose at a 10% concentration.   The incorporation of 10% benzyl alcohol into candy base is difficult but achievable since this material is a liquid at room temperature.   Adequate (5–7%) ground salvage must be used to prevent separation during mixing and to effect proper addition and distribution.   Forming lozenges is difficult because of reduced elasticity of the resultant candy base (due to the presence of the large quantities of ground salvage.)   Also, reproducibility of benzyl alcohol content between batches depends on addition of this material at a uniform temperature to minimize losses from volatilization.   Adequate ventilation is required during processing.   The stability of benzyl alcohol in lozenges is acceptable.   It is compatible with most flavors, although lozenges will discolor (to an orange hue) with age.

Dyclonine

Usual dose: 2–3 mg per lozenge: melting point 173–178°C, 1 g soluble in 60 ml water and 24 ml alcohol.   Dyclonine products are not difficult to flavor because of its low dose and lack of bitter taste.   The lozenge base should be adjusted to a pH between 3 and 5 to effect optimum stability of the medicament [91,92].   Some reactivity with aldehyde-containing flavor components.   Dyclonine has a slow onset of anesthetic activity (5–6 min) but a long duration of action (45–60 min).   Combinations with 5–10 mg benzocaine or menthol per lozenge will effect a rapid onset of anesthetic activity until the dyclonine begins to work.

C.   Antihistamines

Chlorpheniramine Maleate

Usual dose: 2.0 mg per lozenge; melting point: 130–135°C; 1 g soluble in 35 ml water; 1 g soluble in 10 ml alcohol. This material lends itself to satisfactory incorporation and physicochemical stability in candy base. The usual dosage range (2–4 mg); safety and the acceptable stability profiles of this material with most flavorants make chlorpheniramine maleate an ideal ingredient when an antihistamine is required in the lozenge type of dosage form. Use of chlorpheniramine maleate does not produce problems with flavoring since this material has very little flavor of its own.

Phenyltoloxamine Dihydrogen Citrate

$CH_2C_6H_5$

—$OCH_2CH_2N(CH_3)_2$ • $C_6H_8O_7$

Usual dose: 22.0 mg per lozenge; melting point: 138–140°C; soluble in water. The usual therapeutic dose (22.0 mg) along with a high melting point makes the incorporation of phenyltoloxamine dihydrogen citrate in candy base difficult. This material exhibits a bitter and anesthetic taste along with considerable grittiness. The stability of this ingredient in candy base is acceptable.

Diphenhydramine Hydrochloride

C_6H_5
$CHOCH_2CH_2N$ — CH_3 • HCl
C_6H_5 CH_3

Usual dose: 10.0 mg per lozenge; melting point: 166–170°C; 1 g soluble in 1 ml water; 1 g soluble in 2 ml alcohol. Diphenhydramine HCl is a potent antihistamine. Incorporation of 5–10 mg of this ingredient in candy base is not difficult because of its good solubility. Diphenhydramine HCl also possesses antitussive action. It has a bitter, numbing taste that is best masked with citrus flavors. Lozenges tend to discolor (browning) with age.

D. Antitussives

Dextromethorphan Hydrobromide

CH_3O

• HBr

NCH_3

Usual dose: 7.5 mg per lozenge; melting point: 122–124°C; 1.5 g soluble in 1000 ml water; 25 g soluble in 100 ml alcohol. The usual dosage range of dextromethorphan HBr in lozenges is 5–15 mg. Incorporation of this

ingredient in candy base is not difficult because of its melting point and
solubility; addition with liquid salvage is feasible as this compound is not
subject to heat degradation or steam distillation problems. It is compatible
with most flavors and is stable over a wide pH range. Dextromethorphan
HBr has a bitter taste, an anesthetic mouth-feel, and an unpleasant aftertaste. Masking greater than 2.0 mg per lozenge is difficult.

Dextromethorphan HBr is supplied as a 10% adsorbate (10% of dextromethorphan HBr adsorbed on 90% magnesium trisilicate) to avoid flavoring
difficulty [71–75]. This adsorbate, which releases the dextromethorphan
HBr at the pH of stomach fluids, renders the active ingredient almost tasteless. This results in a medicament that is easy to flavor but difficult to
incorporate in candy base, as 10 times the amount of material must be
added to achieve an equivalent dose of the regular dextromethorphan HBr.
The magnesium trisilicate, being insoluble and having a melting point above
that of candy base, will not readily incorporate in the candy mass. The
material that does incorporate produces a grainy, rough lozenge texture
with an unpleasant mouth-feel.

One method of incorporating the adsorbate into candy base is to prepare a granulation (Figure 7) of the dextromethorphan HBr adsorbate with
either glycerin or propylene glycol. A ratio of one part solvent to three
parts dextromethorphan HBr produces a free-flowing granulation. The
resulting lozenge can be easily flavored and has a smooth mouth-feel. Use
of the adsorbate limits incorporation of dextromethorphan HBr to 10 mg or
less (usual range 5.0–7.5 mg per lozenge) unless a 4.0 g or higher weight
lozenge is produced or an alternate manufacturing procedure is used. The
product can be flavored as desired since dextromethorphan HBr will not
degrade in the presence of flavor components, but the use of acidulants
is contraindicated if the tasteless nature of the adsorbate is to be preserved. The adsorbate cannot be added with liquid salvage as the salvage
pH would be 8.0 and addition of acid to lower pH would change the lozenge
taste and mouth-feel. This is because a portion of the dextromethorphan
HBr will be released from its magnesium trisilicate carrier.

E. Analgesics

Aspirin

COOH
OOCCH₃

Usual dose: 175.0 mg per lozenge; melting point: 135°C; 1 g soluble in
300 ml water; 1 g soluble in 5 ml alcohol. A direct addition of the aspirin
or a mixture of flavor and aspirin to candy base allows ready incorporation
of 175.0 mg into a 2.5–3.5 g hard candy lozenge. This medicated candy
possesses an acceptable mouth-feel and can be easily flavored without
danger of medicament–flavor interaction. The candy base must be prepared at a very low moisture content (less than 0.5%), and all flavors and
alternate raw materials must be moisture-free, as incorporation of even a
small quantity of water will result in rapid hydrolysis of aspirin into acetic
and salicylic acids.

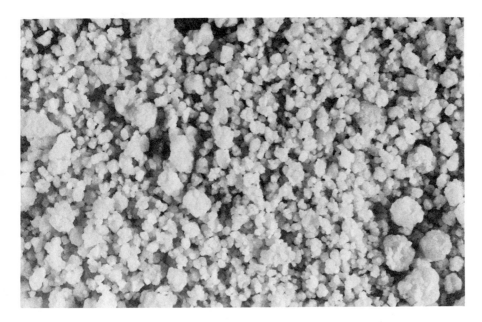

Figure 7   Preparation of a free-flowing granulation of insoluble or high melting point medicaments with a suitable solvent and ground salvage eases incorporation into the candy base.

The hygroscopic nature of the candy base requires that protective packaging be employed if a reasonable product shelf life is to be expected. Use of lozenge rejects as salvage without filtration is not practical, as dissolving the salvage in water results in rapid decomposition of the aspirin.

Acetaminophen

$CH_3-CO-NH-\langle\rangle-OH$

Usual dose: 175.0 mg per lozenge; melting point: 169–170°C; very slowly soluble in water; soluble in alcohol.   It is difficult to incorporate this medicament in candy base because of its poor solubility and high melting point. Preparation of 4.5 g candy lozenges with up to 175.0 mg of acetaminophen requires preparation of a granulation with either 1–2% glycerin or propylene glycol.   The resulting lozenge has a bitter taste with a metallic aftertaste.

Acetaminophen does not decompose when combined with most flavoring agents, but the p-aminophenol, present as an impurity in acetaminophen, will react with low levels of iron to cause the formation of a pink color. Addition of a chelating agent (citric acid) will improve acetaminophen color stability in candy base, but the iron content of the candy base (derived from the iron in corn syrup) should be kept below 2.0 ppm.

F. Decongestants

Phenylpropanolamine HCl

NH$_2$ • HCl
|
HOCH–CH–CH$_3$

I

Usual dose: 18.5 mg per lozenge; melting point: 190–194°C; freely soluble in water and alcohol. The incorporation of 18–20 mg phenylpropanolamine HCl into 2.5–3.0 g lozenges results in a product with an acceptable mouth-feel. The formulation is not difficult to flavor because of the low level of medicament aftertaste. Phenylpropanolamine HCl will degrade via the aldol condensation in the presence of the aldehydes in candy base or with flavors containing aldehydes.

Aldol Condensation

Under alkaline conditions, phenylpropanolamine hydrochloride (I) is stripped of HCl and loses its hydroxy hydrogen to form the anion (II). This anion is then capable of rearranging to a more stable ketone (III). The ketone, however, contains an active α hydrogen which can be extracted in the presence of −OH⁻ to form the anion (IV), which can go on to react with aldehydes or ketones already present in the candy base or with flavors containing aldehydes or ketones.

H NH$_2$
⊖ | |
O–C–CHCH$_3$

II $\xrightarrow{-H^{\ominus}}$

O NH
‖ |
C–CHCH$_3$
α

III $\xrightarrow{{}^{\ominus}OH}$

O NH$_2$
‖ |
C–C–CH$_3$
⊖

IV   +

R$_1$
\   C=O →
R$_2$

O   CH$_3$ OH
‖ | |
C – C – C–R$_1$
    | |
   NH$_2$ R$_2$

(R$_1$, R$_2$ may be aryl, alkyl, H)

The addition of acidulent sufficient to lower the candy base pH to the range of 2.5–3.0 will improve phenylpropanolamine HCl stability in the lozenge—although even with this modification, the medicament will decompose if the lozenge is exposed to moisture during storage. Phenylpropanolamine HCl cannot be added to candy base with salvage solutions because of the reactivity of this medicament with the aldehydic portions in the candy base.

d-Pseudoephedrine Hydrochloride

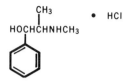

Usual dose: 18.5−25.0 mg per lozenge; melting point: 181−182°C; soluble in water and alcohol. This compound is less bitter than phenylpropanolamine HCl and less reactive in the presence of candy base and with exposure to moisture.

II. PROCESSING

A. Cooking

Water is required to dissolve the sugar and to obtain the proper quantity of invert sugar. The batch then has to be boiled to remove the water. The higher the cooking temperature, the less water remains in the batch (Figure 8) [23,24].

Candy base cookers are divided into three classes: (a) fire cookers; (b) high-speed atmospheric cookers; and (c) vacuum cookers.

Fire Cookers

Cooking on an open fire (Figure 9) is the oldest method for preparing hard candy base. The fire cooker comes in two types: (a) the atmospheric gas cooker (Figure 10 and 11), which is a slow cooker and (b) the draft cooker (Figure 12), which cooks the candy at a faster rate. The use of fire cookers is declining in the United States but is still used for specialized items to produce a particular flavor, texture, or color.

In the tranditional method of manufacturing candy base on a fire cooker, the desired quantity of sugar is dissolved in at least one-third the amount of water by heating and stirring in a copper kettle until all sugar granules are dissolved. The sides of the pan are kept clean during the cooking operation by washing them continuously with water or by placing a lid on the pan so that the steam washes down any crystals above the level of the liquid. Corn syrup or inverting agent is added when the cooking temperature reaches 110°C. Cooking is then continued until a final temperature of 145−156°C is achieved, depending on the final solids and moisture content desired [23].

The formulator must add the correct quantity of water to the sugar, as insufficient water may result in incomplete dissolution of the sugar crystals, while addition of too much water may result in excessive sugar inversion because of increased cooking time. When boiling or dissolving sugar, a fundamental principle is that all solutions be heated and stirred until they are clear of residual crystals. Any undissolved sugar in the mass might act as a seed for crystallization or graining in the finished product. Heat is transmitted through the copper kettle into the sugar solution during

Assume it is desired to find the absolute (vapor) pressure at which a cooker should be operated in order to obtain finished candy with 88 percent solids and a final cook temperature of 75° C. (165° F.). An extended straight-edge is placed at this solids content on scale C-C' (called point 2) and moved up or down until the sum of the values on scale B-B' (called point 1) and scale D-D' (called point 3) equals 75° C. (165° F.). This occurs at 58° C. (136.5° F.) (point 1) on scale B-B' and 11° C. (19.9° F.) (point 3) on scale D-D', and this shows there would be an 11° C. (19.9° F.) boiling point rise and a vapor temperature of 58° C. (136.5° F.). To determine the absolute (vapor) pressure or vacuum under which the cook would have to be operated, merely extend the 58° C. value on scale B-B' across to scale A-A', and this equals 135 mm Hg (point 4). This in turn corresponds to a vacuum of 24.6 inches Hg.

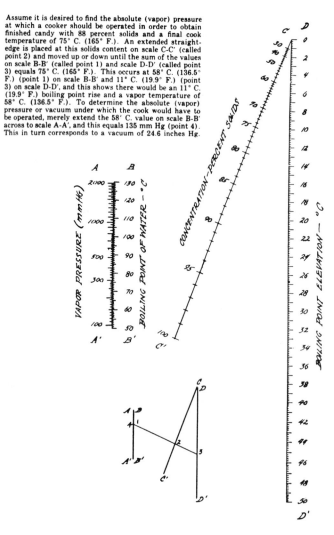

Figure 8   Calculating temperature, vacuum, and moisture content in candy cooking.   (The Manufacturing Confectioner, Vol. 70, No. 7, July, 1970.)

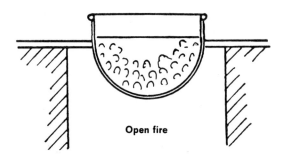

Open fire

Figure 9   Schematic of open-fire cooking method for manufacturing hard candy base.   Cooking temperature determines final candy base moisture content.   (Robert Bosch GmBH, Div. Hamac-Höller.)

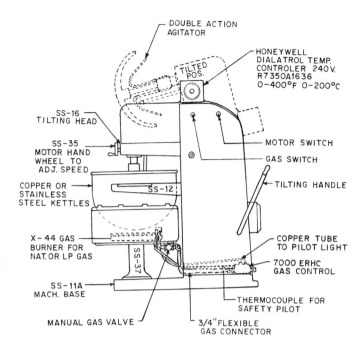

Figure 10   Schematic of atmospheric fire mixer.   (Savage Brothers Co.,
Elk Grove Village, Ill.)

the cooking process. As cooking proceeds, the solution becomes more
viscous until eventually the sugar particles near the wall of the pan are
unable to change places rapidly enough with the cooler ones in the interior
of the batch. As a result, the surface particles are overheated and burned, while particles in the interior are still below the necessary cooking
temperature. This accounts for the yellowing or browning of open-fire-
cooked batches. Browning also occurs if the fire is too hot; so when the
temperature of the batch exceeds 125°C, the fire level should be reduced.
Conversely, if the batch is cooked too slowly, it also becomes yellow and
may become overinverted, particularly if an inverting agent is present.
Use of large kettles with mechanical mixing action improves the efficiency
of the fire-cooking process by increasing the rate of sugar particle movement, thus reducing the incidence of candy base yellowing or browning.

High-Speed Atmospheric Cookers

The high-speed atmospheric cooker (Figure 13) uses an efficient heat exchange surface and a swiftly rotating scraper, which spreads an almost
microscopic film of candy on a heat exchange surface [4]. This results in
a rapid exchange between the heated surface and the batch, the latter
boiling more quickly and producing a lighter candy with controlled and
lower inversion rate than when candy base is cooked on a fire cooker [25].

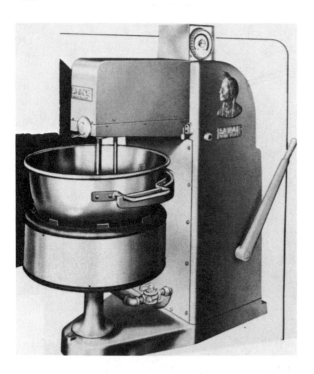

Figure 11   Atmospheric gas furnace.   Features: single or double action agitation with scraping action; 30 to 60 rpm stirring speed; thermostatic control; 110,000 to 286,000 BTU heat output; removable agitator; copper kettle 24 in. × 12 1/2 in. × 16 in. deep.   (Savage Brothers Co., Elk Grove Village, Ill.)

The steam developed by this type of boiling is flashed off to the atmosphere. The candy is brought up to 165–170°C in just a few minutes; however, candy cooked in this way comes out of the cooker at 160°C and must be cooled as rapidly as possible by being dropped onto a cooling slab where it is generally brought down to 100–120°C, so that it can be worked as a plactic-like mass, making it convenient for incorporation of flavor, color, acidulent, and medicaments.

Vacuum Cookers

Vacuum cooking was developed to overcome the disadvantages of cooking candy base on an open fire.   The rationale for vacuum cooking is based on the principle that water at atmospheric pressure boils at 100°C but will boil at about 40°C under a high vacuum; therefore, a sugar solution can be boiled at a lower temperature and still result in removal of the water.   With this process, a sugar solution and corn syrup are boiled to 125–132°C, vacuum is applied, and (owing to the heat in the batch) additional water is boiled off without extra heating.   The resulting vapor is condensed and removed by the cooling water of the vacuum pump.   Today vacuum cooking is the process of choice for manufacturing hard candy base [23].

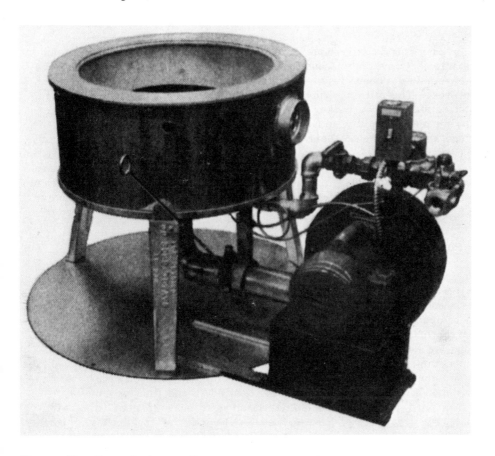

Figure 12   Forced-air gas furnace. Produces fast, high heat; can be used with mixed propane, or natural gas; 3,000-rpm blower speed; 25-in. outer diameter; 25-in. height. (Savage Brothers Co., Elk Grove Village, Ill.)

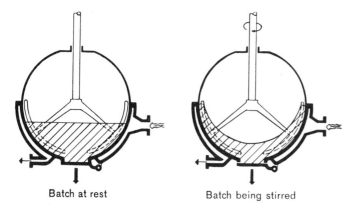

Batch at rest   Batch being stirred

Figure 13   Schematic of high-speed atmospheric cooker with mixer. (Robert Bosch GmBH, Div. Hamac-Höller.)

B. Batch Cookers

Candy base that is stirred at a constant or falling temperature will tend to crystallize. Conversely, candy base stirred at a rising temperature will not crystallize. There is an advantage to stirring a batch at rising temperatures. The stirring will spread a thin film of sugar solution onto the heated surface of the cooker, resulting in the heated sugar particles changing places rapidly and causing a quicker heat exchange between the surface and the batch. This produces a lighter, more reproducible product (Figure 14).

Vacuum batch cookers have two major subgroups: (1) those that are capable of cooking 100% pure sugar down to about 65% sugar in the formulation, and (2) others which will cook 65% sugar down to about 10% sugar [4].

C. Pure Sugar Cookers

Pure sugar cookers are made to be operated in several ways. There is the Hamac-Hansella (Figures 15 and 16), Solich, or Hohberger types, which have a cooking kettle built above a vacuum kettle. The components separate to open with the bottom section dropping down and tilting. The second type of pure sugar kettle is the simplex cooker. These cookers have a separate kettle for precooking the hard candy formula, which is then dumped into the vacuum chamber where the vacuum is drawn on the chamber and the candy base is dried for a specified number of minutes. The time depends on the moisture content desired in the final product.

The pure sugar cookers lend themselves to easy washout (dissolving what sugar crystals may have formed on the sides of the kettles or in the

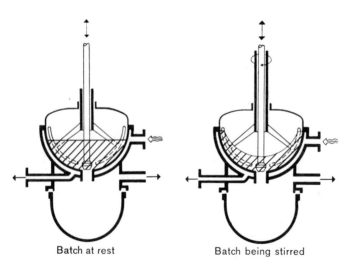

Batch at rest   Batch being stirred

Figure 14   Schematic of batch vacuum cooker with mixer and receiving kettle. (Robert Bosch GmBH, Div. Hamac-Höller.)

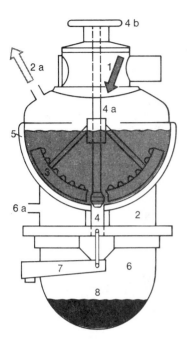

Figure 15 Schematic of Universal Batch Vacuum Cooker. (1) Filling (water, sugar, glucose, and possibly milk and fat), (2) batch cooker, (2a) boiling vapro, (3) beater, (4) valve, (4a) valve rod, (4b) valve operating wheel, (5) steam heating, (6) vacuum chamber, (6a) vacuum connection, (7) swivel device, and (8) delivery pan with boiled sugar mass. (Robert Bosch GmBH, Div. Hamac-Höller.)

vacuum chamber). It is essential that all crystals be dissolved and removed; otherwise the batch being cooked may grain in the kettle—or soon afterward on the cooling or tempering table.

D. Standard Vacuum Cookers

Standard vacuum cookers are designed to cook candy base formulations containing 65% sugar or less. The two types of standard vacuum cookers are the continuous batch process cooker and the continuous process cooker.

Continuous Batch Process Cooker

The installation normally consists of an automatic sugar dissolver, sugar syrup and corn syrup storage kettles, metering pumps, precooker, sugar feed pumps, the actual cooker, a vacuum pump, and a collection kettle. When a precooker kettle is used, it is common to have an intermediate holding tank between it and the cooker, and a pipeline connected to the sugar feed pump from this tank. This system requires an automatic dissolving machine which will continuously meter and dissolve sugar and add corn syrup [26].

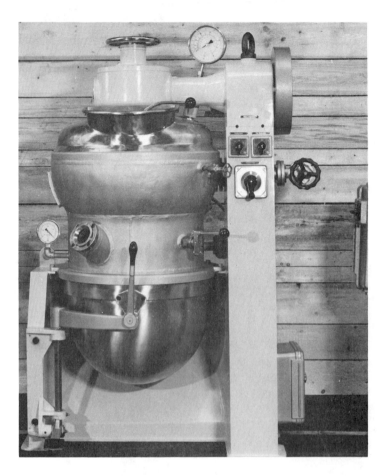

Figure 16   Universal batch vacuum cooker.   Suitable for production of high- and low-boiled sugar masses up to 85 to 90% sugar.   Output: 275 to 350 lb./hr.; batch size up to 90 lb.   (Robert Bosch GmBH, Div. Hamac-Höller.)

Precookers

Precookers are steam-jacketed kettles equipped with celerity cookers (additional heat exchangers) placed in the unit in such a way that more energetic circulation can be obtained than when only the normal heat exchange surfaces are being used [4].

There are also continuous precookers which are called dissolvers (e.g., Solvomat-Hamac-Hansella) whereby an efficient heat exchange surface is used to boil, first, water and sugar which are added on a continual basis, and then the corn syrup which is also added to the machine on a continuous basis along with candy base salvage, if desired (Figure 17).   Each component is added to the dissolver by way of a gear-metering system which is controlled by one gearing system so that the finished, precooked syrup can be brought up to the proper temperature (110−120°C) and used within 1 min or less of reaching this temperature.   The short dwell time in the dissolver reduces the quantity of invert sugar developed and reduces the browning action (Maillard browning) that occurred in the older type of precooking kettles. In the older models, cooking times necessary to bring the batch to temperature were as long as 15—20 min with another 10—15 min needed to use up the product. The hot mass in the precooking kettle could be inverted as much as an additional 1—2%. An optional gearing system can be installed for the continous, accurately metered addition of medicated salvage solutions, which must be added in a uniform and controlled manner. Quantities of salvage added can be altered by incorporating different change gears that can adjust the quantity of salvage solution added to the candy from a little as 1.5% to as much as 25% on a dry weight basis. Slip-on change gears enable the formulator to adjust the mixing ratio of sugar and corn syrup from 80% sugar:20% corn syrup to 45% sugar:55% corn syrup.

Sugar may be metered into the dissolver in a granulated form and mixed with water, or in a liquid syrup form (Figure 18). The sugar is continuously and automatically metered into the precooking chamber where it is cooked by a steam coil that passes almost completely around the bottom

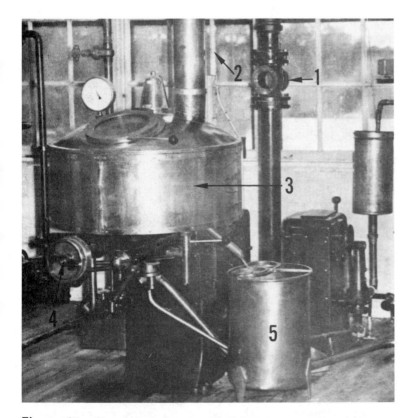

Figure 17 Precooker for production of 650 to 2750 pounds of sugar plus glucose per hour. (1) Corn syrup line; (2) liquid sugar line; (3) precooker; (4) syrup flow valve; (5) intermediate holding container. (Robert Bosch GmBH, Div. Hamac-Höller.)

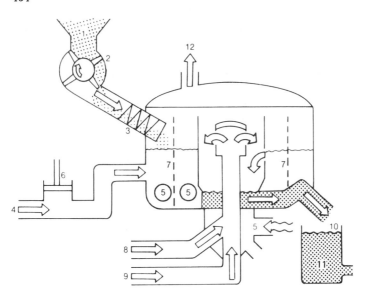

Figure 18   Schematic drawing of Hansella Solvomat precooker. Liquid
sugar feed has replaced the granulated sugar feed and dissolving process.
(1) Granulated sugar feed, (2) metering wheel, (3) worm, (4) water feed,
(5) steam, (6) water pump, (7) sugar-water mixture, (8) glucose feed,
(9) feed for other ingredients, (10) preboiled glucose-sugar solution, (11)
intermediate container, and (12) boiling vapor discharge. (Robert Bosch
GmBH, Div. Hamac-Höller.)

of the compartment, causing the liquid sugar to boil voilently without
mechanical agitation. Liquid sugar precooking temperature can be adjusted
between 100 and 110°C, depending on the desired output. The precooked
liquid sugar then overflows into the central chamber where it is automatically mixed with the preheated corn syrup and any liquid salvage or other
ingredients as desired in the proper proportion (Figure 19). The resulting
precooked liquid sugar, corn syrup, and third ingredient (if required),
after mixing and cooking, flow into an intermediate collection container before further processing (Figure 20). Automatic dissolvers have an output
of 650–1750 lb of sugar per hour.

E. Cooking Machines

The precooked sugar–corn syrup solution, which has been cooked to a
temperature of 100–120°C, now passes through an adjustable output syrup
pump that continuously distributes the candy mass through cooking coils
(Figures 21 and 22). These coils lead to an intermediate chamber where
a thermometer is located, which measures the syrup temperature as it
leaves the coil. The cooking coils and intermediate chamber are never under vacuum since the intermediate chamber is vented to the atmosphere.
This feature enables all vapors from the batches to be vented, resulting

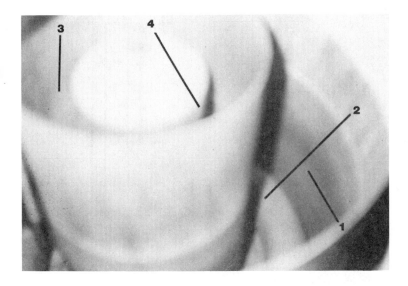

Figure 19　Internal view of Hansella precooker. (1) Precooking chamber; (2) steam coil; (3) central chamber; (4) addition of preheated corn syrup and third ingredient. (Warner-Lambert Co.)

in a dry and smooth-quality product, due to the absence of these vapors in combination with the turbulent vacuum effect that ordinarily exists in the cooking system. This principle also results in a savings of 80–90% in cooling water consumption normally required by the vacuum system to condense these vapors.

From the intermediate chamber, the finished cooked syrup (135–150°C) flows into the vacuum chamber. Flow from intermediate chamber to vacuum chamber is regulated by a metering valve, which is activated by vacuum and only opens when the vacuum chamber and receiving kettle are under full vacuum (635–762 mm Hg). The quantity of cooked syrup in the intermediate chamber must always be sufficient to seal the vacuum.

An adjustable timing device automatically changes the receiving kettles by opening an air valve the moment the required size batch has been cooked to the desired temperature. This action causes a stream of air to flow into the vacuum chamber, thereby breaking the vacuum and automatically closing the metering valve to prevent any syrup from dropping during the receiving kettle exchange. The filled receiving kettle drops from the vacuum hood and swings to the front of the cooker by means of a spring-activated turning device and is replaced by the empty one which, when in position, presses against the vacuum hood and is sealed by the vacuum. The process is repeated without any assistance from an operator (Figure 23).

The automatic kettle-changing timing device works directly from the strokes of the syrup pump; therefore, all batches are uniform in weight and quality and can be regulated from 50 to 100 lb as required. From 300 to 3000 lb of candy base can be prepared per hour of production, depending on the cooker model utilized (Table 3).

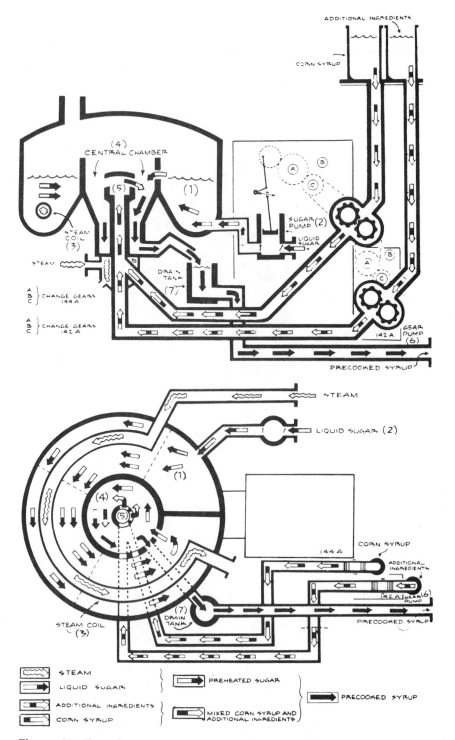

Figure 20 Hansella precooker. (1) Precooking chamber; (2) sugar pump; (3) steam coil; (4) central chamber; (5) preheated corn syrup; (6) third-ingredient pump; (7) intermediate drain tank. (Robert Bosch GmBH, Div. Hamac-Höller.)

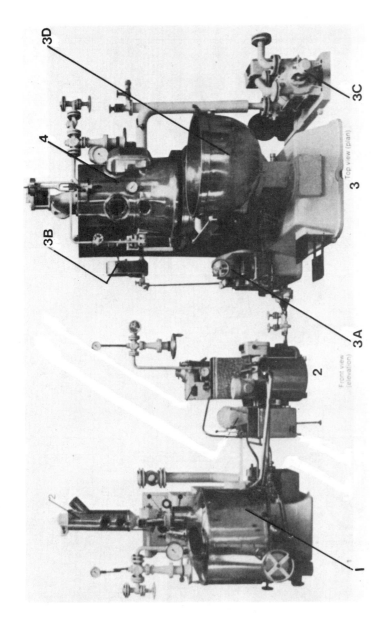

Figure 21 Complete candy base cooking setup. (1) Solvomat precooker; (2) intermediate container; (3) cooker; (3A) pump for sugar and glucose solution; (3B) metering gear; (3C) vacuum pump; (3D) delivery pan; (4) cooking chamber. (Robert Bosch GmBH, Div. Hamac-Höller.)

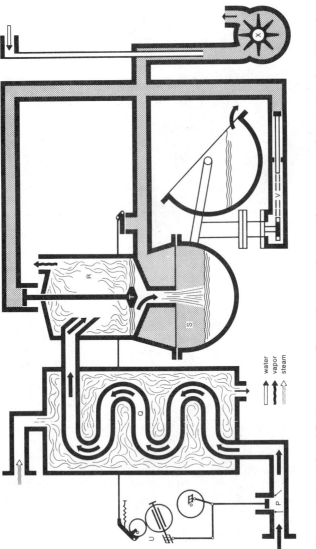

Figure 22   Simplified process flow diagram for continuous cooking system. (P) ad-justable output syrup pump; (Q) cooking coils; (R) intermediate chamber; (S) vacuum chamber; (T) candy base flow metering valve; (U) adjustable timing device to auto-matically change receiving kettles; (V) kettle turning device; (X) rotary type vacuum pump. (Robert Bosch GmBH, Div. Hamac-Höller.)

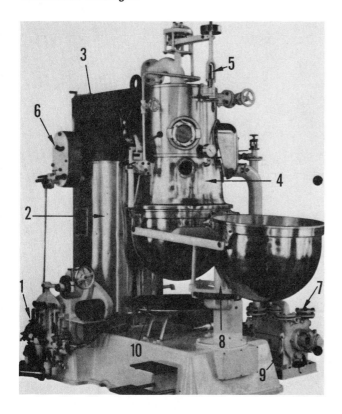

Figure 23 Vacuum cooking machine. (1) Adjustable sugar pump; (2) cooking coil; (3) intermediate chamber; (4) vacuum chamber; (5) flow metering valve; (6) timing device that automatically changes receiving kettles; (7) receiving kettles; (8) kettle turning device; (9) rotary vacuum pump; (10) washing drain. (Robert Bosch GmBH, Div. Hamac-Höller.)

F. Candy Base Manufacturing Principle

The entire cooking unit (Figure 24) is heated to the candy base cooking temperature by passing steam into and around the copper coil. The vacuum system is turned on and the steam pressure in the cooker adjusted by means of a reducing valve. Concurrently, the sugar syrup reservoir of the dissolver is filled and precooking is initiated. The precooking temperature has a considerable effect on the performance of the cooker. If the temperature is too low, more water has to be evaporated in the cooker; too high a temperature can affect the performance of the sugar pump because of the higher viscosity of the precooked mass.

The sugar pump is started and begins pumping the precooked solution into the heated coil where it is boiled and from which it is emptied into the intermediate chamber, where cooking vapors are removed to the atmosphere. The candy base then goes into the vacuum chamber where the final moisture is removed. The lubricated collection kettle is placed under the cooking dome, and the batch-size control mechanism is started. After a predetermined interval, the pan with the cooked batch is swung out.

Table 3   Typical Specifications for Three Hamac-Hansella Candy Base Vacuum Cookers

Specification	Type 135B	Type 145A	Type 155A
Capacity	1200 lb/hr to 3 tons in 8 hr	2000 lb/hr to 6 tons in 8 hr	3000 lb/hr to 10 tons in 8 hr
Drive	2 motors	2 motors	2 motors
For sugar pump	0.5 HP, 1200 rpm	0.5 HP, 1800 rpm	0.5 HP, 1800 rpm
For vacuum pump	7.5 HP, 1800 rpm	10 HP, 1800 rpm	20 HP, 1800 rpm
Steam pressure (permissible pressure)	150 lb/in^2	150 lb/in^2	150 lb/in^2
Working pressure (depending on output)	Up to 120 lb/in^2	Up to 120 lb/in^2	Up to 120 lb/in^2
Steam consumption	220 lb/hr max.	440 lb/hr max.	750 lb/hr max.
Water consumption	105 ft^3 per 8-hr day	210 ft^3 per 8-hr day	350 ft^3 per 8-hr day
Steam connection	1 in.	1 1/4 in.	1 1/4 in.
Condensed water connection	3/4 in.	3/4 in.	1 in.
Space requirements			
Width	6 ft 7 in.	7 ft. 5 in.	9 ft
Depth	8 ft	8 ft	8 ft 8 in.
Height	7 ft 5 in.	7 ft 10 in.	9 ft
Weight	Approx. 3650 lb (net)	Approx. 4500 lb (net)	Approx. 7340 (net)

Source: Robert Bosch GmBH, Div. Hamac-Höller.

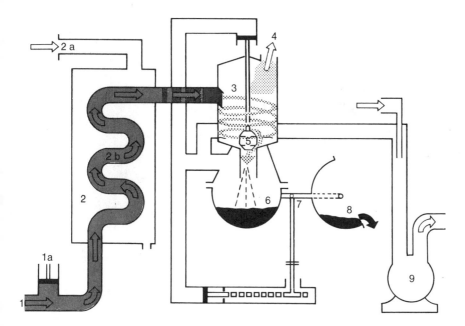

Figure 24   Schematic of candy base vacuum cooking sequence.   (1) Pre-cooked sugar—glucose solution; (1a) feed pump; (2) steam chamber; (2a) steam supply; (2b) cooking coil; (3) vapor space; (4) extraction of vapors; (5) valve; (6) vacuum chamber; (7) pan swiveling device; (8) discharge pan; (9) vacuum pump.   (Robert Bosch GmBH, Div. Hamac-Höller.)

The sugar-corn syrup mixture boils violently as it moves along the relatively narrow coil surrounded by steam.   The heating surface is large; therefore, rapid heat exchange results, and the mass is cooked for a very short time, through very intensely.   This results in a lighter and clearer product with the potential for increased shelf life.

If the output of candy base production is increased, the steam pressure must be increased because more water must be removed over the same length of coil.   Cookers should produce a candy with a final moisture content of about 1% after vacuum treatment (Figure 25).

The sugar pumps must always run in a water bath, insuring against the formation of crystals from friction.   Such crystals could enter the batch and cause premature graining.

The advantages of continuous vacuum cooking are (1) a low final moisture content with little inversion—less than 2% (the inversion is kept even throughout the production run because cooking is rapid); (2) avoidance of caramelizing; and (3) a more pliable consistency of batches for subsequent processing.

G.   Mixing

After the collection kettle is charged with the predetermined weight of candy base, the vacuum is broken and the kettle makes a 180° revolution, placing the second kettle in position for collection of the cooked candy base.   The

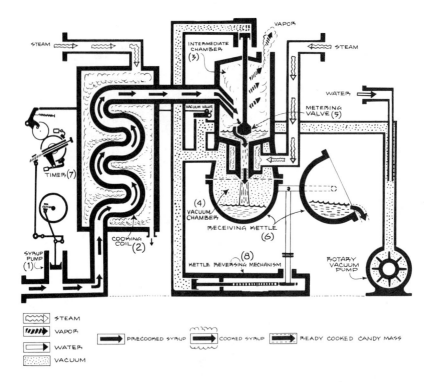

STEAM

VAPOR

WATER

VACUUM

PRECOOKED SYRUP   COOKED SYRUP   READY COOKED CANDY MASS

Figure 25 Complete process flow diagram for cooking system used in continuous and automatic cookers. (1) Adjustable sugar pump; (2) cooking coil; (3) intermediate chamber; (4) vacuum chamber; (5) flow metering value; (6) receiving kettle; (7) timing device that automatically changes receiving kettles; (8) kettle turning device. (Robert Bosch GmBH, Div. Hamac-Höller.)

filled kettle, heavier by the batch weight, presses the empty kettle against the vacuum hood where it is sealed by the vacuum. The cooking cycle may be completed every 3—5 min depending on the number of forming lines being serviced and the weight of the candy base collected per batch. About 1600—2100 lb of candy base can be manufactured per hour under normal batch process manufacturing conditions.

The temperature of the candy base is about 135°C, and the mass is a semisolid, having a plastic-like consistency when it is removed from the cooker. The candy mass is removed from the collection kettle into a lubricated transfer container mounted on a suitable weight-check scale (Figure 26). Here the weight of the candy base is checked and any adjustments for proper batch weight are made to the cooker (Figure 27).

At this point the colors, as solutions, pastes, or color cubes, are added and mixed into the candy base. Addition of the colors at this point (if the colors are heat-stable) allows for maximum retention time in the hot mass, assuring complete melting of the color into the base.

The candy base containing color is then transferred to a water-jacketed stainless steel cooling table for the mixing operation (Figure 28). This mixing can be either manual, using two or more operators, or mechanical, using either a series of plows and rollers or a mixer consisting of two mixing arms, a mixing plunger, and a slowly rotating table top (e.g., Berks mixer; Figure 29). (The plow and roller mixing is used by the continuous process cooker and will be discussed later.) The Berks batch mixing machine can mix from 60 to 130 lb of candy base (Figure 30) while an experienced manual operator can efficiently mix only between 40 and 75 lb.

Throughout the mixing cycle, the temperature of the mixing table is maintained between 40 and 50°C. A table that is too hot will cause the candy base to stick, whereas a cold table will cause premature hardening. Premature hardening will shorten the effective mixing time, increase the tendency to grain, and reduce the efficiency of mixing. This will lessen the uniform incorporation of flavors and medicaments into the candy mass. With both the manual and Berks-type mixers, the operator uses a stainless steel mixing bar (Figure 31) to assist mixing and to speed the incorporation of medicament and flavors in the mass. The mechanical and manual mixing compresses the candy, thus presenting warm sides to the cool table surface for uniform cooling (Figure 32). When mixing cycles are short (less than 5 min), parts of the cooling table may become hot enough to make the candy base stick to the slab. Hydrogenated vegetable oil-based lubricant is spread onto the table surface to alleviate this condition.

Flavor, drug, and ground salvage mixture are added to the candy mass when mixing is initiated. The medicament can be dissolved in the flavor oils, then added to the ground salvage with the flavor, and mixed until uniformly distributed; or it can be added separately—with salvage or directly—to the candy mass, depending on solubility and stability characteristics of the medicament in flavor oils. The flavor, drug, acidulent (if required), and salvage mixture can be prepared on an individual batch basis

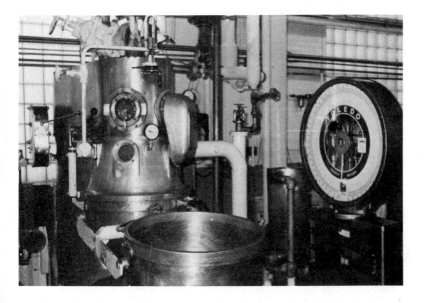

Figure 26 Candy base vacuum cooker. Scale is available to check weight each batch of candy base. (Warner-Lambert Co.)

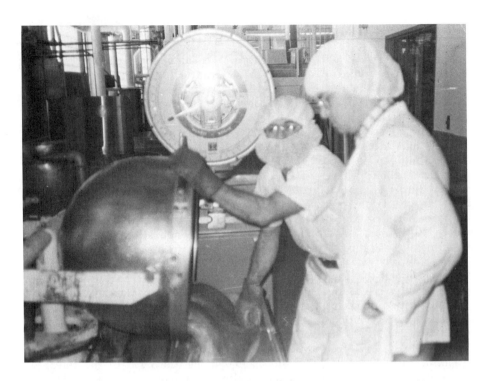

Figure 27 Completed candy base being transferred to weighing container. All batch weights are double-checked. (Warner-Lambert Co.)

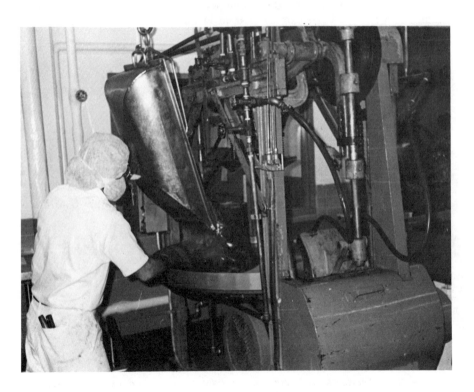

Figure 28 Operator transferring cooked candy base to mixer. (Warner-Lambert Co.)

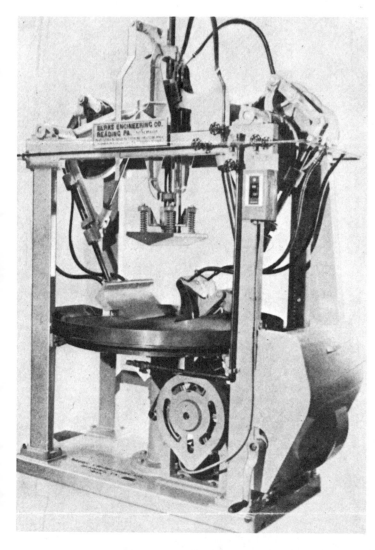

Figure 29   Plow-type batch mixing machine.   Berks Co. mixer is capable of mixing 60 to 130 lb. of candy base.   (Berks Engineering Co. , Reading, Pa.)

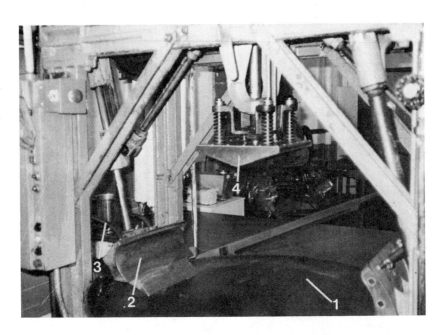

Figure 30   Plow-type mixer.   (1) Water cooled and heated table that rotates one-quarter turn per mixing cycle; (2) mixing plow; (3) water inlet to plows; (4) top plow that flattens mixed candy mass.   (Warner-Lambert Co.)

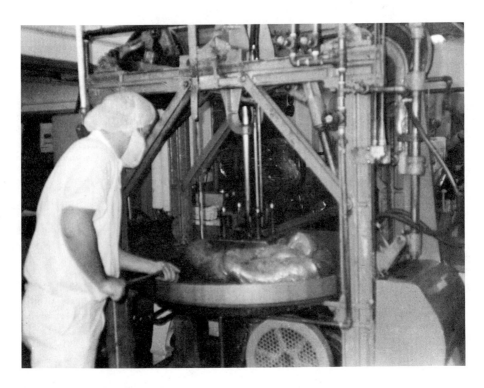

Figure 31   Operator-assisted mixing utilizing a stainless steel mixing bar. (Warner-Lambert Co.)

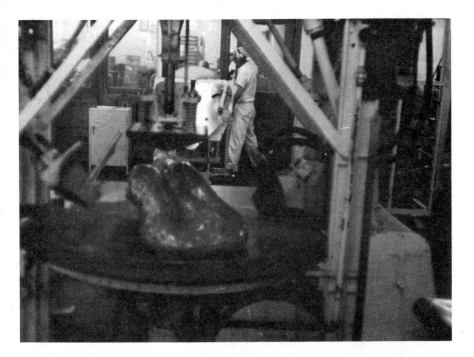

Figure 32   Candy base after side plows have compressed the mass.   Top
plow is now lowering to flatten the base.   (Warner-Lambert Co.)

(Figure 33) or as a master premix (Figure 34) suitable for subdivision into
individual premixes (Figure 35).   This master premix can be prepared using
either planetary, sigma blade, or ribbon blender.   When premixes are prepared on a master batch basis, ground salvage [69] should be milled to a
particle size range of 20–50 mesh (Figure 36).   This produces granules
that will adsorb the liquid mixture to prevent flavor and medicament segregation during granulation preparation and storage before use.   If salvage
is milled to a finer mesh size, the granulation will set or harden during
storage, making distribution into the candy mass more difficult and requiring more operator assistance.   Particles milled to the coarser mesh size
will not adsorb flavor oils; such nonadsorption of flavor oils would result
in problems of segregation and nonuniform distribution of flavor and medicament throughout the salvage mixture.

The medicament cannot be added to the salvage granules in solution
with the flavor oils because of incompatibility or solubility characteristics,
either a direct addition of medicament to candy base on the mixing table can
be made, or a separate solution of the drug in a compatible solvent can be
granulated into a second salvage mixture and added to the candy mass before adding the flavor granulation.   A slurry or free-flowing granulation
with ground salvage using solvents such as glycerin or propylene glycol
added in a ratio of one part solvent to three, four or even five parts medicament may be utilized for addition of insoluble medicaments.

The optimum mixing required to uniformly mix the flavor, salvage, and
medicament into the candy base during the routine manufacture of medicated

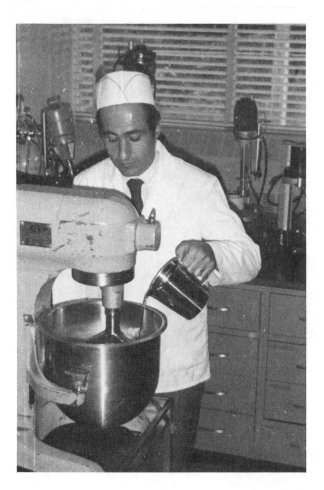

Figure 33 Preparation of flavor, medicament, and ground salvage mixture on an individual batch basis. Sufficient material is contained in the premix for incorporation into 100 lb. of cooked candy base. This procedure can be used to prepare experimental as well as production batches. Here the flavor is added to the ground salvage and medicament mixture. (Warner-Lambert Co.)

hard candy lozenges is determined by the time required to effect a uniform distribution of the materials in candy base. The time period required to cool the mass—or the speed of the cooker—determines how soon the next batch will be available for processing. The normal mixing cycle is 4–6 min.

   After mixing is complete, the candy base is transferred to a warming table (Figure 37) where the batch is covered with a canvas cloth and allowed to temper (equilibrate so that it reaches a uniform temperature). This eliminates hot or cold spots in the mass, which hinder the lozenge-forming operation. Once tempered, the batch is divided into 35- to 50-lb portions that can be readily handled by the operators as they transfer the candy base to the batch former.

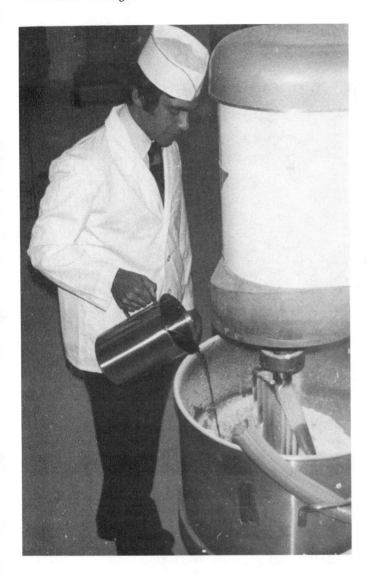

Figure 34   Preparation of flavor, medicament, acidulent, and ground salvage mixture as a master premix that can be subdivided into quantities
suitable for incorporation into individual 100–lb. cooked candy base portions.
The formulator is adding the flavor to the ground salvage, acidulent, and
medicament mixture.   This is followed by sufficient mixing to assure a uniform distribution throughout the batch.   (Warner-Lambert Co.)

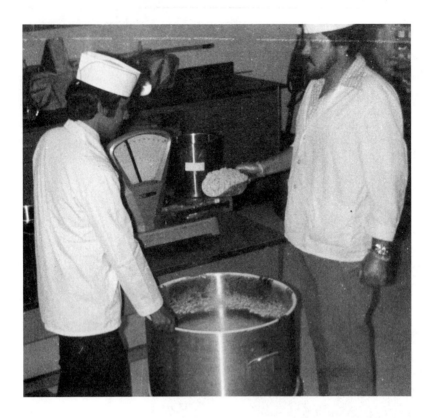

Figure 35   Flavor, ground salvage, acidulent, and medicament mixture being subdivided into quantities suitable for incorporation into the individual cooked candy base. All weights are checked during the subdivision procedure. Depending on the quantity of salvage required per batch, material sufficient for addition into 30 to 75 batches of candy base can be prepared as a single premix.

H.   Batch Forming

After the candy mass has been properly tempered and cut into workable portions, it is transferred to the batch former (Figure 38) which is capable of holding 110–160 lb of candy base. The plastic-like sugar mass is formed by four rollers into a sugar cone that is tapered toward the front of the former (Figure 39). A pair of draw-off rollers in the rope sizer (Figure 40) draws the sugar cone from the batch former·and transfers it at a uniform and predetermined rate to the sizing rollers. The operation of the batch former is synchronized with that of the rope sizer (Figure 41).

The four cone rollers are heated, usually by electricity or steam, to maintain the temperature of the batch (80–90°C) so that the outer jacket of the candy will not crack and will be uniformly shaped by the former. The rollers move in a counterrotating pattern that rolls the batch backward and forward so as not to distort any portion of the candy base in the former, expecially in the area where new material is added.

I. Rope Sizing

The delivery rate of candy coming from the batch former to the sizing rollers is determined by the height to which the batch former is adjusted, by the amount of material in the former, or by a combination of these two variables. The diameter of the sugar rope as it leaves the lower end of the former is adjusted by a hand wheel.

The rope sizer draws the sugar rope out of the batch former by means of the two draw-off rollers. The speed of the individual pairs of sizing rollers is matched so that a smooth and uniform material flow to the successive pairs of rollers is ensured.

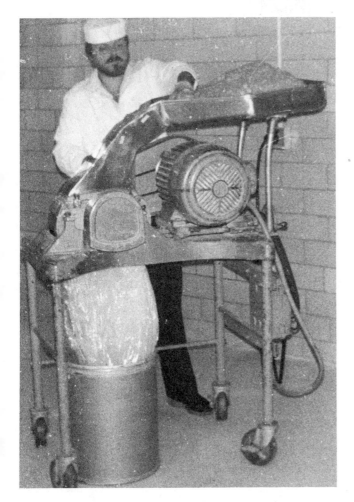

Figure 36 Lozenges rejected due to manufacturing difficulties are milled to a particle size range of 20 to 50 mesh. This produces granules that will absorb the liquid-flavor mixture, to prevent flavor and medicament segregation during medicament-flavor premix preparation and storage. (Warner-Lambert Co.)

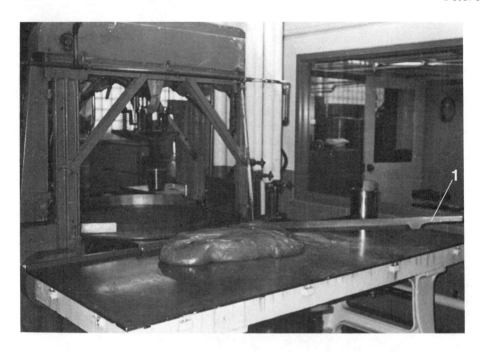

Figure 37 Mixed candy base on tempering table prior to batch forming. Cutting blade on right (1) is used to cut the mass into equal portions for ease of handling. (Warner-Lambert Co.)

The first pair of sizing rollers transports the candy rope, while each successive set reduces the diameter of the candy rope to the proper size (Figure 42). As the candy rope becomes smaller in diameter, the speed of the subsequent roller is increased. The thickness of the rope is determined by the diameter of the sizing rollers and by the gap between rollers. Any thickness of candy rope can be achieved by modifying the five pairs of

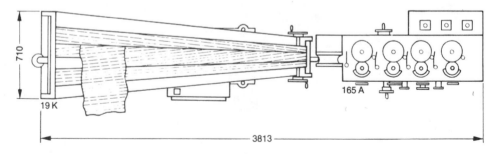

Figure 38 Schematic of batch forming operation. Candy base is fed into batch former. Between 100 and 160 lb. can be mixed. Formed batch is then passed through the 165A rope sizer to produce candy rope of uniform diameter. (Robert Bosch GmBH, Div. Hamac-Höller.)

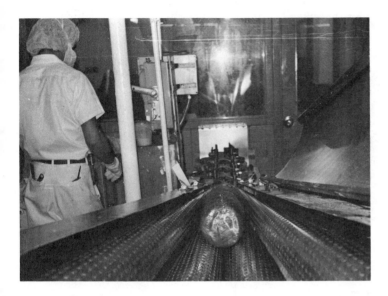

Figure 39   Candy base after forming is fed into sizing rollers from batch former.   Note that candy mass has been formed into a cylinder.   (Warner-Lambert Co.)

successively smaller forming rollers.   The rollers are profiled to ensure satisfactory travel of the rope through the sizer.   Electric heaters under the sizing rollers are thermostatically controlled to maintain the roller temperature a few degrees below the temperature of the batch (between 50 and 60°C).   This prevents cracking at the surface of the rope.

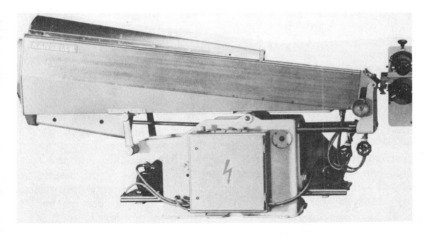

Figure 40   Hansella candy base batch former.   Capacity 165 lb. of unpulled candy.   Initial hand-adjusted sizing wheel is pictured at right.   (Robert Bosch GmBH, Div. Hamac-Höller.)

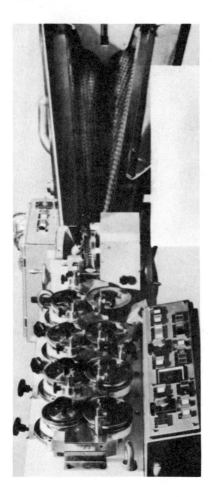

Figure 41   Batch former and rope sizing unit. Rollers are heated a few degrees below temperature of candy base to prevent premature surface cooling. (Robert Bosch GmBH, Div. Hamac-Höller.)

The weight of the final piece is determined by the adjustment of the sizing rollers. Batch forming and sizing are critical operations if each lozenge is to have the same weight. The operator must continually check that the quantity of candy base in the batch former is kept constant and that the height of the batch former is adjusted to compensate for weight changes. The temperature of the batch must be held constant and the temperature of the sizing rollers must be monitored to prevent rapid cooling of the batch surface, which results in cracking as well as reducing the plasticity and forming ability of the candy mass. The rate of heat loss in the batch is reduced by covering the candy mass in the batch former with either the metal cover supplied with the former or a lubricated canvas cover. This also keeps the batch in a plastic-like state that is optimum for forming.

The speed of each set of sizing rollers should be individually adjusted throughout the sizing operation so that the candy rope is conveyed from

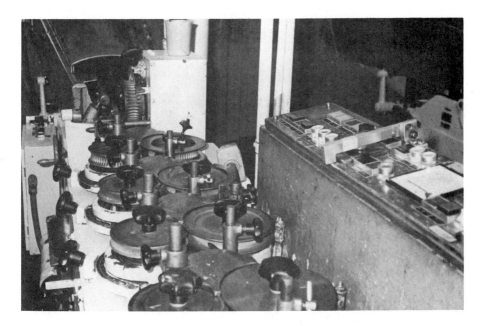

Figure 42   Candy rope is fed through the sizing rollers. Diameter of candy rope determines final lozenge weight. (Warner-Lambert Co.)

one set of sizing rollers to another rather than actually sized down. The sizing operation should taper the rope in such a granual manner as to not produce any unwarranted stretching or bulging of the candy rope. Over-stretching or bulging may result from a sudden change in rope temperature (nontempered candy), candy base consistency or elasticity (undissolved or excessive solid salvage or medicament addition), or improper feed rate (too fast or slow) of candy from batch former to sizing rollers. These inconsistencies will cause the formation of a candy rope with a nonuniform diameter, resulting in the production of lozenges that are either overweight or underweight, as the weight of lozenges formed is determined by the diameter of the candy rope. The piece weight will remain uniform and within product specifications if the diameter of the rope is fixed (Figure 43).

J. Role of the Plastics Operator

Adjustments to the final lozenge weight can be effected only by altering the diameter of the candy rope or by changing the size or configuration of the lozenge dies. Manufacture of product with a uniform weight is assured when each of these conditions is held constant. The dies in the forming machine remain fixed for each product under normal production conditions. Therefore, the major concern is with maintaining a candy rope with a uniform and reproducible diameter. This function is the concern of the plastics operator, so-named because at the time the candy base leaves the batch former, it is in a doughy, plastic-like state. This operator must perform the initial and all subsequent adjustments to the sizing rollers based

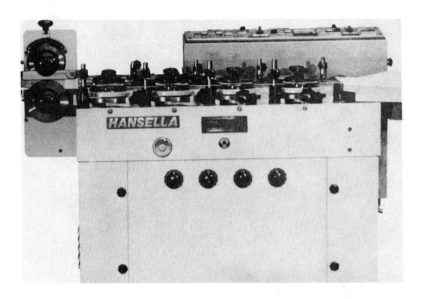

Figure 43   Hansella rope sizer. Feed capacity is variable from 28 to 400 ft. of candy rope per min. A clutch enables the operator to stop or slow the sizing rollers while the motor is running. (Robert Bosch GmBH, Div. Hamac-Höller.)

on the weight of the lozenges desired and by the condition of the candy base. The operator must also adjust the speed of the sizing rollers, depending on the temperature and flow of candy base from the batch former to the sizing rollers. The plastics operator, depending on the quantity of material present in the batch former, is required to adjust the height of the batch former to maintain a uniform flow rate to the sizing rollers. The operator, as the candy leaves the sizing rollers, must initiate the feed into the lozenge-forming machine as well as adjust the forming machine molding speed and pressure.

The plastics operator, monitoring the batch-forming, rope-sizing, and lozenge-forming operations, must be well trained, aware of all the variables that may affect production, and able to diagnose and remedy problems as they arise. Any efficient lozenge-making operation can be severely limited by an inefficient or untrained plastics operator. The efficiency of the forming operator is directly relatable to the quantity of lozenge rejects formed.

K. Lozenge Forming

The candy rope is fed into a final set of sizing rollers after it is discharged from the batch former and rope sizer (Figure 44), and from there into the rotating die head furnished with plungers and guiding cams (Figure 45) for the stamping and formation of the individual lozenges (Figures 46 and 47) [83]. The formed lozenges are then fed onto a distributor belt (Figure 48) which gives the lozenges their initial intensive cooling and shaking, in order to prevent any deformation of the still-plastic lozenges.

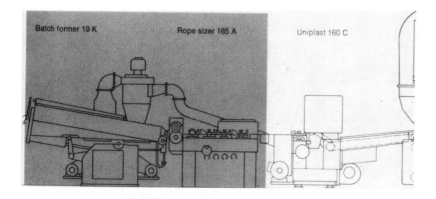

Figure 44   Schematic of batch forming, rope sizing, and lozenge forming operation.   (Robert Bosch GmBH, Div. Hamac-Höller.)

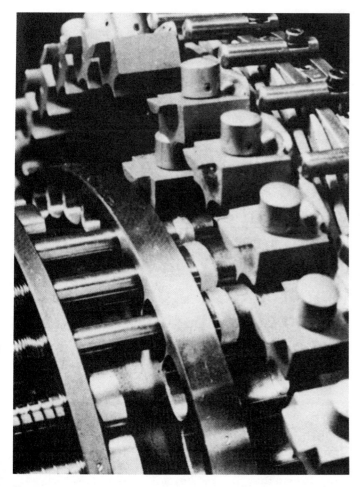

Figure 45   Lozenge forming dies furnished with plungers and guiding cams.
(Robert Bosch GmBH, Div. Hamac-Höller.)

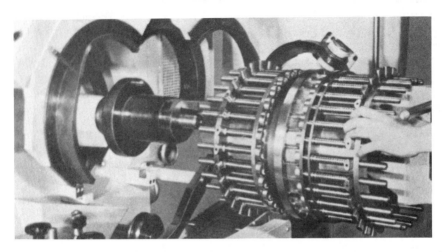

Figure 46   Installation of lozenge forming dies into Uniplast automatic lozenge forming machine.   (Robert Bosch GmBH, Div. Hamac-Höller.)

Various forming machines produce candy at speeds ranging from 450 to 3000 lb/hr (Figures 49–52) depending on the lozenge weight, and in a multitude of shapes depending on the die configuration.   The pressure on the dies is increased gradually and carefully as the forming operation commences, until well-shaped pieces of the desired gauge are formed.   Extreme pressure must be avoided as this will cause premature wearing of the dies and the forming unit.   Such excessive pressure may also cause expansion of the molded piece, with resultant distortion or cracking.   Attempts to obtain a lower weight per piece by increasing the pressure without reducing the diameter of the rope results in failure, since candy piece weight can only be reduced by decreasing the rope diameter.   Before the molding cycle begins, the dies must be warmed to prevent the surface of the formed piece from cooling too quickly and developing cracks (Figure 53).

L.   Cooling

The candy piece must be cooled as rapidly as possible after it is formed to prevent it from losing its shape [4].   The cooling temperature should not fall below 15°C during this operation because air that is too cool will cause the lozenge surface to cool faster than the inside, a situation that places stresses and strains on the lozenge resulting in cracking and formation of air pockets.

After forming, the lozenges are ejected from the forming machine onto a cooling belt (Figure 54). This cooling line may either be a single- or multiple-belt conveyor [4]. Multiple-belt conveyors are preferred because they conserve space (Figure 55). The multiple belts are designed so that the first narrow belt (6–8 in. wide) will run as rapidly as the forming machine. At the end of this belt there is a breaker which will break up the candy if it is held together—and at the same time distribute the lozenges uniformly across a second belt (2–3 ft wide) that travels at a much slower speed than the first. At the end of the second belt, the product is transferred to a third belt, which is wider than the second (3–4 ft) and which travels at a still slower speed. The travel time for lozenges on the cooling belts is calculated so that when product reaches the end, it is cooled to below 35°C. The length of cooling time afforded the product depends on the thickness of the candy, as heat must be extracted from the inside to the outside. The thicker the product, the slower the release of heat. The cooling temperature must be controlled and the relative humidity should also be maintained at 35%. Any deviations from this value should also be

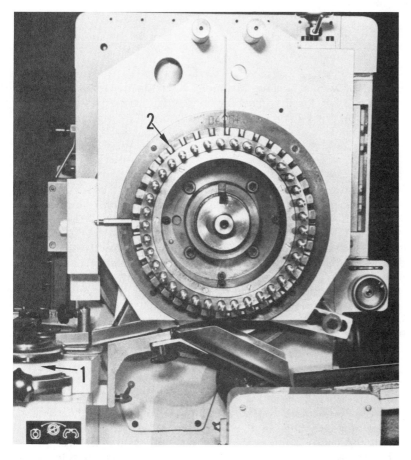

Figure 47 Uniplast 160C: automatic lozenge forming machine, open view. (1) Final rope-sizing rollers; (2) candy forming dies. (Robert Bosch GmBH, Div. Hamac-Höller.)

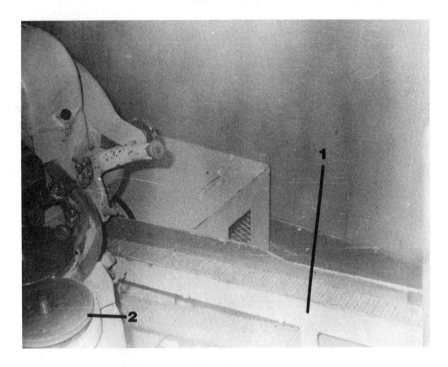

Figure 48 Automatic lozenge forming machine. (1) Ejection chute that carries lozenges away from forming machine to cooling tunnel; (2) final rope-sizing rollers positioned before candy base enters forming machine. (Warner-Lambert Co.)

considered when adjusting the cooling belt speed. All three aspects (lozenge thickness, cooling air temperature, and relative humidity) must be considered to produce lozenges with a minimum of flattening or stress cracking.

Air is blown over the product at a temperature of 15–20°C, at a velocity of 1500–3500 ft/min (normal velocity 2000 ft/min) as the lozenges pass through the cooling belts [4]. A gradual cooling temperature gradient along the belt can also be used instead of a uniform 15–20°C. This gradual reduction in temperature reduces lozenge stress cracking. The relative humidity in the cooling area should be maintained between 35 and 40%. Large differences in relative humidity may increase the incidence of moisture condensation on the surface of the lozenges.

M. Lozenge Sizing

Lozenge sizing is the operation whereby all oversized and undersized material is removed, leaving only that of the specified size. The sizing procedure (along with the candy base mixing process, which determines the uniformity of medicament distribution throughout the mass) is considered an extremely important operation, since proper lozenge weight dictates how much medicament is delivered to the patient per unit dose.

As described in Section II.K, the diameter of the candy rope, and not the force of compression, determines the final lozenge weight. Adjustments in compression force can modify the lozenge thickness (gauge) within certain narrow limits; but (unlike the preparation of tablets) adjustments for weight and size cannot be made on the lozenge former during the forming operation, as the forming machine will mold the candy rope into the shape of the die as it passes through—regardless of diameter. Stretching or compressing the candy during the rope-sizing operation before entrance into the forming machine results in the production of lozenges either too light or too heavy. Since the forming operation molds lozenges to size, control of the lozenge weight depends on control of the size of the piece. Lozenges formed in the desired size range also will be formed in a specified weight range. This relationship is the basis for the sizing operation; lozenge weight is related to its size.

The sizing operation consists of collecting the product as it leaves the cooling belt and transferring it (Figure 56) to a series of counterrotating rollers that are separated via a caliper adjustment (Figure 57). The first

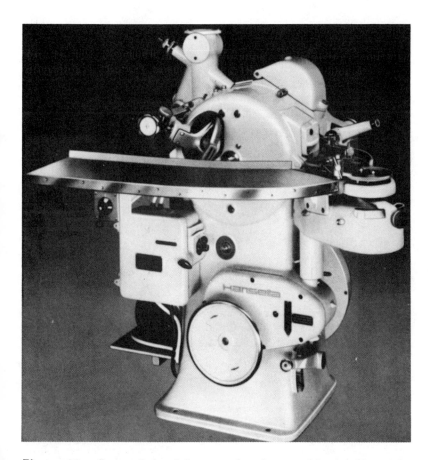

Figure 49 Super Robust lozenge forming machine produces lozenges of all shapes and sizes without seams. (Robert Bosch GmBH, Div. Hamac-Höller.)

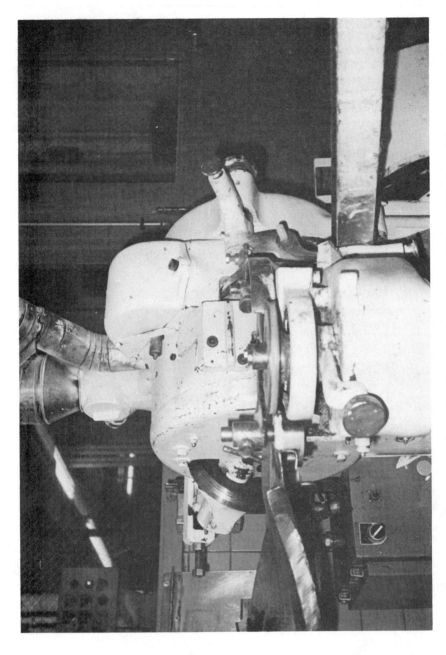

Figure 50 Super Robust lozenge forming machine. From 925 to 1675 lb. of lozenges can be formed per hour. The Super Robust has a 3-speed drive. (Warner-Lambert Co.)

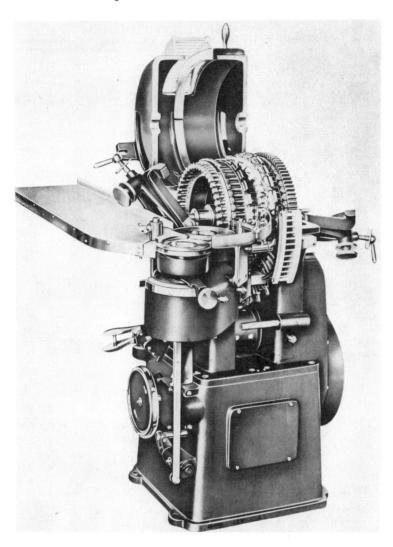

Figure 51   Super Rostoplast forming machine produces lozenges in a wide range of sizes and shapes.   Output: 450 to 700 lb/hr.   (Robert Bosch GmBH, Div. Hamac-Höller.)

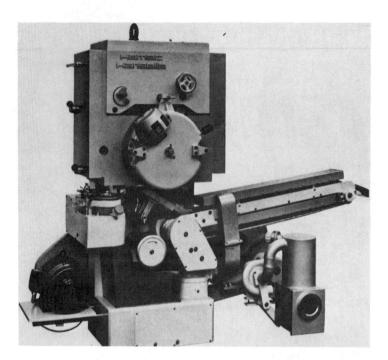

Figure 52 Uniplast 160C: automatic lozenge forming machine, closed view. Lozenge output: 745 to 2200 lb/hr; 4-speed motor. (Robert Bosch GmBH, Div. Hamac-Höller.)

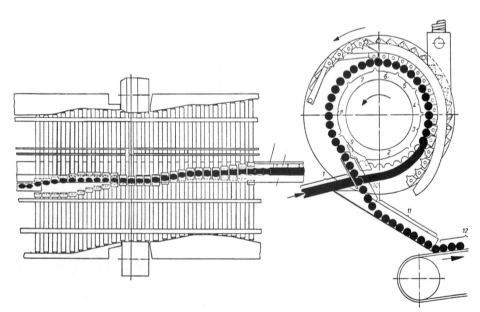

Figure 53 Schematic of lozenge forming operation. (1) Rope feed, (2) rope entry, (3) preforming of rope, (4) separation, (5) sweet preforming in flaps, (6) insertion into the die ring, (7) stamping in the die ring, (8) stress relief, (9) ejection, (10) chute, (11) feed trough to distributor belt, and (12) distributor belt. (Robert Bosch GmBH, Div. Hamac-Höller.)

484

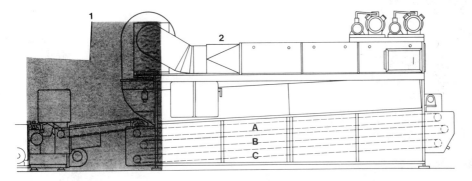

Figure 54 Schematic of lozenge forming and cooling operation. (1) Lozenge forming machine; (2) multiple-belt conveyor cooling tunnel. Belt A moves at the speed of the forming machine. Belts B and C each move at slower rates. The overall belt speed is dependent on the time necessary to cool the product. (Robert Bosch GmBH, Div. Hamac-Höller.)

portion of the rollers where the lozenges are deposited is separated only slightly, thus allowing only undersized lozenges to drop through, where they are collected in salvage containers. Scraps of broken or incompletely formed pieces are also collected, as is stretched candy rope. The opening between the rollers is gradually widened as the lozenges continue down the

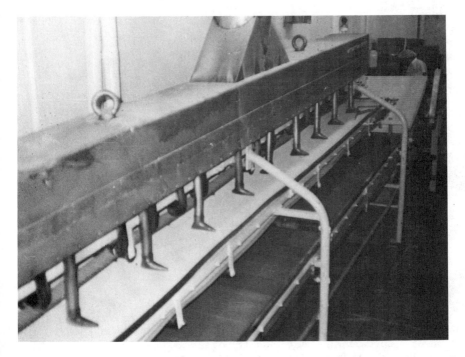

Figure 55 Multiple belt lozenge cooling tunnel. (Warner-Lambert Co.)

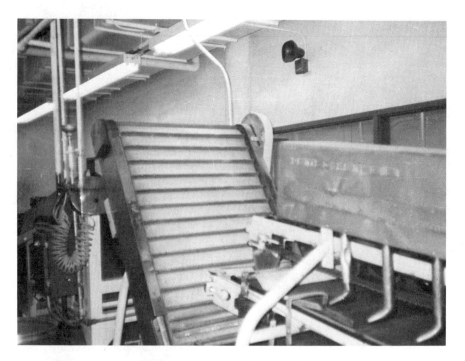

Figure 56   Cooled lozenges are transferred to an elevator for movement to the sizing rollers.   (Warner-Lambert Co.)

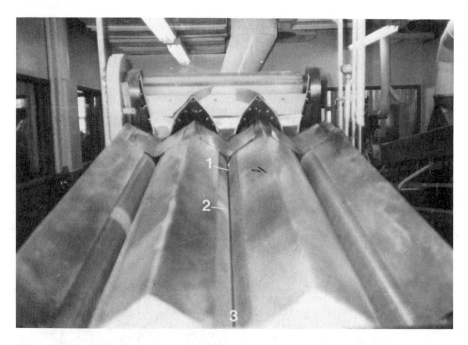

Figure 57   Lozenge sizing operation.   (1) Undersized lozenges removed; (2) lozenges in specification collected; (3) oversized lozenges removed. (Warner-Lambert Co.)

length of the roller so that, in an area beginning about one-third the distance down the roller, the distance between the rollers is opened enough to allow lozenges within desired size specifications to drop through—whereupon they are collected in pans, identified as to batch designation, and held for assay and packaging. Lozenges that are oversized continue down the roller where they are collected at the end in another salvage drum. Lozenges that are distorted with surface air bubbles or with sugar granules adhering to the surface, lozenges with bubbles formed because of dieseling, "doubles" or any large, deformed pieces are also collected in this drum. The speed at which the lozenges are passed down the length of the sizing rollers must be adjusted so that undersized pieces are not carried over to the area where the properly sized product is collected and the lozenges of proper size are not carried out with oversized pieces.

N. Lozenge Storage

The properly sized lozenges are collected on an individual, identified batch basis in labeled containers. They are transferred to a conditioning area that is maintained at a temperature of 15–20°C and controlled relative humidity of 25–35%, for storage until the product is cleared for packaging by the quality control department.

O. Continuous Process Cooker

A recent modification of the continuous batch process cooker involves removal of the collection kettle and its replacement with a continually moving stainless steel belt calibrated to carry the candy base away from the cooker at a predetermined rate in a steady and unbroken stream (Figure 58).

Method of Operation

Figure 59 illustrates schematically the operation of the continuous process cooker.
    Preparation of candy base—from the initial gear metering of sugar and corn syrup, precooking, collection in the center pot, pumping through the cooking coil in the steam chest, cooking and vapor draw-off in the intermediate chamber, to the vacuum drying—is identical to the process described for the continuous batch process method of candy base preparation. Unlike the candy base in the batch process, instead of being collected in a stainless steel or copper kettle, the candy base is continuously drawn off in a thin (6– to 8–in.-wide) strip by passage through two polished counterrotating draw-down rollers onto a heated delivery chute (Figure 60). The mass acts as a sealing agent between the vacuum chamber and the atmosphere as the candy base exits the cooker. It is through this design that a continual vacuum is maintained even through material is being released from the chamber. Concurrent with the removal of cooked candy base from the vacuum chamber, flavor is injected into the center of the candy base ribbon as it leaves the cooker, via two to four metered dosing pumps.
    Precise adjustment of the injection ports is critical to assure surrounding the flavor with candy base, in order to minimize flavor losses through flash-off. The flavored candy base drops from the cooker onto a variable-speed rotating cone head, which effects an initial mixing of flavor into the candy

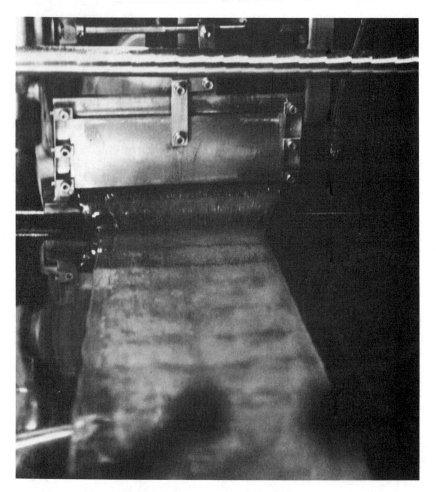

Figure 58   Continuous process cooker. Candy base entering cooling and mixing belt. (Robert Bosch GmBH, Div. Hamac-Höller.)

base. The speed of the cone head is adjusted according to the quantity of flavor added and the efficiency of flavor incorporation in the candy base. The candy, after this initial mixing is completed, slides down the steam-heated delivery chute onto a lubricated and continually moving stainless steel belt, where it is again mixed and sized by a series of three sets of plows and rollers (Figure 61). The candy is uniformly tempered as it moves down the conveyor belt, by the mixing action as well as by a spray of temperature-controlled water on the underside of the belt. Temperature gradients can be controlled by adjusting the water temperature.

The temperature of the base is 130–135°C as the candy leaves the cooker. The candy at this temperature is in a fluid state, so that after initial mixing via the cone head it is uniformly distributed along the width (18–24 in.) of the heated chute before being transferred to the belt. An acidulent (if desired) may be deposited onto the candy during its passage down the length of the steam-heated chute (4–5 ft) by way of a precalibrated

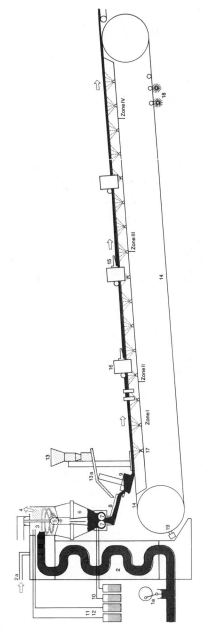

Figure 59 Schematic of continuous process cooker. Cooker: (1) precooked sugar-glucose solution, (1a) pump, (2) steam chest, (2a) steam feed, (2b) cooking coil, (3) intermediate chamber, (4) vapor draw-off, (5) valve, (6) vacuum chamber, (7) continuous sugar draw-off unit, (8) heated delivery chute, (9) mixing container, (10) dosing pump (addition, draw-off unit), (11) dosing pump (addition, intermediate chamber), (12) dosing pump (addition, intermediate chamber, (13) powder feeding unit, (13a) addition, delivery chute. Kneading conveyer band; (14) steel band (conveyor), (14a) profile ledge, (14b) mounting, (14C) guide wheel, (15) plough, (16) kneading station (reversing and kneading), (17) tempering device (water jets), (18) washing station, and (19) greasing station. (Robert Bosch GmBH, Div. Hamac-Höller.)

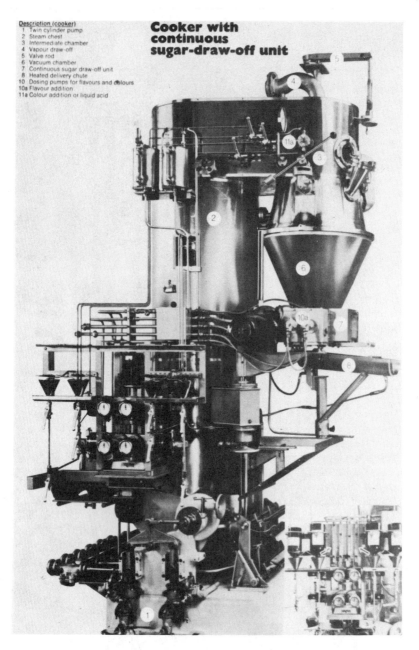

Description (cooker)
 1 Twin cylinder pump
 2 Steam chest
 3 Intermediate chamber
 4 Vapour draw-off
 5 Valve rod
 6 Vacuum chamber
 7 Continuous sugar draw-off unit
 8 Heated delivery chute
10 Dosing pumps for flavours and colours
10a Flavour addition
11a Colour addition or liquid acid

Cooker with continuous sugar-draw-off unit

Figure 60   Cooker with continuous sugar draw-off unit. (Robert Bosch GmBH, Div. Hamac-Höller.)

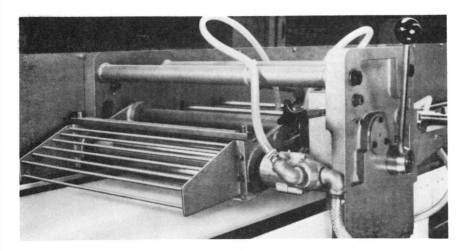

Figure 61 Plow and roller mixer. The unit is cooled by circulating water. The plows are fitted at their bottom edges with exchangeable Teflon strips to prevent damage to the steel belt. The rollers are adjustable in order to obtain a sugar mass of predetermined thickness. (Robert Bosch GmBH, Div. Hamac-Höller.)

vibratory dosing auger [27]. Once the candy base is on the moving and lubricated stainless steel belt, the acidulent and flavor are mixed and folded into it by way of series of three sets of plows and rollers stationed at uniformly spaced intervals along the belt. The ribbon is 6–10 in. wide when mixing has been completed, and the candy base is at the end of the belt where it is continually deposited into the batch former (Figure 62). All steps from this point until the end of the procedure are identical to those described for the batch process mode of manufacture. Lozenges are collected on a routine basis in storage hoppers labeled according to that portion of the batch from which the lozenges were manufactured. They are then held in a quarantine area until analytical and microbiological testing is complete.

Plow and Roller Mixing

Lozenges produced on the continuous process cooker are brighter in color and clearer in appearance than those produced by the batch process because the plow and roller mixing is more gentle. The mass is mixed at a higher temperature, thus entrapping less air than is associated with manual mixing or the Berks mixer type of mechanical mixing. Also, no solid, ground salvage is mixed into the batch—a procedure that rapidly cools the candy base and increases the incidence of air entrapment and candy base opacity. Conversely, the thoroughness of mixing resulting from the plow and roller combination is less than that obtained with batch process manual or mechanical procedures. This is not a disadvantage in instances where only flavor and acidulent (if needed) are added to the candy base after cooking is complete. The less energetic type of mixing encountered with plow and roller limits the quantity and consistency of material that can be efficiently mixed into the candy base (watery materials or materials

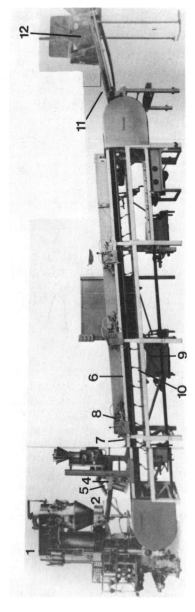

Figure 62 Continuous process cooker. (1) Continuous cooker; (2) heated delivery chute; (3) powder feeding unit; (4) mixing container; (5) powder delivery chute; (6) steel band (conveyor); (7) plow; (8) kneading station; (9) water-cooled tempering device; (10) water jets; (11) elevator to transfer candy base to batch former; (12) candy base entering batch former. (Robert Bosch GmBH, Div. Hamac-Höller.)

that are tacky are difficult to incorporate). To help alleviate this limitation, medicaments and colors are added with salvage through the cooker
or pumped into the intermediate chamber. However, alternative methods
of addition must be investigated if medicaments or colors are heat-sensitive
or react with candy base.

Color and Medicament Addition Procedures

When the formulator must add dyes that exhibit color distortion or fading
because of heat sensitivity or reactivity with candy base components, the
dyes can be dissolved or suspended in glycerin and added to the candy
base after cooking, through one of the metered dosing pumps available,
to inject flavor into the mass as it leaves the cooker (see insert, Figure
60).

The addition of medicaments in the same manner as the addition of
acidulents (sprinkling onto the surface of the candy base) is not practical
because of lack of adequate control or sensitivity in the vibratory dosing
auger mechanism. If the dosage of the medicament is at a low level (less
than 5.0 mg per dose) and the solubility or dispersibility of the medicament
lends itself to preparation of a high-solids but free-flowing solution or dispersion (solution or dispersion addition "rate" of medicament to candy base
must be less than 2 lb/100 lb of finished candy base), the drug may be
added through one of the metered dosing pumps, as the candy base leaves
the cooker or slightly after the point of flavor addition. This reduces
possible medicament−candy base or medicament−flavor interactions. Addition of active ingredients through the pumping system requires a pump
that possesses a high degree of sensitivity to assure homogeneous addition
of medicament into the candy base. This guarantees a uniform drug distribution throughout the manufacturing run. A flow meter or indicator
for the liquid additions should be attached in order to control the consumption of the drug mixture, if the dosing pumps supplied with the continuous
process cooker are to be used to deliver medicaments to the candy base.

The solution or dispersion containing the medicament, as well as any
color solutions or suspensions, should be heated to 110−120°C before addition to prevent localized crusting or hardening of the candy mass at the
point of injection. This crusting can result in a nonuniform distribution of
color or medicament and can clog the pump injection ports, resulting in a
retardation of medicament or color solution flow. Flavors need be heated
only to 50−60°C (a flavor-heating glycerin system has been incorporated
into the machine) before addition, since the quantities added are lower
and the flavor components easier to incorporate in the candy base without
the problems of crusting.

Candy Base Output

The speed of the forming machine and the size of the candy piece formed
determine the speed at which the cooker and the belt are set. The candy
base production rate and the speed of the belt are adjusted to deliver 20−
25 lb of candy base per minute if one forming machine is being supplied.
Up to 42 lb of candy base per minute can be manufactured if two forming
lines are supplied. It is possible to divide the sugar rope by a cutting
device in such a way that two batch formers, and consequently two forming
lines, can be supplied with a single candy line.

Advantages of Continuous Process Cooker

Production of large quantities of candy base (10 tons/8 hr) is feasible using the continuous process cooker because components of the candy manufacturing and forming operation are used close to their designated capacities. The number of production workers (12 vs. 4), forming machines (4 vs. 2), candy base cookers (2 vs. 1), and cooling lines (4 vs. 2) needed to produce a given quantity of product in an 8-hr shift using the batch system is at least double whatever may be required to produce identical quantities on the continuous setup. The appearance of the finished lozenge is elegant since an almost clear piece, free from haze or air bubbles, results. Colors are vivid, and air entrapment and defects are reduced because of a uniform tempering of the batch, and deletion of solid salvage (plows and rollers cannot efficiently incorporate solid salvage) results in the formation of lozenges with a greater resistance to graining. This is because the base is not seeded with sugar dust or sugar crystals before the lozenges are formed. The result is the manufacture of a product that will maintain its original appearance from two to three times longer when stored under identical conditions and packaged in the same containers as batch process manufactured lozenges.

Disadvantages of the Continuous Process Cooker

The manufacture of medicated lozenges on the continuous process cooker is not without its drawbacks. The most severe fault—the one that requires rectification before a medicinal product can be manufactured using this process—is the lack of adequate controls during production and the ramifications that may result before human or machine errors are detected.

Unlike the batch system, which produces a predetermined quantity of candy base that is weighed and checked before the addition of flavors, colors, or medicaments, the continuous process cooker produces an unbroken stream of candy. The only adequate method for determining the quantity of candy base produced during any specified period of time is to break the candy ribbon before it enters the batch former and collect the product for a predetermined period of time, weigh it, and calculate the output of candy base per minute. Adjustments in cooker or belt speed are made as required. Normal quality-control compliance checking is carried out every 15–20 min throughout the run. An increase or decrease in candy base output during any specific time period will be reflected in a change in the concentration of flavor or acidulent present in the candy (a change in the organoleptic presentation), if medicament or color is added with salvage during cooking. If medicament or color is added after the candy base is formed, any significant increase or decrease in candy base output may result in production of lozenges with undersirable color or product that is out of specification when assayed for the desired medicament concentration. The manufacture of 30–40 lb of candy base per minute could result in 450–600 lb of lozenge rejects being formed before remedial actions are initiated—even though the routine checking of candy base output is mandatory. The production team responsible for maintenance of the cooker assembly must take precautions necessary to mitigate the chances of a nonuniform or faulty candy base output due to cooker, pump, valve, steam line, or vacuum malfunction or failure.

A second disadvantage associated with the production of lozenges via the continuous process cooker is the method of flavor addition. Injection of the liquid flavors at the point where the candy base leaves the cooker exposes the flavor to the candy at a temperature exceeding 130°C. The ideal situation is to inject the flavor into the center of the candy ribbon as it leaves the cooker, by positioning the metered dosing-pump injection ports into the center of the mass. This would, in theory, surround the flavor with candy base, thus reducing flavor flash-off tendencies. In practice, though, it is not always possible to maintain the position of the injection ports in the center of the cooked candy mass, or to prevent portions of the flavor from leaking out of the base or being injected through the mass and being lost. (Generally such loss is prevalent when high concentrations, greater than 50.0 g/min, are being injected.) There is a tendency for the candy to separate or tear away from the injection ports, resulting in raw flavor being sprayed onto the surface of the mass. The incidence of flavor loss from this occurrence is greater than 75%. It is not practical to add flavors farther down the belt where temperatures are lower, as the mixing action of the plows and rollers is not energetic enough to assure uniform incorporation of the flavor in the base. The initial mixing as candy drops onto the chute as well as the action of the rotating cone head produces an acceptable initial mixing that complements the plow and roller action when flavor is injected at the point where the candy leaves the cooker. Flavor tends to collect on the surface of the base if it is added farther down the belt and is only folded into the center of the ribbon, thus increasing the percentage loss and producing lozenges with pockets of liquid flavor trapped in the center. Incorporation of flavors as a mixture with ground salvage and addition to the mass in the same manner that is used for citric acid powder (vibratory auger feed) is not practical since the wetted salvage will not flow uniformly from the auger. Agglomeration of the flavor-salvage mixture occurs in the hopper. Also, the material that is delivered by the powder-feeding unit will not be completely mixed into the base because of the inability of the plows and rollers to give the vigorous mixing required to incorporate the salvage mixture in the candy base.

The addition of selected solvents (benzyl alcohol, glycerin, propylene glycol) to flavors in order to raise the boiling point of the mixture will aid in reducing flavor flash-off, but the concentration of solvent necessary to achieve this condition will range between half to four times the required flavor quantity. The addition of sufficient solvent to lower flavor losses might not be a practical solution to the problem unless the quantity of flavor added to the base is low (less than 1.0 g/lb). This is because as the quantity of flavor added per minute increases, so does the percentage of flavor loss increase due to the inability of the mixing system to efficiently incorporate the liquid into the mass. The addition of 0.5−1.0 g of flavor per pound of candy base results in a loss of less than 10%, whereas addition of 1.0−2.0 g/lb produces 15−20% flavor loss, and more than 3.0 g of flavor added per pound could result in flavor loss in the range of 40−60%.

Lozenge Rejects

There are two reasons for the formation of higher levels of lozenge rejects when medicated products are manufactured on the continuous process cooker than when they are produced by the batch process: (a) difficulties of flavor addition, and (b) the possibility that nonuniform candy base production may produce lozenges with drug, flavor, or color levels out of specification. As much as 1000–1500 lb of lozenges may be produced before a potential problem is detected or diagnosed and remedial actions are taken, since the cooker output is usually in the range of 40–42 lb of candy base being manufactured per minute. If an analysis of lozenges determines that high or low drug contents have resulted—that place the drug concentration out of the acceptable tolerances, through either improper weighing of medicaments, pump failure, or decomposition—it is possible that 12,000–20,000 lb of finished lozenges could be produced before analytical results determine that the lozenges are rejected for out-of-specification drug concentration.

The lozenge-forming and cooling operation probably produces the highest percentage of rejects on an ongoing basis. Product rejection during forming and cooling is an inherent weakness in all lozenge production, regardless of the type of candy base production, but it is proportional to the output of product manufactured per minute [69].

Forming equipment capable of manufacturing up to 2500 lb of candy lozenges per hour was developed concurrently with candy base cooking equipment capable of producing up to 2700 lb of candy base per hour. This high-speed production demands an unbroken supply of candy base, properly tempered and fed through the sizing rollers at a uniform rate. Any cold or hot spots that may develop in the mass, or any reduction in candy base elasticity from high concentrations of medicament or solvent or from improper positioning of the batch former (rate of feed into the sizing rollers), or any temperature variation in the rollers or batch former will place stress on the candy rope and form lozenges that are out of the specified range. Adjustments can be made to remedy this situation, but until this is done, as much as 200–300 lb of undersized or oversized lozenges can be formed. Continued variations in the quality of candy base produced will result in lozenge-forming problems, with an increase in the number of adjustments and rejects. The high-speed forming machinery also increases the incidence of lozenge chipping and sticking, as well as breaking of finished product during the cooling operation. The speed at which the lozenges pass through the final sizing rollers also produces a higher incidence of rejected lozenges. The quantities of lozenges that must be sized require that the sizing rollers be set at a high speed. This rate results in 5–10% of proper weight and proper size product being carried over the desired "drop-through area"—and out with the oversized lozenges. A time-consuming resizing operation is the only way to reclaim these lozenges.

Summary

The quantity of lozenge salvage produced may exceed the amount that can be readily returned to the process (18–22%) unless close controls can be instituted over all aspects of medicated lozenge production on the continuous process cooker. When this situation occurs, it is not practical—from a cost or raw materials standpoint—to manufacture medicated lozenges with this procedure. The quantity of salvage formed should not exceed 10% of product produced if rigid controls are maintained on the quantity of the candy base produced per minute, flavor, color, and medicament addition rates, as well as on the lozenge forming, cooling, and sizing operations.

The continuous process cooker offers many advantages in the high-speed production of medicated lozenges possessing improved organoleptic characteristics with extended shelf life. This method of manufacture requires a closer surveillance over all aspects of product manufacture than does the batch method, since a human or mechanical error during production can turn 15,000–20,000 lb of finished product into that much lozenge salvage.

III. FORMULATIONS (HARD CANDY LOZENGES)

The following formulations represent various methods of manufacturing medicated hard candy lozenges.

A. Medicament-Flavor-Ground Salvage Method of Addition

Example 1: Antihistamine Lozenges (4.0 mg/2.5-g lozenge)

Ingredient	Quantity
A. Liquid sugar (67.5% w/w solids)	88.9 lb
B. Corn syrup 43°Baumé (80.5% w/w solids)	49.7 lb
C. Ground candy salvage (20–50 mesh)	3.0 lb
D. Chlorpheniramine maleate	72.75 g
E. Wild cherry flavor, imitation	75.0 g
F. Benzyl alcohol NF	75.0 g
G. Citric acid fine granular	300.0 g
H. Red color cubes	10.0 g

Liquid sugar and corn syrup are gear-metered into the dissolver and precooked at 125°C. Final cooking is performed at 148°C with a vacuum of 710 mm Hg to produce 100 lb of candy base with a 60:40 sugar/corn syrup ratio. The chlorpheniramine maleate is dissolved in a mixture of wild cherry and benzyl alcohol with the aid of heat. The mixture is uniformly mixed with the citric acid and ground candy salvage. Color is added to the cooked candy base in the collection kettle; flavor-drug-salvage mixture is added on the mixing table. Candy base is mixed, tempered, formed, rope-sized, molded, cooled, and sized.

B. Direct Medicament Addition

Example 2: Analgesic Lozenges (162.5 mg/4.0-g lozenge)

Ingredient	Quantity
A. Liquid sugar (67.5%) w/w solids)	88.9 lb
B. Corn syrup 43°Baumé (80.5% w/w solids)	49.7 lb

Example 2: (Continued)

Ingredient	Quantity
C. Ground candy salvage (20—50 mesh)	2.0 lb
D. Aspirin 100-mesh crystals	1.85 kg
E. Imitation orange flavor	35.0 g
F. Menthol crystals	50.0 g
G. Orange color paste	12.0 g

Liquid sugar and corn syrup are gear-metered into the dissolver and precooked at 120°C. Final cooking is performed at 148°C with a vacuum of 73 mm Hg to produce 100 lb of candy base with a 60:40 sugar/corn syrup ratio. The menthol is dissolved in the orange flavor and uniformly mixed into the ground salvage. Color is added to candy base in the collection kettle; the aspirin is added in the transfer kettle and folded into the mass; and the flavor-salvage mixture is added on the mixing table. Candy base is mixed, tempered, formed, rope-sized, molded, cooled, and sized.

C. Medicament Addition via Granulation

Example 3: Antitussive-Decongestant Lozenges (7.5 and 18.5 mg/3.5-g lozenge)

Ingredient	Quantity
A. Liquid sugar (67.5% w/w solids)	88.9 lb
B. Corn syrup 43°Baumé (80.5% w/w solids)	49.7 lb
C. Ground candy salvage (20—50 mesh)	4.0 lb
D. Dextromethorphan HBr, 10% adsorbate	1.0 kg
E. Pseudoephedrine HCl	241.0 g
F. Eucalyptus oil NF	150.0 g
G. Menthol crystals	170.0 g
H. Glycerin USP	2.0 lb

Liquid sugar and corn syrup are gear-metered into the dissolver and precooked at 125°C. Final cooking is performed at 150°C with a vacuum of 736 mm Hg to produce 100 lb of candy base with a 60:40 sugar/corn syrup ratio. The menthol is dissolved in the eucalyptus oil and uniformly mixed into a mixture of ground salvage, dextromethorphan HBr, adsorbate, and pseudoephedrine HCl. Glycerin is added and mixed until a free-flowing granulation results. The granulation is added to the candy base on the mixing table. Candy base is mixed, tempered, formed, rope-sized, molded, cooled, and sized.

D. Dual-Granulation Addition to Reduce Chemical Incompatibilities

Example 4:   Decongestant Lozenges (15.0 mg/4.0-g lozenge)

Ingredient	Quantity
A. Liquid sugar (67.5% w/w solids)	88.9 lb
B. Corn syrup 43°Baumé (80.5% w/w solids)	49.7 lb
C. Ground candy salvage (20—50 mesh)	7.0 lb
D. Phenylpropanolamine HCL	172.0 g
E. Artificial berry-mint flavor	150.0 g
F. Berry shade color paste blend	15.0 g
G. Benzyl alcohol NF	100.0 g

Liquid sugar and corn syrup are gear-metered into the dissolver and precooked at 125°C.   Final cooking is performed at 147°C with a vacuum of 736 mm Hg to produce 100 lb of candy base with a 60:40 sugar/corn syrup ratio.   The phenylpropanolamine HCl is dissolved in benzyl alcohol with the aid of heat and uniformly mixed with 4 lb of ground salvage.   The berry-mint flavor is separately and uniformly mixed with 3 lb of ground salvage.   Color is added to candy base in the collection kettle.   The phenylpropanolamine HCl-salvage mixture is added in the transfer kettle and folded into the mass, and the flavor-salvage mixture is added to the candy base on the mixing table after 60 sec of mixing has been completed.   Candy base is mixed, tempered, formed, rope-sized, molded, cooled, and sized.

E.   Addition of Liquid Salvage with Color (10% Salvage)

Example 5:   Antihistamine Lozenges (10.0 mg/2.5-g lozenge)

Ingredient	Quantity
A. Liquid sugar (67.5% w/w solids)	80.00 lb
B. Corn syrup 43°Baumé (80.5% w/w solids)	44.75 lb
C. Liquid salvage (70% w/w solids)	14.30 lb
D. Ground candy salvage (20—50 mesh)	4.00 lb
E. Diphenhydramine HCl	185.00 g
F. Artificial wild cherry flavor	125.00 g
G. Citric acid USP, fine granular	325.00 g
H. FD&C Red No. 40	8.50 g

The FD&C Red No. 40 is dissolved in the liquid salvage. Liquid sugar, corn syrup, and salvage solution are

Example 5:   (Continued)

---

gear metered into the dissolver and precooked at 125°C.
Final cooking is performed at 150°C with a vacuum of 736
mm Hg to produce 100 lb of candy base with a 60:40 sugar/
corn syrup ratio and 10% salvage-color mixture. The diphenhydramine HCl is dissolved in the flavor, added to
a mixture of citric acid and ground salvage, and mixed
until uniformly incorporated. The flavor-drug-ground
salvage mixture is added to the color-salvage-candy
base mixture on the mixing table. Candy base is mixed,
tempered, formed, rope-sized, molded, cooled, and sized.

F. Addition of Liquid Salvage with Color and Medicament (20% Salvage)

Example 6:   Anesthetic Lozenges (2.4 mg/3.5-g lozenge)

Ingredient	Quantity
A. Liquid sugar (67.5% w/w solids)	71.1 lb
B. Corn syrup 43°Baumé (80.5% w/w solids)	88.6 lb
C. Liquid salvage (70% w/w solids)	88.6 lb
D. Hexylresorcinol	43.75 g
E. FD&C Yellow No. 5	2.5 g
F. FD&C Green No. 3	2.5 g
G. Natural and artificial spearmint blend	100.0 g
H. Menthol crystals	75.0 g
I. Ground candy salvage (20–50 mesh)	4.0 lb

The FD&C Yellow No. 5, FD&C Green No. 3, and the hexylresorcinol are dissolved in the liquid salvage. Liquid sugar,
corn syrup, and salvage solution are gear-metered into the
dissolver and precooked at 125°C. Final cooking is performed at 146°C with a vacuum of 710 mm Hg to produce
100 lb of candy base with a 60:40 sugar/corn syrup ratio
and 20% salvage-medicament-color mixture. The menthol
crystals are dissolved in the flavor, added to a mixture
of ground salvage, and mixed until uniformly incorporated.
The ground salvage-flavor mixture is added to the medica-
ment-color-salvage-candy base mixture on the mixing table.
Candy base is mixed, tempered, formed, rope-sized, molded,
cooled, and sized.

IV. CENTER-FILLED HARD CANDY LOZENGES

Incorporation of soft or liquid centers into hard candy lozenges enables
the product formulator to modify the presentation of medicament to the
patient. The rationale for preparation of a product of this type normally
would fall into the same categories as those presented for developing two-
layer tablets (elimination of drug incompatibilities). In the case of liquid-
center hard candy products, the major criteria cannot be met since preparation of a pharmaceutically acceptable filled lozenge cannot be realized due
to unacceptable content uniformity variations which result when centers are
placed in lozenges. While most centers will fall within the desired 10% fill,
an unacceptable number will fall outside this range and some will be as far
off as ±50% from theory.

Eliminating the separation of medicaments in either the shell or the center, the major advantage for formulating medicated center-filled products
is aesthetics. A different flavor can be placed in the center than in the
shell. High-impact flavors can be incorporated in the center that will contrast with subtle flavorings presented in the shell. Aromatics can give a
burst of flavor or perceived efficacy to the user, thus increasing the overall organoleptic presentation of the product. However, medicament must
be uniformly distributed between the shell and the center to eliminate the
problem of nonuniformity of center fill.

A. Types of Center Fills

Four major categories of center fill are now utilized [84].

Liquid Fill

This type of center is utilized when a high-impact type of filling is desired.
The liquid is presented in a very short concentrated burst after the user
breaks through the shell. This results in a noticeable sensation of liquid
coating the throat. Normal percentage fill (w/w) ranges from 10 to 20%.
Due to the low viscosity of the material and the low specific gravity, higher
fill percentages result in a thin shell wall which if cracked or ruptured will
contaminate surrounding lozenges or the product container. Some of the
materials utilized for this type of filling include fruit juice, sugar syrup,
hydroalcoholic solutions, and sorbitol solution. Flavor and colors can be
incorporated in the center or the center can be left unaltered.

Two major disadvantages of liquid center include (1) the tendency for
the product to leak if the shell cracks or the ends of the tablet are not
properly sealed, (2) reduced product shelf life due to the liquid center.
The liquid center material, being highly aqueous, will cause the lozenge to
grain from the inside out. Water in contact with sugar and corn syrup
actually melts the product from within. Eventually, the shell wall weakens
and the liquid material leaks out of the center. Average shelf life for
liquid centers is 6—9 months. Storage in heated environments will shorten
this time span.

Another problem with the use of liquid center material is leakage during processing. If the aqueous material should leak onto forming rollers or shell material, the candy base will become sticky thus making processing difficult.

Fruit Centers

Fruit center fillings are prepared when highly confectionary-type products are desired. This type of center is richly flavored, sweet, and full bodied. Jams and jellies, whose viscosity has been adjusted with corn syrup or liquid sucrose, are most frequently utilized in this type of center. While the impact of this material is not as pronounced as with liquid center, the rich flavor and sweetness help differentiate the center from the shell. The average fill weight of fruit centers is 20—25%. The lower moisture content of fruit center along with higher viscosity helps retard the internal graining and melting characteristics, thus increasing the shelf life to 12—15 months. Leakage during processing is a problem since the more viscous fruit will coat rollers and make processing extremely difficult.

Paste Centers

Paste centers are not utilized to a great extent since they are more difficult to fill and afford the poorest differentiation between shell and center. The high specific gravity allows for fill of up to 40% w/w and the high viscosity reduces the tendency for the center material to leak out of the lozenge should cracking occur. The same problems of processing difficulty, if leaking should occur during filling, are applicable here. Paste formulations contain granular or crystal-sized materials such as nuts or fruits. The lower moisture content of the paste center helps retard graining and internal candy base melting, so typical shelf life of paste centers can be as long as 24 months.

Fat Centers

The fill material most applicable to medicated lozenges is the fat-based center fill. Here, the medicament and/or flavor can be suspended or dissolved in hydrogenated vegetable oil and incorporated in the lozenge center. During processing, if leakage should occur, the fat will act as a lubricant that will not impede production or cause the sticking of candy base to the rollers or the faces of candy dies.

Utilization of a high melting point fat (85—100°F) will reduce the tendency for center to leak out of the tablet during packaging or storage since at room temperature the center is a solid or semisolid. When the lozenge is placed in the mouth, body heat melts the center material thus releasing a liquid when the shell is broken. Fats can be incorporated in lozenges at 25—32% w/w fill. The projected shelf life of a fat-filled lozenge is 3—5 years since the candy base is insoluble in the oil and will not grain or melt from the inside. If the lozenge is protected from atmospheric moisture, the shelf life can be extended indefinitely.

A disadvantage of the fat filling is presentation of flavors from the matrix. Vegetable oil retards the impact of flavor to the taste buds so the true impact and goodness of flavors is markedly reduced. Even high aromatic flavors such as menthol and eucalyptus do not retain their usual organoleptic characteristics. This is a problem when different flavors are

incorporated in the shell and center. The lower flavor impact reduces
the differentiation of shell from center.

One formulation modification used to circumvent this problem is to form
an emulsion of glycerin or propylene glycol with the vegetable oil, flavors,
and medicaments. This emulsion is less oily, more hydrophilic, and gives
an improved presentation of flavor to the mouth. While the emulsion will
make the candy base more sticky if leakage should occur during processing,
in most instances this is not severe enough to discontinue production.
Fill volumes with the emulsion are about 3—5% lower than with the fat alone.

Since the candy base is also insoluble in glycerin and propylene glycol,
the shelf life is not compromised when the emulsion is filled into hard candy.
Addition of glycerin or propylene glycol to the vegetable oil will lower the
melting point of the fat but in most cases the center will still be a semisolid that will not readily leak out of the shell. If the center does become
fluid after formation of an emulsion center, use of a higher melting point
fat should alleviate the problem. Fats with a melting point above 102°F
should not be used under any circumstances since they will leave a fatty-
oily taste in the mouth.

A summary of type of filling vs. shape and center fill percentage is
summarized in Table 4.

B. Processing

Candy base is prepared in the normal manner described for hard candy
lozenges. Ideally, candy base at 60:40 or 55:45 sugar—corn syrup ratio
should be used since higher sugar ratios tend to crystallize too fast and
do not stretch properly when center material is injected. Sugar ratios below 55:45 are too elastic and do not hold their shape.

Candy base is cooked and medicament, flavor, and color are added in
the normal manner. The candy is tempered and transferred to the batch
former.

In the batch former is a hollow Teflon-coated fill pipe attached to a
jacketed pump (Figure 63). The candy base is added to the batch former
which converts the mass to a sugar cone. The candy during forming is
wrapped around the Teflon-coated pipe in the former (Figure 64).

With the candy in the batch former, but prior to reaching the draw-
down rollers, the end of the Teflon pipe is positioned so that the center
fill material can be pumped into the candy rope. At the position immediately beyond the pipe, a hollow cavity is formed. The liquid is pumped
into this void. The speed of the rope determines the diameter of the hollow space and thus the quantity of center material available for filling.
If the rope is pulled or pushed, the cavity diameter changes and the percent center fill is compromised. Immediately after the center fill is deposited into the rope, it is sized through the rollers and formed into tablets, cooled, sized, and collected (Figure 65).

The temperature of the center fill material should be close to that of
the candy base at the point of filling (85—95°C) [60]. This will prevent
crystallization and premature hardening of the candy should cold center fill
come in contact with hot candy. If this occurs, control of tablet weight will
be affected and the cooked candy will become brittle when formed thus increasing the number of center fill leakers. If the center material is too hot,
cooling is delayed and the number of deformed lozenge rejects increases.

Table 4 Type of Filling vs. Shape and Typical Percentage Center Fill[a]

Type	for machine	for candy	Filling percentage			
			Liquid	Fruit	Fat	Paste
97 A	Superrostoplast 96 A	>14 mm Ø	20	25	32	43
67 B	Superrobust 85 A	>14 mm Ø	–	–	–	–
67 C	Superrobust 85 A	Ring tablet	–	–	–	–
67 D	Superrobust 85 A	>14 mm Ø	–	–	–	–
161 H	Uniplast 160 A B C D	>14 mm Ø	18	22	28	43
161 K	Uniplast 160 A B C D	>18 mm Ø	20	25	32	–
161 L	Uniplast 160 A B C D	Pillow, waffle	–	25	32	–
161 M	Uniplast 160 A B C D	Humbug	–	–	–	–
161 N	Uniplast 160 C D	Center-ring tablet	–	–	–	–
161 P	Uniplast 160 D	>18 mm Ø	20	25	32	–
161 S	Uniplast 160 C D	Chewable candy	20	–	22	–
161 SO	Uniplast 160 C D	Toffee	–	–	22	–
161 T	Uniplast 160 D	>18 mm Ø	18	22	28	32

[a]The oval shape lozenge configuration lends itself to the best geometry for center filling.
Source: Robert Bosch, GmBH, Division of Hamac-Höller.

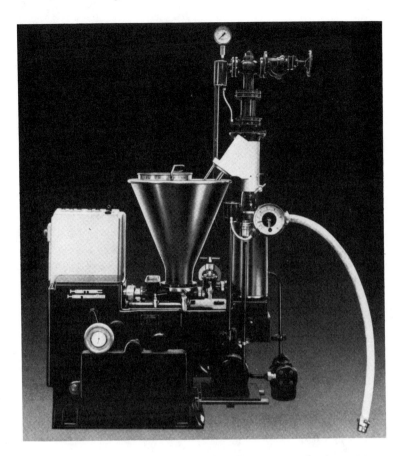

Figure 63 Hansella 148A center fill machine. Hopper is jacketted to maintain center fill temperature. Product is recirculated to maintain uniformity. (Robert Bosch GmBH, Div. Hamac-Höller.)

The diameter of the feed pipe, speed of forming, center fill flow rate, and pressure all must be coordinated to produce finished lozenges with a uniform center fill. The candy rope must not be stretched. This could result in breakage of the rope around the fill pipe resulting in leakage of center fill material onto the batch former rollers, candy base, or around the sizing rollers. If the candy base becomes sticky when coated with center fill material, lozenges will stick to the dies during forming (Figure 66). Cleanup after a center fill leak is laborious.

Adequate crimping pressure must be used to cut the lozenges during forming. This prevents tearing of the candy or incomplete closure of the tablet thus allowing fill material to leak from the center.

Much progress has been made in improving center fill procedures. Utilization of extruders to feed candy base and improved center fill material delivery systems have increased the percentage center fill, but the technology has not progressed to the stage where centers are uniform to the extent that pharmaceutical content uniformity values can be met should segregation of medicaments between shell and center be attempted.

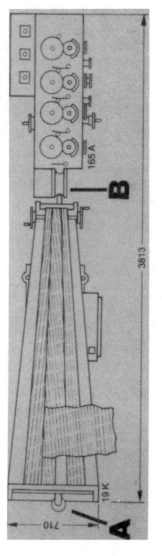

Figure 64 Tempered candy base is added to the batch former as a thin ribbon to assure that a uniform encasement of the teflon coated fill pipe is achieved. Center fill pump is attached at point A. Center fill material fills hollow space in candy rope at point B where the center fill pipe ends. Candy passes through the first draw down roller and then to the rope sizer. (Robert Bosch GmBH, Div. Hamac-Höller.)

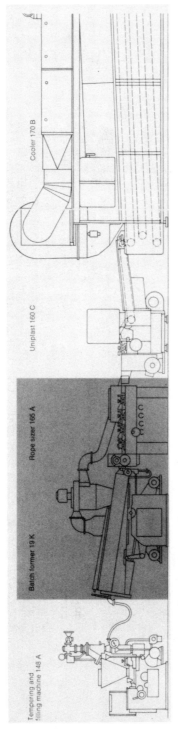

Figure 65 Typical hard candy lozenge center fill production line. The center fill machine stores, maintains temperature, recirculates fill material and pumps the center into the formed candy rope as it exits the batch former. The rope is then sized to the proper diameter, formed into lozenges in the uniplast and cooled prior to final tablet sizing and packaging. (Robert Bosch GmBH, Div. Hamac-Höller.)

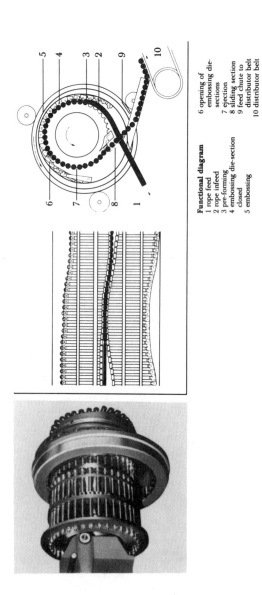

Functional diagram

1 rope feed
2 rope infeed
3 pre-forming
4 embossing die-section
  closed
5 embossing

6 opening of
  embossing die-
  sections
7 ejection
8 sliding section
9 feed chute to
  distributor belt
10 distributor belt

Figure 66   Uniplast tablet dies and a functional diagram showing the lozenge forming operation. Pressure at embossing step 5 must be controlled to assure complete closure of the tablet to avoid, leakage of center fill from the center.   (Robert Bosch GmBH, Div. Hamac-Höller.)

V. FORMULATIONS (CENTER-FILLED LOZENGES)

The following formulations represent various methods of manufacturing center-filled medicated confections.

Example 7: Decongestant (15.0 mg/4.5 g) Medicated Lozenges
with Liquid Center—Direct Medicament Addition, 15% w/w
Center Fill

Ingredient	Quantity
A. *Shell*	
Liquid sugar (67.5% w/w solids)	88.90 lb
Corn syrup 43°Baumé (80.5% w/w solids)	49.70 lb
Ground candy salvage (20—50 mesh)	2.00 lb
Pseudoephedrine HCl USP	155.00 g
Spearmint flavor	50.00 g
Green color cubes	10.00 g
B. *Center*	
Pseudoephedrine HCl USP	152.00 g
Peppermint flavor	75.00 g
Menthol	100.00 g
Liquid sugar (67.5% w/w solids)	74.10 lb
Corn syrup 58—62 DE	62.25 lb

Liquid sugar and corn syrup are gear-metered into the dissolver and precooked at 125°C. Final cooking is performed at
148°C with a vacuum of 736 mm Hg to produce 100 lb of candy
base with a 60:40 sugar/corn syrup ratio. The flavor is uniformly mixed into the ground salvage. Color is added to candy
base in the collection kettle. The pseudoephedrine HCl is
added in the transfer kettle and folded into the mass and the
flavor-salvage mixture is added on the mixing table. Candy
base is mixed and tempered. The mass is transferred to the
batch former containing the center fill pipe where it is formed
to a candy rope around the pipe. Center fill sugar and corn
syrup are mixed and heated to 105°C. Pseudoephedrine HCl
and flavor are dissolved and the mixture added to the reservoir
of the pump. Center fill material is cooled to 95°C, then pumped
into the rope prior to sizing. The filled rope is sized, molded,
cooled, and lozenges are collected for packaging.

Example 8: Anesthetic (10.0 mg/5.0 g) Medicated Lozenges
with Fat Emulsion and Direct Medicament Addition—25% Center
Fill Weight

Ingredient	Quantity
A. *Shell*	
Liquid sugar (67.5% w/w solids)	81.50 lb
Corn syrup 43°Baumé (80.5% w/w solids)	56.04 lb
Ground candy salvage (20—50 mesh)	2.00 lb
Benzocaine NF	93.00 g
Spearmint flavor	35.00 g
B. *Center*	
Benzocaine NF	93.00 g
Hydrogenated vegetable oil 98°F mp	50.00 lb
Glycerin USP	50.00 lb
Glyceryl monostearate	1.00 lb
Menthol	150.00 g
Eucalyptus oil	75.00 g
Green color paste	20.00 g

Liquid sugar and corn syrup are gear-metered into the dissolver and precooked at 120°C. Final cooking is performed at
148°C with a vacuum of 736 mm Hg to produce 100 lb of candy
base with a 55:45 sugar/corn syrup ratio. The flavor is uniformly mixed into the ground salvage. The benzocaine is
added in the transfer kettle and folded into the mass and the
flavor-salvage mixture is added on the mixing table. Candy
base is mixed and tempered. The mass is transferred to the
batch former containing the center fill pipe where it is formed
to a candy rope around the pipe. The glycerin and vegetable
oil are each heated separately to 90°C. Emulsifier is added and
dissolved in the oil. Add glycerin to the oil and mix until a
smooth emulsion is formed. Add menthol dissolved in flavor
and benzocaine. Cool to 90°C. The center fill emulsion is
added to the reservoir of the pump, then pumped into the
rope prior to sizing. The filled rope is sized, molded,
cooled, and the formed lozenges are collected for packaging.

VI. PACKAGING

Hard candies are hygroscopic and prone to absorbing atmospheric moisture. Confections, when exposed to humid conditions, are susceptible to graining and sticking, resulting in a product with reduced consumer appeal. Moisture absorption in medicated lozenges can also result in drug decomposition because of interaction of medicament with the candy base, flavor, or acidulent.

Confectionary products which are marketed for mass appeal and rapid turnover are produced with an expected shelf life of 8–12 months. Medicated lozenges, on the other hand, should be expected to have a shelf life of 3–5 years. The location in the home where the material is stored is another factor that governs the integrity of both medicated and nonmedicated products. Confections are usually stored in the kitchen, whereas medicated lozenges are stored in the medicine cabinet—a location that exposes the product to cycles of extreme temperature and moisture.

The hygroscopic nature of the candy base, the storage conditions to which medicated lozenges are exposed, the length of time they are stored, and the potential for drug interactions (because of the reactivity of candy base components) require that packaging offer the product more than just an aesthetic surrounding that presents product to consumer.

A. Individual Bunch Wrap

The majority of medicated lozenge products are individually bunch-wrapped with either cellophane or aluminum foil laminated with tissue paper impregnated with a wax or FDA food-approved release agent (Figure 67). This covering is provided for aesthetics rather than as a protective moisture barrier, as bunch wrap offers only minimal moisture protection in that open

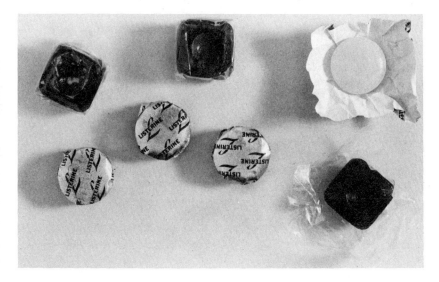

Figure 67 Individually bunch wrapped lozenges. Laminated aluminum foil or cellophane wraps are most commonly used.

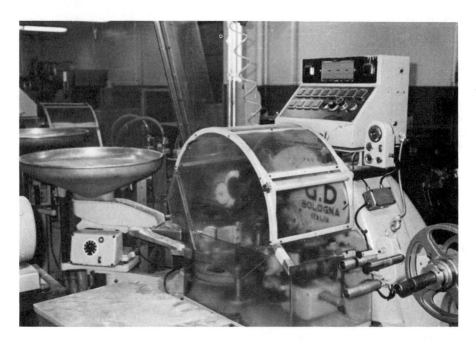

Figure 68   G. D. (Bologna, Italy) lozenge bunch wrapping machine.   Un-
wrapped lozenges are stored in the hopper prior to mechanical aligning
and passage into the bunch wrapping machine.   (Warner-Lambert Co.)

spaces result when the foil or cellophane is folded around the lozenge.
Production of a completely moisture-proof bunch wrap is not practical from
the standpoint of cost, machine speed, or efficiency.   The major advantage
is that bunch wrap prevents lozenges from sticking together and from becoming dusty or breaking during shipping, shelving, or storage.   Bunch
wrap also aids in keeping the lozenges sanitary before use, expecially if
the product is handled or carried individually in the pocket or purse [28].

Two disadvantages associated with the use of bunch wrap are (a) a
tendency of the cellophane portion of the foil laminate to stick to the lozenge during prolonged storage at elevated humidity (lozenges that grain
more than 40% become increasingly more sticky and prone to adhering to
the bunch wrap); (b) the extra time that bunch wrapping adds to the
packaging operation.   The bunch wrapping process is the slowest of all
the packaging procedures because each lozenge must be mechanically aligned
and handled individually (Figures 68 and 69).   Conversely, the benefits
derived from bunch wrapping by increasing consumer appeal and confidence
in the product—by professionalizing the mode of presentation, eliminating
the sticking together of lozenges, and reducing the dusting or chipping
of lozenges during transit and storage, as well as presenting a uniform
appearance inside the box regardless of the physical state of the lozenges—
indicates that bunch wrap should be considered as an integral part of the
medicated lozenge package.

B. Container

The container offers the lozenges protection from breakage during transit
(Figure 70) and provides a convenient vehicle for transportation. The
more portable the container, the easier it is for the user to maintain a uniform dosage schedule (Figure 71).

The container does not offer complete protection from moisture because
the end folds of the package are not airtight. A sealed, waxed paper
lining will increase moisture protection, but in general the carton is used
only as a means of protecting, displaying, and transporting the lozenges.
A plastic tube may offer greater moisture protection than a paper carton
depending on the type of plastic resin, thickness, and the seal integrity
of cap to body.

C. Carton Overwrap

Overwrapping the container with cellophane, foil, or waxed paper will improve the resistance to moisture penetrating the package. A carboard carton overwrapped with nitrocellulose cellophane or Saran Wrap and stored at
25°C with a relative humidity of 80% will contain lozenges with an average
grain of 40% after 90 days, while the same package stored without the cellophane overwrap will contain lozenges grained to an average of 90−95%.

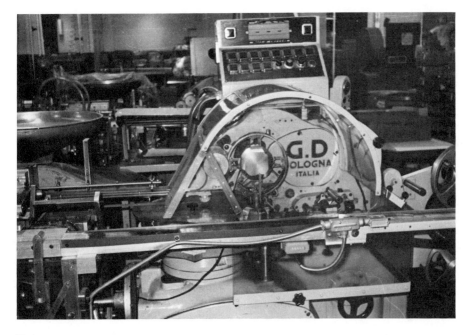

Figure 69   G. D. (Bologna, Italy) bunch wrapping machine.   Wrapped
lozenges ready for packaging.   (Warner-Lambert Co.)

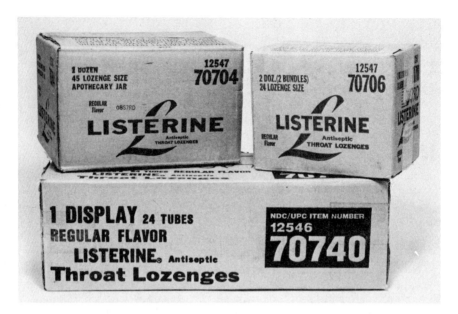

Figure 70   Outer cardboard box offers the trade containers protection during warehouse storage and shipping.

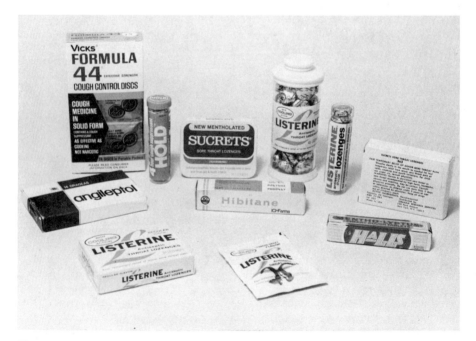

Figure 71   Production trade packages. Cardboard box, foil pouch, styrene tube, metal box, strip-pack, and roll are the most common in use.

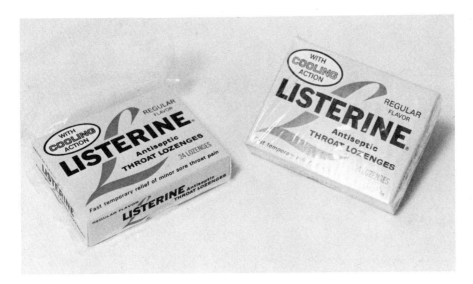

Figure 72   Carton overwrap. Moisture protection afforded the contents depends on the quality of seal and the moisture-transmission values of the wrap.

Sticking to the bunch wrap dramatically increases after the lozenge has grained 40% or more. The sticking is so intense after 80% graining occurs that the laminate will separate from the foil and stick to the lozenge surface. Lozenges that have maintained drug potency and flavor integrity become so physically unattractive when this condition does occur that they are unusable to the patient (Figure 72).

D. Bundle Wrap

A portion of any product's shelf life is spent in a warehouse. A medicated lozenge may at times experience 12–24 months of warehouse storage before reaching the consumer. Warehouse conditions vary from location to location, but in many instances warehouses are not climate-controlled. Prolonged storage in the ambient environment may cause product graining and decomposition even before the product is placed on store shelves. A means of mitigating this condition is to wrap a moisture-resistant covering around groups of boxes. This bundle wrap acts as a primary barrier to prevent moisture damage or premature graining before the product is placed on the retail shelves. The bundle wrap is removed before displaying the product since its only function is to protect the product during warehouse storage. Typical bundle wrap materials include waxed aluminum foil, Saran Wrap, polypropylene, waxed paper, or other materials with low-water-vapor transmission values. Routine checking of the seal integrity throughout the bundle-wrapping operation is carried out by either water submersion or vacuum-testing procedures. Incomplete sealing, folds, creases, or holes can negate much of the protection offered by the bundle wrap. An efficient bundle wrap (Figure 73) should offer medicated lozenges adequate

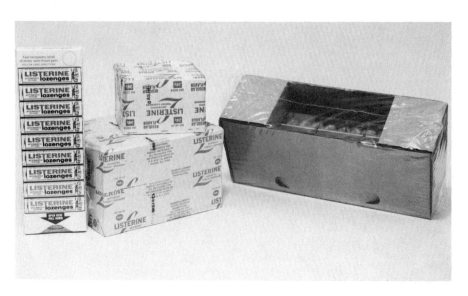

Figure 73   Bundle wrap. Vital for moisture protection during warehouse storage.

ambient shelf life storage, free from graining, for a minimum of 24 to as many as 36 months.

E. Foil Pouches

Perhaps the best protection that can be afforded a medicated lozenge product is packaging in a sealed aluminum foil, heat-sealable pouch [29]. This package employs aluminum foil as thin as 0.0008 in. laminated with polyethylene and tissue paper, and impregnated with wax to aid in sealing the pouch. As few as one and as many as four pieces can be packaged in one pouch, depending on the pouch and lozenge sizes. The product is guaranteed an indefinite shelf life free from the disadvantages associated with moisture permeation, as this type of package has a moisture transmission value approaching zero.

A quality control check of seal integrity is performed on a routine basis during the foil-pouching operation. A method both rapid and efficient for determining seal integrity is to place a group of five pouches in a container (a desiccator is suitable) under vacuum (380 mm Hg) in water for 60—120 sec; break the vacuum; open the pouches; and observe whether moisture has entered the pouch. Use of a colored water solution highlights moisture permeation, rendering pinhole imperfections more visible. The vacuum test, while efficient, is destructive to the pouches. Testing via a destructive procedure results in waste of a significant number of pouches, expecially when extended packaging runs or frequent interval testing is involved.

A second test, classified as nondestructive, is the carbon dioxide permeation test. Here the pouches are placed in a carbon dioxide atmosphere for a predetermined time, then checked with a carbon dioxide-sensing device for the presence of the gas in the packet. The packages that pass this test are suitable for inclusion as salable production material. Testing of foil integrity is more fully described in Chapter 5.

Packaging lozenges in foil pouches eliminates the need for individually bunch-wrapping the product. The lack of moisture penetration through the foil laminate removes the tendency for lozenges to stick together. Lozenges will not break or cause excessive dusting in the pouch during transit since excessive movement with resulting attrition is limited by the tight fit of the lozenge in the packet (Figure 74).

A drawback of not bunch-wrapping foil pouched lozenges is the dusting that occurs during the packaging operation. The attrition in the storage hopper and delivery chutes as lozenges are fed into the pouches results in increased dusting of the lozenge surface. This does not affect product efficacy, stability, or surface texture; but from the standpoint of aesthetics, the quality of the product's appearance has been reduced. Lozenges in pouches can be sold as individual units of two to four lozenges per pouch or boxed in groups of pouches and sold in cartons.

Examples of some typical carton wrap and bundle wrap materials with their physical characteristics are contained in Table 5 [30]. Examples of graining characteristics of lozenges stored in various containers with different overwraps are present in Table 6 and Figure 75.

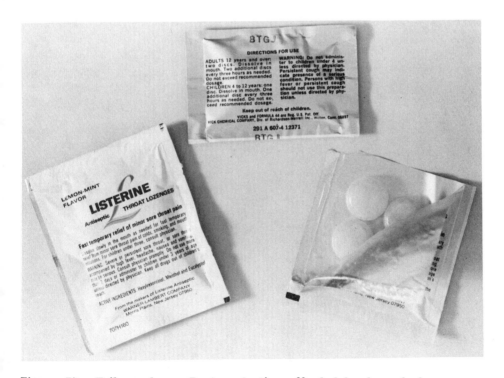

Figure 74 Foil pouches. Best protection afforded hard candy lozenges.

Table 5   Physical Properties of Selected Packaging Films

Product/opacity	Water vapor transmission rate in $g/m^2/100°F$, 95% RH/24 hr	Sealing properties	Machine performance	Printability	Heat shrinkability	Grease/oil resistance
Waxed glassine paper/opaque	4	Heat	Excellent	No	No	Excellent
Polymer-coated cellophane (1 mil)/transparent	6–14	Heat or adhesive	Excellent	Excellent	No	Excellent
Unoriented polypropylene (1 mil)/transparent	8–10	Heat	Fair to good	Good if treated	No	Excellent
Vinyl (1 mil)/transparent to translucent	8 and higher	Heat or adhesive	Fair to good	Special inks	Some types	Excellent
Propylene medium density (0.926–0.940 mil)/transparent to translucent	8–15	Heat	Fair to good	Good if treated	Some types	Good

Table 6   Effect of Wrap on Graining of Stored Lozenges

Container	Percent of lozenge exhibiting graining						
	Months at 25°C/80% RH				Months at 37°C/80% RH		
	1	2	3	6	1	2	6
Unprotected lozenges	70	90	100	100 (Liquefied)	82	100	100 (Liquefied)
Cardboard box without overwrap	52	78	93	100	72	93	100 (Liquefied)
Cardboard box with nitrocellulose cellophane overwrap	14	22	36	50	28	47	72
Cardboard box with polyethylene film overwrap	7	16	29	45	14	38	69
Cardboard box with nitrocellulose cellophane overwrap and waxed aluminum foil bundle wrap	0	0	0	<5	0	0	<10
Cardboard box with nitrocellulose cellophane overwrap and polypropylene shrink film (1.0 mil) bundle wrap	0	0	5	17	0	<10	25
Foil lozenge pouch—pouch paper/polyethylene (1 mil)/foil (0.0008")	0	0	0	0	0	0	0

Note: Lozenge studied was medicated hard candy.

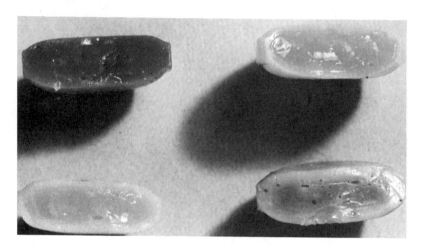

Figure 75   Grained lozenges. Top left: ungrained lozenge; top right:
25% grained lozenge; bottom left: 50% grained lozenge; bottom right: 75%
grained lozenge.

VII.   CHEWY OR CARAMEL BASE MEDICATED TABLETS

An alternative to the conventional "suck-type" hard candy lozenge is incorporation of medicament into a caramel base which can be chewed instead of
dissolved in the mouth. Caramel is the general term for all chewy candies
[78]. There are two main types: caramels and toffees. Toffees are not
prepared by pulling (mechanical air incorporation) and are considered high-
quality confectionary items. The term *toffee* came from the word *toughy*
and in the United States it is called taffy [23]. This dosage form is more
suitable for systemic vs. mucous membrane-active drugs since the dwell
time of the active ingredient in the oral cavity is significantly less than is
experienced with throat lozenges.
    Many of the raw materials utilized in the preparation of chewy candies
parallel those found in high-boiled sweets, but the method of preparation
and the final product composition result in a dosage form that can be chewed
or, if desired, slowly dissolved in the mouth. By changing the ratios of
certain ingredients, the consistency of the product and the type of chew
obtained can be significantly altered.

A.   Raw Materials

Candy Base

Typical confectionary-based chewy tablets contain from 40 to 80% candy base.
This is a mixture of sugar and corn syrup, with a ratio of 50:50 to 75:25
sugar to corn syrup. As this ratio approaches 50:50 the resultant product
becomes more chewy and taffy-like while at 70:30 sugar—corn syrup, a
grained, soft, and dry chew results. In between lies a large variety of
alternative chew possibilities that can suit the overall desire of the product
formulator.
    The size of the tablet vs. the concentration of medicament will also help
dictate the ratio of sugar to corn syrup. As the concentration of drug

present in the matrix increases, the softer will be the chew and the faster the time for graining. If a firmer chew is desired, more corn syrup is added, but if more structure (body) is needed, the sugar concentration must be increased. The candy base is the frame around which the product is built.

Sugar-Corn Syrup Ratio

As mentioned above, the ratio of sugar to corn syrup is critical in determining the type of product chew. Higher corn syrup-to-sugar ratios form a hard, sticky, taffey-like chew, while increasing sugar concentrations favor a dry, grainy chew associated with after-dinner mints.

Candy base is cooked in a manner similar to that described for hard candy lozenges. The major differences occur in the cook temperature and level of vacuum applied during processing. Whereas hard candy base has an average moisture content of 0.5—1.5%, chewy confections are prepared in the range of 3—5% moisture. This increased moisture lowers the viscosity of the corn syrup vehicle thus allowing for the softer consistency. The lower viscosity also allows for more sugar crystal movement in the base, thus explaining the increase in graining tendencies and the formation of a softer and drier chew when the product is prepared with higher sugar contents.

As the candy base content of the product increases, so does its effect on the overall processability of the tablet. Chewy candies with a high candy base content (greater than 65%), high moisture (above 3.5%), and high corn syrup-to-sugar ratio (50—55% corn syrup) will tend to "cold-flow" (stick, droop, and flatten out even at room temperature) and have a taffy-like chew. Products with a high sugar-to-corn syrup ratio (60—70% sugar) and high moisture (above 3.5%) will grain rapidly (sugar crystallization), have a dry, soft chew and be difficult to process. This is because the product will lack the elasticity for acceptable forming and shaping. Graining gives the product structure but also a brittleness that reduces stretch and causes the candy rope to break and tear instead of stretching. Reduction of moisture in this situation will result in a harder, more brittle chew. Increased moisture will cause cold flow and increase stickiness.

The sugar, corn syrup, and moisture contents of the chewy product must be well controlled if a tablet with optimum chew characteristics, processability, and shelf life is to be formulated.

The use of high-maltose corn syrup tends to produce a tablet with a somewhat harder chew. This raw material, at equivalent moisture, will produce candy base with a higher viscosity which will be harder and less grained than candy prepared under identical conditions utilizing regular 42— to 43-DE corn syrup. The dextrose equivalent of the corn syrup will also affect the chew characteristics of the final tablet. Reduction of dextrose content below 36 DE will result in product with a tougher, taffy-like chew, while use of corn syrup with a DE above 46 increases the incidence of cold flow, product browning, and atmospheric moisture intolerance. Except for the browning problem, the use of 42- to 43-DE regular grade corn syrup is indicated when preparing medicated chewy confections.

Aeration

Air must be incorporated in toffee-based confections in order to attain the desired, distinctive type of soft chew. Since a pulling machine is not used [67,81], aeration must be accomplished by using a whipping agent that will entrap air and lower the density of the final product. This aeration, with resultant reduction in density, makes the product more chewy and gives the impression of a more meltaway type of chew. Utilization of a pulling machine reduces the efficiency of product manufacture, especially when high-speed forming equipment is employed.

Raw materials such as milk protein, egg albumin, gelatin, xanthan gum, starch, pectin, algin, carageenin as well as combinations of these materials have all been used successfully to lower the density of the candy. The whipping agent is prepared as a separate mixture before incorporation in the product.

One or more of the whipping agents are suspended in hot water and rapidly mixed with cooling until a highly aerated, foamlike mixture is produced. Gums are often mixed with the whipping agent in order to give body to the mass and allow for the entrapment of more air. The gum will impart extended stability to the whip thus enabling longer storage of this component and more efficient reduction of the final tablet density. This stabilized mass will also hold the air better when incorporated in the candy base.

Addition of the whipping agent must be accomplished at a temperature low enough to prevent the destruction of the whip but high enough to allow incorporation of cold materials in the hot mass without causing crystallization. The whip should be added at a temperature somewhere between 90 and 120°F. During the addition procedure, a gentle kneading action is indicated. This will assure a uniform incorporation of the whip in the candy base without destroying its air retention characteristics.

Humectants

Addition of humectants to the chewy base enables the product to meet two criteria. First, the addition of humectant lowers the equilibrium relative humidity (ERH) [61] of the formulation, while at the same time improving the chew and mouth-feel characteristics of the product.

Many toffee-based formulations have an equilibrium moisture level of 45–55%. Products with higher corn syrup levels may even test at 55–70%. The significance of equilibrium relative humidity value means that at times, when the ambient relative humidity is below the ERH of the formulation it will surrender moisture to the atmosphere. On the other hand, when stored in environments above the ERH, the product will pick up ambient moisture and become sticky. Ideally, when the product is formulated, it should be targeted at a 35–40% equilibrium level. Achieving this concentration means that if the ambient conditions are maintained at 35–40% RH, the product will maintain its integrity. Should the product be exposed to higher humidity conditions, it will pick up some moisture but rapidly lose it when the conditions are again favorable. In the winter, when the relative humidity is low, the product may lose water at the surface but will regain its integrity when exposed to favorable humidity conditions. Formulation of a product with this type of equilibrium moisture tolerance results in one that is much less apt to harden in the package, since it is easier to protect a product from moisture pickup than it is to protect it from drying out and hardening. If the product is hard, the customer will consider the chew totally unacceptable, but a tablet that softens and becomes slightly sticky in most cases is still consumer-acceptable. Chewy-based confections that are formulated at a high ERH are most always subject to hardening.

Glycerin is the best of the food-acceptable, humectant materials. It has a bland taste, good mouth-feel, and is completely inert. Propylene glycol is bitter and sorbitol tends to crystallize and make the tablet harder to chew. The humectant can be added to the product after incorporation of the whip. If desired, any colorants can be suspended or dissolved in the humectant and added at the same time. Normal concentrations of humectant run between 1.5 and 5% of the batch weight.

Lubricants

Addition of a lubricant to a chewy product helps prevent the candy from sticking to the teeth during chewing. Since most lubricants are oils and do not incorporate well in candy base, care must be taken to use the lowest concentration that will give the desired effect. In most instances 3—7% will properly lubricate the candy. If higher concentrations are needed, emulsions may be required to prevent oil separation.

Vegetable oils and fats are used as lubricants in chewy candies. When selecting a proper lubricant, the melting point of the fat and the concentration must be evaluated. Incorporation of the oil in the chewy candy base is most easily accomplished as a simple mixture and not by preparing an emulsion. In either case, the oil tends to express out of the candy when the product is placed under stress. Heat or mixing may cause the oil to separate from the product. When this occurs, the candy loses some of its elasticity and becomes more difficult to process. Another problem of oil separation is product flavor change since the oil occludes the flavor. The tablet chew may become grainy and nonhomogeneous.

Reduction of oil content below 5% or the use of a higher melting point fat or oil can remedy this problem. Oils with a melting point of 98—105°F are well suited for this type of product. Below 95°F the oil is still a solid or a semisolid, which reduces the chances of migration. When chewed, the oil rapidly softens and melts in the mouth thus allowing it to perform its function of lubricating the product to prevent sticking on the teeth. Fats above 105°F are not recommended because they do not melt in the mouth. This will produce a confection that, when chewed, will have a fatty sensation in the mouth, since the candy will dissolve and the unmelted fat remains on the teeth.

Any of the bland hydrogenated vegetable oils (cottonseed, palm, soy, etc.) that fall in the desired melting point range are acceptable lubricants for this type of product.

Addition of the hydrogenated vegetable oil should take place below 90°C and after the whipping agent has been thoroughly incorporated. If the oil is added too soon after addition of the whipping agent it will cause the whip to deaerate and lose its density reduction characteristics.

Medicaments

Whereas hard candy lozenges can accommodate only 2—4% medicament, the chewy tablet can take up to 35—40% material. The soft tablets are not difficult to chew; therefore preparation of 4.0- to 5.0-g tablets is not unreasonable. This means that as much as 1.5—2.0 g of certain medicaments can be delivered per dosage unit.

Addition of medicament to chewy base poses a unique problem to the formulator. As the patient chews the tablet and releases the drug, it is solubilized or suspended in the saliva. Therefore, any off-taste, bitterness, or anesthetic characteristics are accentuated both during and after chewing. Medicated syrups are quickly swallowed, and hard candy lozenges release the medicament slowly and it is quickly swallowed. Chewable compressed tablets keep some of the medicament entrapped in the granules where it is partially masked, but the chewy dosage brings out the worst flavor and bitterness characteristics of all active ingredients. Even flavor oils appear bitter when used at concentrations that would normally help mask an unacceptable taste, since the flavor oils are picked up by the saliva and retained in the mouth.

Utilization of adsorbate technology [70–75] helps to mitigate this problem. Preparation of 5–20% medicament adsorbates on carriers such as magnesium trisilicate or Veegum [63,70] renders many bitter principles palatable in the mouth. Once swallowed, the adsorbate readily releases the drug at the low pH of the stomach. Use of powder coating and microencapsulation techniques are also procedures that will make many drugs palatable when incorporated in the confectionary mass.

Based on the heat stability of the medicament, the drug addition can take place anywhere between 105°C and 65°C with 95–105°C being optimum addition temperatures. This allows for adequate mixing time and sufficient candy base fluidity to assure a uniform incorporation of drug throughout the product.

Seeding Crystals

Under normal circumstances, after cooling, the chewy base will crystallize [62,82] into a pliable mass that can be processed into individual dosage units. Depending on the ratio of sugar to corn syrup, this crystallization may take from 24 to 72 hr and may be variable depending on atmospheric conditions. A method utilized to speed up this crystallization and allow the base to be formed into tablets in a much shorter time is a process called *seeding* [82]. Here fine sugar crystals are added to the warm candy mass. These crystals become a seed which stimulates crystallization of other sugar crystals and thus the formation of product with sufficient strength to withstand final tablet processing. Ideally, sufficient seed should be added to the product to produce a rapid and coarse graining. A coarse grain when broken down by extrusion will result in formation of tablets with a very fine grain. The fine-grained tablets are softer, have more resistance to cold flow, and have a more acceptable chew characteristic.

Fine-powdered sugar at 3–10% is used as seed material. If the sugar is too course, the resultant tablets tend to be gritty. If the sugar is too fine, the seeding characteristics are diminished. If properly seeded, the product should be fully grained within 3–6 hr after addition. Seed material should be added to the base at a temperature not exceeding 85°C. Above this temperature the sugar will melt into the product and lose its crystalizing characteristics. The seeding material should not be mixed for more than 5–10 min since excessive mixing will also tend to melt the seed into the product.

Flavors

Flavors may be added to the chewy base at the same time as the seed material. Temperatures should be below 90°C to prevent excessive flavor flashoff. Rapid incorporation of the flavor in the base will also reduce flavor loss. Liquid or powdered flavors are suitable for use in this type of product.

The concentration of flavor used in chewy products should be kept to a minimum. The flavor itself can impart bitterness to the base when chewed out of the tablet since it will be rapidly solubilized and mixed with saliva. In most cases flavor concentration should not exceed 0.5%. When developing the product flavor, the formulator should taste flavored and unflavored candy base to determine how much of the product bitterness is contributed by the flavor oils.

B. Processing

Many of the procedures utilized in the manufacture hard candy lozenges are incorporated into the preparation of the chewy dosage form.

Hard Candy Base

Candy base is prepared in the same manner as described for medicated lozenges. Cooking temperatures and vacuum parameters are lower in order to prepare base with a higher moisture content (3–5%). This increased water lowers the viscosity of the corn syrup phase, which helps avoid the brittle glassy candy that results when base is manufactured at 0.5–2.0% moisture [77].

The candy base, after cooking, is transferred to a suitable mixer (Figure 76). Planetary or sigma blade configuration is acceptable. The vessel must be heated to a temperature of 95–125°C in order to avoid rapid cooling and crystallization of the candy when it contacts a cool surface. If the vessel surface is too cool and the candy crystallizes, lumps of hard candy will be dispersed throughout the product. If the mixer temperature is set too high (above 130°C), the extra mixing time required to cool the batch will result in a condition whereby candy base is cooled with extended mixing. The friction generated onto the candy base along with cooling causes a seeding of the batch that results in a rapid fine crystallization of the sugar from the base. This is nonreversible and, if allowed to continue, will form a solid mass of grained candy in the vessel. Ideally, the container temperature must be high enough to prevent candy base sticking to the walls and blades but low enough to minimize the mixing time required to cool the base to the initial desired processing temperature (Figure 77).

Once the candy base has been cooled to a temperature below 120°C, the whipping agents may be added. These ingredients include milk solids, egg albumin, gelatin, starches, gums, or a combination of these materials all whipped and hydrated before addition. This is critical because the foaming and air-holding qualities of the whip are diminished when added to hot candy base. For optimum effect, maximum air must be entrapped into the whipping agents during the hydration procedure. The thicker whipped mass will entrap more air into the candy. A negative is that too much gum or protein will result in a hard, taffy-like chew.

The whipping agent should be added to candy base that is below 105°C. This allows for optimum retention of air in the product and formation of a good protein matrix. If the candy base is too hot (above 120°C), aeration is lost and the protein matrix collapses. Addition of this material at too low a candy base temperature (below 90°C) results in product sticking and candy base crystallization.

Colors and Humectants

Any colorants may be added by dispersing them in the humectant. Color addition to the humectant must be accompanied by efficient mixing to assure

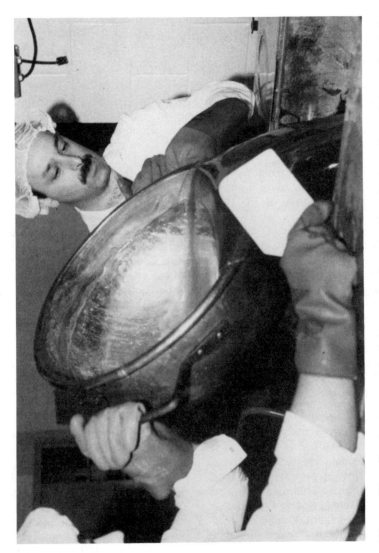

Figure 76   Candy base cooked to proper temperature is transferred to preheated mixer.   Mixer temperature should be no more than 20°C below that of the candy base to avoid rapid cooling and crystallization.   (Warner-Lambert Co.)

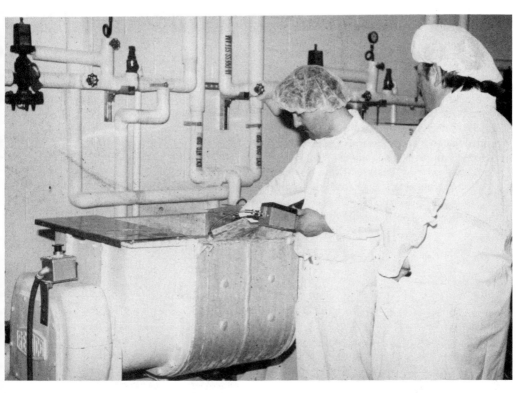

Figure 77   Candy base is mixed to a temperature below 120°C. At this point the whipping agents may be added. (Warner-Lambert Co.)

uniform particle distribution and prevention of dye lumps which results in mottled tablets. Dyes suspended in glycerin, dextrose, or propylene glycol may be used and added directly to the product. Color addition (Figure 78) can take place at any time during the process and is limited only to the stability of the dye component in the presence of hot candy base.

Humectants should be added at a temperature above 90°C to avoid rapid and uncontrolled cooling of the product in the mixing kettle.

Medicaments

Medicament addition (Figure 79) to the product is governed by the heat stability of the drug in the presence of candy base. The earlier in the process the medicament can be added, the longer the mixing time and the better the distribution. Conversely, heat-sensitive drugs may be added at the lowest workable product temperature and mixed for a time period sufficient to achieve content uniformity.

Drugs such as dextromethorphan HBr, chlorpheniramine maleate, calcium carbonate [76], acetaminophen, carbetapentane citrate, aluminum, or magnesium hydroxide and diphenhydramine HCl are heat-stable. They can be added at any time in the process (after aeration) and mixed until the product is cooled. Other medicaments such as benzocaine, pseudoephedrine HCl, phenylpropanolamine HCl, dyclonine, aspirin, and dimenhydrinate are subject to rapid heat degradation. These ingredients are added at temperatures ranging from 65 to 75°C and are mixed for as little as 5 min to achieve proper distribution. Medicaments should be added after the addition of aeration ingredients to avoid interference with the air entrapment

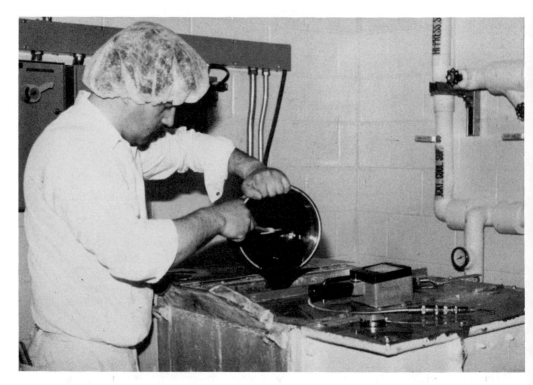

Figure 78   Color addition.   Dyes are suspended in propylene glycol or glycerin to aid distribution.   (Warner-Lambert Co.)

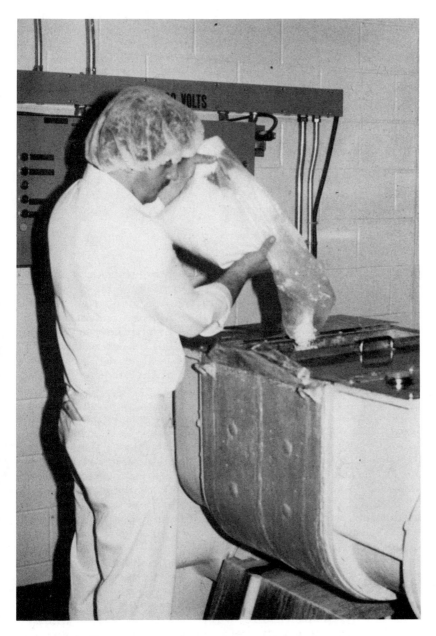

Figure 79 Medicament addition. Heat stability of the drugs determines at what temperature they may be added. (Warner-Lambert Co.)

procedure but added before addition of flavors to avoid interaction of medicament and flavor. Optimum medicament addition temperature is 95—105°C.
Addition temperatures below 70°C increase distribution problems due to the
high viscosity of the product.

Lubricants

Lubricants (vegetable oils) should be added away from the whipping agent.
The oil acts as a defoaming agent, which lessens the aeration characteristics of the whip and results in a product with a hard chew. Lubricant, if
added after the medicament, causes the lowest degree of product deaera-
tion. Addition of lubricant below 80°C is not recommended since the candy
base will not completely incorporate the oil when it gets too thick. Addition at temperatures below 80°C may result in a phase separation of the
lubricant causing the final tablet to lose elasticity and have an oily texture with a fatty taste.

Flavor and Seeding Crystal Addition

Incorporation of the flavor into the seeding crystals prevents excessive
flash-off from the hot product and aids incorporation of the oil or powder
in the batch. Seeding crystals should be added to the product at a temperature not exceeding 85°C (Figure 80). This will prevent the melting
of the seed crystals, thus lessening the product's crystallizing characteristics. The seed should not be mixed for more than 10 min after addition
to prevent crystal melting. If the batch temperature is too low (less than
60°C), premature crystallization will make removal of the product from the
mixing vessel difficult.

    Product is removed from the mixing kettle after seed addition (Figure
81). Ideally, the product should have a viscosity low enough to allow the
material to slowly flow out of the mixer without operator assistance. The
higher the viscosity, the more difficult and time consuming is this step.
Product that is too fluid at this stage, even if in the desired temperature
range (60—85°C), may have been overmixed thus allowing the seed to melt
back into the base. When the seed is lost, the time for the candy to grain
is markedly increased. Properly seeded base can be processed 3—4 hr
after cooling while unseeded or improperly seeded candy may take 1—3
days at controlled temperature and humidity conditions to reach an acceptable level of product grain.

    Graining gives the tablet structure and body. Incomplete grain re-
sults in cold flow, or drooping and flattening of the product. The inability to hold the desired shape occurs when the incomplete candy base
structure allows movement of the corn syrup in the vehicle. Proper
graining will allow for a solid structure so that tablets are formed with a
soft chew and a resistance to cold flow even under elevated temperature or
humidity conditions.

Tablet Forming

As the candy base cools to room temperature (Figure 82), the combination
of high (3—5%) moisture content, seed, and falling temperature results in
the formation of a rapid, coarse-grained product. The coarse-grained
material is hard to chew and very brittle. Coarse graining gives the
product extreme strength and resistance to cold flow.

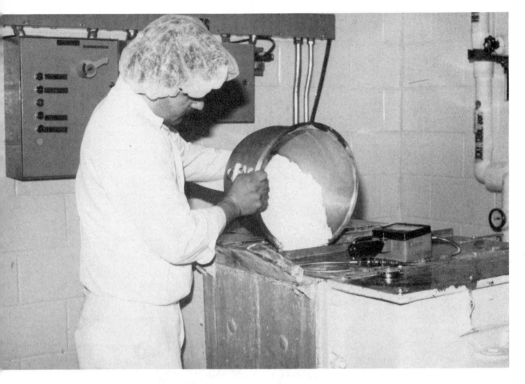

Figure 80 Flavor and seeding crystal addition. Seed should not be mixed for more than 10 minutes to avoid melting of the seed crystals into the batch. (Warner-Lambert Co.)

In as little as 3–4 hr after cooling, the product has grained to an extent that individual tablets may be formed. Depending on the type of equipment available, product may be cut and wrapped or formed in a manner similar to that utilized for hard-boiled candy lozenges.

Since the product is now hard, brittle, and cooled to room temperature, it must be worked into a pliable state that will allow the formation of individual dosage units. This must be done regardless of the type of tablet-forming operation. The method of choice is extrusion [79]. Here the mass is broken down to a more flexible state by passing the product through an extruder (Figure 83). The course-grained mass is broken down so that a more elastic and workable base is produced. This is accomplished by reducing the coarse-grained matrix into a fine-grained state (Figure 84). This fine grain has more elasticity, a softer chew, but sufficient structure to restrict the tendency toward cold flow.

The work of extrusion adds heat to the product. To control sticking and prevent expression of the vegetable oil lubricant, the candy base temperature should be kept between 30 and 45°C during the extrusion and

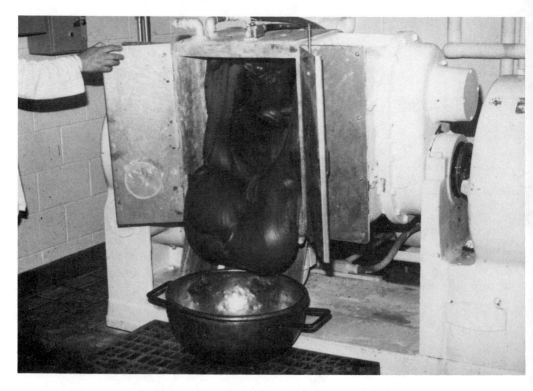

Figure 81   Removal of the medicated candy mass from the mixer. Ideally the product should have a viscosity low enough to allow the material to flow out of the mixer without operator assistance. Some manual cleaning around the blades may be required. (Warner-Lambert Co.)

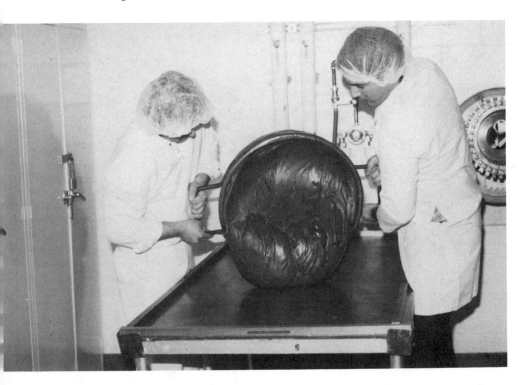

Figure 82 Medicated caramel base is deposited onto a cooling table. During this rapid cooling period a product with a coarse grain is formed. At least 3 to 4 hours cooling is required to enable the product to properly grain before extrusion. (Warner-Lambert Co.)

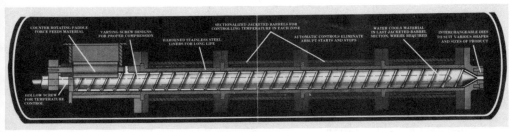

Figure 83 Schematic of jacketted extruder. The screw design of the extruder can be varied to obtain the desired compression and mixing force. (The Bonnot Company, Kent, Ohio.)

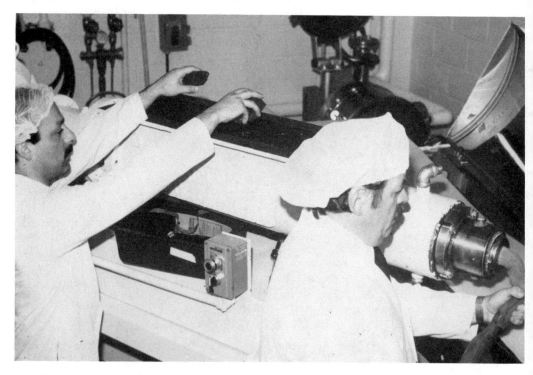

Figure 84 Grained caramel mass is extruded into a flexible candy rope.
Diameter and shape of the rope can be adjusted by changing the exit die
configuration. (Warner-Lambert Co.)

forming operations (Figures 85 and 86). Should the base exceed this temperature, oil separation is noted, sticking of tablets to the punch faces
occurs, and the formed tablets are soft, thus increasing the incidence of
tablets sticking together or deforming. If the product temperature falls
below 30°C, the candy mass is brittle and nonelastic. This results in a
nonuniform candy rope and difficulty in maintaining an acceptable tablet
weight variation. Tablets prepared from a cold rope are also difficult to
form thus increasing the tendency for fissures and imperfections on the
tablet surface.

The candy base is extruded into a 1- to 2-in. round rope (diameter
depends on final tablet weight) (Figure 87). The candy rope temperature
is maintained at a level that allows for adequate elasticity to assure uniform
weight tablets. The temperature must not reach the point that sticking to
the punch faces or sticking of tablets together after forming or deformation
of product while cooling results. After extrusion, the rope, tablet-forming,
cooling, and collection operations are the same as described for hard candy
lozenges (Figures 88 and 89).

An alternative to forming tablets utilizing hard candy lozenge procedures
is passing extruded rope through a cutting and wrapping machine (Figure
90). Here the extruded candy rope (square instead of round) is cut into
chunks using a knife, then wrapped in the desired bunch wrap. The

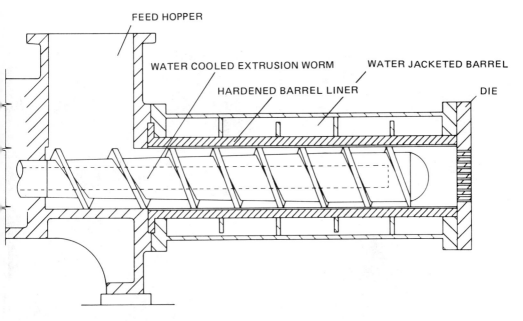

Figure 85 Schematic of jacketted extruder. More than one pass or a series of extruders may be required to obtain a product rope with the proper consistency. (The Bonnot Company, Kent, Ohio.)

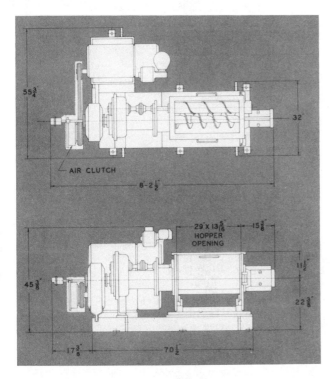

Figure 86 Schematic of extruder hopper and screws. (The Bonnot Company, Kent, Ohio.)

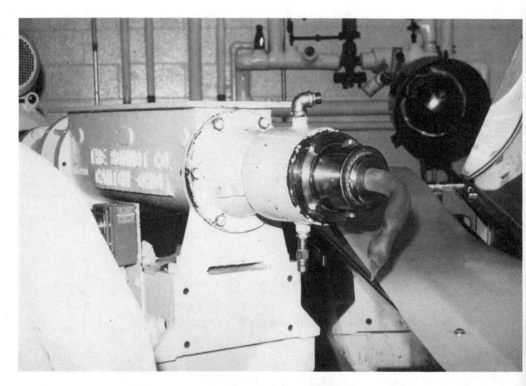

Figure 87 The diameter and shape of the candy rope is governed by the die configuration placed on the end of the extruder. Tablets weighing 4 to 5 grams require a 1-1/2 to 2 inch rope. This rope must then be sized to the proper diameter prior to the tablet forming operation. (Warner-Lambert Co.)

advantage of cut and wrap is that it is a single-step operation. Disadvantages include speed of tablet preparation and the limited shapes available.

C. Packaging

Control of moisture both in and out of the package is a major consideration when choosing a primary package for chewy tablets.

If the final product is prepared at an equilibrium moisture content of 35%, transmission of water into the product in summer months is more of a problem than release of moisture from the tablets in the winter. If properly formulated, unprotected tablets in low-humidity conditions will case-harden forming a tough crust at the surface. Prolonged exposure to a low-humidity environment will result in a gradual hardening of the tablet. Conversely, at elevated humidity conditions, moisture will be drawn into the product resulting in softening and sticking. Once the tablets are returned to normal humidity conditions (30–50% RH), the product will return to its original condition. To circumvent these moisture-related phenomena the product may be packaged in glass, high-density polyethylene bottles, fin-sealed pouches, or fin-sealed sticks (Figure 91).

Summary

Chewy type confectionary-base tablets can be prepared using many of the raw materials and processes utilized for hard candy. Regulation of candy base moisture and addition of aerating ingredients, humectants, lubricants, and seed control the product texture and give the desired chew characteristics.

Higher quantities of medicament can be delivered in this dosage form that can be incorporated into hard candy lozenges, but flavor masking of bitter principles is more of a problem.

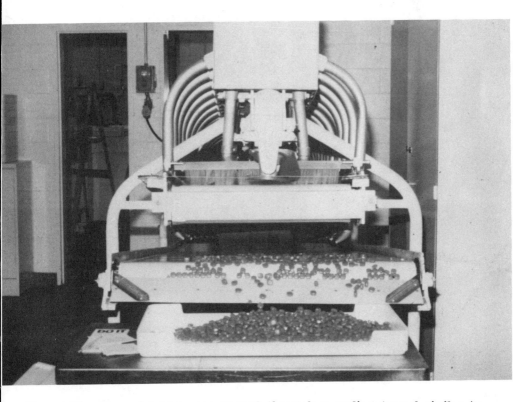

Figure 88 Formed tablets are passed through a cooling tunnel similar to that used for hard candy lozenges. This prevents sticking or deforming of the tablets. (Warner-Lambert Co.)

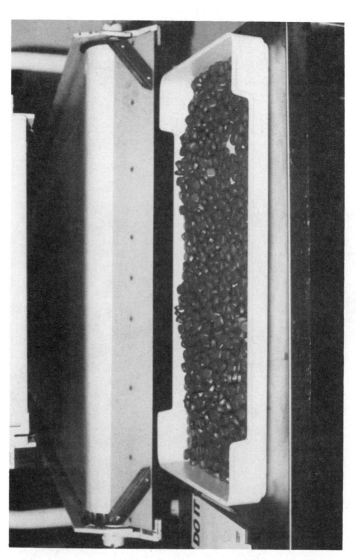

Figure 89   Cooled tablets are collected in trays.   The tablets should not be stored more than one deep to prevent sticking of flattening of the product. (Warner-Lambert Co.)

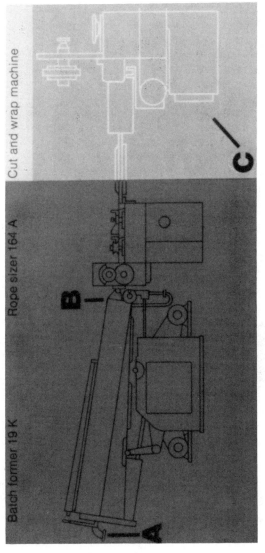

Figure 90 Cut and wrap machine. The candy mass is formed and rope sized in the same manner as Uniplast formed lozenges. Instead of tablet forming, the candy rope is passed through a cut and wrap machine that cuts the rope with a knife and wraps the product as a continuous operation. (Robert Bosch GmBH, Div. Hamac-Holler.)

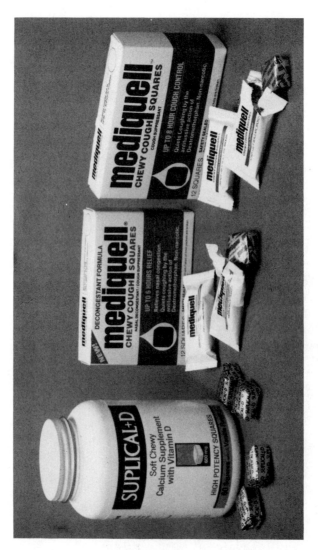

Figure 91 Chewy or caramel base medicated tablets can be bunch wrapped and packaged in glass or plastic bottles or foil wrapped and placed into fin-sealed pouches. (Warner-Lambert Co.)

VIII. FORMULATIONS (CHEWY-BASED CONFECTIONS)

The following formulations represent various methods of manufacturing medicated chewy-based confections.

Medicament—Egg Albumin—Cut-and-Wrap Process

Example 9: Decongestant Tablets (30.0 mg/4.0 g)

Ingredient	Quantities
Liquid sugar (67.5% w/w solids)	88.9 lb
Corn syrup 43°Baumé (80.5% w/w solids)	47.9 lb
Pseudoephedrine HCl 15% adsorbate	4280.0 g
Egg albumin	250.0 g
Gelatin USP	100.0 g
Water	450.0 g
Sorbitol solution	450.0 g
Hydrogenated vegetable oil 98°F MP	3000.0 g
FD&C Yellow No. 6	10.0 g
Glycerin USP	1500.0 g
Citric acid USP anhydrous	65.0 g
Imitation orange flavor	50.0 g
Fine-granulated sugar	1000.0 g

Liquid sugar and corn syrup are gear-metered into the dissolver and precooked to 125°C. Final cooking is performed at 143°C with a vacuum of 15 in. Hg. to produce 100 lb of candy base with a 60:40 sugar/corn syrup ratio.

The egg albumin and gelatin are dissolved in a mixture of water and sorbitol solution and heated with mixing to 65°C. Heat is removed and rapid mixing continued until an aerated mass is formed.

Candy base is transferred to a jacketed mixer that has been prewarmed to 125°C. Add egg albumin mixture and mix until temperature is 110°C. Add glycerin and dye mixture and mix until temperature falls to about 90°C. With mixing add pseudoephedrine adsorbate. Cool to 80°C and add hydrogenated vegetable oil. Mix until temperature falls to 70°C and add flavor, sugar, and citric acid. Mix for 5 min and remove from the mixer.

The mass is cooled for 4 hr, extruded into a 2-in. square rope, and passed through a cut-and wrap-machine to form 4.0-g square pieces.

Medicament—Milk Solids—Lozenge-Forming Equipment

Example 10:   Antitussive Tablets (15.0 mg/4.0 g)

Ingredient	Quantity
Liquid sugar (67.5% w/w solids)	96.30 lb
Corn syrup 43° Baumé (80.5% w/w solids)	43.57 lb
Nonfat dry milk solids high heat	400.00 g
Xanthan gum	200.00 g
Water	500.00 g
Dextromethorphan HBr 10%, adsorbate	2075.00 g
Sorbitol solution	350.00 g
Hydrogenated vegetable oil 98°F MP	2500.00 g
FD&C Red No 40	25.00 g
Glycerin USP	2000.00 g
Menthol USP	50.00 g
Wild cherry flavor	60.00 g
Fine-granulated sugar	1500.00 g
Citric acid USP anhydrous	75.00 g

Liquid sugar and corn syrup are gear-metered into the dissolver and precooked to 125°C. Final cooking is performed at 140°C with a vacuum of 12 in. Hg to produce 100 lb of candy base with a 65:35 sugar/corn syrup ratio.

The milk solids and xanthan gum are dissolved in a mixture of water and sorbitol solution and heated with mixing to 60°C. Heat is removed and rapid mixing continued until an aerated mass is formed.

Candy base is transferred to a jacketed mixer prewarmed to 125°C. Add milk solids and mix until temperature is 115°C. Add glycerin and dye mixture and mix until temperature falls to about 100°C. Add dextromethorphan 10% adsorbate. Cool to 85°C and add hydrogenated vegetable oil. Mix until temperature falls to 70°C and add flavor, sugar, and citric acid. Mix for 5 min and remove from the mixer.

The mass is cooled for 3 hr, extruded into a 2-in. round rope, and passed through an extruder to a series of sizing rollers, molded, and cooled. Formed pieces are individually bunch-wrapped before packaging.

IX. COMPRESSED-TABLET LOZENGES

This section, devoted to describing the preparation of compressed-tablet lozenges, includes many facets covered in other chapters of this text. The general guidelines to be set forth—for wet and dry granulations, milling, and drying, as well as for tablet compression—are analogous to those for regular compressed tablets. The major deviations occur in the specific types of raw materials most applicable to this type of dosage form, the non-routine lozenge disintegration requirements, tablet press and granulation considerations associated with preparing a tablet of the diameter and guage of a compressed lozenge—as well as certain specific organoleptic peculiarities unique to this specialized route of drug administration.

Whereas the typical tablet is designed for rapid disintegration and dissolution characteristics, compressed-tablet lozenges, with the desired area of activity on the mucous membrane of the mouth and pharynx, are usually large-diameter tablets (5/8 to 3/4 in.), compressed in a weight range of 1.5−4.0 g and formulated with a goal of slow, uniform, and smooth disintegration or erosion over an extended time period (5−10 min). The formulator performing product development should remain cognizant of any deviations from normally occurring medicament bioavailability profiles that may result from the addition of binders or excipients to the formulation.

As previously discussed, the emphasis in the case of the lozenge is on the slow, uniform release of medicament directly onto the affected mucous membrane. This increased dwell time in the oral cavity places an added burden on the formulator to develop flavor blends that will effectively mask unpleasant principals contributed by the medicaments, while at the same time maintaining a smooth lozenge surface texture as the tablet slowly disintegrates. This attribute enhances the patient acceptance and desire to hold the tablet in the mouth until it is completely dissolved. The tablet should erode (not disintegrate) while in the oral cavity, as the presence of particulate matter can be extremely disconcerting to the patient. For maximum drug efficacy, the product must not be chewed; thus a tablet with hardness approximating that of the boiled candy lozenge (30−50 kg in.2) should be compressed.

A. Rationale for Preparation of Compressed-Tablet Lozenges

Hard candy base is the most widely used vehicle for administration of medicaments that act by direct contact on mucous membrane of the oral cavity or are ingested by first dissolving the dose slowly in the mouth. Along with its sweet taste and pleasing appearance, the candy base imparts a demulcent effect of its own, increasing the efficacy of anesthetics or other materials added to relieve the discomfort of inflamed or abraded tissue. From an aesthetic aspect, adults and children find the hard candy base a pleasant and palatable vehicle for medicament administration, expecially when multiple dose or prolonged administration is indicated.

Four primary characteristics associated with preparation and storage of hard candy preclude the universal incorporation of medicaments in this type of vehicle. These factors include (a) the high temperature (135−150°C) necessary to drive off water and prepare hard candy. (b) The reactivity of candy base with medicaments—from the base itself as well as from flavors and acidulents that may be added to the formulation. (The intimate combination of ingredients may lead to drug instability problems since hard candy base, with its 0.5—1.5% moisture content and hygroscopic characteristics, more closely follows the kinetics of liquid rather than solid dose.) (c) The required therapeutic dose of medicament or combination of medicaments may be at a level sufficiently high as to preclude the incorporation of adequate material into either a single or two-lozenge dose. (The larger the number of doses the patient is required to take to achieve a therapeutic response, the greater the chance of noncompliance with a proper dosage schedule. Also, because of its physical nature, the drug may produce a lozenge with a rough surface texture when combined with candy base, thus reducing the organoleptic appeal of the product.) (d) Suitable candy base and lozenge-forming equipment may not be available, or the volume of sales does not warrant the capital expenditures required to set up a candy line. (A company that is already manufacturing tablets may feel that the production of a compressed lozenge is a more logical extension of its technology than entrance into the boiled candy lozenge area).

A suitable formulation alternative may be the compressed-tablet lozenge if one or more of the above situations apply, and the category of medicament and mode of drug administration require contact with the mucous membrane of the oral cavity, thus indicating a lozenge type of vehicle. This type of dosage form can fulfill all the parameters of the hard candy version, but can be manufactured in the conventional mode of pharmaceutically acceptable dosage forms.

The incorporation of medicaments into a compressed tablet lozenge may pose fewer problems than are associated with hard candy base. Whereas the type of medicament, quantity, reactivity, particle size, heat sensitivity, moisture sensitivity, and melting point are critical to the ultimate success of producing a hard candy lozenge with medicament, many of these same aspects are of minor concern when preparing the compressed tablet version. Much of the appeal that the medicated hard candy lozenge offers to the patient comes from the organoleptic presentation of the drug in a pleasing and somewhat demulcent vehicle. Incorporation of medicament into tablet base makes the drug no more or less efficacious. From a vehicle presentation aspect, with proper blending of ingredients a base with the same pleasing and demulcent characteristics can be formulated.

The compressed lozenge can be prepared by the historical wet granulation technique or by direct compression. For maximum efficacy and prolonged dwell time in the mouth, the tablet should be of sufficient size (1.5—4.0 g) and hardness (30—50 kg in.^{2}) to dissolve slowly and posses the organoleptic appeal of the hard candy version.

Raw Materials

Use of tablet compression techniques open up a myriad of raw materials that may be suitable for incorporation in this type of base. Previous discussions centered around the proper ratios of sugar and corn syrup that would produce a controlled crystallization rate and a resultant product with maximum clarity, smoothness, and resistance to graining or sticking. Addition of raw materials to compressed lozenges is determined by the effects of the raw materials on tablet compression, disintegration, erosion, mouthfeel, and powder or granulation flow characteristics.

The following materials are essential to the preparation of a pharmaceutically elegant product when formulating a compressed-tablet lozenge [31]:

1. Tablet base or vehicle
2. Binder
3. Flavor
4. Colors
5. Lubricants
6. Medicaments

A working knowledge of the principles of tablet base preparation and compression are essential if the formulator is to produce any compressed lozenge product. The art and science of tablet manufacture is complicated and beset with many pitfalls and potential problem areas, mainly in the selection of raw materials, granulation preparation, comminution, mixing, and compression. Chances of preparing an acceptable product—unless the formulator has had previous tableting experience—are as remote as the chances of the uninitiated successfully manufacturing the hard candy lozenge version.

Tablet Base or Vehicle

This is the basis of any tablet formulation. The materials chosen for incorporation in the tablet base will determine the overall method of tablet preparation (wet granulation or direct compression) [66] as well as the final physicochemical characteristics that may be associated with the product.

Sugar

Perhaps the simplest tablet formulation would involve the use of sugar as the base. Sugar, in this case, is pulverized by mechanical comminution to a fine powder (40–80 mesh), blended with medicament, granulated with either a sugar syrup or corn syrup binding solution in order to prepare medium- to large-size (2–8 mesh) granules, dried, milled to smaller and more uniform particle size (20–30 mesh), flavored, lubricated, and compressed into tablets of desired shape and size.

Sugar is inexpensive and lends itself to the formation of tablets with acceptable compression and mouth-feel characteristics. The resultant mouth-feel will be creamy in texture with an unabrasive and smooth surface if the final particle size of the sugar granulation is controlled at 20 mesh or finer.

Dextrose- and Sucrose-Modified Vehicles

The use of dextrose by itself, as well as dextrose- and sucrose-modified materials in combination with or in place of sucrose, can produce tablets as acceptable as those prepared with sucrose—in terms of compression characteristics, mouth-feel, and appearance, and in some cases at a cost lower than is possible with sucrose alone. Some examples of modified tablet vehicles now available are included here.

Dextrose is produced by a number of different manufacturers under a variety of trade names and is supplied as a white crystalline sugar (a pure monosaccharide) that is 100% fermentable and available in either a hydrated or anhydrous form [32]. Dextrose possesses a negative heat of dissolution, which imparts a more cooling mouth-feel characteristic to tablets than does sucrose.

Dextrose exhibits good flow and compression characteristics but is more suited to wet granulation procedures as opposed to direct compaction, expecially where high-weight tablets or tablets with a high percentage of active ingredient are involved. Dextrose tablets tend to exhibit browning at elevated temperatures (37°C and above) as well as in direct sunlight.

Emdex is a highly refined, total-sugar product composed of free-flowing crystallized maltose-dextrose porous spheres of 92% dextrose, 2—5% maltose, and a portion of higher glucose saccharides [33]. Emdex has good flow and compression characteristics, and while it does contain 8—10% moisture, it is not hygroscopic. Emdex is not as reactive as dextrose, but some evidence of reactivity with primary amino groups does exist.

Mor-Rex is a white, bland-tasting, low-density maltodextrin with lower hygroscopicity than corn syrup and a moisture content of about 5%. The composition of Mor-Rex includes 82% hexasaccharide, 4% disaccharide, and 1% monosaccharide. The total reducing sugar content is 10—13% [34].

Mor-Rex, while not suitable as a primary compression vehicle because of its bland taste and marginal flow properties, possesses good binding character, inertness, and resistance to moisture pickup, all of which make it an acceptable filler, expecially where hygroscopic, deliquiscent, or sticky materials must be added to the vehicle. Because of its binding qualitites, Mor-Rex cannot be used in large quantities in wet-granulated formulations, as the resultant tabet will either be too hard or possess a gummy consistency. Mor-Rex is a valuable ingredient for slowing disintegration time and for binding tablets that tend to exhibit unacceptable compression quality.

Royal-T Dextrose with Malto-dextrin is a specially compounded agglomerated dextrose containing maltodextrin [35]. This material is supplied as white agglomerated crystals with a moisture content of 8.5% and a dextrose equivalent of 96. Royal-T is suitable for both direct compression and wet granulation procedures. The resultant tablets have the organoleptic advantages associated with dextrose (cooling mouth-feel), but improved compression characteristics due to the presence of the maltodextrin.

Nu-Tab is a directly compressible tablet vehicle composed of processed sucrose, invert sugar (equimolecular mixture of levulose and dextrose), starch, and a small quantity of magnesium stearate. Nu-Tab can be supplied in a range of controlled particle sizes [36]. It possesses better flow, compression, and mouth-feel characteristics than sucrose alone. Nu-Tab is primarily used in direct-compression tableting and can accept up to 30% medicament and still produce tablets of acceptable quality. Nu-Tab is resistant to moisture pickup, thus making it an acceptable vehicle for moisture-sensitive medicaments. This vehicle is resistant to elevated temperature darkening.

Di-Pac represents a cocrystallization of 3% highly modified dextrins with sucrose to produce a tablet vehicle with improved flow, compression, and a mouth-feel similar to that of sucrose. Di-Pac contains less than 1% moisture, less than 1% reducing sugar, and is resistant to moisture pickup [37]. This vehicle is intended for directly compressible tablets where low to medium concentrations of active ingredients (less than 20%) are to be incorporated. Di-Pac is resistant to discoloration and its low moisture content makes it ideal for reactive or moisture-sensitive medicaments.

Sugartab is a white, free-flowing agglomerated sugar product recommended for direct compression of tablets. Sugartab contains approximately 90—93% sucrose, with the balance being invert sugar. The moisture content is less than 1% [38]. Sugartab is composed almost entirely of coarse particles—offering a typical distribution of 30% retained on 20-mesh screen and 3% passing through an 80-mesh screen. The coarse mesh size makes it a good carrier for certain materials that may have inherent compression problems of a type that may be alleviated by combining with a controlled particle size excipient milled to the optimum size range for the formulation.

Care must be taken when evaluating this material to ascertain if medicament distribution or segregation problems will occur after milling of the large Sugartab particles to a finer mesh size. Browning has occurred upon storage at elevated temperature (37–45°C).

Sweetrex is a directly compressible tablet base containing a special blend of natural sugars possessing a sweetness factor greater than that of sucrose. Sweetrex contains dextrose, levulose (fructose), maltose, isomaltose, and other higher polysaccharides in a blend with a binding capacity of up to 50% active ingredients [39]. This material will pick up moisture to a certain extent, but its major drawback is a tendency toward darkening at elevated temperature (37–45°C) and upon exposure to sunlight when combined with certain medicaments.

Mola-Tab is a directly compressible tablet vehicle containing 60% molases solids, 30% whole wheat flour, and 10% wheat bran. Mola-Tab contains about 4% moisture. This material is a deep-brown-colored, free-flowing granule with good compressibility. Tablet products containing this material have a good mouth-feel and a noticeable molasses flavor which helps mask some of the medicament bitterness. Because of the high quantity of reducing sugar and 4% moisture, a noticeable increase in product darkening is noted at elevated temperature storage conditions. Tablets compressed with this material exhibit slow erosion and a smooth surface texture. Tablets will pick up moisture but are not hygroscopic. Mola-Tab is a source of natural molasses and dietary fiber [86–87].

Hony-Tab is a directly compressible tablet vehicle containing 60% honey solids, 30% whole wheat flour, and 10% wheat bran. Hony-Tab contains about 4% moisture. This material is a straw-colored, free-flowing granule with good compressibility. Compressed tablets containing this material have a good mouth-feel with a noticeable sweetness and honey flavor which helps mask medicament bitterness. Because of the high quantity of reducing sugar and 4% moisture, a noticeable increase in product darkening is noted at elevated temperature storage conditions. Tablets compressed with this material exhibit slow erosion and a smooth surface texture. Tablets will pick up moisture but are not hygroscopic. Hony-Tab is a source of natural honey and dietary fiber [86,88].

Sugar-Free Vehicles

Manufacture of a sugar-free compressed tablet lozenge is more readily achievable than the counterpart hard candy lozenge. Sugar-free candy lozenges of sorbitol or sorbitol-mannitol combinations cannot be prepared on high-speed lozenge-manufacturing equipment due to the length of time it takes for crystallization to occur (0.5–14 hr). The long crystallization time relegates the preparation of sugar-free lozenges to that of a molding operation; thus manufacturing plants geared for conventional lozenge production cannot be readily adapted to the molding procedures unless a change of equipment is instituted. This is one reason medicated sugar-free lozenges have not gained wide acceptance in products containing medicaments.

Conversely, compressed sugar-free lozenges do not require any special handling, manufacturing procedures, or equipment, thus lending themselves to this type of manufacturing process. The most commonly used sugar-free tablet base vehicles include the three described below:

Mannitol is a naturally occurring sugar alcohol, an isomer of sorbitol but with a different chemical configuration and a different set of physical properties [40]. Mannitol is available as a fine powder, primarily for use in wet granulations, and in granular form for use in direct-compression tablets where the need for improved flow and compression characteristics exists. Mannitol contains less than 0.3% moisture and is nonhygroscopic. Its flow and compression characteristics are good, as are its chemical inertness and resistance to discoloration. Mannitol is only 50% as sweet as sugar, but its negative heat of solution enables it to impart a pleasant, cooling sensation in the mouth as the lozenge dissolves. Mannitol is noncariogenic.

Sorbitol is a chemical isomer of mannitol that is 50% as sweet as sugar, noncariogenic, nonreactive with most medicaments, but extremely hygroscopic [41]. Its flow, compression, and mouth-feel characteristics are similar to those of mannitol, and its negative heat of solution helps it impart a pleasant, sweet, cooling sensation in the mouth. Sorbitol is better able to carry high quantities of active ingredients than most excipients, especially in a wet-granulated tablet base, since formulations containing greater than 20% sorbitol tend to be tacky and adhesive with good compression characteristics; but its hygroscopic nature makes it undersirable where extended shelf life is required or when moisture-sensitive medicaments are incorporated in the granulation. Moisture-resistant packaging is essential with sorbitol-containing compressed lozenges. Sorbitol is available as a crystalline powder or as free-flowing granules [65]. Tablets prepared with sorbitol are less resistant to discoloration because of the presence of higher quantities of moisture picked up from the atmosphere during storage in containers that are resistant to moisture [68]. The incidence of formulation discoloration is minimal when sorbitol formulations are protected from moisture.

Polyethylene Glycol 6000 and 8000 are polymers of ethylene oxide with the generalized formula $HOCH_2(CH_2OCH_2)_nCH_2OH$, with n representing the average number of oxyethylene groups. Polyethylene glycols (PEGs) are designated by a number roughly representing their average molecular weight. Most polyethylene glycols in the molecular range of 1000–8000 are white, waxy solids, soluble in water and in many organic solvents, and resistant to hydrolysis [42]. PEG 6000 has a melting range of 53–56°C, while PEG 8000 has a melting range of 60–63°C. PEGs 6000 and 8000 are best suited for use in tablet formulations since lower molecular weight polyethylene glycols, with their reduced melting points (less than 50°C), increase the incidence of tablet binding and picking during compression. The punch faces, die walls, and table become heated during the manufacture of tablets because of friction. This increase in temperature is sufficient to soften a granulation and increase its tackiness, expecially if low-melting-point materials are present in the formulation. The higher the percentage of low-melting-point materials in the product, the greater the propensity for sticking and picking. Conversely, higher molecular weight polyethylene glycols exhibit no advantage over PEG 6000 or 8000 in improving compression characteristics of the granulations to which they are added, or in reducing picking or sticking. Addition of the high molecular weight material (PEG 20,000) may produce brittle tablets or tablets with unpleasant mouth-feel characteristics.

Polyethylene glycols are not intended to be incorporated in tablet granulations as the primary excipient or vehicle but are added in quantities ranging from 5 to 35% of the final tablet weight. The major benefits derived from addition of PEG to tablet granulations include prolonging disintegration time and improving the tablet surface texture in instances where the addition of certain medicaments to the formulation might result in a tablet with a rough or pitted surface. The inclusion of varying percentages of PEG 6000 or 8000 to a formulation aids in increasing the attainable hardness of many directly compressible tablet vehicles as well as improving the compres- pressibility of some marginally acceptable granulations. Also, the PEG 6000 or 8000 does not have any discernible flavor or mouth-feel character- istics of its own. Polyethylene glycol, being inert, is compatible with most medicaments that may be incorporated in the tablet formulation. This ma- terial can be added to a powder mixture before wet-granulating, added with flavors and lubricants after the granulation is dried, or added to a direct- compression vehicle prior to mixing.

The quantity of PEG added to direct-compression tablet bases is deter- mined by the physical characteristics of each individual vehicle. Some formulations possess a slow disintegration profile of their own and compress to a hardness sufficient to give the desired 5- to 10-min dwell time in the oral cavity. This desired, slow, in vivo disintegration is not possible with some bases because of the rapid disintegration characteristics of the tablet components. Addition of PEG (20—30%) will, in many instances, slow disin- tegration (erosion) to the desired time interval [43]. Incorporation of PEG in tablets containing medicament in the 30+ percentage range may improve particle cohesive forces, compression characteristics, and tablet hardness values in those instances where addition of the medicament results in a poor or marginally acceptable product.

Addition of polyethylene glycol to a wet-granulated tablet base will also aid binding and improve the organoleptic quality of the product, but its use in this type of granulation is mostly relegated to the latter function, as tablet disintegration can be controlled by the incorporation of different binders or binder concentrations. The resulting tablet will have a soft, wet, and spongy consistency, difficult to compress, susceptible to picking and binding, as well as possessing an exceptionally long (20—30 min) in vivo disintegration time if the quantity of PEG added to a wet-granulated vehicle is excessive. Polyethylene glycol is best added externally with flavor and lubricants when incorporated in a wet granulation tablet base.

Other Fillers

Other fillers suitable for inclusion into compressed lozenge tablet base in- clude *dicalcium phosphate (Emcompress* [89]), *calcium sulfate (powder* or *Compactrol* [90]), *calcium carbonate*, and *lactose* [44]. These materials, when added in varying percentages, aid in the densification of the granu- lation to improve flow and die fill characteristics. Dicalcium phosphate, Compactrol, and lactose can be used in either wet granulations or direct- compression vehicles, while powdered calcium sulfate and calcium carbonate are most suitable for wet-granulated tablet bases.

Microcrystalline cellulose (Avicel) is another filler suitable for incorpo- ration into both wet and direct-compression granulations, as an aid in im- proving marginal compression characteristics of a formulation. Avicel is available in a variety of particle sizes as well as in anhydrous form, and is suitable for moisture-sensitive medicaments or for materials that are sticky or hygroscopic [45]. Some disadvantages of microcrystalline cellulose

re tablet base include (a) diminution of granulation flow character-
.en this material is incorporated in concentrations above 20%; (b)
in lozenge disintegration time due to the exceptional disintegration
s of Avicel; (c) production of a particulate disintegration instead
th erosion of the lozenge; (d) reduction in organoleptic appeal
due to the starchy, fibrous, and drying mouth-feel imparted to the lozenge
as it dissolves in the oral cavity. Avicel added in concentrations of less
than 20% can improve the compression of marginally compressible tablet
granulations without imparting many of the above-mentioned negative characteristics to the product. A summary of tablet vehicle components is presented in Table 7.

Binders

The function of a binder in a wet-granulated tablet base is to hold together
as discrete granules the particulate matter that forms as a result of the
granulating procedure. The binder is also the major contributor to final
tablet hardness, since the type and concentration of binder present will
enhance the *intragranular* forces in each individual granule as well as the
intergranular forces, which are the bonding forces between granules [31].
    When preparing a tablet granulation, if the intragranular force is great-
er than the intergranular force, the tablet will break, leaving an irregular
and rough surface on the fracture line; but if the intergranular force or
forces are greater, the fracture will be smooth. When compressing quantities of active ingredients into direct-compression vehicles, the intergranular
forces must be maintained at a level sufficient to produce tablets with acceptable hardness and compression characteristics of their own. As these
materials are added to a direct-compression tablet base, the level and efficiency of the intergranular forces of the tablet base are reduced, resulting in a lessening of tablet hardness, compression, and, in some instances, flow characteristics. At a certain critical concentration (different
for each medicament in each individual tablet vehicle), the compression
quality or attainable hardness values fall out of the acceptable range. Additional binder is required when this situation occurs, to form particles
possessing sufficient intergranular force to produce a tablet within the required hardness and compression parameters.
    Remedial actions required to improve direct-compression granulations
may include (a) the addition of more tablet base to lower medicament concentration; (b) the incorporation of adjunct materials designed to improve
the compression quality (e.g., PEG 6000 or 8000). A major disadvantage
of adding more tablet vehicle is an increase in final tablet size and weight.
The alternative, if neither of the above approaches proves acceptable, may
be conversion to the preparation of a wet-granulated tablet base.
    Since the compressed-tablet lozenge weight is in the range of 1.5–4.0 g,
medicament concentration usually will not exceed 20%, a level that is suitable for compression into most directly compressible granulations. Use of
wet granulation is reserved for improvement of organoleptic quality of the
tablet, prolonging disintegration time, or the preference of the formulator
for the wet granulation method of tablet base preparation.
    Binders that are most effective in the wet granulation of compressed-
tablet lozenges include acacia, corn syrup, sugar syrup, gelatin, polyvinylpyrrolidone, tragacanth, and methylcellulose. These ingredients are effective in increasing the intergranular forces while at the same time helping
to improve the demulcent and surface texture characteristics of the lozenge
when it is dissolving in the oral cavity.

The effects of binders on the resultant tablets can only be determined by a series of compression trials. The preparation of tablets with optimum compression and organoleptic characteristics is greatly influenced by the selection of the proper binder at an optimum concentration. Therefore, the formulator is required to screen a number of different granulations and binder combinations at various levels to determine which binder is best for any particular medicament or medicament combination. Other factors, such as particle size and distribution, moisture content, and granulation milling conditions, must be evaluated as they are also an integral part in optimizing final tablet compression and mouth-feel qualities.

Flavors

The selection of flavors is a vital aspect in the development of compressed-tablet lozenges. When formulating chewable tablets, as opposed to lozenges, the formulator must consider the critical aspect of mouth-feel after a tablet has been chewed. In contrast, the long dwell time of lozenges in the oral cavity requires that the formulator develop not only a pleasantly flavored product, but also a product whose flavor masks bitter principles that may be present in the formulation. The chemistry of the flavors incorporated in medicated lozenge tablet base must be evaluated by the formulator to minimize the possibility that interactions will occur between flavor components and the medicaments present in the lozenge.

Unlike the problems encountered in the hard candy lozenge base, where surface grittiness and possible nonuniform distribution result if flavors are not added in the liquid state, flavors are best added to compressed-tablet lozenges almost exclusively in spray-dried or liquid forms adsorbed onto a suitable diluent (Cab-O-Sil or Microcel). Spray-dried flavors cause fewer problems than liquid flavors because addition of liquid flavors to a wet granulation along with the granulating solution results in potentially high and nonuniform flavor losses occurring during the drying operation. If liquid flavors are added subsequent to the comminution of a granulation, or if they are added to a direct-compression granulation, the result is the formation of sticky and wet powders with a tendency to nonuniform distribution of flavor through the product. A secondary result of the addition of liquid flavors to the completed tablet granulation is a reduction in the cohesive characteristics of the granules because of the presence of the oily flavor adsorbed onto the surface of the granules. The net result is a lessening of tablet hardness and a reduction in compression quality characteristics.

The probability of medicament—flavor interactions is lessened with the addition of spray-dried flavors to the medicated granulation. This allows for the use of a greater variety of flavors than can be incorporated into the hard candy lozenge version.

Colors

Water-soluble and Lakolene dyes* can be used to color compressed tablet lozenges. Water-soluble dyes can be added to the powder mixture during

---

*An FD&C Lakolene dye is any *lake* made by extending on a substrate of alumina, a salt prepared from a certified FD&C water-soluble straight color by combining such a certified color with the basic aluminum or calcium ions.

Table 7   *Physical Characteristics of Components Utilized as Base Filler*

Material	Composition	Form	Tablet base	Accepts >20% medicament into base	Granulation flow characteristics
Sucrose	Derived from sugar cane or beet root	Coarse crystals to fine powder	Wet granulated	Excellent	Very good
Dextrose	Complete hydrolysis of cornstarch	Coarse crystals to fine powder	Wet granulated	Excellent	Good
Emdex	92% Dextrose 2—5% Maltose	Crystals	Direct compression	Fair	Decrease with tablet weight >3.5 g
Mor-Rex	82% Hexasaccharide 4% Disaccharide 1% Monosaccharide	Fine powder	Direct compression; Wet granulation (not a primary component)	—	—
Royal-T dextrose	Agglomerated dextrose with maltodextrin	Fine crystals	Direct compression	Very good	Good
Di-Pac	97% Sucrose 3% Modified dextrins	Fine to coarse crystals	Direct compression	Fair	Decrease with tablet weight > 3.5 g
Sugartab	90—97% Sucrose Invert sugar	Coarse particles	Direct compression	Very good	Very good
Sweetrex	Dextrose Levulose Maltose	Fine crystals	Direct compression	Fair	Good
Mannitol	Sugar alcohol	Fine powder to coarse granules	Direct compression; wet granulation	Fair; very good	Fair; very good
Sorbitol	Chemical isomer of mannitol	Fine crystals	Direct compression; wet granulation	Very good; excellent	Good
Polyethylene glycols	Polymer of ethylene oxides	Coarse crystals to fine powder	Direct compression; wet granulation (not a primary component)	—	—

Disintegration characteristics	Mouth-feel	Surface texture	Compression quality	Stability under moist conditions	Resistance to discoloration
Controlled with selected binders	Good; fine particle size produces creamy feel	Smooth	Excellent	Fair	Good
Rapid, but can be controlled with binders/other fillers	Very good; cooling mouth-feel	Smooth	Very good	Fair	Poor
Rapid but can be controlled with binders/other fillers	Very good; slight cooling mouth-feel	Good	Good	Excellent	Fair
Slows disintegration of rapidly soluble medicaments and exipients	–	–	–	Excellent	Good
Maltodextrin content slows disintegration	Very good; slight cooling mouth-feel	Smooth	Very good	Fair	Poor
Hard tablets slow disintegration	Good	Smooth	Very good	Excellent	Good
Hard tablets with slow disintegration	Good	Good	Very good	Fair	Fair
Rapid, but can be controlled with binders/other fillers	Very good; slight cooling mouth-feel	Good	Very good	Fair	Poor
Rapid, but can be controlled with binders/other fillers	Very good; slight cooling mouth-feel	Smooth	Very good	Excellent	Good
Hard tablets slow disintegration	Very good; cooling mouth-feel	Smooth	Excellent	Poor	Good
Slows disintegration of rapidly soluble medicaments and excipients	–	–	–	Very good	Good

Table 7   (Continued)

Material	Composition	Form	Tablet base	Accepts >20% medicament into base	Granulation flow characteristics
Dicalcium phosphate	Produced by various chemical means	Fine powder to coarse granules	Direct compression; wet granulation	Good; good	Improves granulation flow qualities
Calcium sulfate	Natural form	Fine powder to coarse granules	Wet granulation Direct compression	Fair	Improves granulation flow qualities
Calcium carbonate	Various chemical means	Fine powder	Wet granulation	Fair	improves granulation flow qualities
Lactose	Milk sugar	Fine powder to coarse granules	Direct compression; wet granulation	Good; excellent	Improves granulation flow qualities
Avicel	Microcrystalline cellulose	Fine powder	Direct compression; wet granulation	Good; very good	Fair Very good
Mola-Tab	60% Molasses 30% Wheat flour 10% Wheat bran	Fine to coarse crystals	Direct compression	Very good	Very good
Hony-Tab	60% Honey 30% Wheat flour 10% Wheat bran	Fine to coarse crystals	Direct compression	Very good	Very good

Disintegration characteristics	Mouth-feel	Surface texture	Compression quality	Stability under moist conditions	Resistance to discoloration
Slows disintegration of rapidly soluble medicaments and excipients	Poor	Chalky	Good	Very good	Good
Slows disintegration of rapidly soluble medicaments and excipients	Poor	Chalky	Fair	Excellent	Good
Slows disintegration of rapidly soluble medicaments and excipients	Poor	Chalky	Fair	Excellent	Good
Hard tablets with slow disintegration	Good	Good	Very good	Fair	Fair
Rapid—difficult to control with binders/other fillers	Poor	Chalky	Very good	Very good	Good
Slow disintegration	Very good	Smooth	Very good	Fair	Fair
Slow disintegration	Very good	Smooth	Very good	Fair	Fair

the preparation of wet-granulated vehicles prior to granulation in combination with the excipients and medicaments, or they can be dissolved in the granulating solution and added with the binder. Either soluble or Lakolene dye may be used if color is added to the powder mixture prior to granulation, although the appearance of the final tablet (mottled rather than uniform color distribution) will determine which type of dye is best suited for a particular granulation. Replacement with a soluble dye is indicated should incorporation of a Lakolene dye cause the final tablet to appear mottled. If a situation occurs where a dye (soluble or Lakolene) is added internally (with excipients and medicaments) to the granulation before adding binder, and the resulting tablets have a mottled appearance after compression, addition of small quantities (0.01–0.05%) of Lakolene dye with the external portion of the granulation (lubricant, flavor, or glidant) may alleviate the problem.

Incorporation of Lakolene dyes is indicated in the manufacture of direct-compression granulations since no logical step exists in the process where water-soluble dyes can be added [31]. Before its addition to the powder mixture, the Lakolene dye is mixed with an equal portion of one of the granulation components to prevent dye particle agglomeration—a situation that occurs if the dye is added to the powder mixture as a single portion. Mixing with another powder separates dye particles and prevents agglomeration. The powder-dye mixture can be passed through a 60-, 80-, or 100-mesh screen to further distribute the dye.

A method that can be used to add water-soluble dyes to direct-compression granulations in situations where the use of Lakolene dyes is contraindicated (chemical incompatibility with the substrate) involves the preparation of a wet granulation of the soluble dye on cornstarch. The mixture is dried (moisture content less than 0.5%), milled, and incorporated in the direct-compression granulation in the same manner as the Lakolene dyes.

Lubricants

The function of a lubricant as a component of the tablet granulation is divided into three specific areas: (a) lubrication of the individual particles to aid in the release of the tablet from the die wall; (b) antiadhesive properties which facilitate the release of the tablet material from the faces of the lower and upper punches; (c) glidant properties to improve material flow from the powder hopper onto the machine table and into the dies [31].

While many ingredients employed as lubricants fulfill one, two, or (in a few instances) even three of the required functions of a tablet lubricant, some materials function specifically to alleviate problems only in certain areas. Addition of magnesium stearate, zinc stearate, calcium stearate, stearic acid, Sterotex (a mixture of selected triglycerides), PEG, or combinations of these materials will usually alleviate most of the granulation deficiencies associated with die face and sidewall sticking or release problems. When the situation of die wall sticking or incomplete release from punch faces does occur, and addition of excessive quantities of lubricant (concentrations greater than 5%) does not improve the condition, an examination of the granulation binder concentration, particle size distribution, or moisture content (levels greater than 2.5% increase granulation tackiness) should be initiated.

An addition of specialized materials (glidants) that will improve powder or granule flow properties is indicated when a level of lubricant is reached that imparts effective lubrication characteristics to the granulation but unacceptable flow or nonuniform die fill problems still remain. Ingredients such as fire-dried fumed silica (Cab-O-Sil) or talc when added at levels up to 0.25% should improve granulation flow and die fill efficacy. Densification of the granulation should be evaluated if glidant addition does not alleviate the situation. The formulator, when selecting the types of lubricants most suitable for inclusion in the formulation, should be aware of the specific lubrication problem involved and choose the materials best suited to remedy the situation. An addition of Cab-O-Sil or talc will not alleviate the problem if the lubrication difficulty is with sidewall adhesion, whereas a slight increase (or addition) of as little as 0.01% alkaline stearate (e.g., magnesium stearate) may improve the condition.

One aspect associated with ingredients added to relieve granulation lubrication difficulties is that more is not always better. Addition of lubricats above certain critical concentrations (different concentrations for each individual granulation) reduces cohesive forces among granules, thus lessening granulation compression characteristics and, in some instances, medicament bioavailability. Incorporation of glidant at levels above 0.5% may form a granulation with reduced bulk density and die fill properties. When lubricant concentrations need be added at levels that begin to adversely affect granulation efficacy, the formulator should examine the base granulation for the reasons why the base does not possess acceptable lubricant or flow characteristics.

Medicaments

The compressed-tablet lozenge granulation, because of its bulk and compression characteristics, will accept from 20 to 60% active ingredient as part of the vehicle. Incorporation of almost any desired dosage of medicament or combinations of medicaments into a single tablet does not pose the difficulties encountered with the hard candy lozenge version. For maximum benefits from the flavor and for best mouth-feel and organoleptic characteristics, no more than 25–30% of the final tablet weight (1.5–4.0 g) should be medicament (0.45–1.2 g). Higher quantities of drugs can be compressed into the base but may adversely affect lozenge flavor, aftertaste, and disintegration (erosion) characteristics.

Anesthetics such as benzocaine (5–10 mg), hexylresorcinol (2.4–4.0 mg); decongestants such as phenylpropanolamine HCl (15–25 mg), pseudoephedrine HCl (15–30 mg); antihistamines such as chlorpheniramine maleate (1–4 mg) and phenyltoloxamine citrate (18–22 mg); antitussives such as dextromethorphan HBr, 10% adsorbate (50–150 mg) and diphenhydramine HCl (10–25 mg); and analgesics such as aspirin and acetaminophen (130–325 mg) are well tolerated in compressed-lozenge base.

Many of the active ingredient incompatibilities, in terms of both medicament (e.g., aspirin-antihistamine, benzocaine-decongestant) and flavor or lozenge base components, are either reduced or eliminated by controlling lozenge base moisture content at low levels (less than 0.5%), by diluting reactants in a nonreactive vehicle, and, in extremely reactive situations, by manufacturing a two-layer tablet to effect maximum separation of reactive components. Other methods utilized by the formulator to minimize drug interactions—in order to present to the patient combinations of drugs with flavors that heretofore were not feasible in candy or lozenge base—include altering the method of granulation preparation (wet method instead of direct-compression base), use of spray-dried flavors, and proper dilution of medicaments.

X. MANUFACTURING: COMPRESSION SEQUENCE

Manufacture of a compressed-tablet lozenge follows all the basic guidelines
of tablet compression on a rotary tablet press [46]. When compressing a
granulation of any type, the formulator should become familiar with the
potential and actual problem areas and be able to take remedial action at
any point in the manufacturing sequence of the dosage form. The basic
steps of tablet compression include the following steps (Figure 92).

A. Die Filling

Die filling is the step in the compression operation where the granulation
leaves the storage hopper and is transferred by gravity or forced-flow feed
to the feed frame. At this point the granulation is made available to fill the
die cavity as it passes under the feed frame. Except for the final compression step, this is probably the most critical operation in the compression
cycle, since an incomplete or nonuniform die fill affects tablet hardness,
friability, weight, drug delivery, and uniformity.

Unlike the manufacture of a regular compressed tablet (0.2−0.75 g) or
chewable tablet (0.5−1.5 g), the required higher weight (1.5−4.0 g) of
the compressed-tablet lozenge requires more material to fill a die cavity

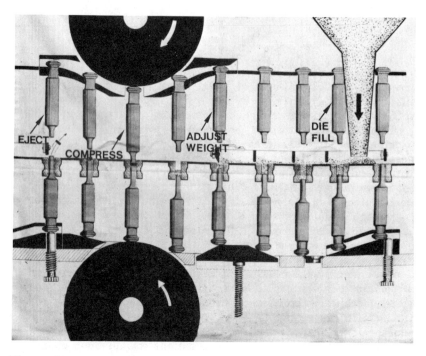

Figure 92   The basic steps of tablet compression. (Sharples-Stokes Div.,
Pennwalt Corp.)

that has the same dwell time under the granulation in the feed frame. The formulator should take appropriate measures to control particle size distribution and density in order to ensure that the granulation will possess a uniform and complete die cavity fill characteristic. Each individual formulation will require different adjustments to optimize the die fill conditions, some of which include the following: (a) Addition of lactose, dicalcium phosphate, calcium sulfate, or sucrose to a direct-compression granulation; addition of extra binder or use of a coarser milling cycle in the case of a wet granulation, to improve die fill quality in cases where the aforementioned problems of nonuniform tablet hardness, friability, or weight adjustments are die fill-related. (b) The bulk density of the various ingredients added to the granulation should be maintained as closely as possible, expecially when formulating direct-compression products. This prevents powder segregation during the blending operation or during the dwell time in the hopper or in the feed frame. Powder segregation results in nonuniform drug distribution, impairment of flow and die fill characteristics, as well as nonuniformity of tablet lubrication or medicament bioavailability. (c) The quantity of fine powder present in a granulation (fines are those granulation particles that pass through an 80-mesh sieve) should be controlled (less than 15%) to minimize segregation or sifting of excessive powder around the bottom punch and onto the barrel. This accumulation of powder may cause binding of the lower punch in the punch guide. The result is that the punch may not drop to its lowest depth to receive sufficient granulation for a complete die fill. The required weight of granulation will not enter the die and without a complete die fill the desired tablet weight cannot be attained. A granulation that exhibits acceptable flow, density, and die fill characteristics will lend itself to compression on high-speed tablet presses.

B. Weight Adjustment

The depth at which the lower punch is set to produce a specified volume of die cavity is the weight adjustment of the tablet press. The bottom punch is set at maximum depth as it passes under the granulation in the feed frame to allow for the greatest die fill. The lower punch, just before leaving the feed frame area, rides along an adjustable weight adjustment cam track. The height at which this cam is adjusted determines the volume of die cavity and the weight of granulation contained in the die cavity. Excess granulation that was contained in the die cavity before the weight adjustment is scraped off and remains in the feed frame.

The tablet machine weight adjustment is determined by the desired product weight, the quality of granulation flow, and the formulation density. A lower volume is needed to contain the desired weight of granulation if the granulation is dense or the flow is good. The parameters discussed under die fill pertain to weight adjustment, since the better the granulation flow and die fill, the lower the volume necessary to achieve a desired weight. Additionally, the lower the required volume of fill, the more uniform will be the die fill and the lower the tablet weight variation. This aspect is especially critical where large-diameter and high-weight tablets are compressed on a high-speed tablet press. The lower the volume of die cavity that must be filled, the lower the resultant variation in tablet weight.

C. Compression Hardness

The prerequisite for any tablet granulation, whether prepared by wet granulation or by the direct-compression method, is that the granulation should bond together under pressure [47]. The ideal granulation is one that will bond with a minimum of pressure applied for the shortest time. The greater the bonding forces of the particles, the closer to optimum is the hardness achieved. Tablet granulations possessing bonding forces that produce hard tablets with a minimum of pressure applied for a short period of time are most suitable for production on high-speed tablet presses (Figure 93–95) [48–51]. Low-compression forces reduce wear on tablet tooling and on the tablet press (Figure 96).

The phenomenon referred to as *capping* or *lamination* results when particles fail to bond under compression. Capping, a less severe condition than laminating, refers to the tablet when its top is cracked at the edge or is loose—as a cap. Laminating is associated with capping but refers to the tablets that are split or cracked on the sides by expansion when the pressure is released [52]. The three major reasons for the occurrence of capping or lamination are the following.

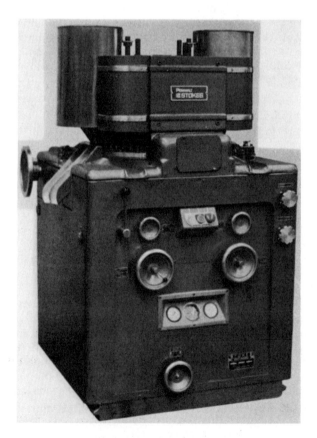

Figure 93   Stokes Model 551 rotary tableting press.   (Sharples-Stokes Div., Pennwalt Corp.)

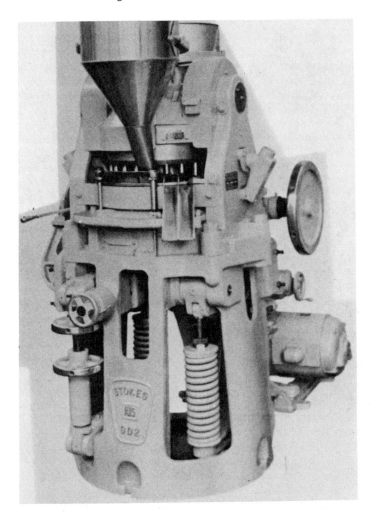

Figure 94   Stokes Model DD-2 double-sided rotary tableting press.
(Sharples-Stokes Div., Pennwalt Corp.)

Insufficient Binder, Moisture, or Cohesive Forces Among Granules

Binder

When preparing wet-granulated formulations, addition of insufficient
quantities of binder will result in production of granules lacking proper
intragranular or intergranular forces which, upon compression, produce
tablets with granules that do not bond in areas of high stress.

Moisture

Each indicidual tablet granulation possesses a certain critical moisture-
content range which aids in producing granules with optimum cohesive
forces. Most granulations perform well when the moisture content falls in
the 0.75—2.0% range, but the exact range (both upper and lower limits)

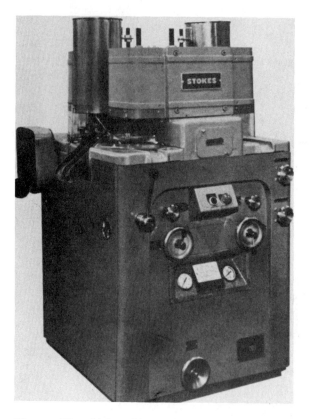

Figure 95   Stokes Model 328 rotary tableting press.   (Sharples-Stokes Div.,
Pennwalt Corp.)

should be determined and included as part of the manufacturing specifications.   Moisture content below the critical range cause particles to rapidly
lose cohesiveness and the tablets to lose their sheen.   However, moisture
content above the critical range cause granulations to become sticky and
tablets to harden with age.   The incidence of medicament reactivity with
flavors or tablet base ingredients is increased with the addition of excessive moisture to medicated granulations.

Cohesive Forces

The addition of quantities of medicaments or fillers possessing minimal
cohesive forces of their own into direct-compression granulations can reduce
overall granulation cohesive forces to the extent that the tablet compression
quality is no longer acceptable.   Milling a granulation in such a manner as
to produce an excessive quantity of fine or coarse particles can affect the
compression quality of a granulation to the extent that capping or lamination
results.

Excessive Pressure During Compression

Application of forces during compression of the granulation in excess of
the optimum particle bonding pressure results in destruction of the

intergranular bond. This pressure effect, as a cause of capping and lamination, can be determined by reducing the pressure of compression in gradual increments until an acceptable tablet is formed or until one that is too soft is compressed. Should a soft tablet result before capping is alleviated, the formulator can eliminate this as a cause of unacceptable tablet compression characteristics.

Since compression of lozenges requires high-compression forces to produce a product with extended disintegration time, the granulation must either be able to withstand the high forces of compression (30−50 kg in.^{2}) or possess sufficient particle bonding forces to produce a hard tablet with only a moderate degree of compression pressure.

Air Entrapment

Air entrapment is a common source of capping problems with high-weight tablets. Should the nature of the granulation (flocculent or containing many coarse particles) result in entrapment among granules of excessive air which is unable to escape during compression, the air will collect in layers and cause separation. This cause of tablet lamination is usually remedied by *densifying* the granulation—which is accomplished by the addition of more binder in a wet-granulated product or the incorporation of diluents such as lactose, calcium carbonate, or dicalcium phosphate (where applicable) in a direct-compression tablet.

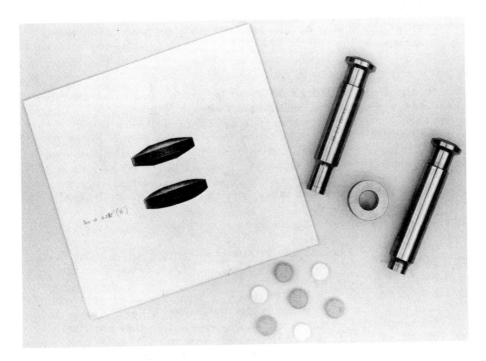

Figure 96 Compressed tablet lozenges. Left: schematic of lozenge punch shape; right: lozenge punches and dies; center: compressed tablet lozenges.

D. Tablet Ejection

The pressure goes outward toward the die wall while the granulation is under compression, making it necessary to use a lubricant to reduce the friction between the tablet and the die wall to permit effective release of the tablet from the upper and lower punch faces and the die walls. The tablet must then be forcibly removed from the die cavity upon completion of the compression operation.

   Many of the problems associated with tablet ejection are lubricant-related and fall into two major categories: (a) lubricant failure because of incorporation of insufficient or improper type of lubricant, and (b) sticking.

Lubricant Failure

The tablet ejection difficulties resulting from lubricant failure are usually indicated by the presence of irregular lines on the side band of the tablet. Continued compression under conditions of lubricant failure results in a squeaking or popping sound during tablet ejection, as the die becomes heated by the friction caused by pressure against the die sidewalls. Side-wall pressure will increase if compression is continued and results in a condition where the tablet will not be completely ejected from the die wall at the point of tablet scrape-off. This results in broken tablets and, in extreme conditions, a scoring of the die sidewalls, or even a release of the die from the die lock (a condition that will result in damage to the tablet press or feed frames). Conversely, the presence of regular lines on successive tablets from the same punch and die set may indicate a worn die. The incomplete release of a tablet from a single punch (especially associated with ellipsoidal punches) may indicate a worn or bent lower punch.

Sticking

Sticking results from the failure of the antiadhesive function of the lubricant and usually results from an improperly dried or lubricated granulation. This phenomenon refers to the punch faces and occurs when tablets do not leave the punch faces clean. The tablet faces become dull or pitted (perhaps both) during compression, and the condition progressively worsens to the point where the tablets chip and break and are hard to remove form the lower punch or pull apart from the upper. The moisture analysis of the granulation should be reevaluated, and the alkaline stearate content should be increased (0.05–0.1%).

   Two additional forms of sticking are:

   1. *Filming*, a form of sticking that is slow forming and caused mostly by the loss of the highly polished finish of the punch faces—from moisture associated with high humidity (greater than 50%) in the compression area. Punch faces become coated by a film that can become so thick that tablets from concave and bevel-edge punches may eventually fill and appear flat. Control of atmospheric moisture content should alleviate this condition.

   2. *Picking*, a form of sticking to punch faces when specks appear to be lifted or "picked up" from the tablet faces. This condition is usually caused by moist granules in the granulation or increased tackiness because of the presence of excessive binder. Picking also may be caused by the

incorporation of excessive quantities of lubricant or tablet components with low melting points. The punches become heated during extended compression runs, causing the low-melting-point components to soften and adhere to punch faces. A modification of the lubricating system or a slight (0.01– 0.1%) increase in lubricant concentration may eliminate this situation.

XI. TYPICAL FORMULATIONS (COMPRESSED-TABLET LOZENGES)

The following formulations represent various methods of manufacturing compressed-tablet lozenges.

A. Wet Granulation Techniques

Example 11:   Antitussive-Anesthetic Lozenges (2.5-g Tablet)

Ingredient	Quantity
Dextromethorphan HBr 10% adsorbate	4.0%
Benzocaine	2.0%
Filler	
Confectioners sugar 6x (3% corn starch)	58.0%
Polyethylene glycol 8000 (powdered)	15.0%
Cornstarch USP	12.0%
Binder	
Gelatin USP	3.0%
Flavor	
Spray-dried powder	As desired
Color	
Lakolene color	As desired
Lubricant	
Magnesium stearate USP	0.5%
Polyethylene glycol 8000 powdered	1.0%

A 15–20% gelatin granulating solution is prepared and cooled to 25°C. Medicaments and fillers are blended. Any lumpy materials are milled in order to prepare powders with a uniform particle size. The medicament-filler mixture is granulated with the binder solution and mixed until uniform granules are formed. The granulation is oven-dried to a moisture content of 1.0–1.5%. The lubricant, color, and flavor are mixed into the dried granulation, which is then mechanically

Example 11:   (Continued)

comminuted to a mesh size of 40—80. The granulation is blended to uniformly mix all components. Tablets of 2.5 g each are compressed on a suitable rotary press.

B. Direct-Compression Techniques (Analgesic-Antihistamine Lozenge 3.0 g)

Example 12:   First Layer (1.0 g) of Two-Layer Analgesic-Antihistamine Lozenge (3.0 g)

Ingredient	Quantity
Medicament	
Aspirin (100-mesh crystals)	16.25%
Filler	
Polyethylene glycol 8000 powdered	16.25%
Microcrystalline cellulose	15.00%
Mannitol (granular)	50.00%
Flavor	
Spray-dried powder	As desired
Color	
Lakolene color	As desired
Lubricant	
Polyethylene glycol 8000 (powdered)	1.50%
Stearic acid powder	0.50%

Example 13:   Second Layer (2.0 g) of Two-Layer Analgesic-Antihistamine Lozenge (3.0 g)

Ingredient	Quantity
Medicament	
Chlorpheniramine maleate	0.25%
Phenylpropanolamine HCl	0.93%

Example 13:   (Continued)

Ingredient	Quantity
Filler	
Confectioners sugar 6x (3% cornstarch)	15.0%
Polyethylene glycol 8000 (powdered)	20.0%
Mannitol (granular)	45.0%
Microcrystalline cellulose	10.0%
Flavor	
Spray-dried powder	As desired
Color	
Lakolene color	As desired
Lubricant	
Magnesium stearate USP	0.5%
Polyethylene glycol 8000 (powdered)	3.0%
Stearic acid (powdered)	0.25%
Cab-O-Sil M-5	0.1%

The medicament, filler, flavor, color, and lubricant are mixed
and milled to a uniform mesh size. The powder mixture is
blended and compressed on a two-layer tablet press.

XII.   QUALITY CONTROL PROCEDURES

Since the basis of the lozenge dosage form is sugar and corn syrup, quality
control testing begins with the analysis of candy base raw materials and
continues through to the final packaging operation [53,64].

A.   General Checks: Candy Base Manufacturing

As the manufacture of the candy base is initiated, a final check of the
corn syrup and sugar delivery gears, as well as any third ingredient delivery systems, is made to assure the proper ratios of candy base ingredients
are delivered to the precooker. Continual checks are also made on the
temperature, steam presure, and cooking speed of the precooker as well
as the steam pressure, temperature, vacuum, and cooking speed of the
candy base cooker. The cooker speed is adjusted according to the speed
of the lozenge-forming machine.

Moisture Analysis

Determination of candy base moisture content, regardless of the method
used, is a critical procedure in quality control testing to verify that the

metering devices and vacuum settings on the candy cookers are performing correctly. Production of candy base with moisture content exceeding 1.0–1.5% increases candy lozenge-manufacturing difficulties, incidence and rate of graining, as well as medicament—flavor and medicament—candy base interactions, all of which tend to shorten product shelf life. For optimum shelf life, moisture content should range from 0.75 to 1.25% with 1.0% generally the normal manufacturing parameter. A number of different testing procedures are available to determine the percentage of moisture in candy base [54]. Chewy or caramel candy bar-moisture content should range between 3.0–5.0%.

Gravimetric Method (Vacuum Oven)

The sample (usually about 1.0 g) is weighed accurately into a tared weighing container and placed in a vacuum oven at 60–70°C for 12–16 hr. The sample is removed from the oven, weighed, and the difference in moisture calculated.

Titrimetric Method

The titrimetric determination of water depends on the fact that a solution of sulfur dioxide and iodine in pyridine and alcohol (Karl Fischer reagent) reacts with water stoichiometrically. The entire operation requires the rigid exclusion of atmospheric moisture. This method permits the determination of candy base moisture content in a very short period of time (less than 5 min). With this procedure, a sample calculated to contain 10–250 mg of water is added to the titration flask and titrated with Karl Fischer reagent. The end point can be determined visually in colorless solutions; in colored solutions an electronic method is used.

Azeotropic Distillation Method (Toluene or Xylene)

A measured quantity of pulverized candy (10–12 g) is placed into a 500-ml glass flask. Between 150 and 200 ml of toluene is added to the flask, which is connected to a trap with connecting tube and a reflux condenser fitted with a granuated 5-ml-capacity receiving tube. The flask is heated for 1–2 hr, refluxing until all water has come over to the receiving tube—where the percentage that was present in the candy can be calculated from the volume of water present in the receiving tube (Figure 97). During the distillation procedure, care must be taken not to allow the solvent and the residue candy to become discolored (brown or even yellow) because this is certain indication that caramelizing has occurred. Caramelizing of sugar, with the loss of water from the sugar, would give a high reading.

Determination of Sugar and Corn Syrup Ratios

In order to ascertain if pump settings are correct for delivering the desired ratios of sugar and corn syrup to the formulation, or if the candy cooking and delivery systems are functioning properly, a determination of the percentage of sugar, corn syrup, and other ingredients is carried out on a routine basis.

Dextrose Equivalent Method: Lane Eynon Titration Method

The use of dextrose equivalent methods of analysis before and after inversion will determine the percentage of sugar and corn syrup as well as the percentage of inversion due to cooking or due to the types of materials

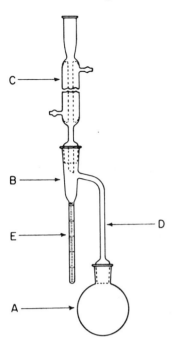

Figure 97 Toluene moisture apparatus. A = 500-ml glass flask; B = trap; C = reflux condenser; D = connecting tube; E = receiving tube of 5-ml capacity. (U.S. Pharmacopeia XXI.)

used in the manufacture of hard candy. One dextrose equivalent is derived from the candy while another portion of candy is inverted so that all sugars will read as dextrose equivalents. The difference will be the noninverted sugars or regular sugar. A correction factor is also used. The first dextrose equivalent will be the portion of sugar inverted by cooking along with the dextrose equivalent from the corn syrup [4].

Calculation of the candy base, corn syrup dextrose equivalent, on a dry basis before cooking, the cooked candy base moisture content, and the dextrose equivalent before and after inversion will determine the percent invert formed during cooking as well as the composition of the original candy-base. A *cook invert* (inversion during cooking) above 2.5% will increase candy base moisture pickup tendencies, whereas a cook invert below 2.0% will increase sugar crystallization.

Percentage Reducing Sugars

Standard

A 3-g portion of anhydrous dextrose is dissolved in 500 ml water. A 25-ml volume of alkaline cupric tartrate solution (Fehling's solution) is titrated with the dextrose solution to within 1−2 ml of the expected end point. The solution is boiled for 2 min and then two drops of methylene blue indicator is added and titrated to a yellowish red end point. Controlling boiling and titrating times is important for reproducible results.

The calculation is as follows:

$$\frac{(3.0 \text{ g}) \times [\text{volume of standard dextrose solution consumed by Fehling's solution}]}{500} = \begin{bmatrix} \text{Reducing sugar} \\ \text{factor (F) for} \\ 3.0 \text{ g dextrose} \end{bmatrix}$$

Sample

A 10-g sample of candy base is dissolved in 250 ml water. A 25-ml volume of alkaline curpic tartrate solution (Fehling's Solution) is titrated in the same manner as the standard. The calculation is as follows:

$$\frac{\text{Reducing sugar factor} \times 100}{\frac{\text{Sample weight}}{250} \times \begin{bmatrix} \text{Volume of sample} \\ \text{solution consumed by} \\ \text{Fehling's solution} \end{bmatrix}} = [\text{Percent reducing sugars}]$$

Reducing sugar analysis should be carried out on a routine basis as a check for proper cooking times, temperatures, integrity of components, and corn syrup content, and to check whether salvage solutions have been adusted to the proper pH.

Salvage Solutions

Salvage solutions manufactured with and without medicaments must undergo a series of quality control procedures before incorporation in the candy base cooking cycle. Immediately upon dissolution of the lozenge salvage, the solution pH is adjusted within the range of 4.5–7.5 by addition of either citric acid or sodium carbonate monohydrate to prevent excessive sugar inversion when the solution is cooked with the other candy base components. When the salvage solution has been adjusted into the desired pH range, the solids content is determined. The optimum solids content for salvage solutions is in the 65–74% range, with 70 ± 2% the most suitable concentration. Salvage solutions that exceed the upper limit of the solids content range become progressively thicker and more difficult to pump. This will result in nonuniform delivery of product to the cooker. Solutions that are prepared below the desired lower limit of solids content contain quantities of water that will lengthen cooking times, thus resulting in the formation of higher invert sugar levels and increased yellowing of the candy.

Solids content of salvage solution is determiend by using a refractometer calibrated in Brix (a saccharometer scale of measurement used to designate the concentration of sugar in water solution, with the weight of the solids being expressed as a percentage of the total weight). A hand-held refractometer (Figure 98) can be used to determine the approximate solids content, but for quality control purposes an Abbé refractometer (Figure 99) with a temperature-controlled bath (20 or 25°C) should be employed.

Once the salvage solution pH and solids content have been determined and adjusted to the required range, colors and medicaments (if desired) are added, mixed, and assayed for concentration levels in the salvage. (An assay is performed at this time to assure that the proper quantity of color and medicament will be delivered to the candy base. Improper drug or color content in the salvage solution will produce finished lozenges out of specification for medicament or out of the acceptable color range. Failure

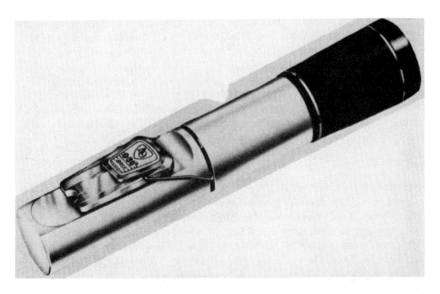

Figure 98   Hand refractometer. Designed for rapid field-determination of.
dissolved sugar content. The instrument automatically compensates for
temperatures from 16 to 38°C. (American Optical Co.)

to determine the drug or color content in salvage may result in 60–200
batches of lozenges being rejected.)

In instances where drug or colors present in salvage cannot be passed
through the cooker after solution pH and solids content have been adjusted
(Sec. I.A), activated charcoal or diatomaceous earth is suspended in the
solution and filtered in order to remove color and/or medicament as required [20,69]. When no medicament or color need be added to the salvage
solution or removed due to incompatibility, the material is ready for use
after pH and solids content have been adjusted to the desired ranges.

Forming Checks

While lozenges are being formed, a continuous weight check progresses in
order to ascertain whether the candy rope is of the proper diameter. Adjustments to the rope diameter are made by adjusting the clearance between
the sizing rollers. The operator checks the weights of groups of 10 or 20
lozenges as well as the weight of individual lozenges. At the same time,
the operator checks the guage (thickness) of the lozenges being formed,
using a micrometer guage. Adjustments to the forming machine molding
pressure can be made in order to increase or decrease the lozenge guage
as required.

The finished lozenge weight check reduces the quantity of rejects
formed as oversized or undersized, as well as detecting any inconsistencies
in lozenge weight (rope diameter) resulting from improper candy base manufacture, incomplete mixing of raw materials into the base, nontempering or
overcooling, improper adjustment of the batch former height, or lozenge-
forming machine molding difficulties. Lozenge weight checks must conform
to the USP XXI test for tablet weight variation:

Weigh individually 20 whole tablets and calculate the average weight: the weights of not more than 2 of the tablets differ from the average weight by more than the percentage listed and no tablet differs by more than double that percentage.

The average lozenge weight usually exceeds 1.0 g. In this weight range, if two tablets fall outside the weight range, a resample of 80 lozenges is taken. If the resample has five or fewer lozenges outside the acceptable limits, the batch is considered satisfactory.

Cooling Checks

Lozenges are visually examined during and after the cooling operation [55] in order to determine whether (a) any stress cracking is occurring because of too rapid cooling; (b) excess air bubble formation has resulted because of prolonged mixing; (c) surface cracking is occurring due to excessive cooling of the candy base before forming or due to low temperatures of

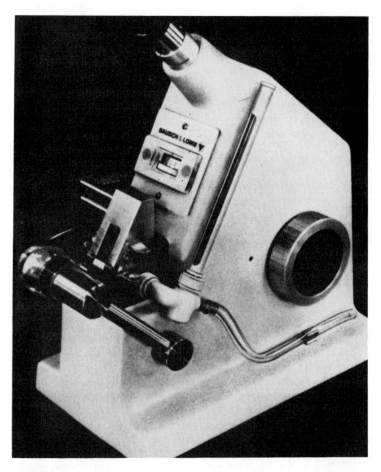

Figure 99   Abbé-3L refractometer. This instrument is accurate to ±0.05% for Brix measurements (0 to 85% sucrose). For precision temperature control, an external water bath can be connected into the refractometer case. (Bausch and Lomb, Analytical Systems Div.)

forming rollers, tempering table, or die faces; (d) lozenges are broken, chipped, or brittle because of low reducing sugar content or premature graining of the lozenge base; (e) black specks and air bubbles have resulted because of dieseling resulting from terpene-containing flavor oils; (f) color is correct; (g) organoleptic presentation is satisfactory.

Lozenges that fail the visual test are rejected and remedial actions initiated to remedy the situation. Twenty lozenge samples are taken at random from various portions of each batch. If more than one defect is found, a second sample of 125 lozenges is taken. The resample is considered satisfactory if seven or fewer major defects are found.

Sizing Checks

Oversized and undersized lozenges are routinely checked for diesels, excessive sugar dust formation, or breaking. On a regular basis, the oversized or undersized salvage is resized in order to determine if the sizing operation speed is correct. If the operation is proceeding too rapidly, undersized lozenges will appear in the production material and properly sized lozenges will appear in the oversized salvage.

Sampling

Lozenges are sampled from different sections of each batch. At least one sample is taken for each 30–35 lb of lozenges sized. After lozenges are manufactured, they are stored on a batch basis in temperature- and humidity-controlled areas (15–20°C at 25–30% relative humidity) until quality control testing of physical and chemical (flavor and medicament) parameters is complete. Such testing would include:

Description: Physical examination
Taste: Organoleptic comparison to type sample
Hardness for compressed or chewy caramel tablets: Meets specifications for compression or chew
Color: Comparison to type sample
Thickness: Meets specifications for packaging and appearance
Weight variation: Described above
Drug content and content uniformity

Groups of 10 lozenges are assayed for drug content. Analytical procedures used should be stability-indicating in nature (gas-liquid chromatography or liquid chromatography) [56,57]. ...the content of each of 10 tablets is within the limits of 85.0 percent and 115.0 percent of the average of the limits specified in the potency definition. If not more than one result falls outside the limits of 85.0 to 115.0 percent and if none of the tablets falls outside the limits of 75.0 percent to 125.0 percent of the average, assay each of the remaining tablets. The requirements are met if the content of each of the additional 20 tablets falls within the limits of 85.0 percent and 115.0 percent of the average of the limits specified. . . .

B. Microbiological Testing

While a continual check is made on the physical and chemical properties of the hard candy lozenges both during and after processing, another problem

area that must be considered is microbiological contamination [58,59].
During the candy base cooking cycle, temperatures are high enough to
sterilize the raw materials, but addition of contaminated raw materials on
the mixing table, contaminated cooling air, contaminated utensils, or improper hygiene by the production workers can cause bacteria, mold, or
spore contamination of the candy. The high solids content will not in itself support bacterial growth, but as the lozenge picks up surface moisture, conditions may be suitable for an increase in bacterial or mold counts.
A strain of *Salmonella typhosa* can persist in hard candy under proper conditions for more than 12 months. The presence of any bacterial, mold, or
spore contamination is indicative of a lack of adequate housekeeping or
hygiene among the production workers. If microbiological contamination becomes evident, a complete evaluation of all possible problem areas must be
carried out until the source is located and eliminated.

Routine microbiological testing is as critical as routine analytical evaluation. The quality control department must develop a microbiological
sampling plan to effectively determine areas of possible contamination. Raw
materials, finished products, machinery, cooling tunnels, environmental conditions, and storage drums are all sources of microbiological contamination.
Production workers should be educated toward proper hygiene, and sufficient washing facilities must be provided.

Laboratory microbiological testing should include the following counts:
(a) total plate; (b) total coliform; (c) yeast and mold; (d) *Escherichia coli*;
(e) *Staphylococcus*; (f) *Salmonella*.

C. Product Release

Once the finished lozenge is determined to be within the physical, chemical,
and microbiological specifications set for the product, it is approved for
packaging and distribution.

D. Stability Testing

The previous section described the routine quality control tests necessary
to determine if the product is being manufactured according to a series of
predetermined formulation guidelines. If these guidelines are followed and
the product is within specifications, then an acceptable product will result.
Stability testing is not a *routine* quality control test, but rather an analytical tool to determine the effective product shelf life.

Shelf life determination, or product storage stability testing, is initiated
upon completion of the first laboratory prototypes when production begins
and at periodic intervals during routine production, and continues for a
minimum of 5 years. The purpose of this series of tests is to determine
the physical and chemical stabilities of medicament, flavor, candy base,
and color—both under accelerated temperature and humidity conditions
and at ambient storage conditions. This testing will enable the formulator
to predict the acceptable shelf life of the product in a relatively short
period of time and make changes as required to eliminate any incompatibilities that may influence product stability.

E. Arrhenius Relationship

The chemical kinetics of medicament, flavor, and color in hard candy base
is directly applicable to the Arrhenius relationship [24]. This relationship is valid only as long as it is possible to linearize a property of the
degradation (drug concentration, flavor content, color loss) with time.
By plotting the property vs. time on arithemetic or semilog graph paper,
it is possible to determine whether the degradation is proceeding according
to zeroth-order, first-order, or pseudo-first-order reaction. Most materials in candy base degrade by first-order or pseudo-first-order reactions,
permitting a measure of the degradation rate from a plot of the logarithm
of residual drug concentration vs. time. The slope of the resultant
straight line represents the rate of degradation. Plots that do not result
in a straight line indicate that the drug is degrading through a more
complex reaction.

Once the rates of degradation are determined for the medicament in
candy base at three or more elevated temperature storage conditions, it is
possible to estimate the rate of degradation at room temperature through
the use of the Arrhenius relationship. If, by plotting the logarithm of
the rates of degradation vs. the reciprocal of the absolute temperature, a
linear relationship results, it is possible to determine degradation at room
temperature. This makes it possible to calculate the shelf life of the product which, for medicinals, is generally the time it will take for the dosage
form to retain 90% of its labeled drug content [24].

F. Elevated Temperature and Elevated Humidity Testing

Elevated temperature and elevated humidity testing is initiated as soon as
product is manufactured. While the choice of time and temperature storage
conditions is left to the discretion of the formulator, an effective stability
program should include product storage for 1−2 months at 60°C, 3−6 months
at 45°C, 9−12 months at 37°C, and 36−60 months at 25 and 4°C. These
conditions are suitable for determining the initial Arrhenius plot relationship and the follow-up confirmatory medicament stability values.

As soon as possible, product should be tested in the proposed trade
package both at elevated temperature and elevated humidity conditions.
Testing conditions generally utilized by the product development laboratory
include 25°C at 80% relative humidity for 6−12 months, 37°C at 80% relative
humidity for 3 months, and 25°C at 70% relative humidity for 6−12 months.
The elevated humidity studies are carried out both at constant humidity
and in humidity cabinets with day and night cycling. Elevated humidity
tests are vital for ascertaining medicament stability, candy stickiness, sur-
face-graining characteristics, clouding, and development of cold flow. At
the same time the moisture protection characteristics that different packaging materials offer to the lozenge are evaluated. Bunch wrap, cartons,
carton overwrap, shipping boxes, and bundle wrap are tested. Materials
that offer the product maximum protection from moisture are chosen so that
optimum warehouse, store, and in-home protection from moisture penetration
are afforded the product.

G. Flavor Stability

Volatile oils in medicated candies are not only responsible for taste but may also contribute to the antiseptic action of the lozenge. The quantity of volatile oils in the medication can be determined quantitatively or by subjective taste response. The method of choice for determining the loss of flavor oils with time is gas-liquid chromatography [57]. Using the data in accordance with the Arrhenius relationship will enable an estimation of the loss rate of the oils under normal shelf storage conditions [24].

H. Physical Stability

Concurrent with the chemical stability evaluation, a physical stability study is carried out on the product in order to determine what factors will detract from the organoleptic appeal of the product and how long these changes will take to occur. A routine physical stability evaluation includes the following:

Color. Lozenges are placed in direct sunlight, in a fadeometer, and at elevated temperature to determine if the colors are light-fast. Lozenges are also tested for color changes occurring due to the presence of medicaments, flavors, or acidulents in the formulation.

Odor. Changes in the odor of flavors stored at elevated temperature conditions are evaluated by sealing the lozenges in glass bottles and determining if any off-odors result.

Taste. The product is tasted and compared to production controls in order to determine if any flavor changes have occurred. Many small flavor changes that cannot be detected via gas-liquid chromatography can be ascertained when the lozenge is tasted. Any changes in the surface texture are also evaluated during the taste evaluation.

Hardness. Compressed tablet lozenges are tested for proper hardness using an instron or schleuniger hardness tester. Chewy caramel products are tested for hardness using an instron or a penetrometer. The force required to penetrate the tablet is used as a measure of chewiness, surface hardness, and stability.

Grain. Lozenge sticking is noted. When graining occurs, the degree is recorded. The lozenge is broken in half and the grain is measured with an eyepiece fitted with a micrometer guage. The degree of lozenge graining is usually reported as *percentage of lozenge grained*.

Bunch wrap appearance. Color changes that may occur on the paper surface due to medicament or color reaction with the bunch wrap material, sticking of bunch wrap to the surface of the lozenge, or splitting of the laminate from the foil are evaluated.

REFERENCES

1. Lozenges, Mouthwashes, and Gargles. *Drug Ther. Bull.* 10:33 (1972).
2. A. H. Kutscher and E. V. Zegarelli, A New Long Lasting Lozenge: Properties and Uses. *J. Oral Ther. Pharmacol.*, 4:6 (1968).
3. E. W. Martin and J. E. Hoover, *Husa's Pharmaceutical Dispensing*, 5th Edition. Mack Publishing, Easton, PA, 1959.
4. Simon Schnitzer, *Hard Candy*. NCESF Short Course in Candy Technology. University of Wisconsin, 1970.

5. E. W. Martin, E. F. Cook, et al., *Remington's Practice of Pharmacy*, 16th edition. Mack Publishing, Easton, PA, 1980.

6. J. M. Newton, *Properties and Functional Uses of Corn Syrup*. From Symposium Proceedings, Products of the Wet Milling Industry in Food, 1970.

7. *A Formulary for Better Candies*. Technical Information sheet, A. E. Staley Manufacturing Company, Decatur, IL.

8. W. J. Hoover, *Corn Sweeteners*. NCESF Short Course in Candy Technology. University of Wisconsin, 1970.

9. E. E. Fauser, J. E. Cleveland, et al., Baumé–Dextrose Equivalent–Dry Substance Tables for Corn Syrup and Corn Sugar. *Industrial and Engineering Chemistry*, 15:3 (March 15, 1943.)

10. S. E. Allured, A Most Unique Hard Candy. *The Manufacturing Confectioner*, 51:6 (1971).

11. R. Lees, High Boiled Sweets; Simple in Composition But Physical Structure Is Complex; *Confectionary Production*, 38:9 (1972).

12. Fred Janssen, *Invert Sugar as a Doctor in Candy Making*. Presented at a Northern California Section of American Association of Candy Technologists, November 1968.

13. R. E. Henry, Versatility of Corn Syrups Expands with Wider Research. *Candy and Snack Industry*, 141:6 (1976), pp. 748–752.

14. M. E. Schwartz, *Confectionary and Candy Technology*. Noyes Data Corporation, 1974, pp. 9–15, 298–299.

15. R. Lees, High Boiled Sweets; Products Should Not Grain Nor Become Sticky. *Confectionary Production*, 38:10 (1972).

16. B. R. Suri, Stabilization of pH of Corn Syrup for Hard Candy. *The Manufacturing Confectioner*, 47:7 (1967).

17. G. Richardson, Coloring Matters: Their Addition to Different Types of Confectionary. *The Manufacturing Confectioner*, 53:10 (1973).

18. R. R. Frey, et al., Process of Incorporating Volatile Aromatics in Hard Candy. South African Patent Application 112,856, May 1971.

19. G. Fellows, Confectionary Flavors. *The Manufacturing Confectioner*, 52:4 (1972).

20. W. T. Clarke, The Re-use of Chocolate and Confectionary Rejects. *The Manufacturing Confectioner*, 55:6 (1975).

21. M. A. Cherkas, et al., Medicated Hard Candy, U.S. Patent 3,439,089 (1969).

22. P. Kabasakalian, et al., Fractional Experimental Design. Study of the Incompatibility of Benzocaine in Throat Lozenges, *Journal of Pharmaceutical Sciences*, 58:1 (1969).

23. Eberhard Berten, *Hard Candy and Caramels*, 3rd Revised Edition. Hamac-Hansella Machinery Corporation, Piscataway, NJ, 1965.

24. L. Lachman, H. A. Lieberman, and G. Richardson, Medicated Candies, *Drug and Cosmetic Industry*, 99, Nos. 1, 2, and 3 (July, August, and Sept. 1966).

25. C. D. Pratt, et al., *Twenty Years of Confectionary and Chocolate Progress*, AVI, Westport, CT, 1970.

26. A. B. Cramer, Hard Candy and Continuous Cooking—8 Years Later—A Reappraisal, *The Manufacturing Confectioner*, 51:5 (1971).

27. A. Meiners, Incorporating Flavor and Acid in Continuous Manufacturing Systems, *The Manufacturing Confectioner*, 53:10 (1973).

28. Anonymous: Hard Candy Packaging: Moisture Content, Humidity are Factors in Selection of Wrapping Materials and Styles, *Candy and Snack Industry*, 141:11 (1976).

29. Anonymous: Chocolate Packaging Roundup: Product Composition Affects Material Selection, *Candy and Snack Industry*, 141:10 (1976).

30. *Modern Packaging 1976—77 Encyclopedia and Buyer's Guide*, 49:12 (1976).

31. W. Vink, Tabletting: Manufacture of Compressed Candies, *The Manufacturing Confectioner*, 56:1 (1976).

32. Cerelose Dextrose, *Technical Bulletin*, CPC International, Englewood Cliffs, NJ.

33. A Series of Unique Chemicals for the Pharmaceutical Manufacturer, *Technical Bulletin*, Edward Mendell Co., Carmel, NY.

34. Mor-Rex Hydrolyzed Cereal Solids, *Technical Bulletin*, CPC International, Englewood Cliffs, NJ.

35. Royal-T Dextrose with Malto-Dextrin 2031, *Technical Bulletin*, CPC International, Englewood Cliffs, NJ.

36. NuTab A direct Compression Binder, *Technical Bulletin* Sucrest Pharmaceutical Division, Pennsauken, NJ.

37. Di-Pac, *Technical Bulletin*, American Sugar Company, NY.

38. SugarTab, *Technical Bulletin*, Edward Mendell Co., NY.

39. Sweetrex, *Technical Bulletin*, Edward Mendell Co., NY.

40. Mannitol, USP, Tablet Excipient, *Technical Bulletin*, ICI America. Wilmington, DE.

41. Crystalline Sorbitol Tablet Type, *Technical Bulletin 615*, Pfizer Chemical Division, NY.

42. Carbowax Polyethylene Glycols, *Technical Bulletin*, Union Carbide Corporation, NY.

43. H. N. Wolkoff and G. Pinchuk, Throat Lozenge Vehicle, U.S. Patent 3,511,914 (1970).

44. Lactose, USP Fast-Flo: The Perfect Excipient, *Technical Bulletin*, Formost Foods Company, San Francisco, CA.

45. Avicel in Direct Compression Tabletting, *Technical Bulletin PH-9*, FMC Corporation, Marcus Hook, PA.

46. Tablet Making, *Technical Bulletin 14-100.500A*, Pennwalt-Stokes, Warminister, PA.

47. Factors Determining the Hardness of Tablets, *Technical Bulletin 11-100.621B*, Pennwalt-Stokes, Warminister, PA.

48. J. P. Malle, Compacted Candy Concepts, *The Manufacturing Confectioner* 56:5 (1976).

49. Model 541 Rotary Tableting Press, *Technical Bulletin 551-A*, Pennwalt-Stokes, Warminister, PA.

50. Model 328 Rotary Tableting Press, *Technical Bulletin 374*, Pennwalt-Stokes, Warminister, PA.

51. Model DD-2 Double-Sided Rotary Tableting Press, *Technical Bulletin 358*, Pennwalt-Stokes, Warminster, PA.

52. Binding, Capping, Laminating and Sticking of Tablets: Cause and Remedy Charts, *Technical Bulletin 8-100.652A*, Pennwalt-Stokes, Warminster, PA.

53. E. J. Abeling, Finished Goods Quality Assurance, *The Manufacturing Confectioner*, 52:7 (1972).

54. *The United States Pharmacopeia, Twenty-First Revision*, United States Pharmacopeial Convention, January 1, 1985.

55. R. Lees, High Boiled Sweets: Suggested Data Sheet for Remedying Faults, *Confectionary Production*, 38:11 (1972).

56. Derek McManua, Candy Laboratory Use of Gas-Liquid Chromatography, *The Manufacturing Confectioner*, 50:2 (1970).

57. M. M. Hussein, Gas Chromatography: Superior Method for Determining Flavor Content in Finished Candy, *Candy and Snack Industry, 141*:8 (1976).

58. B. Ostergren, Practical Biological Testing in Confectionary Plants, *The Manufacturing Confectioner, 54*:6 (1974).

59. I. I. Kazi, "Plant Sanitation," *The Manufacturing Confectioner, 56*:4 (1976).

60. H. Becker, Filled Hard Candy Production Requires Precise Control of Unit Quality, Uniformity and Temperature, *Candy and Snack Industry, 142*:3 (1977).

61. S. H. Cakebread, The Shelf Life of High Boilings. V. Calculating the E.R.H., *The Manufacturing Confectioner, 50*:1 (1970).

62. H. E. Horn, Crystallization Guidelines Provide Criteria and Control for Panning Process, *Candy and Snack Industry, 142*:11 (1977).

63. Veegum, *Technical Bulletin*, R. T. Vanderbilt Company, NY.

64. A. J. Chalmers, Hard Candy Processing: Problems and Solutions, *The Manufacturing Confectioner, 63*:10 (1983).

65. J. DuRoss, Modified Crystalline Sorbitol, *The Manufacturing Confectioner, 62*:11 (1982).

66. D. Caton, Direct Compression, *The Manufacturing Confectioner, 62*:11 (1982).

67. J. Schleuter, Aeration of Hard Candies, *The Manufacturing Confectioner, 62*:6 (1982).

68. R. Calliari, Sorbitol for Confections, *The Manufacturing Confectioner, 63*:11 (1983).

69. A. J. Chalmers, Reclaiming Hard Candy Reworks, *The Manufacturing Confectioner, 65*:10 (1985).

70. J. Denick, D. Peters, and A. K. Talwar, Medicament Adsorbates of Decongestants with Complex Aluminum Silicate and Their Preparation, U.S. Patent 4,758,424 (1988).

71. J. Denick, D. Peters, and A. K. Talwar, Magnesium Trisilicate Suitable for Preparation of Medicament Adsorbates of Decongestants, U.S. Patent 4,632,821 (1986).

72. D. Peters, J. Denick, and A. K. Talwar, Magnesium Trisilicate Suitable for Preparation of Medicament Adsorbates, U.S. Patent 4,581,232 (1986).

73. D. Peters, J. Denick, and A. K. Talwar, Magnesium Trisilicate Suitable for Preparation of Medicament Adsorbates of Antihistamines, U.S. Patent 4,642,231 (1987).

74. D. Peters, J. Denick, and A. K. Talwar, Confectionary Compositions Containing Magnesium Trisilicate Adsorbates, U.S. Patent 4,647,459 (1987).

75. D. Peters, J. Denick, and A. K. Talwar, Magnesium Trisilicate Suitable for Preparation of Medicament Adsorbates of Analgesics, U.S. Patent 4,643,892 (1987).

76. D. Peters and J. Denick, Chewable Mineral Supplement, U.S. Patent 4,582,709 (1986).

77. J. Hume, Notebook of a Practical Confectioner. I. Preparing, Cooking and Making Toffees and Caramels, *Confectionary Products, 43*:385– 386 (Sept. 1977).

78. E. Pyrz, Caramel: A Review, *The Manufacturing Confectioner, 56*:6 (1976).

79. B. W. Minifie, Extrusion: Caramel, Fudge and Chewing Sweets, *The Manufacturing Confectioner*, 55:11 (1975).

80. B. Vospalek, Sugar in the Confectionary Industry, *The Manufacturing Confectioner*, 66:5 (1986).

81. P. W. Jung, Aeration of Hard Candy, *The Manufacturing Confectioner*, 67:5 (1985).

82. R. W. Hartel, Sugar Crystallization in Confectionary Products, *The Manufacturing Confectioner*, 67:10 (1987).

83. T. Long, Forming Hard Candy, Pennsylvania Manufacturing Confectioners Association, April 1980.

84. H. R. Riedel, Hard Candy Fillings, *The Manufacturing Confectioner*, 56:9 (1976).

85. C. J. DeBlaez, Buccal Residence Time of Lozenges, *Pharm. Acta Helv.* 52:5 (1977).

86. S. D. Uko-nne and R. W. Mendes, Directly Compressible Molasses and Honey, *Pharmaceut. Technol.* 6:11 (1982).

87. Mola-Tab, *Technical Bulletin*, Ingredient Technology Corporation, Woodbridge, NJ.

88. Hony-Tab, *Technical Bulletin*, Ingredient Technology Corporation, Woodbridge, NJ.

89. Encompress, *Technical Bulletin*, Edward Mendell Co., Carmel, NY.

90. Compactrol, *Technical Bulletin*, Edward Mendell Co., Carmel, NY.

91. P. A. Lane and B. A. Brown, Anesthetic lozenges, U.S. Patent 4,139,627 (1979).

92. J. E. F. Reynolds and A. B. Prasad, *Martindale: The Extra Pharmacopoeia*, 28th Edition. The Pharmaceutical Press, London, England, 1982.

SUGGESTED READING*

Ahrens, G. W.: Sugar-free Compounded Tablet or Lozenge Base Material for use in the Preparation of Suckable, Structurally Sound and Hard at Room Temperature Nonhygroscopic Noncaries Forming Tablets or Lozenges, U.S. Patent 3,525,795 (1970).

Barnett, C. D.: *Candy Making as a Science and Art*, Don Gussow Publications, NY.

Barry, R. H., Weiss, M.: Dextromethorphan and Benzyl Alcohol Hard Candy Lozenges Free From Opaqueness and/or Tiny Entrapped Air Bubbles, U.S. Patent 3,427,379 (1969).

Bornberg, John D.: Practical Quality Control in the Confectionery Industry, *The Manufacturing Confectioner*, 51:6 (1971).

Burlinson, H.: The Evolution of the Compressed Tablet, *Aust. J. Pharm.*, 49:738—752 (October 1968).

Bush, J. W. and Pyrz, E. Z.: Lower Calorie Candies, U.S. Patent 3,809,756 (1974).

Cakebread, S. H.: Chemistry of Candy I, *The Manufacturing Confectioner*, 49:2 (1969).

---

*References included in this list are intended as general sources of information regarding the various aspects of confectionary manufacture.

Cakebread, S. H.: The Shelf-Life of High Boilings, *The Manufacturing Confectioner*, 49:9–12 (1969).

Cakebread, S. H.: Deriving Recipes From Analytical Figures—Complex High Boilings II, *The Manufacturing Confectioner*, 50:3–4 (1970).

Cakebread, S. H.: The Chemistry of Candy Part V: Mainly Arithmetic, *The Manufacturing Confectioner*, 51:6 (1971).

Cakebread, S. H.: Requirements for Production of Grained Confections, *The Manufacturing Confectioner*, 52:3 (1972).

Candy Industry Catolog and Formula Book, 23rd Annual Edition (1969–1970), Magazines for Industry, New York.

Candy and Snack Industry Buying Guide 1975, Magazines for Industry, NY.

Carle and Montanari Spa., Lanzillo, A., Candy Mass Production, U.S. Patent 4,054,271.

Chalmers, A. J.: Hard Candy Processing and Quality Observations, *The Manufacturing Confectioner*, 63:5 (1983).

Christenson, G. L. et al: Long Lasting Troche, U.S. Patent 3,594,467 (1971).

Confectionary Production 37:12, 1981, pp. 528–529, 546.

DuRoss, J. W.: Sugar Free Hard Candy, German Patent 2,409,107 (1974).

Frey, R. R.: Additives for use in the Preparation of Cooked Candies, U.S. Patent 3,738,843 (1973).

Gillies, Martha T.: *Candies and Other Confections*, Noyes Data, Park Ridge, NJ, 1979.

Gobba, A. H. et al: In Vitro Effects of Separate Ingredients and Combinations Proposed to be used as Oropharyngeal Lozenges on Different Bacterial Flora and Yeasts, *Drug Res. J.*, 1:111–128, No. 1 (1968).

Gotsch, G.: Hard Caramels II, *Dragoco Report*, 1 (1979).

Gott, P. P. et al: *All About Candy and Chocolate*, National Confectioners Association, Chicago, 1978.

Griffenhagen, G. B. and Hawkins, L. L., ed., *Handbook of Non-Prescription Drugs*, American Pharmaceutical Association, Washington, D.C., 1973.

Gutterson, M.: *Confectionary Products Manufacturing Processes 1969*, Noyes Development, Park Ridge, NJ.

Hohberger, N.: Continuous Cooking with a Batch System, *The Manufacturing Confectioner*, 63:11 (1983).

Horn, H. E.: Crystallization Guidelines Provide Criteria and Control for Panning Process, *Candy and Snack Industry*, 142:12 (1977).

IPT Standard Specifications for Tableting Tools, *Tableting Specification Manual*, American Pharmaceutical Association Academy of Pharmaceutical Sciences, 1971.

Kuzio, W.: Flavor Enhancers Broaden Product Appeal, *Candy and Snack Industry*, 141:8 (1976).

Laino, J. M.: Quality Control—or Quality Assurance? *The Manufacturing Confectioner*, 53:5 (1973).

Leighton, A. E.: A Text Book on Candy Making, *The Manufacturing Confectioner* (1952).

Liebrand, J. T.: Process for the Manufacture of Sugarless Confections, U.S. Patent 3,738,845 (1973).

Minifie, B. W.: Pectin: Its Use in Candy Technology, *The Manufacturing Confectioner*, 51:11 (1971).

Norrish, R. S.: Selected Tables of Physical Properties of Sugar Solutions, *Scientific and Technical Surveys*, 51 (July 1967).

Pariser, E. R.: How Physical Properties of Candy Affect Taste, *The Manu-facturing Confectioner, 41*:5 (1961).

Products of the Wet Milling Industry in Food, *Symposium Proceedings,* Washington, D.C., Corn Refiners Association, (1970).

Richmond, W.: *Choice Confections,* Manufacturing Confectioner Publishing Company, Glen Rock, NJ (1976).

Ross, J. W.: Sugarless Confection, U.S. Patent 3,438,781 (1969).

Slawatycki, A.: Producing Lozenges Automatically, *The Manufacturing Confectioner, 50*:11 (1970).

Toscano, V.: The Use of Fructose in Confections, *The Manufacturing Con-fectioner, 55*:5 (1975).

Vink, W.: Continuous Processing of Hard Candy: A Different Approach, *The Manufacturing Confectioner, 66*:10 (1988).

Vrana, P.: New Machinery for Confectionary Cooking and Processing, *The Manufacturing Confectioner, 64*:12 (1984).

Index